Thoracic Emergencies

Guest Editor

JOEL P. TURNER, MD, MSc, FRCP

EMERGENCY MEDICINE CLINICS OF NORTH AMERICA

www.emed.theclinics.com

Consulting Editor
AMAL MATTU, MD

May 2012 • Volume 30 • Number 2

SAUNDERS an imprint of ELSEVIER, Inc.

W.B. SAUNDERS COMPANY

A Division of Elsevier Inc.

1600 John F. Kennedy Boulevard • Suite 1800 • Philadelphia, Pennsylvania 19103-2899
http://www.theclinics.com

EMERGENCY MEDICINE CLINICS OF NORTH AMERICA Volume 30, Number 2
May 2012 ISSN 0733-8627, ISBN-13: 978-1-4557-3855-7

Editor: Patrick Manley
Developmental Editor: Donald Mumford

Emergency Medicine Clinics of North America (ISSN 0733-8627) is published quarterly by Elsevier Inc., 360 Park Avenue South, New York, NY, 10010-1710. Months of issue are February, May, August, and November. Business and Editorial Offices: 1600 John F. Kennedy Boulevard, Suite 1800, Philadelphia, PA 19103-2899. Customer Service Office: 6277 Sea Harbor Drive, Orlando, FL 32887-4800. Periodicals postage paid at New York, NY, and additional mailing offices. Subscription prices are $142.00 per year (US students), $281.00 per year (US individuals), $478.00 per year (US institutions), $201.00 per year (international students), $404.00 per year (international individuals), $576.00 per year (international institutions), $201.00 per year (Canadian students), $347.00 per year (Canadian individuals), and $576.00 per year (Canadian institutions). International air speed delivery is included in all *Clinics'* subscription prices. All prices are subject to change without notice. **POSTMASTER:** Send address changes to *Emergency Medicine Clinics of North America*, Elsevier Periodicals Customer Service, 11830 Westline Industrial Drive, St. Louis, MO 63146. Customer Service (orders, claims, online, change of address): Elsevier Periodicals Customer Service, 11830 Westline Industrial Drive, St. Louis, MO 63146. Tel: 1-800-654-2452 (U.S. and Canada); 314-453-7041 (outside U.S. and Canada). Fax: 314-453-5170. E-mail: journalscustomerservice-usa@elsevier.com (for print support); journalsonline support-usa@elsevier.com (for online support).

Reprints. For copies of 100 or more of articles in this publication, please contact the Commercial Reprints Department, Elsevier Inc., 360 Park Avenue South, New York, NY 10010-1710. Tel.: 212-633-3812; Fax: 212-462-1935; E-mail: reprints@elsevier.com.

Emergency Medicine Clinics of North America is covered in *MEDLINE/PubMed (Index Medicus), Current Contents/Clinical Medicine, EMBASE/Excerpta Medica, BIOSIS, SciSearch, CINAHL, ISI/BIOMED,* and *Research Alert.*

Printed and bound by CPI Group (UK) Ltd, Croydon, CR0 4YY

Transferred to Digital Print 2012

Contributors

CONSULTING EDITOR

AMAL MATTU, MD, FAAEM, FACEP
Program Director, Emergency Medicine Residency; Professor, Department of Emergency Medicine, University of Maryland School of Medicine, Baltimore, Maryland

GUEST EDITOR

JOEL P. TURNER, MD, MSc, FRCP
Faculty Lecturer, McGill Emergency Medicine; Director, Royal College Emergency Medicine Residency Training Program; Director, Emergency Medicine Ultrasound Training Program, McGill University; Attending Staff, Emergency Department, Jewish General Hospital, Montreal, Quebec, Canada

AUTHORS

MARC AFILALO, MD, MCFP(EM), FACEP, CSPQ, FRCP(C)
Associate Professor, Faculty of Medicine, McGill University; Director, Emergency Department, Jewish General Hospital, Montreal, Quebec, Canada

PATRICK M. ARCHAMBAULT, MD, MSc, FRCPC
Assistant Professor, Department of Family Medicine and Emergency Medicine; Division of Critical Care, Department of Anesthesiology, Université Laval, Quebec City; Emergency and Critical Care Medicine Specialist, Department of Emergency Medicine; Department of Anesthesiology, Centre de santé et services sociaux Alphonse-Desjardins (CHAU de Lévis), Lévis, Quebec, Canada

BRUNO BERNARDIN, MD
Assistant Professor, Department of Medicine, McGill University, Royal Victoria Hospital; Director, Emergency Trauma Fellowship; Trauma Coordinator, Emergency Department, Montreal General Hospital, McGill University Health Center, Montréal, Quebec, Canada

CORY A. BRULOTTE, MD, FRCPC
Department of Emergency Medicine, Alberta Health Services: Calgary Zone, Calgary, Alberta, Canada

JOSEPH CHOI, MD
Resident, McGill University FRCP Emergency Medicine Residency Program, Royal Victoria Hospital, Montreal, Quebec, Canada

JERRALD DANKOFF, MDCM, CSPQ
Assistant Professor, Attending Staff, Emergency Department, Jewish General Hospital, McGill University, Montreal, Quebec, Canada

SALEH FARES, MD, MPH, FRCPC, FACEP
Consultant, Emergency Medicine, Zayed Military Hospital, Abu Dhabi, United Arab Emirates; Adjunct Faculty, Harvard-Affiliated Disaster Medicine/EMS Fellowship Program, Department of Emergency Medicine, Boston, Massachusetts

CHRIS HALL, MD, FRCPC
Clinical Lecturer, Division of Emergency Medicine, Foothills Medical Centre, University of Calgary, Calgary, Alberta, Canada

FURQAN B. IRFAN, MBBS
Research Associate, Department of Surgery, Medical College, Aga Khan University, Karachi, Pakistan

SARA KAZIM, MD
Division of Emergency Medicine, Montreal General Hospital, McGill University Health Center; Resident, Emergency Medicine Residency Training Program, McGill University, Montreal, Quebec, Canada

EDDY S. LANG, MDCM, CCFP(EM), CSPQ
Senior Researcher and Associate Professor, University of Calgary; Department of Emergency Medicine, Alberta Health Services: Calgary Zone, Calgary, Alberta, Canada

GARY L. LEE, MD, CCFP-EM, FRCPC, FACEP
Attending Physician, Faculty Lecturer, Department of Emergency Medicine, Montreal Children's Hospital, Montreal General Hospital, McGill University, Montreal, Quebec, Canada

PATRICK M. LING, MD, MPH
Program Director, Division of Emergency Medicine, Royal University Hospital, University of Saskatchewan, Saskatoon, Saskatchewan, Canada

NISREEN MAGHRABY, MD
Division of Emergency Medicine, Montreal General Hospital, McGill University Health Center; Resident, Emergency Medicine Residency Training Program, McGill University, Montreal, Quebec, Canada

ARIANA MURATA, MD
Emergency Resident, Division of Emergency Medicine, Royal University Hospital, University of Saskatchewan, Saskatoon, Saskatchewan, Canada

JOE NEMETH, MD
Assistant Professor, Division of Emergency Medicine, Montreal General Hospital, McGill University Health Center, Montreal, Quebec, Canada

DAVID W. OUELLETTE, MD, FRCPC
Assistant Professor of Medicine, Department of Medicine, Schulich School of Medicine and Dentistry, University of Western Ontario; Emergency Medicine Consultant, Division of Emergency Medicine, Department of Medicine, London Health Sciences Centre, London, Ontario, Canada

MATTHEW OUGHTON, MD, FRCP(C)
Assistant Professor, Faculty of Medicine, McGill University; Attending Physician, Department of Medicine, Division of Infectious Diseases, Jewish General Hospital, Montreal, Quebec, Canada

CATHERINE PATOCKA, MDCM
Senior Emergency Medicine Resident, McGill Emergency Medicine Residency Program, Royal Victoria Hospital, McGill University, Montréal, Quebec, Canada

KAREN SCHIFF, MD, FRCPC
Division of Emergency Medicine, McMaster University, Hamilton, Ontario, Canada

MAUDE ST-ONGE, MD, MSc, FRCPC
Emergency Medicine Specialist, Department of Emergency Medicine, Centre hospitalier universitaire de Quebec, Quebec City, Quebec; Resident, Adult Critical Care Medicine Residency Program, University of Toronto, Sunnybrook Health Sciences Center, Toronto, Ontario, Canada

ERROL STERN, MD, FACEP, CSPQ, FRCP(C)
Assistant Professor, Faculty of Medicine, McGill University; Attending Physician, Emergency Department, Jewish General Hospital, Montreal, Quebec, Canada

PAUL D. TOURIGNY, MD, FRCPC
Clinical Assistant Professor, Division of Emergency Medicine, Foothills Medical Centre, University of Calgary; Flight Physician, Shock Trauma Air Rescue Society, Calgary, Alberta, Canada

JEAN-MARC TROQUET, MD
Director, Emergency Department, Montreal General Hospital, McGill University Health Center; Faculty Lecturer, Department of Family Medicine, McGill University, Montréal, Quebec, Canada

JOEL P. TURNER, MD, MSc, FRCP
Faculty Lecturer, McGill Emergency Medicine; Director, Royal College Emergency Medicine Residency Training Program; Director, Emergency Medicine Ultrasound Training Program, McGill University; Attending Staff, Emergency Department, Jewish General Hospital, Montreal, Quebec, Canada

SUNEEL UPADHYE, MD, MSc, FRCPC
Division of Emergency Medicine, McMaster University, Hamilton, Ontario, Canada

ERIN WELDON, MD, FRCPC (EM)
Assistant Professor, Department of Emergency Medicine, University of Manitoba, Winnipeg, Manitoba, Canada

JEN WILLIAMS, BScPT, MDCM, FRCPC (EM)
Emergency Physician, Kingsway Emergency Agency, Royal Alexandra Hospital, Edmonton, Alberta, Canada

KAREN G.H. WOOLFREY, MD, FRCP(C), FACEP
Associate Professor and Clinical Educator, Department of Medicine; Director, Royal College Emergency Medicine Residency Training Program, University of Toronto; Director, Postgraduate Education, Department of Emergency Medicine, Sunnybrook Health Sciences Centre, Toronto, Ontario, Canada

Contents

Ariana Murata and Patrick M. Ling

Asthma is a chronic inflammatory airway disease that is commonly seen in the emergency department (ED). This article provides an evidence-based review of diagnosis and management of asthma. Early recognition of asthma exacerbations and initiation of treatment are essential. Treatment is dictated by the severity of the exacerbation. Treatment involves bronchodilators and corticosteroids. Other treatment modalities including magnesium, heliox, and noninvasive ventilator support are discussed. Safe disposition from the ED can be considered after stabilization of the exacerbation, response to treatment and attaining peak flow measures.

Cory A. Brulotte and Eddy S. Lang

Chronic obstructive pulmonary disease (COPD) is a significant cause of morbidity and mortality worldwide. Acute exacerbations of COPD (AECOPDs) are a common presentation to emergency departments and are an important cause of respiratory failure. This article discusses the disease process and diagnosis of COPD and AECOPD. A further in-depth discussion is undertaken of evidence-based treatments, palliation, and disposition of patients who present to emergency departments with AECOPD.

Karen G.H. Woolfrey

In those patients who are hospitalized with pneumonia, mortality is 15%. Close to 90% of deaths attributed to pneumonia are in patients older than 65 years. This article provides the emergency physician with an understanding of how to make the diagnosis, initiate early and appropriate antibiotic therapy, risk stratify patients with respect to the severity of illness, and recognize indications for admission. The discussion is balanced with an emphasis on cost-effective management, an understanding of the changing spectrum of pathogenesis, and a cognizance toward variable and less common presentations.

Seasonal influenza causes significant morbidity and mortality, primarily due to increased complication rates among the elderly and patients with chronic diseases. Timely diagnosis of influenza and early recognition of an outbreak or epidemic are crucial in preventing complications, hospitalizations and deaths. Emergency departments serve as frequent points-of-entry into the healthcare system for most influenza cases, and thus well positioned to promptly identify and manage influenza. Early treatment initiated within six hours of symptom onset provides the greatest benefit. Specific infection control measures implemented by emergency departments can curb the spread of influenza in hospitals during influenza season.

Acute aortic dissection in the emergency department (ED) remains one of the riskiest clinical and medicolegal challenges facing ED physicians. The variability in clinical presentations and mimics, the unreliability of clinical assessments and initial screening tools, and the need for advanced imaging all present obstacles in making an accurate and timely diagnosis for this entity. This article reviews available information and evidence regarding pathophysiology, risk factors, clinical variations in presentation, the usefulness of different diagnostic testing modalities, and management options in the ED when considering this diagnosis. Key recommendations from recent guidelines are reviewed in the context of ED practice.

Pulmonary embolism (PE) remains one of the most challenging medical diseases in the emergency department. PE is a potentially life threatening diagnosis that is seen in patients with chest pain and/or dyspnea but can span the clinical spectrum of medical presentations. In addition, it does not have any particular clinical feature, laboratory test, or diagnostic modality that can independently and confidently exclude its possibility. This article offers a review of PE in the emergency department. It emphasizes the appropriate determination of pretest probability, the approach to diagnosis and management, and special considerations related to pregnancy and radiation exposure.

Severe chest trauma, blunt or penetrating, is responsible for up to 25% of traumatic deaths in North America. Respiratory compromise is the most frequent dramatic presentation in blunt trauma, while injuries to the heart and great vessels pose the greatest risk of immediate death following penetrating trauma. More than 80% of patients will be managed with interventions that can be performed in the emergency department. This article reviews the presentation, diagnosis, and management of the most important thoracic injuries. A structured approach to the acutely unstable patient is proposed to guide resuscitation decisions.

Patients requiring airway management in the emergency department present an enormous challenge. It requires not only a firm concept of techniques for securing the airway but also of dealing with the potential difficult airway (DA) in which establishing a definite airway is not possible with techniques routinely used. This article highlights the importance of recognition and management of the DA in emergent situations. Both awake and nonawake intubation are discussed, and indications and guidelines are given for the use of nonsurgical and surgical airway interventions.

This article reviews invasive and noninvasive ventilation for emergency physicians. It presents an overview of respiratory physiology principles that will help emergency physicians adapt their ventilation strategies to any clinical situation. The basic modes of ventilation are summarized. The advantages and limitations of certain novel modes of ventilation are presented. This review highlights a variety of ventilation strategies to be used for patients with normal lung mechanics and gas exchange, acute hypoxemic respiratory failure, decreased lung compliance, airflow obstruction, and weakness or restriction of the chest wall. This article will help clinicians prevent, recognize, and treat complications of mechanical ventilation.

Dyspnea and hypotension often present a diagnostic challenge to the emergency physician. With limitations on traditional methods of evaluating these patients, lung ultrasound has become an essential assessment tool. With the sensitivity of lung ultrasound approaching that of CT scan for many indications, it is quickly becoming a fundamental technique in assessing patients with thoracic emergencies. This article reviews the principles of thoracic ultrasound; describes the important evidence-based sonographic features found in pneumothorax, pleural effusion, pneumonia, and pulmonary edema; and provides a framework of how to use thoracic ultrasound to aid in assessing a patient with severe dyspnea.

Emergency department presentations of pleural-based diseases are common, with severity ranging from mild to life threatening. The acute assessment, diagnosis, and treatment of pleural disease are critical as urgent invasive maneuvers such as thoracocentesis and thoracostomy may be indicated. The emergency physician must have a systematic approach to these conditions that allows for rapid recognition, diagnosis, and definitive management. This article focuses on nontraumatic pleural disease, including diagnostic and treatment considerations of pleural effusion, empyema, primary spontaneous pneumothorax, secondary spontaneous pneumothorax, pediatric pneumothorax, spontaneous hemothorax, and spontaneous tension pneumothorax.

Physiologic sequelae from increasing ambient pressure in underwater activities, decreasing ambient pressure while at altitude, or the consequences of drowning present a unique set of challenges to emergency physicians. In addition, several environmental toxins cause significant respiratory morbidity, whether they be pulmonary irritants, simple asphyxiants, or systemic toxins. It is important for emergency physicians to understand the pathophysiology of these illnesses as well as to apply this knowledge to the clinical arena either in the prehospital setting or in the emergency department. Current treatment paradigms and controversies within these regimens are discussed.

Pediatric respiratory illnesses are a huge burden to emergency departments worldwide. This article reviews the latest evidence in the epidemiology, assessment, management, and disposition of children presenting to the emergency department with asthma, croup, bronchiolitis, and pneumonia.

With the increasing prevalence of human immunodeficiency virus/AIDS patients and patients receiving chemotherapy for various malignancies, the numbers of immunosuppressed patients who present to the emergency department is on the increase. Thoracic-related emergencies in these vulnerable patients are serious and challenging to diagnose for the emergency physician, due mainly to atypical presentations, atypical pathogens, and to the often tenuous state of health of the patient. This article addresses a variety of cardiovascular, pulmonary, and esophageal emergencies that are seen specifically in immunocompromised patients presenting to the emergency department. Epidemiology, clinical presentation, investigations, prognosis, management, and evidence-based recommendations are discussed.

GOAL STATEMENT

The goal of *Emergency Medicine Clinics of North America* is to keep practicing physicians up to date with current clinical practice in emergency medicine by providing timely articles reviewing the state of the art in patient care.

ACCREDITATION

The *Emergency Medical Clinics of North America* is planned and implemented in accordance with the Essential Areas and Policies of the Accreditation Council for Continuing Medical Education (ACCME) through the joint sponsorship of the University of Virginia School of Medicine and Elsevier. The University of Virginia School of Medicine is accredited by the ACCME to provide continuing medical education for physicians.

The University of Virginia School of Medicine designates this enduring material activity for a maximum of 15 *AMA PRA Category 1 Credit*(s)™ for each issue, 60 credits per year. Physicians should claim only the credit commensurate with the extent of their participation in the activity.

The American Medical Association has determined that physicians not licensed in the US who participate in this CME enduring material activity are eligible for a maximum of 15 *AMA PRA Category 1 Credit*(s)™ for each issue, 60 credits per year.

The Emergency Medicine Clinics of North America CME program is approved by the American College of Emergency Physicians for 60 hours of ACEP Category I Credit per year.

Credit can be earned by reading the text material, taking the CME examination online at http://www.theclinics.com/home/cme, and completing the evaluation. After taking the test, you will be required to review any and all incorrect answers. Following completion of the test and evaluation, your credit will be awarded and you may print your certificate.

FACULTY DISCLOSURE/CONFLICT OF INTEREST

The University of Virginia School of Medicine, as an ACCME accredited provider, endorses and strives to comply with the Accreditation Council for Continuing Medical Education (ACCME) Standards of Commercial Support, Commonwealth of Virginia statutes, University of Virginia policies and procedures, and associated federal and private regulations and guidelines on the need for disclosure and monitoring of proprietary and financial interests that may affect the scientific integrity and balance of content delivered in continuing medical education activities under our auspices.

The University of Virginia School of Medicine requires that all CME activities accredited through this institution be developed independently and be scientifically rigorous, balanced and objective in the presentation/discussion of its content, theories and practices.

All authors/editors participating in an accredited CME activity are expected to disclose to the readers relevant financial relationships with commercial entities occurring within the past 12 months (such as grants or research support, employee, consultant, stock holder, member of speakers bureau, etc.). The University of Virginia School of Medicine will employ appropriate mechanisms to resolve potential conflicts of interest to maintain the standards of fair and balanced education to the reader. Questions about specific strategies can be directed to the Office of Continuing Medical Education, University of Virginia School of Medicine, Charlottesville, Virginia.

The faculty and staff of the University of Virginia Office of Continuing Medical Education have no financial affiliations to disclose.

The authors/editors listed below have identified no professional or financial affiliations for themselves or their spouse/partner:

Marc Afilalo, MD, MCFP(EM), CSPQ, FRCP(C); Patrick M. Archambault, MD, MSc, FRCPC; Bruno Bernardin, MD; Cory A. Brulotte, MD, FRCPC; Joseph Choi, MD; Jerrald Dankoff, MDCM, CSPQ; Saleh Fares, MD, MPH, FRCPC; Chris Hall, MD, FRCPC; Furgan B. Irfan, MBBS; Sara Kazim, MD; Eddy S. Lang, MDCM, CCFP(EM), CSPQ; Gary L. Lee, MD, CCFP-EM, FRCPC; Patrick M. Ling, MD, MPH; Nisreen Maghraby, MD; Patrick Manley, (Acquisitions Editor); Amal Mattu, MD, (Consulting Editor); Ariana Murata, MD; Joe Nemeth, MD; David W. Ouellette, MD, FRCPC; Catherine Patocka, MDCM; Karen Schiff, MD, FRCPC; Errol Stern, MD, CSPQ, FRCP(C); Maude St-Onge, MD, MSc, FRCPC; Paul D. Tourigny, MD, FRCPC; Jean-Marc Troquet, MD; Joel P. Turner, MD, MSc, FRCP (Guest Editor); Suneel Upadhye, MD, MSc, FRCPC; Eric Weldon, MD, FRCPC (EM); Jen Williams, BScPT, MDCM, FRCPC (EM); William A. Woods, MD (Test Author); and Karen G.H. Woolfrey, MD, FRCP(C).

The authors/editors listed below identified the following professional or financial affiliations for themselves or their spouse/partner:
Matthew Oughton, MD, FRCP(C) is on the Advisory Board for Sunovion.

Disclosure of Discussion of Non-FDA Approved Uses for Pharmaceutical Products and/or Medical Devices

The University of Virginia School of Medicine, as an ACCME provider, requires that all faculty presenters identify and disclose any off-label uses for pharmaceutical and medical device products. The University of Virginia School of Medicine recommends that each physician fully review all the available data on new products or procedures prior to clinical use.

TO ENROLL

To enroll in the Emergency Medicine Clinics of North America Continuing Medical Education program, call customer service at 1-800-654-2452 or visit us online at www.theclinics.com/home/cme. The CME program is available to subscribers for an additional fee of $190.00.

Foreword

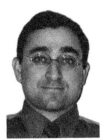

Amal Mattu, MD
Consulting Editor

"The unofficial mantra of the specialty of emergency medicine is 'A-B-C: airway, breath sounds, circulation.'"[1] This mnemonic emphasizes the well-accepted priority in the approach to managing unstable patients. The *Emergency Medicine Clinics* series has addressed airway as well as circulation issues considerably in recent months and years. This should serve as no surprise to anyone who keeps up with the emergency medicine literature … airway and cardiovascular issues always attract great notoriety and excitement. The "B" in our traditional mantra, however, often tends to be neglected or relegated to being of secondary importance. Yet nothing could be further from the truth. The "B" represents the lungs, which form the vital link between the celebrated airway and cardiovascular system. Poor lung function compromises every other vital organ in the body by depriving them of the body's primary nutrient, oxygen. Poor lung function also allows the rapid buildup of the body's most dangerous poison, carbon dioxide, which can impair virtually every vital organ and metabolic process. It should be clear to everyone that the "B," though less eminent than "A" and "C," certainly deserves its rightful place within our specialty's mantra.

In this month's issue of *Clinics*, Dr Joel Turner and a distinguished group of his colleagues have provided us with a series of articles that bring the "B" back to preeminence. They address the whole gamut of acute pulmonary diseases that emergency physicians face on a regular basis, including asthma, chronic obstructive pulmonary disease, pulmonary embolism, and pneumonia. They also address newer entities such as H1N1 influenza. They address emergencies that occur in special populations as the young, the elderly, and patients with HIV. Additionally, they address some issues pertaining to trauma and vascular conditions of the thorax. They also address critical management issues pertaining to invasive and noninvasive mechanical ventilation. Finally, they discuss the various imaging modalities, including cutting-edge uses for bedside ultrasound in diagnosing and managing patients with thoracic emergencies.

This issue of *Clinics* represents an important contribution to education and clinical practice in emergency medicine. In itself, this issue constitutes a full reading curriculum pertaining to pulmonary and thoracic emergencies. Our thanks go to Dr Turner and his

Emerg Med Clin N Am 30 (2012) xiii–xiv
doi:10.1016/j.emc.2012.01.002   **emed.theclinics.com**

colleagues for reminding us so clearly that the lungs truly are the vital link between the "A" and the "C."

Amal Mattu, MD
Department of Emergency Medicine
University of Maryland School of Medicine
110 S. Paca Street, 6th Floor, Suite 200
Baltimore, MD 21201, USA

E-mail address:
amattu@smail.umaryland.edu

REFERENCE

1. Mattu A, Olshaker JS. Preface: respiratory emergencies. Emerg Med Clin North Am 2003;21:xv–xvi.

Preface

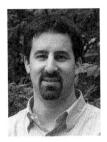

Joel P. Turner, MD, MSc, FRCP
Guest Editor

Airway, Breathing Circulation … Airway, Breathing Circulation …. This mantra has been ingrained into every medical student, resident, and attending staff as THE priority in assessing medical and trauma patients presenting to the emergency department. As such, any condition, be it infectious, traumatic, or vascular, which compromises the thoracic cavity can result in profound and deleterious effects on a patient's airway, respiratory, and cardiovascular status, and, by extension, his/her morbidity and mortality.

The patient presenting with complaints of dyspnea and/or chest pain is so ubiquitous in our daily practice that not an hour goes by that we are not assessing a patient's thoracic region for the presence of pathology. In 2007, there were 2.7 million visits by adults (>15 years of age) to an American emergency department with a complaint of shortness of breath and 5.9 million visits for chest pain.[1] In patients over the age of 64, chest pain and dyspnea are the leading reasons for visiting an ED.

This issue of *Emergency Clinics* will provide an evidence-based review of a variety of thoracic emergencies found in the adult and pediatric population. Specifically, these will include the assessment and management of the difficult airway, the use of varying noninvasive and invasive ventilator strategies, a systematic approach in managing the patient with major thoracic trauma, pleural diseases, and vascular emergencies, as well as a variety of infectious and environmental conditions affecting the thoracic/respiratory system.

In the past 10 years, we have seen significant advances in the diagnosis, treatment, and overall understanding of well-known medical conditions (COPD, asthma, pneumonia, HIV-related illnesses, pulmonary embolism). The shear number of original articles addressing these conditions is staggering. In addition, we have also been witness to the appearance of "new diseases" such as the H1N1 influenza pandemic.

Finally, we have also seen the emergence of a "new" technology available to the emergency physician—thoracic ultrasound—which has revolutionized our ability to assess, diagnose, and monitor a multitude of thoracic pathologies rapidly.

Emerg Med Clin N Am 30 (2012) xv–xvi
doi:10.1016/j.emc.2012.01.001
0733-8627/12/$ – see front matter © 2012 Elsevier Inc. All rights reserved.

emed.theclinics.com

It has been a distinct pleasure to edit this issue of *The Clinics*. I would like to thank all the dedicated authors who have contributed so much of their time to write their articles. I would like to thank Patrick Manley and Amal Mattu for their support and guidance through this journey. I would like to thank my wife and family especially for their support and patience during the editing and writing phases of this issue.

Joel P. Turner, MD, MSc, FRCP
Department of Emergency Medicine
Jewish General Hospital
3755 Côte-Sainte-Catherine Road, Room D-010
Montreal, Quebec, Canada H3T 1E2

E-mail address:
joel.turner@mcgill.ca

REFERENCE

1. Niska R, Bhuiya F. National hospital ambulatory medical care survey: 2007 emergency department summary. Natl Health Stat Report 2010;26:1–31.

Asthma Diagnosis and Management

Ariana Murata, MD, Patrick M. Ling, MD, MPH*

KEYWORDS

- Asthma • Emergency • Diagnosis • Management

EPIDEMIOLOGY

Asthma is one of the most common chronic diseases in adults, affecting 300 million people worldwide.[1] Asthma affects 7% to 8% of people in North America,[2–4] including more than 24 million Americans[4] and 3 million Canadians.[2,3] The prevalence of asthma in older adults is 6% to 10%.[4,5] The number of elderly patients will increase in the future as this segment of the population continues to grow. Currently, the highest prevalence of asthma is seen in English-language countries and Latin America.[6] Asthma rates steadily increased from the 1960s to 1990s, with most ongoing gains seen in developing countries and older adults.[5,7,8] Since the late 1990s, the prevalence of asthma has been either stabilizing or declining in higher income countries.[6,7,9–12]

Asthma accounts for 2 million visits to emergency departments (EDs) annually in the United States.[13] Between 6% and 13% of those with asthma exacerbations require hospital admission.[14,15] Older adults have higher rates of hospitalization. In a large-scale study, older adults were twice as likely (14%) to be hospitalized as younger adults (7%).[16] Asthma accounts for around 4000 deaths annually in the United States[4,13] and 500 deaths in Canada.[3] Mortality from asthma has been decreasing since the 1990s.[3,17] However, mortality remains highest in elderly patients, accounting for two-thirds of deaths from asthma.[5] Asthma exacerbations are potentially fatal and should be treated seriously, although death occurs in a minority of asthmatics.[17–19]

PATHOPHYSIOLOGY

Asthma is a chronic inflammatory disorder that is characterized by bronchial hyperresponsiveness and airway obstruction.[20] Bronchospasm is the key feature of asthma, and is triggered by allergens or other stimuli. Mast cells are activated through immunoglobulin E receptors to release inflammatory mediators that directly target bronchial smooth muscle.[21,22] Bronchodilators are usually effective in reversing these symptoms, and are the recommended first-line treatment of asthma.[20,23,24]

The authors have nothing to disclose.

Division of Emergency Medicine, Royal University Hospital, University of Saskatchewan, Room 2684, 103 Hospital Drive, Saskatoon, Saskatchewan S7N 0W8, Canada

* Corresponding author.

E-mail address: patrick.ling@usask.ca

Emerg Med Clin N Am 30 (2012) 203–222

doi:10.1016/j.emc.2011.10.004

Inflammation is central to the pathophysiology of asthma, and can lead to permanent changes in airway structure and pulmonary function, in a process known as airway remodelling.[25,26] Inflammatory cells involved in asthma include lymphocytes,[27,28] mast cells,[21] eosinophils,[29,30] neutrophils, dendritic cells,[31] macrophages,[32] and epithelial cells.[33] Research into the inflammatory nature of asthma is leading to advances in therapy, in areas such as immunotherapy and leukotriene receptor modulators.

HISTORY AND PHYSICAL EXAMINATION

The classic triad of asthma includes chronic cough, wheeze, and dyspnea. However, patients often present with only 1 of these symptoms, which can make diagnosis challenging. In studies of patients presenting solely with wheeze, chronic cough, or dyspnea, only 24% to 35% were eventually diagnosed with asthma.[25,34,35] Symptoms of asthma are typically worse at night or early in the morning. A personal history of atopy and family history of asthma favor the diagnosis.

Asthma symptoms are typically variable and worsen with exposure to triggers. Common precipitants include house dust mites,[36,37] animal dander, cockroaches,[36] *Alternaria*,[38] pollens, and molds. Air pollutants and sulfites can cause exacerbations.[39] In a recent multicenter study of 654 asthmatics, exposure to environmental tobacco smoke was associated with worse lung function, higher acuity of exacerbations, and increased health care use.[40] Viral respiratory infections are the most common causes of asthma exacerbations in children and infants.[41,42] Aspirin and other nonsteroidal antiinflammatory drugs (NSAIDs) can trigger attacks in up to 20% of asthmatics.[43] Occupational exposure to chemicals and dust should be considered.[44] Strong emotional expression,[45,46] exercise,[47] and menstrual cycles may worsen the symptoms of asthma.[48,49]

Risk factors for severe, uncontrolled asthma should be assessed, including previous intubations or intensive care admissions, 2 or more hospitalizations for asthma in the past year, 3 or more ED visits for asthma in the past year, hospitalization or ED visit for asthma in the past month, using more than 2 canisters of short-acting β-agonist monthly, and lack of a written asthma action plan.[20] Difficulty perceiving the severity of asthma symptoms is a worrisome sign.[20] Low socioeconomic status, inner-city residence, illicit drug use, and major psychosocial problems are risk factors for death from asthma.[20]

A history of compliance with medications, prehospital care, and types and doses of asthma maintenance medications should be obtained. Prolonged symptoms are more difficult to treat, given the inflammatory nature of asthma. Differential diagnoses should be ruled out by careful history taking. Comorbidities that could aggravate asthma should be identified, including allergic bronchopulmonary aspergillosis, gastroesophageal reflux disease, obesity, rhinosinusitis, obstructive sleep apnea, and depression.[20]

Asthma is often underdiagnosed and undertreated in older adults.[5,50] The elderly asthmatic suffers from the typical symptoms of asthma, but is more likely to have reduced perception of bronchoconstriction.[51–53] This may lead to delay in seeking medical care and increased risk of severe asthma attacks.[53–55] Older adults are more likely to have comorbidities or use medications (eg, β-blockers, acetylsalicylic acid, NSAIDs) that may exacerbate asthma.[43,56]

The severity of an asthma exacerbation can be assessed by quantitative measurements of lung function, such as peak expiratory flow (PEF). Patients with mild asthma (PEF ≥70% of predicted) present with dyspnea on exertion and increased respiratory rate. They are able to speak in sentences and to lie down. Moderate wheeze may be heard on auscultation. The patient suffering from a moderate asthma exacerbation (PEF 40%–69%) has dyspnea at rest, and is more comfortable sitting than lying down. Loud wheeze is commonly heard throughout exhalation. Suprasternal retractions and use of accessory respiratory muscles are commonly seen.

Clinical signs of severe asthma (PEF <40%) include use of accessory respiratory muscles, inability to speak or lie supine because of dyspnea, and pulsus paradoxus (decrease in systolic blood pressure of ≥12 mm Hg with inspiration). In particularly severe attacks, pulsus paradoxus can be greater than 25 mm Hg. Respiratory rate is often more than 30 breaths per minute. The patient is most comfortable sitting up and can be agitated. Loud wheeze is heard throughout inspiration and expiration. Cyanosis, decreasing level of consciousness, and respiratory muscle fatigue are markers of impending respiratory arrest. Failure of severe symptoms to respond to initial treatment is particularly worrisome.

DIFFERENTIAL DIAGNOSIS

Wheezing is characteristic of asthma, but can be a presentation of many different diseases. Physicians should be aware that "all that wheezes is not asthma; all that wheezes is not obstruction." The clinical diagnosis of asthma should be confirmed by quantitative measurements of lung function.[20] Spirometry is the preferred diagnostic test, and can be done in pulmonary function laboratories, or alternatively in the primary care office. Spirometry measures the forced vital capacity (FVC; the maximal volume of air that can be exhaled from maximal expiration) and the FEV_1 (volume of air exhaled during the first second). Spirometry assesses obstruction and potential reversibility of symptoms, and can be done in patients older than 5 years of age.[20] Additional pulmonary studies, methacholine bronchoprovocation, or chest radiography may be needed if the diagnosis is in doubt. Allergy testing may be indicated. Biomarkers of inflammation, such as sputum eosinophils[57,58] and fractional exhaled nitric oxide,[59] are currently being evaluated as adjunctives for the diagnosis of asthma.

More than 50% of older adults with obstructive disease may share features of both asthma and chronic obstructive pulmonary disease (COPD).[60] Overlap syndrome of asthma and COPD is characterized by evidence of incompletely reversible airway obstruction (COPD) and increased variability of airflow. This subgroup of patients is still poorly recognized and is typically excluded from current therapeutic trials. A recent study of 1546 patients showed that those with overlap syndrome had lower quality of life than those with either disease alone.[61] These patients would benefit from further studies to clarify optimal treatment strategies **Box 1**.

ED EVALUATION

Asthma exacerbations are characterized by obstruction to expiratory airflow, and can be assessed by quantitative tests of lung function. These measurements include PEF and spirometry, and are more reliable indicators of the severity of acute asthma than clinical symptoms alone.[20] PEF is the most commonly used test in the ED to assess the degree of obstruction. PEF readings are safe, quick, and cost-effective. They can be used to monitor a patient's response to treatment over time. Normal PEF values vary with gender, height, age, and ethnicity. A value less than 200 L/min usually indicates severe obstruction. Repeated PEF or FEV_1 measurements at ED presentation and 1 hour after treatment are the strongest predictors of hospitalization in asthmatics.[62,63]

Box 1
Differential diagnosis of wheezing in adults

- Asthma
- COPD
- Congestive heart failure
- Pulmonary embolism
- Pneumonia
- Tumors
- Cough secondary to drugs (eg, angiotensin-converting enzyme [ACE] inhibitors)
- Foreign body in trachea or bronchus
- Aspiration pneumonitis
- Allergic rhinitis and sinusitis
- Postnasal drip
- Gastroesophageal reflux
- Vocal cord dysfunction
- Recurrent cough not caused by asthma

Clinicians should educate patients in the early recognition and treatment of asthma exacerbations. Patients should start immediate treatment at home with inhaled bronchodilators if they recognize symptoms or if PEF decreases to less than 80% of predicted. PEF should be reassessed after initial bronchodilator treatment (eg, up to 2 treatments 20 minutes apart of 2–6 puffs by metered-dose inhaler [MDI] or nebulizer treatments). Initial PEF or FEV_1 is used to classify the severity of asthma in patients in the ED. Signs, symptoms, and clinical course vary with the different levels of asthma severity (**Table 1**).

Pulse oximetry is a reliable way to monitor for hypoxemia in the asthmatic patient. It is recommended for patients in severe distress, PEF or FEV_1 less than 40% of normal, or if the patient cannot perform lung function measurements.[20] Arterial blood gas measurements are rarely done, and are indicated only in patients with PEF less than 25% of predicted, because this group alone is at risk for significant hypercapnia or acidosis.[64] Increased or normal arterial carbon dioxide pressure ($Paco_2$) is a worrisome sign, because it indicates that obstruction is so severe that the patient cannot respond to the increased respiratory drive that typifies acute asthma. When indicated, venous blood gases are strongly correlated with arterial blood gases and can reliably be used to measure pH and CO_2 pressure (pco_2).[65] Respiratory failure can develop from further progression of symptoms. Blood gases can also be considered in patients who are unable to perform pulmonary function tests.

Chest radiographs are generally not useful in the setting of acute asthma, and most commonly show pulmonary hyperinflation.[66] They should only be used to evaluate other suspected causes of the patient's symptoms (eg, pneumonia, pneumothorax, congestive heart failure). Electrocardiograms should be done in patients with suspected cardiac disorders.

TREATMENT

Early recognition and treatment of the asthma exacerbation is essential for success in overall management. Patients presenting to the ED with acute asthma should be

Table 1
Classifying severity of asthma exacerbations in the urgent or emergency care setting

	Symptoms and Signs	Initial PEF (or FEV₁)	Clinical Course
Mild	Dyspnea only with activity (assess tachypnea in young children)	PEF ≥70% predicted or personal best	Usually cared for at home Prompt relief with inhaled SABA Possible short course or oral systemic corticosteroids
Moderate	Dyspnea interferes with or limits usual activity	PEF 40%–69% predicted or personal best	Usually requires office or ED visit Relief from frequent inhaled SABA Oral systemic corticosteroids; some symptoms last for 1–2 d after treatment is begun
Severe	Dyspnea at rest; interferes with conversation	PEF <40% predicted or personal best	Usually requires ED visit and likely hospitalization Partial relief from frequent inhaled SABA Oral systemic corticosteroids; some symptoms last for >3 d after treatment is begun Adjunctive therapies are helpful
Subset: life threatening	Too dyspneic tospeak; perspiring	PEF <25% predicted or personal best	Requires ED/hospitalization; possible ICU Minimal or no relief from frequent inhaled SABA Intravenous corticosteroids Adjunctive therapies are helpful

Abbreviations: FEV₁, forced expiratory volume in 1 second; ICU, intensive care unit; SABA, short-acting β2-agonist.

Reproduced from National Asthma Education and Prevention Program. Expert panel report III: Guidelines for the diagnosis and management of asthma. Bethesda (MD): National Heart, Lung, and Blood Institute; 2007 (NIH publication no. 08-4051).

quickly evaluated for the adequacy of airway, breathing, and circulation. This evaluation should include a complete set of vital signs, pulse oximetry, respiratory rate, and an assessment of respiratory effort. Treatment should be started immediately.

Current recommendations are outlined in the 2007 National Asthma and Education and Prevention Program (NAEPP) Expert Panel Report (EPR-3) (coordinated by the National Heart, Lung, and Blood Institute of the National Institutes of Health) and the 2005 Canadian Asthma Consensus Guidelines.[20,23,24] Goals of therapy include correction of hypoxemia, rapid reversal of airway obstruction, and treatment of inflammation. Begin treatment by giving oxygen to keep the oxygen saturation at more than 90%. The adequacy of the patient's airway, breathing, and circulation should be carefully assessed. The offending stimulus, if known, should be removed. β-Agonists are given to achieve rapid reversal of airflow obstruction. Anticholinergics are added for the treatment of severe exacerbations. Administration of systemic corticosteroids should be considered early in the treatment of those with moderate or severe asthma exacerbations, or those who do not respond quickly and completely to β-agonists. Response to therapy should be monitored with serial measurements of lung function.[20]

β2-AGONISTS

β2-Agonists are potent bronchodilators that act on β receptors to quickly and effectively relax bronchial smooth muscle. Short-acting β-agonists are the recommended first-line therapy for the acute asthma exacerbation.[20] Albuterol is the most commonly used β2-agonist for acute asthma.

β2-Agonists can be administered in multiple forms, including MDI, nebulizer, subcutaneous injection, and intravenous injection. Traditionally, aerosolized bronchodilators have been administered by continuous-flow nebulization. However, multiple studies have found little difference in efficacy between MDI and nebulizer therapy.[67–69] Hospital admission rates are equivalent between the 2 modalities.[69] MDI is more cost-effective and time-effective than nebulizer therapy,[67,70] but must be administered with proper inhaler technique using a holding chamber or spacer device (eg, Aerochamber). MDI/spacers result in significantly shorter stays in the ED, greater improvements in PEF, and lower cumulative dose of albuterol.[67] MDIs can be administered easily in the patient's own home. An additional concern with aerosolized or nebulized medication is its potential to spread infectious agents.[71] Recommendations suggest the use of personal protective devices and N95 masks by health care providers for suspected influenzalike illnesses.[72] Barriers to widespread administration of MDI/spacers in the ED include lack of leadership for change, lack of consensus about the benefits of this modality, perceived resistance from patients and parents, and perceived increased in cost and workload.[73,74]

For acute asthma, 2 to 6 inhalations of albuterol are given with MDI and spacer device. Therapy is repeated every 20 minutes for up to 4 hours until there is maximal improvement in respiratory symptoms. Alternatively, if MDI is unavailable or if the patient is unable to use proper techniques, 2.5 to 5.0 mg of nebulized albuterol is given every 20 minutes to a total of 3 doses (maximum of 15 mg in one hour). Albuterol can also be given as a continuous nebulization at a rate of 10 to 15 mg over 1 hour. A Cochrane Review reported a number needed to treat (NNT) of 10 for the use of continuous versus intermittent β-agonists in the treatment of acute asthma to prevent 1 hospital admission.[75] Therapy should be titrated to an objective measure of airflow obstruction (eg, FEV_1 or PEF) and clinical response.

β-Agonists should only be used for relief of acute symptoms. If used on a chronic basis, they can cause desensitization and tolerance. Adverse effects associated with β-agonists include tremor, tachycardia, palpitations, hyperglycemia, and hypokalemia.

Current evidence does not support the use of intravenous β2-agonists for the treatment of acute severe asthma.[76] Long-acting β-agonists (LABAs) have no role in acute asthma management. LABAs can be used in combination with inhaled corticosteroids for long-term treatment of moderate or severe persistent asthma. They should not be used as monotherapy.[20]

Short-term side effects of β-agonists include tachycardia and hypokalemia. Long-term adverse effects include sinus and ventricular tachycardia, syncope, atrial fibrillation, congestive heart failure, myocardial infarction, cardiac arrest, and sudden death.[77] In long-term use, compared with placebo, β-adrenergic-agonists significantly increased the risk for cardiovascular events (relative risk, 2.54; 95% confidence interval, 1.59–4.05).

ANTICHOLINERGICS

Anticholinergics block the action of acetylcholine on the parasympathetic autonomic system. They decrease vagally mediated smooth muscle contraction in the airways, leading to bronchodilation. Anticholinergics are recommended for the treatment of severe asthma, in combination with short-acting β-agonists.[20,78] The synergistic effects of these 2 agents decrease hospitalization rates and improve lung function.[78–80] Ipratropium bromide is the most commonly used anticholinergic agent for the treatment of asthma.

Ipratropium has a slow onset of action, reaching its peak effect in 90 minutes. In contrast, the onset of action for albuterol is less than 5 minutes. In addition, ipratropium is not as potent a bronchodilator as albuterol. For these reasons, ipratropium should not be used alone for acute asthma management. For the acute exacerbation, 0.5 mg of ipratropium is given by nebulization every 20 minutes for 3 doses. Alternatively, 8 puffs with MDI and spacer can be given every 20 minutes for up to 3 hours.

A recent study showed the benefit of a multiple-dose protocol of ipratropium combined with albuterol in patients with severe asthma exacerbations (FEV <50%). Both medications were administered through MDI every 10 minutes for 3 hours. Patients had significant improvements in pulmonary function and decreased admission rates. The most benefit was seen in those with more severe obstruction (FEV ≤30%) and long duration of symptoms (≥24 hours before ED presentation).[80] In a 2008 Cochrane Review, the addition of multiple doses of anticholinergics to β2-agonists decreased the risk of hospital admission by 25% in children with moderate and severe asthma. The NNT using multiple additional doses of anticholinergics plus β-agonists for the treatment of asthma exacerbation to prevent 1 hospital admission is 12.[78]

Anticholinergics are not recommended for hospitalized patients.[20] Two randomized controlled trials did not show significant benefit from ipratropium for hospitalized patients with severe asthma.[81,82]

CORTICOSTEROIDS

Acute asthma is characterized by airway edema, mucus hypersecretion, and cellular infiltration, in addition to bronchospasm. This inflammatory reaction can lead to persistent airway obstruction, and is the target of corticosteroids. Corticosteroids are the most potent and effective antiinflammatory agents available for the treatment of asthma. Their onset of action can take up to 6 hours to become clinically apparent.[83]

Early systemic corticosteroids in the ED are recommended for moderate or severe asthma, or if β-agonists do not fully correct the decline in pulmonary function.[20] A 2001 Cochrane Review of 863 patients showed a significant reduction in hospital admission rates when corticosteroids were given within 1 hour of ED presentation; absolute risk reduction was 12.5% (NNT of 8).[84] In addition, a short course of corticosteroids for asthma exacerbations significantly decreases relapse rates and use of short-acting β2-agonist.[85] Current guidelines recommend that systemic corticosteroids be added immediately if there is an incomplete (PEF 50%–79% of best or predicted) or poor (<50% PEF) response to β-agonist therapy. The patient's response to β-agonists is established by administering up to 2 treatments 20 minutes apart, either by MDI or nebulizer. Systemic corticosteroids can also be considered in those with a good (≥80% PEF) response to short-acting β2-agonists (SABAs).[20] Following ED discharge, a course of corticosteroids should be given for 3 to 10 days to prevent relapse.[20,85]

Systemic corticosteroids come in multiple forms, including oral, intravenous, and intramuscular. The efficacy of oral corticosteroids is equivalent to the intravenous form.[86–88] Oral steroids are preferred, because they are less invasive.[20] Prednisone is administered orally at a dose of 40 to 60 mg. A recent randomized controlled trial showed that adults treated in the ED with 2 days of dexamethasone (16 mg daily) had equivalent outcomes to those treated with 5 days of prednisone (50 mg daily). In this study, 104 subjects receiving dexamethasone and 96 subjects receiving prednisone were assessed. The outcomes measured included return to normal level of activity and prevention of relapse.[89]

Intravenous corticosteroids are recommended for critically ill patients and those intolerant of the oral form.[20] Hospitalized patients are given 40 to 60 mg of methylprednisolone intravenously every 12 to 24 hours. For patients who require critical care admission, higher doses of 60 to 80 mg of methylprednisolone are given every 12 hours. Several studies have shown that intramuscular corticosteroids are as effective as oral treatment.[85,90] A randomized controlled trial of 190 adult patients in the ED showed that subjects treated with a single dose of 160 mg intramuscular methylprednisolone had similar relapse rates to those treated with 160 mg of oral methylprednisolone tapered over 8 days.[90]

Long-term use of systemic corticosteroids should be avoided; it is indicated only for the most severe cases of asthma. Side effects of chronic corticosteroid use can be significant, and include immune suppression, adrenal suppression, growth suppression, Cushing syndrome, cataracts, and glucose imbalances.[20] Conversely, inhaled corticosteroids are the recommended first-line therapy for long-term treatment of mild, moderate, and severe persistent asthma.[20,23,24] They are absorbed locally and have a minimal side effect profile.

MAGNESIUM SULFATE

There is evidence that magnesium inhibits the influx of calcium into smooth muscle cells, causing bronchodilation.[91] In addition, magnesium acts on neutrophils to decrease inflammation.[92] A 2009 Cochrane Review found that intravenous magnesium sulfate significantly improved pulmonary function and decreased hospital admission rates in patients suffering from severe asthma. There was no significant effect noted for all asthmatics in general.[93] Side effects of intravenous magnesium were minimal.

Current guidelines recommend that magnesium be given for life-threatening exacerbations of acute asthma, or if the exacerbation remains severe (PEF <40%) after 1 hour of conventional therapy.[20] For these indications, 2 g of intravenous magnesium sulfate should be administered.

Limited studies have shown variable efficacy of nebulized inhaled magnesium in combination with β2-agonists for the treatment of acute asthma. The benefit seems to be greatest in the subgroup of severe asthma.[94] More data are needed to support definitive conclusions.

HELIOX

Heliox is a blend of 70% to 80% helium and 20% to 30% oxygen, which has a lower gas density than air. Heliox can potentially decrease resistance to airflow and enhance delivery of nebulized bronchodilators.[95,96] The role of heliox in asthma management remains unclear. Currently, it is not recommended as an initial treatment of asthma.[20,97] There have been few controlled studies and the optimal duration of heliox treatment is unknown. Current guidelines recommend that heliox-driven albuterol nebulization should be given for life-threatening exacerbations or if the exacerbation remains severe (PEF <40%) after 1 hour of conventional therapy.[20]

A 2006 Cochrane Review concluded that heliox improved pulmonary function only in the subgroup of patients with the most severe obstruction. However, this conclusion was based on a small number of studies.[97] A recent randomized trial of 59 adults with severe asthma found significant improvements in FEV_1 in those treated with nebulized bronchodilators with heliox. The largest gains were in those who sat upright and leaned the trunk forward at an angle of 50° to –60°.[98] A randomized controlled trial of 80 adults showed the greatest benefit in older adults and those with the lower pretreatment PEFs.[99] A randomized controlled trial of 30 children with moderate to severe asthma showed a greater degree of clinical improvement in those treated with heliox-driven albuterol nebulization. Eleven patients (73%) in the heliox group were discharged in less than 12 hours, compared with 5 (33%) in the control group.[100]

Since the 2006 Cochrane Review, 2 small studies have been conducted in children with moderate to severe asthma comparing heliox-powered albuterol therapy versus controls; these did not show a statistical difference in clinically important outcomes (admission rate, need for intubation, hospital length of stay).[101,102]

LEUKOTRIENE MODIFIERS

Leukotrienes are potent inflammatory mediators. Leukotriene modifiers improve lung function and decrease asthma exacerbations.[103,104] Three leukotriene modifiers are currently available for long-term therapy for asthma: montelukast, zafirlukast, and zileuton. However, many studies have found that overall efficacy of inhaled corticosteroids is superior to that of leukotriene modifiers for the long-term control of asthma.[103,104] Leukotriene modifiers are an alternative chronic treatment of patients with mild persistent asthma, who are unable to use inhaled corticosteroids.[20]

Leukotriene modifiers have not been used traditionally in the emergent setting. However, promising new research shows that leukotriene modifiers may have a future role in the ED. A randomized multicenter trial evaluated the effects of oral zafirlukast in 641 acute asthmatics. Those receiving zafirlukast in the ED had significant improvement in dyspnea and FEV_1, decreased risk of relapse, and decreased need for extended hospital care.[105] Intravenous leukotriene modifiers have also shown promise in the setting of acute asthma. A randomized controlled trial of 201 asthmatics showed significant improvements in FEV_1 in the first 20 minutes after treatment with intravenous montelukast.[106]

IMMUNOTHERAPY

Immunotherapy is an emerging area of asthma treatment that targets allergen triggers of asthma. It is the only treatment modality that modifies the underlying disease process. Immunotherapy has no role in the acute management of asthma but can be used for long-term maintenance therapy. Injection immunotherapy should be considered when the allergic component is well documented, and when asthma control remains inadequate.[23,24,107]

METHYLXANTHINES

Theophylline and aminophylline are widely prescribed for asthma worldwide, and have been used for more than 50 years. However, current evidence shows that this medication class does not produce additional bronchodilation when combined with standard β-agonist therapy, and results in more adverse effects.[108] Currently, the methylxanthines are not recommended as therapy for the acute exacerbation of asthma. Sustained-release theophylline can be considered for the treatment of mild persistent asthma.[20]

CROMOLYN SODIUM AND NEDOCROMIL

Cromolyn sodium and nedocromil are alternative treatments for mild persistent asthma. These medications block chloride channels and modulate mast cell mediator release.[109] They can be used as preventive treatment before exercise or allergen exposure.[20] These agents have no role in the acute management of asthma.

MANAGEMENT OF STATUS ASTHMATICUS

Status asthmaticus is an acute, severe exacerbation of asthma that does not respond to conventional treatment. It can progress to respiratory failure and death. All patients presenting to the ED with severe asthma should be started on early intensive therapy. This therapy includes β2-agonists, anticholinergics, and systemic corticosteroids. If patients fail to respond to initial therapy, they should be moved to a more closely monitored setting.

Heliox-driven nebulization of bronchodilators and intravenous magnesium sulfate are recommended adjunctive treatments for life-threatening asthma exacerbations, or for severe exacerbations that fail to respond to conventional therapy within the first hour.[20] Subcutaneous epinephrine (0.01 mg/kg to maximum dose of 0.3–0.5 mg) or nebulized epinephrine can be considered. A meta-analysis of 6 studies (including 161 adults and 121 children and adolescents) compared the efficacy of nebulized epinephrine with nebulized β2-agonists. Patients receiving nebulized epinephrine had a nonsignificant improvement in lung function.[110]

Ketamine is a dissociative agent that dilates bronchial smooth muscle and increases circulating catecholamines. Ketamine reduces bronchospasm and can help delay the need for intubation.[111,112] Several case reports of patients with status asthmaticus treated with intravenous ketamine have shown promising results. In these studies, ketamine was given as an intravenous bolus of 0.5 to 1 mg/kg, then as an infusion of 0.5 to 2 mg/kg over 1 hour. These patients failed to improve with conventional therapies, but responded successfully to ketamine.[113,114] However a double-blind randomized controlled trial comparing ketamine bolus and infusion with placebo in moderately severe asthma exacerbations in children did not show improvement in pulmonary index score.[115]

If the patient continues to deteriorate despite maximal medical therapy, noninvasive ventilation or endotracheal intubation with mechanical ventilation should be considered.

NONINVASIVE VENTILATION

Noninvasive ventilation is a promising area of acute asthma treatment. The goal of this modality is to support and reduce the patient's respiratory effort, giving enough time to allow other treatments to take effect and possibly avoid intubation.[116] Small studies have supported its use for acute asthma.[117,118] Noninvasive ventilation can be considered for the stable asthmatic who is tiring from the high respiratory demand, and who is expected to recover in the next few hours.[116] A recent Cochrane Review and guidelines do not support the routine use of noninvasive ventilator support.[119–122]

INTUBATION AND MECHANICAL VENTILATION

A minority of severe asthmatics require invasive ventilation in a critical care setting. Endotracheal intubation should be considered in the patient with impending respiratory failure, despite maximal medical therapy. Risk factors for death from asthma include previous intubations or intensive care admissions, or recent history of poorly controlled asthma.[123-127] Four percent of patients hospitalized for asthma require endotracheal intubation and mechanical ventilation.[128]

Mortality among those requiring ventilation is around 8%.[129] Death is multifactorial, and can be caused by severe obstruction, extreme hyperinflation, complications of acute asthma, failure by the patient or clinician to appreciate the severity of the disease, and failure to optimally control asthma.

Warning signs that a patient will need intubation include decreasing level of consciousness, cyanosis, deterioration of FEV_1 or PEF, inability to maintain oxygenation by mask, respiratory muscle fatigue, and cardiac instability.[116] There is no evidence to support a specific pH or P_{CO_2} for intubation, and the decision should be made on clinical grounds. Intubation should be done by the most experienced clinician available, ideally with a large-bore endotracheal tube ($\geq$8.0 mm).[20] Rapid-sequence intubation (RSI) is the preferred approach, because the patient is typically exhausted with little physiologic reserve. The clinician should anticipate rapid oxygen desaturation with RSI, and use preoxygenation or positive pressure ventilation to optimize respiratory status.

Ketamine is the induction agent of choice for sedation and intubation of an asthmatic patient, because of its bronchodilating properties.[111,112] Intravenous ketamine is given at a dose of 1 to 2 mg/kg at a rate of 0.5 mg/kg/min and results in general anesthesia without respiratory depression.[130] Propofol induces bronchodilation and is an alternative induction agent, but can cause hypotension.[131,132]

Ventilator settings should be adjusted to minimize the risk of dynamic hyperinflation, caused by air trapping because of insufficient time for exhalation. Dynamic hyperinflation can lead to cardiovascular collapse and barotrauma. Asthmatics are particularly at risk for this complication, because the nature of the disease causes airflow obstruction that significantly affects expiratory flow. Respiratory rate settings should be decreased to give the patient more time to exhale. Initial tidal volume should be set at less than 8 mL/kg, to decrease the risk of lung inflation.[133]

Bronchodilators and systemic corticosteroids can be administered to the ventilated patient. For the intubated patient with refractory asthma, intravenous ketamine or inhaled isoflurane can be useful adjuncts. Heliox and extracorporeal life support can also be considered.

ASTHMA AND PREGNANCY

Asthma affects 3% to 8% of pregnant women and has a variable clinical course.[134-137] Clinical symptoms improve in one-third of pregnancies, worsen in one-third, and remain unchanged in one-third.[133,138] Clinical severity of asthma during pregnancy seems to follow severity before pregnancy.[139,140] Asthma exacerbations occur in 20% to 36% of pregnancies, most frequently between weeks 14 and 24. Poorly controlled asthma during pregnancy has been linked with increased risk of prematurity, cesarean delivery, preeclampsia, and growth restriction.[135,141-143]

The treatment of asthma during pregnancy can be challenging. The goal of asthma treatment during pregnancy should be to optimize the outcome of both mother and fetus. SABAs, anticholinergics, and inhaled corticosteroids seem to be safe during pregnancy. Budesonide is the long treatment of choice, because it has been extensively studied in pregnancy.[20] Systemic corticosteroids have been linked with prematurity, low birth weight, preeclampsia, congenital malformations, and cerebral palsy, and should be used with caution.[144-147] A meta-analysis of mothers treated with oral corticosteroids in the first trimester showed a significant increase in the risk of oral clefts in their offspring.[146] A recent large-scale study of antenatal steroids showed no difference in body size or survival free of major neurosensory disability in children at 2 years of age.[148] Epinephrine should be avoided during pregnancy, except in cases of anaphylaxis.

DISPOSITION

The goal for discharge from the ED is an FEV_1 or PEF greater than or equal to 70% of predicted, and a response that is sustained for 60 minutes after last treatment. Patient education is a key component to successful asthma management, and should be initiated in the ED.[20] Medications and inhaler techniques should be reviewed. A written asthma action plan that describes early recognition and self-management of exacerbations should be started or reviewed.[20] Patients should be counseled to avoid allergens or other triggers of asthma. Cigarette smoking in asthma is associated with increased disease severity, more frequent hospital admissions, and accelerated lung function decline.[149] Counseling for smoking cessation should be an essential component of asthma management.[150] Patients should seek follow-up asthma care within 1 to 4 weeks.[20]

β-Agonists and corticosteroids should be included in the discharge plan. Many studies have shown that a short course of corticosteroids significantly reduces early relapse rates after treatment of acute asthma in the ED.[151,152] In mild to moderate asthma exacerbations, inhaled corticosteroids and oral corticosteroids were similarly effective in preventing relapse. Patients with significant asthma exacerbations should receive a course of oral corticosteroids for 3 to 10 days. Intramuscular injection of long-acting methylprednisolone can be considered in patients at high risk of medical noncompliance.[90] Compared with oral, intramuscular corticosteroids are equally effective in terms of rates of relapse. A combination inhaled and oral corticosteroids regimen compared with oral corticosteroid treatment alone showed a trend toward reduced asthma relapse rates.[153]

Patients with FEV_1 or PEF 40% to 69% of predicted despite intensive therapy require continued treatment in the ED or hospital admission. Patients with FEV_1 or PEF less than 40% should be admitted to the intensive care unit. Adjunctive therapies and mechanical ventilation should be considered for these patients. Patients who continue to have features of severe exacerbation after initial treatment require admission. Patients who show greater than 75% PEF following one hour of initial treatment are suitable candidates for discharge from the ED.[121]

SUMMARY

Asthma is a chronic inflammatory disease that is commonly encountered in the ED. Early signs of worsening asthma should be recognized and immediate treatment given. β-Agonists, anticholinergics, and corticosteroids are mainstays of treatment of the asthma exacerbation. Magnesium sulfate, epinephrine, and heliox can be considered for life-threatening presentations of asthma. Control of environmental triggers, improvements in daily maintenance therapy for asthma, and increasing patient education should help to reduce the severity and frequency of asthma exacerbations seen in the ED.

REFERENCES

1. Masoli M, Fabian D, Holt S, et al. The global burden of asthma: executive summary of the GINA Dissemination Committee Report. Allergy 2004;59: 469–78.

2. Statistics Canada. Asthma by sex, provinces and territories 2010. Available at: http://www40.statcan.ca/l01/cst01/HEALTH50A-eng.htm. Accessed October 27, 2011.
3. Public Health Agency of Canada. Life and breath: respiratory disease in Canada. 2007. Available at: http://www.phac-aspc.gc.ca/publicat/2007/lbrdc-vsmrc/index-eng.php#tphp. Accessed October 27, 2011.
4. Centers for Disease Control and Prevention. National Health Interview Survey: Asthma. 2009. Available at: http://www.cdc.gov/asthma/default.htm. Accessed October 27, 2011.
5. Gibson P, McDonald V, Marks G. Asthma in older adults. Lancet 2010; 376(9743):803–13.
6. Lai CKW, Beasley R, Crane J, et al. Global variation in the prevalence and severity of asthma symptoms: Phase Three of the International Study of Asthma and Allergies in Childhood (ISAAC). Thorax 2009;64:476–83.
7. Eder W, Ege MJ, von Mutius E. The asthma epidemic. N Engl J Med 2006;355: 2226–35.
8. Bjorksten B, Clayton T, Ellwood P, et al, ISAAC Phase III Study Group. Worldwide trends for symptoms of rhinitis and conjunctivitis: phase III of the International Study of Asthma and Allergies in Childhood. Pediatr Allergy Immunol 2008;19: 110–24.
9. Asher MI, Montefort S, Bjorksten B, et al, ISAAC Phase Three Study Group. Worldwide time trends in the prevalence of symptoms of asthma, allergic rhino-conjunctivitis, and eczema in childhood: ISAAC Phases One and Three repeat multicountry cross-sectional surveys. Lancet 2006;368:733–43.
10. Senthilselvan A, Lawson J, Rennie DC, et al. Stabilization of an increasing trend in physician-diagnosed asthma prevalence in Saskatchewan, 1991 to 1998. Chest 2003;124(2):438–48.
11. Braun-Fahrlander C, Gassner M, Grize L, et al. No further increase in asthma, hay fever and atopic sensitisation in adolescents living in Switzerland. Eur Respir J 2004;23(3):407–13.
12. Ronchetti R, Villa MP, Barreto M, et al. Is the increase in childhood asthma coming to an end? Findings from three surveys of schoolchildren in Rome, Italy. Eur Respir J 2001;17(5):881–6.
13. Moorman JE, Rudd RA, Johnson CA. National surveillance for asthma–United States, 1980-2004. MMWR Surveill Summ 2007;56:1–54.
14. Rowe BH, Bota G, Clark S. Comparison of Canadian versus American emergency department visits for acute asthma. Can Respir J 2007;14:331–7.
15. Lougheed MD, Garvey N, Chapman KR. The Ontario Asthma Regional Variation Study: emergency department visit rates and the relation to hospitalization rates. Chest 2006;129:909–17.
16. Diette G, Krishnan JA, Dominici F, et al. Asthma in older adults: factors associated with hospitalization. Arch Intern Med 2002;162(10):1123–32.
17. Chen Y, Johansen H, Thillaiampalam S, et al. "Asthma". Health Reports. Statistics Canada Catalogue 2005;no. 82-003.16(2):43–6.
18. Restrepo RD, Peters J. Near-fatal asthma: recognition and management. Curr Opin Pulm Med 2008;14(1):13–23.
19. Romagnoli M, Caramori G, Braccioni F, et al. Near-fatal asthma phenotype in the ENFUMOSA Cohort. Clin Exp Allergy 2007;37(4):552–7.
20. National Asthma Education and Prevention Program. Expert panel report III: guidelines for the diagnosis and management of asthma. Bethesda (MD): National Heart, Lung, and Blood Institute; 2007 (NIH publication no. 08-4051).

21. Boyce JA. Mast cells: beyond IgE. J Allergy Clin Immunol 2003;111(1):24–32.

22. Brightling CE, Bradding P, Symon FA, et al. Mast-cell infiltration of airway smooth muscle in asthma. N Engl J Med 2002;346(22):1699–705.

23. Becker A, Lemiere C, Bérubé D, et al. Summary and recommendations from the Canadian Asthma Consensus Guidelines, 2003. CMAJ 2005;173:S3–11.

24. Becker A, Berube D, Chad Z, et al. Canadian Pediatric Asthma Consensus Guidelines, 2003 (updated to December 2004): introduction. CMAJ 2005;173: S12–4.

25. Pratter MR, Curley FJ, Dubois J, et al. Cause and evaluation of chronic dyspnea in a pulmonary disease clinic. Arch Intern Med 1989;149(10):2277–82.

26. Busse WW, Lemanske RF. Asthma. N Engl J Med 2001;344(5):350–62.

27. Cohn L, Elias JA, Chupp GL. Asthma: mechanisms of disease progression and persistence. Annu Rev Immunol 2004;22:789–815.

28. Akbari O, Faul JL, Hoyte EG, et al. CD4+ invariant T-cell–receptor+ natural killer T cells in bronchial asthma. N Engl J Med 2006;354(11):1117–29.

29. Williams TJ. The eosinophil enigma. J Clin Invest 2004;113(4):507–9.

30. Chu HW, Martin RJ. Are eosinophils still important in asthma? Clin Exp Allergy 2001;31(4):525–8.

31. Kuipers H, Lambrecht BN. The interplay of dendritic cells, Th2 cells and regu- latory T cells in asthma. Curr Opin Immunol 2004;16(6):702–8.

32. Peters-Golden M. The alveolar macrophage: the forgotten cell in asthma. Am J Respir Cell Mol Biol 2004;31(1):3–7.

33. Polito AJ, Proud D. Epithelial cells as regulators of airway inflammation. J Allergy Clin Immunol 1998;102(5):714–8.

34. Pratter MR, Hingston DM, Irwin RS. Diagnosis of bronchial asthma by clinical evaluation. An unreliable method. Chest 1983;84(1):42–7.

35. Irwin R, Curley FJ, French CL. Chronic cough. The spectrum and frequency of causes, key components of the diagnostic evaluation, and outcome of specific therapy. Am Rev Respir Dis 1990;141:640–7.

36. Huss K, Adkinson NF Jr, Eggleston PA, et al. House dust mite and cockroach exposure are strong risk factors for positive allergy skin test responses in the Childhood Asthma Management Program. J Allergy Clin Immunol 2001; 107(1):48–54.

37. Htut T, Higgenbottam TW, Gill GW, et al. Eradication of house dust mites from homes of atopic asthmatic subjects: a double-blind trial. J Allergy Clin Immunol 2001;107(1):55–60.

38. Bush RK, Prochnau JJ. Alternaria-induced asthma. J Allergy Clin Immunol 2004; 113(2):227–34.

39. Taylor SL, Bush RK, Selner JC, et al. Sensitivity to sulfited foods among sulfite- sensitive subjects with asthma. J Allergy Clin Immunol 1988;81(6):1159–67.

40. Comhair SA, Gaston BM, Ricci KS, et al, National Heart Lung Blood Institute Severe Asthma Research Program (SARP). Detrimental effects of environmental tobacco smoke in relation to asthma severity. PLoS One 2011;6(5):e18574.

41. Johnston SL, Pattemore PK, Sanderson G, et al. Community study of role of viral infections in exacerbations of asthma in 9-11 year old children. BMJ 1995; 310(6989):1225–9.

42. Martinez FD, Wright AL, Taussig LM, et al. Asthma and wheezing in the first six years of life. N Engl J Med 1995;332(3):133–8.

43. Jenkins C, Costello J, Hodge L. Systematic review of prevalence of aspirin induced asthma and its implications for clinical practice. BMJ 2004; 328(7437):434.

44. Quirce S, Sastre J. New causes of occupational asthma. Curr Opin Allergy Clin Immunol 2011;11:80–5.
45. Furgał M, Nowobilski R, Pulka G, et al. Dyspnea is related to family functioning in adult asthmatics. J Asthma 2009;46(3):280–3.
46. Rosenkranz MA, Davidson RJ. Affective neural circuitry and mind-body influences in asthma. Neuroimage 2009;47(3):972–80.
47. Randolph C. An update on exercise-induced bronchoconstriction with and without asthma. Curr Allergy Asthma Rep 2009;9(6):433–8.
48. Macsali F, Real FG, Plana E, et al. Early age at menarche, lung function, and adult asthma. Am J Respir Crit Care Med 2011;183(1):8–14.
49. Martinez-Moragon E, Plaza V, Serrano J, et al. Near-fatal asthma related to menstruation. J Allergy Clin Immunol 2004;113(2):242–4.
50. Jones SC, Iverson D, Burns P, et al. Asthma and ageing: an end user's perspective - the perception and problems with the management of asthma in the elderly. Clin Exp Allergy 2011;41(4):471–81.
51. Cuttitta G, Cibella F, Bellia V, et al. Changes in FVC during methacholine-induced bronchoconstriction in elderly patients with asthma: bronchial hyper-responsiveness and aging. Chest 2001;119(6):1685–90.
52. Quadrelli SA, Roncorini A. Features of asthma in the elderly. J Asthma 2001; 38(5):377–89.
53. Ekici M, Apan A, Ekici A, et al. Perception of bronchoconstriction in elderly asthmatics. J Asthma 2001;38(8):691–6.
54. Kikuchi Y, Okabe S, Tamura G, et al. Chemosensitivity and perception of dyspnea in patients with a history of near-fatal asthma. N Engl J Med 1994;330(19): 1329–34.
55. Bijl-Hofland ID, Cloosterman SG, Folgering HT, et al. Relation of the perception of airway obstruction to the severity of asthma. Thorax 1999;54(1):15–9.
56. Brooks TW, Creekmore FM, Young DC, et al. Rates of hospitalizations and emergency department visits in patients with asthma and chronic obstructive pulmonary disease taking beta-blockers. Pharmacotherapy 2007; 27(5):684–90.
57. Deykin A, Lazarus SC, Fahy JV, et al, Asthma Clinic Research Network, National Heart, Lung and Blood Institute/NIH. Sputum eosinophil counts predict asthma control after discontinuation of inhaled corticosteroids. J Allergy Clin Immunol 2005;115(4):720–7.
58. Green RH, Brightling CE, McKenna S, et al. Asthma exacerbations and sputum eosinophil counts: a randomised controlled trial. Lancet 2002;360(9347): 1715–21.
59. Smith AD, Cowan JO, Brassett KP, et al. Use of exhaled nitric oxide measurements to guide treatment in chronic asthma. N Engl J Med 2005;352(21): 2163–73.
60. Gibson PG, Simpson JL. The overlap syndrome of asthma and COPD: what are its features and how important is it? Thorax 2009;64(8):728–35.
61. Kauppi P, Kupiainen H, Lindqvist A, et al. Overlap syndrome of asthma and COPD predicts low quality of life. J Asthma 2011;48(3):279–85.
62. Karras DJ, Sammon ME, Terregino CA, et al. Clinically meaningful changes in quantitative measurements of asthma severity. Acad Emerg Med 2000;7(4): 327–34.
63. Kelly AM, Kerr D, Powell C. Is severity assessment after one hour of treatment better for predicting the need for admission in acute asthma? Respir Med 2004;98(8):777–81.

64. Martin TG, Elenbaas RM, Pingleton SH. Use of peak expiratory flow rates to eliminated unnecessary arterial blood gases in acute asthma. Ann Emerg Med 1982;11(20):70–3.
65. Rang LC, Murray HE, Wells GA, et al. Can peripheral venous blood gases replace arterial blood gases in emergency department patients? CJEM 2002; 4(1):7–15.
66. Tsai TW, Gallagher EJ, Lombardi G, et al. Guidelines for the selective ordering of admission chest radiography in adult obstructive airway disease. Ann Emerg Med 1993;22(12):1854–8.
67. Newman KB, Milne S, Hamilton C, et al. A comparison of albuterol administered by metered-dose inhaler and spacer with albuterol by nebulizer in adults presenting to an urban emergency department with acute asthma. Chest 2002; 121(4):1036–41.
68. Idris AH, McDermott MF, Raucci JC, et al. Emergency department treatment of severe asthma. Metered-dose inhaler plus holding chamber is equivalent in effectiveness to nebulizer. Chest 1993;103(3):665–72.
69. Cates CJ, Crilly JA, Rowe BH. Holding chambers (spacers) versus nebulisers for beta-agonist treatment of acute asthma. Cochrane Database Syst Rev 2009:CD000052.
70. Burrows T, Connett GJ. The relative benefits and acceptability of metered dose inhalers and nebulisers to treat acute asthma in preschool children [abstract]. Thorax 2004;59(Suppl 2):ii20.
71. Davies A, Thomson G, Walker J, et al. A review of the risks and disease transmission associated with aerosol generating medical procedures. J Infect Prev 2009;10(4):122–6.
72. Bahadori K, Doyle-Waters MM, Marra C, et al. Economic burden of asthma: a systematic review. BMC Pulm Med 2009;9:24.
73. Scott SD, Osmond MH, O'Leary KA, et al, Pediatric Emergency Research Canada (PERC) MDI/spacer Study Group. Barriers and supports to implementation of MDI/spacer use in nine Canadian pediatric emergency departments: a qualitative study. Implement Sci 2009;4:65.
74. Osmond MH, Gazarian M, Henry RL, et al, PERC Spacer Study Group. Barriers to metered-dose inhaler/spacer use in Canadian emergency departments: a national survey. Acad Emerg Med 2007;14(11):1106–13.
75. Camargo CA Jr, Spooner CH, Rowe BH. Continuous versus intermittent beta-agonists for acute asthma. Cochrane Database Syst Rev 2009:CD001115.
76. Travers AA, Jones AP, Kelly KD, et al. Intravenous beta2-agonists for acute asthma in the emergency department. Cochrane Database Syst Rev 2009:CD002988.
77. Salpeter SR, Ormiston TM, Salpeter EE. Cardiovascular effects of β-agonists in patients with asthma and COPD: A meta-analysis. Chest 2004;125(6): 2309–21.
78. Plotnick L, Ducharme F. Combined inhaled anticholinergics and beta2-agonists for initial treatment of acute asthma in children. Cochrane Database Syst Rev 2008:CD000060.
79. Rodrigo GJ, Castro-Rodriguez JA. Anticholinergics in the treatment of children and adults with acute asthma: a systematic review with meta-analysis. Thorax 2005;60(9):740–6.
80. Rodrigo GJ, Rodrigo C. First-line therapy for adult patients with acute asthma receiving a multiple-dose protocol of ipratropium bromide plus albuterol in the emergency department. Am J Respir Crit Care Med 2000;161(6):1862–8.

81. Craven D, Kercsmar CM, Myers TR, et al. Ipratropium bromide plus nebulized albuterol for the treatment of hospitalized children with acute asthma. J Pediatr 2001;138(1):51–8.
82. Goggin N, Macarthur C, Parkin PC. Randomized trial of the addition of ipratropium bromide to albuterol and corticosteroid therapy in children hospitalized because of an acute asthma exacerbation. Arch Pediatr Adolesc Med 2001; 155(12):1329–34.
83. Hood PP, Cotter TP, Costello JE, et al. Effect of intravenous corticosteroid on ex vivo leukotriene generation by blood leucocyctes of normal and asthmatic patients. Thorax 1999;54(12):1075–82.
84. Rowe BH, Spooner CH, Ducharme FM, et al. Early emergency department treatment of acute asthma with systemic corticosteroids. Cochrane Database Syst Rev 2001;1:CD002178.
85. Rowe BH, Spooner CH, Ducharme FM, et al. Corticosteroids for preventing relapse following acute exacerbations of asthma. Cochrane Database Syst Rev 2007;3:CD000195.
86. Becker JM, Arora A, Scarfone RJ, et al. Oral versus intravenous corticosteroids for children hospitalized with asthma. J Allergy Clin Immunol 2005;103(4):586–90.
87. Barnett PL, Caputo GL, Baskin M, et al. Intravenous versus oral corticosteroids in the management of acute asthma in children. Ann Emerg Med 1997;30(3):355–6.
88. Ratto D, Alfaro C, Sipsey J, et al. Are intravenous corticosteroids required in status asthmaticus? JAMA 1988;260(4):527–9.
89. Kravitz J, Dominici P, Ufberg J, et al. Two days of dexamethasone versus 5 days of prednisone in the treatment of acute asthma: a randomized controlled trial. Ann Emerg Med 2011;58(2):200–4.
90. Lahn M, Bijur P, Gallagher EJ. Randomized clinical trial of intramuscular vs oral methylprednisolone in the treatment of asthma exacerbations following discharge from an emergency department. Chest 2004;126(2):362–8.
91. Gourgoulianis KI, Chatziparasidis G, Chatziefthimiou A, et al. Magnesium as a relaxing factor of airway smooth muscles. J Aerosol Med 2001;14(3):301–7.
92. Cairns CB, Kraft M. Magnesium attenuates the neutrophil respiratory burst in adult asthmatic patients. Acad Emerg Med 1996;3:1093–7.
93. Rowe BH, Bretzlaff JA, Bourdon C, et al. Magnesium sulfate for treating acute exacerbations of acute asthma in the emergency department. Cochrane Database Syst Rev 2009:CD001490.
94. Blitz M, Blitz S, Beasely R, et al. Inhaled magnesium sulfate in the treatment of acute asthma. Cochrane Database Syst Rev 2009:CD003898.
95. Goode ML, Fink JB, Dhand R, et al. Improvement in aerosol with helium-oxygen mixtures during mechanical ventilation. Am J Med 2001;163:109–14.
96. Kress JP, Noth I, Gehlbach BK, et al. The utility of albuterol nebulized with heliox during acute asthma exacerbations. Am J Respir Crit Care Med 2002;165(9): 1317–21.
97. Rodrigo GJ, Pollack C, Rodrigo C, et al. Heliox for non-intubated acute asthma patients. Cochrane Database Syst Rev 2010:CD002884.
98. Brandão DC, Britto MC, Pessoa MF, et al. Heliox and forward-leaning posture improve the efficacy of nebulized bronchodilator in acute asthma: a randomized trial. Respir Care 2011;56(7):947–52.
99. Lee DL, Hsu CW, Lee H, et al. Beneficial effects of albuterol therapy driven by heliox versus by oxygen in severe asthma exacerbation. Acad Emerg Med 2005;12(9):820–7.

100. Kim IK, Phrampus E, Venkataraman S, et al. Helium/oxygen-driven albuterol nebulization in the treatment of children with moderate to severe asthma exacerbations: a randomized, controlled trial. Pediatrics 2005;116(5):1127–33.

101. Rivera ML, Kim TY, Stewart GM, et al. Albuterol nebulized in heliox in the initial ED treatment of pediatric asthma: a blinded, randomized controlled trial. Am J Emerg Med 2006;24(1):38–42.

102. Bigham MT, Jacobs BR, Monaco MA, et al. Helium/oxygen-driven albuterol nebulization in the management of children with status asthmaticus: a randomized, placebo-controlled trial. Pediatr Crit Care Med 2010;11(3):356–61.

103. Garcia-Garcia ML, Wahn U, Gilles L, et al. Montelukast, compared with fluticasone, for control of asthma among 6- to 14-year-old patients with mild asthma: the MOSAIC study. Pediatrics 2005;116(2):360–9.

104. Ostrom NK, Decotiis BA, Lincourt WR, et al. Comparative safety and efficacy of low-dose fluticasone propionate and montelukast in children with persistent asthma. J Pediatr 2005;147(2):213–20.

105. Silverman RA, Nowak RM, Korenblat PE, et al. Zafirlukast treatment for acute asthma: evaluation in a randomized, double-blind, multicenter trial. Chest 2004;126(5):1480–9.

106. Camargo CA Jr, Smithline HA, Malice MP, et al. A randomized controlled trial of intravenous montelukast in acute asthma. Am J Respir Crit Care Med 2003; 167(4):528–33.

107. Abramson MJ, Puy RM, Weiner JM. Injection allergen immunotherapy for asthma. Cochrane Database Syst Rev 2010:CD001186.

108. Parameswaran K, Belda J, Rowe BH. Addition of intravenous aminophylline to beta2-agonists in adults with acute asthma. Cochrane Database Syst Rev 2009:CD002742.

109. Alton EW, Norris AA. Chloride transport and the actions of nedocromil sodium and cromolyn sodium in asthma. J Allergy Clin Immunol 1996;98(5 Pt 2): S102–5.

110. Rodrigo GJ, Nannini LJ. Comparison between nebulized adrenaline and beta2 agonists for the treatment of acute asthma. A meta-analysis of randomized trials. Am J Emerg Med 2006;24(2):217–22.

111. L'Hommedieu CS, Arens JJ. The use of ketamine for the emergency intubation of patients with status asthmaticus. Ann Emerg Med 1987;16(5):568–71.

112. Hemmingsen C, Nielsen PK, Odorico J. Ketamine in the treatment of bronchospasm during mechanical ventilation. Am J Emerg Med 1994;12(4): 417–20.

113. Denmark TK, Crane HA, Brown L. Ketamine to avoid mechanical ventilation in severe pediatric asthma. J Emerg Med 2006;30(2):163–6.

114. Shlamovitz GZ, Hawthorne T. Intravenous ketamine in a dissociating dose as a temporizing measure to avoid mechanical ventilation in adult patient with severe asthma exacerbation. J Emerg Med 2011;41(5):492–4.

115. Allen JY, Macias CG. The efficacy of ketamine in pediatric emergency department patients who present with acute severe asthma. Ann Emerg Med 2005; 46(1):43–50.

116. Hodder R, Lougheed D, FitzGerald M, et al. Management of acute asthma in adults in the emergency department: assisted ventilation. CMAJ 2010;182(3): 265–72.

117. Murase K, Tomii K, Chin K, et al. The use of non-invasive ventilation for life-threatening asthma attacks: changes in the need for intubation. Respirology 2010;15(4):714–20.

118. Soroksy S, Stav D, Shpirer I. A pilot prospective, randomized, placebo-controlled trial of bilevel positive airway pressure in acute asthmatic attack. Chest 2003;123:1018–25.

119. Ram FS, Wellington S, Rowe BH, et al. Non-invasive positive pressure ventilation for treatment of respiratory failure due to severe acute exacerbations of asthma. Cochrane Database Syst Rev 2005;1:CD004360.

120. Bateman ED, Hurd SS, Barnes PJ, et al. Global strategy for asthma management and prevention: GINA executive summary. Eur Respir J 2008;31(1): 143–78.

121. Douglas G, Higgins B, Barnes N, et al. British guideline on the management of asthma: a national clinical guideline. Thorax 2008;63(Suppl 4):iv1–121.

122. Sutton L. Is NIV an effective intervention for patients with acute exacerbations of asthma? BestBETS, 2009. Available at: http://www.bestbets.org/bets/bet.php?id=15529. Accessed October 27, 2011.

123. Dhuper S, Maggiore D, Chung V, et al. Profile of near-fatal asthma in an inner-city hospital. Chest 2003;124(5):1880–4.

124. Mitchell I, Tough SC, Semple LK, et al. Near-fatal asthma: a population-based study of risk factors. Chest 2002;121(5):1407–13.

125. Eisner MD, Lieu TA, Chi F, et al. Beta agonists, inhaled steroids, and the risk of intensive care unit admission for asthma. Eur Respir J 2001;17(2): 233–40.

126. Malmstrom K, Kaila M, Kajosaari M, et al. Fatal asthma in Finnish children and adolescents 1976-1998: validity of death certificates and a clinical description. Pediatr Pulmonol 2007;42(3):210–5.

127. Turner MO, Noertjojo K, Vedal S, et al. Risk factors for near-fatal asthma. A case-control study in hospitalized patients with asthma. Am J Respir Crit Care Med 1998;157(6 Pt 1):1804–9.

128. Krishnan V, Diette GB, Rand CS, et al. Mortality in patients hospitalized for asthma exacerbations in the United States. Am J Respir Crit Care Med 2006; 174(6):633–8.

129. McFadden ER Jr. Acute severe asthma. Am J Respir Crit Care Med 2003;168: 740–59.

130. Papiris S, Kotanidou A, Malagari K, et al. Clinical review: severe asthma. Crit Care 2002;6(1):30–44.

131. Conti G, Ferretti A, Tellan G, et al. Propofol induces bronchodilation in a patient mechanically ventilated for status asthmaticus. Intensive Care Med 1993; 19(5):305.

132. Zaloga G, Todd M, Levit P, et al. Propofol-induced bronchodilation in patients with status asthmaticus. Internet J Emerg Intensive Care Med 2001;5(1).

133. Brenner B, Corbridge T, Kazzi A. Intubation and mechanical ventilation of the asthmatic patient in respiratory failure. J Allergy Clin Immunol 2009; 124(Suppl 2):S19–28.

134. Murphy VE, Gibson PG, Smith R, et al. Asthma during pregnancy: mechanisms and treatment implications. Eur Respir J 2005;25(4):731–50.

135. Namazy JA, Schatz M. Pregnancy and asthma: recent developments. Curr Opin Pulm Med 2005;11(1):56–60.

136. Liccardi G, Cazzola M, Canonica GW, et al. General strategy for the management of bronchial asthma in pregnancy. Respir Med 2003;97(7):778–89.

137. Kwon HL, Belanger K, Bracken MB. Asthma prevalence among pregnant and childbearing-aged women in the United States: estimates from national health surveys. Ann Epidemiol 2003;13(5):317–24.

138. Gluck JC. The change of asthma course during pregnancy. Clin Rev Allergy Immunol 2004;26(3):171–80.
139. Schatz M, Dombrowski MP, Wise R, et al. Asthma morbidity during pregnancy can be predicted by severity classification. J Allergy Clin Immunol 2003; 112(2):283–8.
140. Murphy VE, Gibson P, Talbot PI, et al. Severe asthma exacerbations during pregnancy. Obstet Gynecol 2005;106(5 Pt 1):1046–54.
141. Dombrowski MP, Schatz M. Asthma in pregnancy. Clin Obstet Gynecol 2010; 53(2):301–10.
142. Bakhireva LN, Schatz M, Jones KL, et al, Organization of Teratology Information Specialists Collaborative Research Group. Asthma control during pregnancy and the risk of preterm delivery or impaired fetal growth. Ann Allergy Asthma Immunol 2008;101(2):137–43.
143. Murphy VE, Clifton VL, Gibson PG. Asthma exacerbations during pregnancy. Thorax 2006;61(2):169–76.
144. Schatz M, Dombrowski MP, Wise R, et al, Maternal-Fetal Medicine Units Network, The National Institute of Child Health and Development; National Heart, Lung and Blood Institute. The relationship of asthma medication use to perinatal outcomes. J Allergy Clin Immunol 2004;113(6):1040–5.
145. Schatz M, Zeiger RS, Harden K, et al. The safety of asthma and allergy medications during pregnancy. J Allergy Clin Immunol 1997;100(3):301–6.
146. Park-Wyllie L, Mazzotta P, Pastuszak A, et al. Birth defects after maternal exposure to corticosteroids: prospective cohort study and meta-analysis of epidemiological studies. Teratology 2000;62(6):385–92.
147. Wapner RJ, Sorokin Y, Mele L, et al, National Institute of Child Health and Human Development Maternal-Fetal Medicine Units Network. Long-term outcomes after repeat doses of antenatal corticosteroids. N Engl J Med 2007;357(12):1190–8.
148. Crowther CA, Doyle LW, Haslam RR, et al, ACTORDS Study Group. Outcomes at 2 years of age after repeat doses of antenatal corticosteroids. N Engl J Med 2007;357(12):1179–89.
149. Fattahi F, Hylkema MN, Melgert BN, et al. Smoking and nonsmoking asthma: differences in clinical outcome and pathogenesis. Expert Rev Respir Med 2011;5(1):93–105.
150. Jang AS, Park SW, Kim DJ, et al. Effects of smoking cessation on airflow obstruction and quality of life in asthmatic smokers. Allergy Asthma Immunol Res 2010;2(4):254–9.
151. Chapman KR, Verbeek PR, White JG, et al. Effect of a short course of prednisone in the prevention of early relapse after the emergency room treatment of acute asthma. N Engl J Med 1991;324(12):788–94.
152. Fiel SB, Swartz MA, Glanz K, et al. Efficacy of short-term corticosteroid therapy in outpatient treatment of acute bronchial asthma. Am J Med 1983;75(2): 259–62.
153. Krishnan JA, Nowak R, Davis SQ, et al. Anti-inflammatory treatment after discharge home from the emergency department in adults with acute asthma. J Allergy Clin Immunol 2009;124(Suppl 2):S29–34.

Acute Exacerbations of Chronic Obstructive Pulmonary Disease in the Emergency Department

Cory A. Brulotte, MD, FRCPC[a],*, Eddy S. Lang, MDCM, CCFP(EM), CSPQ[a,b]

KEYWORDS

- Chronic obstructive pulmonary disease • COPD • Exacerbation

Chronic obstructive pulmonary disease (COPD) is recognized as a major cause of morbidity and mortality worldwide. According to the World Health Organization, there were an estimated 210 million persons suffering from the disease in 2007; it is responsible for 5% of all deaths, and it is projected to become the third leading cause of death worldwide by the year 2030 behind ischemic heart disease and cerebrovascular disease.[1] In the United States, acute exacerbations of COPD (AECOPDs) account for more than 1.5 million emergency department (ED) visits annually[2] and more than 125,000 deaths.[3] The Global Initiative for Chronic Obstructive Lung Disease (GOLD) and many other evidence-based practice guidelines have been created and updated to bring light to COPD's burden of disease, provide a working definition of the disease, and disseminate information for its identification, prevention, and treatment.[4–8]

DEFINITIONS

COPD is an umbrella term that is used to describe a heterogeneous group of progressive chronic respiratory diseases. The GOLD consensus definition for COPD[9] consists of 3 key points:

1. The pulmonary component of COPD is characterized by a limitation in airflow that is not fully reversible. It is usually progressive and is associated with an abnormal inflammatory response of the lung to noxious particles or gases.

The authors have nothing to disclose.

[a] Department of Emergency Medicine, Alberta Health Services: Calgary Zone, Foothills Medical Center, 1403 29th Street Northwest, Room C231, Calgary, Alberta, Canada T2N 2T9

[b] University of Calgary, Unit 1633, 1632 14 Avenue NW, Calgary, Alberta, Canada T2N 1M7

* Corresponding author.

E-mail address: corybrulotte@gmail.com

Emerg Med Clin N Am 30 (2012) 223–247

doi:10.1016/j.emc.2011.10.005

0733-8627/12/$ – see front matter © 2012 Published by Elsevier Inc.

2. COPD has significant extrapulmonary effects that contribute to disease severity.
3. COPD is preventable and treatable.

Previous definitions for COPD have included the terms, *emphysema* and *chronic bronchitis*. These terms are no longer used in the definition. Emphysema is a pathology term, not a clinical description. Emphysema describes the destruction of the gas exchange surfaces of the lung[10] yet there are several more pathologic abnormalities seen in patients with COPD.[11] Chronic bronchitis is the presence of cough and sputum production for at least 3 months in each of 2 consecutive years. Chronic bronchitis does not reflect the morbidity and mortality associated with airflow limitation. And many patients develop airflow limitation without chronic cough and sputum production.[9,12,13]

GOLD recommends simple spirometry for diagnosis and classification of COPD (**Box 1**).[9]

The most common presentation of COPD seen in EDs and the primary focus of this article is AECOPD. The classification outlined in Box 1 applies to the diagnosis and classification of baseline stable COPD status and does not apply to AECOPD.

ETIOLOGY AND RISK FACTORS FOR THE DEVELOPMENT OF COPD

Exposure to noxious particulate gases is the greatest risk factor and etiologic group of agents responsible for the development of COPD. Among these, primary and environmental tobacco smoke is most commonly implicated.[14,15] Inorganic and organic

---

Box 1
Spirometric classification of COPD based on postbronchodilator FEV_1

Stage I: mild

    FEV_1/FVC <0.70

    FEV_1 $\geq$80% predicted

Stage II: moderate

    FEV_1/FVC <0.70

    50% $\leq$ FEV_1 <80% predicted

Stage III: severe

    FEV_1/FVC <0.70

    30% $\leq$ FEV_1 <50% predicted

Stage IV: very severe

    FEV_1/FVC <0.70

    FEV_1 <30% predicted or FEV_1 <50% predicted plus chronic respiratory failure

Abbreviations: FEV_1, forced expiratory volume in the first second of expiration; FVC, forced vital capacity; respiratory failure, arterial partial pressure of oxygen (Pao_2) less than 8.0 kPa (60 mm Hg) with or without arterial partial pressure of carbon dioxide ($Paco_2$) greater than 6.7 kPa (50 mm Hg) while breathing air at sea level.

Data from the Global Strategy for the Diagnosis, Management and Prevention of COPD, Global Initiative for Chronic Obstructive Lung Disease (GOLD) 2011. Available from: http://www.goldcopd.org/.

occupational dusts and outdoor air pollution, play a significant but lesser role as etiologic agents for the development of COPD.[16,17] In the developing world, where a large burden of COPD exists, indoor air pollution from heating and cooking with biomass in poorly ventilated dwellings is a significant etiologic agent and risk for the development of COPD.[18–21]

There is a multitude of other risk factors associated with the development of the disease. Incidence increases with age[22] and is inversely related to socioeconomic status.[23] Multiple genes are associated with COPD[24] and specific genetic factors, such as the deficiency of the antiprotease α_1-antitrypsin, contribute to disease progression.[25] Observational data exist suggesting susceptibility in some families to severe COPD[26] and a specific phenotype is linked to an increased risk of COPD exacerbations.[27] Any factors that affect growth, and thus lung growth, during gestation and childhood may affect an individuals' risk of COPD development.[28] The prevalence of disease is almost equal in women and men but women show a greater susceptibility to the damaging effects of tobacco smoke.[29,30] Pulmonary viral and bacterial infection and colonization are associated with airway inflammation and an increased risk of COPD.[31,32] Finally, HIV may accelerate disease development.[33]

PATHOGENESIS, PATHOLOGY, AND PATHOPHYSIOLOGY
Pathogenesis

Current theory holds that the development of the pathologic lung damage and destruction, which characterizes COPD, is the result of an abnormal and amplified host inflammatory response resulting from a primary insult—chronic exposure to noxious particulates and gases.[11,34,35]

In patients with COPD, there is inflammation in the airways, parenchyma, and pulmonary vasculature. There is a mobilization and accumulation of neutrophils, macrophages, and T lymphocytes to various parts of the lung. The accumulation of these inflammatory components and the mediators they release serve as a self-perpetuating stimulus for further immune activation. It is hypothesized that these neutrophils release granules containing proteases that results in a change of the protease-antiprotease environment of the lung. This excess of proteases, such as elastase, goes unchecked and destroys alveolar walls.[11,34] This hypothesis is based on the observation that more than 80% persons who lack the major protease inhibitor α_1-antitrypsin, as seen in α_1-antitrypsin deficiency, develop COPD.[11]

Furthermore, this process of excess inflammation is thought to be accelerated by a change in the oxidant-antioxidant balance of the lung. Normally, the lung contains a healthy complement of antioxidants (superoxide dismutase and glutathione) that keep direct oxidative damage to a minimum. Tobacco smoke and other inhaled particulates contain abundant reactive oxygen species, which deplete these antioxidant mechanisms and inactivate native antiproteases, thereby inciting tissue damage.[11]

Pathology and Pathophysiology

The hallmark of COPD is airflow obstruction that is not fully reversible owing to several pathologic structural abnormalities. Emphysema is seen most commonly in patients with COPD and is characterized by the irreversible enlargement and destruction of the respiratory bronchioles and alveoli without accompanying fibrosis.[10,11,34] The distal airspace enlargement with alveolar destruction decreases the elastic recoil of the lung, results in collapse of the supporting walls of the airway,[35] and decreases expiratory airflow,[34] which result in obstruction and hyperinflation.

The major site of airway obstruction in COPD is in the smaller conducting airways of the lungs less than 2 mm in diameter. In these airways several mechanisms contribute to airflow obstruction. There is a hyperplasia of the mucus-secreting goblet cells of the airways and this results in chronic mucus hypersecretion that can result in plugging of the small airways. There is inflammatory infiltration and resultant thickening of the airway walls with neutrophils, macrophages, B cells, and T cells, which contributes to airflow limitation. Finally, there is thickening of the bronchiolar wall due to smooth muscle hypertrophy and peribronchial fibrosis.[34–36]

Some reversible airflow obstruction caused by airway hyper-responsiveness does take place but it does not occur in all individuals with COPD[37] and has a different biology than asthma.[38] Increasing severity of airway hyper-responsiveness does, however, predict decline in FEV_1[39] and is associated with higher mortality.[40]

Obstruction can result in hyperinflation of the lungs, which in turn can cause flattening of the diaphragm. This hinders ribcage movement during respiration and shortens the diaphragm muscle fibers, reducing its power. This ultimately results in a downward spiral of impaired respiration that worsens as the disease progresses both acutely and over time.[41] The hyperinflation seen in COPD is the main mechanism for a patient's dyspnea.[42]

Gas exchange abnormalities in COPD result in hypoxemia and hypercapnea. The severity of emphysema correlates with decreased Pao_2 and other markers of ventilation-perfusion (V/Q) mismatch. Peripheral airway obstruction also results in V/Q mismatch and combines with ventilatory muscle and diaphragmatic impairment in severe disease to reduce ventilation, leading to carbon dioxide retention. The abnormalities in alveolar ventilation and a reduced pulmonary vascular bed further worsen the V/Q mismatch.[43]

COPD is associated with extrapulmonary pathologies that significantly contribute to morbidity and mortality. The cardiovascular system is affected in several ways. Mild to moderate pulmonary hypertension occurs in patients with COPD. This is associated with decreased survival and is the result of hypoxia-induced vasoconstriction and the pulmonary remodeling that occurs in the disease. This can result in right heart hypertrophy and, over time, right heart failure known as cor pulmonale.[44] Furthermore, atherosclerosis and cardiovascular death are associated with increasing COPD severity.[45]

Neurologic and psychiatric problems, such as disordered sleep, anxiety, depression, and cognitive decline, are all are associated with COPD and result in a decrease in quality of life. Musculoskeletal problems include disuse atrophy, wasting, cachexia from increased energy use, and osteoporosis. Polycythemia or anemia is also common.[44,45]

ACUTE EXACERBATIONS OF COPD AND THEIR ETIOLOGY

An AECOPD is defined as "an event in the natural course of the disease characterized by a change in the patient's dyspnea, cough, and/or sputum that is beyond the normal day-to-day variations, is acute in onset, and may warrant a change in regular medication in a patient with underlying COPD."[46] AECOPDs are common and in one Canadian study they represented 4% of all ED patient visits.[47] AECOPD accelerates decline in FEV_1[48,49] and many patients do not return to their baseline lung function after the exacerbation.[50]

The frequency of AECOPDs has been shown significantly associated with worsening lung function, a history of exacerbations, a history of gastroesophageal reflux, and a poor quality of life.[27] AECOPDs can be complicated by pneumothorax, respiratory failure, and death. Each admission for AECOPD carries a mortality of 2.5%.[51]

The etiology of AECOPD can be broken down into 3 main categories: (1) infection, which causes the vast majority of COPD exacerbations and can be the result of bacterial, viral, or co-infection; (2) increased airway inflammation by a noninfectious source, such as air pollution or occupational gases and particulates; and (3) an alternative pathology that destabilizes COPD, such as pneumothorax, pulmonary embolism, heart failure, mucus plugging causing atelectasis, anxiety/depression, or a cold environment.[52] It does, however, remain undefined in up to one-third of cases.[46] MacDonald and colleagues[52] proposed a mnemonic for the etiology (**Box 2**).

β-Blockers traditionally have been thought to be contraindicated in COPD for fear of worsening respiratory status and causing an exacerbation. A recent Cochrane review has shown that cardioselective β-blockers, given as a single dose or for longer duration, produce no change in FEV_1 or respiratory symptoms compared with placebo and did not affect the FEV_1 treatment response to β_2-agonists.[53]

DIAGNOSIS
History and Physical Examination

In dyspneic patients without a known diagnosis of COPD, the disease should be considered when a patient has any combination of chronic cough, chronic sputum production, dyspnea at rest or with exertion, or a history of COPD risk factors, such as inhalational exposure to tobacco smoke, occupational dust, and chemicals. Physical examination findings may include cyanosis, a barrel chest with increased anteroposterior diameter, pursed lip breathing, decreased breath sounds or wheezing, and in the severely ill signs of right heart failure, including ankle edema and jugular venous distension.[54] The prevalence of Hoover's sign (paradoxic indrawing of the lower rib cage due to a flattened diaphragm) increases with worsening COPD and in one study was observed in up to 76% of those with very severe COPD.[55] The combination of a greater than 40 pack-year history of smoking, age greater than or equal to 45, and a minimum laryngeal height (distance between the suprasternal notch and top of the thyroid cartilage) at end inspiration of less than or equal to 4 cm has a positive likelihood ratio of 58.5 for spirometry-confirmed COPD.[56] Clinicians, however, must always maintain a broad differential because many elements of the history and physical examination are not sensitive or specific for COPD and are seen in other diseases.

Box 2
Etiology of acute exacerbations of COPD

A—Airway viral infection

B—Bacterial infection (including pneumonia)

C—Co-infection

D—Depression and anxiety

E—Embolism (pulmonary)

F—Failure (cardiac or lung integrity in a pneumothorax)

G—General environment

X—No specific cause identified

Data from MacDonald M, Beasley RW, Irving L, et al. A hypothesis to phenotype COPD exacerbations by aetiology. Respirology 2011;16:264–8.

AECOPDs are heralded by increasing dyspnea, worsening exercise tolerance, worsening sputum purulence, and increased sputum production. In patients with severe baseline COPD, an altered mental status may be the only sign of an exacerbation.[54] Physical examination in AECOPD shows many of the findings discussed previously. Moreover, increased work of breathing may lead to tripoding (neck angled forward with upper torso supported on the elbows and arms), accessory muscle use, and diaphoresis. Diaphragmatic muscle fatigue is heralded by paradoxic inward inspiratory abdominal motion (abdominal paradox), which is an ominous sign. As ventilatory failure worsens, patients become increasingly hypercapneic and acidotic, leading to confusion, stupor, hypopnea, and finally apnea.[57]

Laboratory Testing

Standard blood tests should be ordered to help elucidate the cause of an AECOPD or to aid in identifying an alternate cause of a patient's presentation. There is no blood test that is specific to identifying COPD. Sputum testing in not routinely recommended in EDs because it is unreliable, is difficult to distinguish between colonization and infection, and does not result in a change of antibiotic management. It may be considered when tuberculosis is strongly suspected and GOLD recommends sputum collection in AECOPD only if a patient has failed initial antibiotic therapy after admission.[54]

Blood Gas Analysis

Arterial blood gas (ABG) measurement is recommended by guidelines for use in moderate or severe AECOPD, pulse oximetry less than 92% on room air, assessment for home oxygen therapy, and to follow pH, partial pressure of carbon dioxide (Pco_2), and partial pressure of oxygen (Po_2) before and after a patient is put on noninvasive positive pressure ventilation (NIPPV) or a ventilator.[4–8] An ABG may be useful in determining respiratory failure when Po_2 is less than 60 mm Hg or Pco_2 is greater than 50 mm Hg; however, diagnosis and treatments instituted for AECOPD are generally based on clinical examination. The ABG procedure is painful and a local anesthetic, such as lidocaine, should be used if it is performed. If Pco_2 is the sole value required, however, arterialized earlobe gases are less painful and provide accurate Pco_2.[7] Moreover, ABGs can result in complications, such as painful hematomas and vascular injury. Thus, the information gained from the ABG should be weighed against its downside and, if multiple ABGs are needed, an arterial line should be considered. Venous blood gases (VBGs) are less painful and have fewer complications. The correlation of VBG and ABG measurements has been studied in patients with AECOPD. pH and bicarbonate values correlate well but Pco_2 and Po_2 do not. A VBG Pco_2 of 45 mm Hg has been shown to be 100% (95% CI, 94%–100%) sensitive for arterial hypercarbia.[58,59]

Electrocardiogram

There are several common ECG changes that are associated with COPD. Many of the changes seen on the ECG of patients with COPD are also seen in chronic lung disease of many types. In COPD, there is a clockwise rotation of the heart in the longitudinal plane and the right heart chambers hypertrophy and come closer to the chest wall whereas the mass of the left ventricle is pushed back.[60] These changes can lead to

- Right axis deviation
- A P-wave axis >60°, which is 96% sensitive for COPD[61]
- P pulmonale (P waves >2.5 mm in limb leads II, III, or aVF)

- The lead I sign, which is an isoelectric P wave; QRS amplitude <1.5 mm; and T-wave amplitude <0.5 mm in lead I
- S waves in leads I, II, and III
- Low-voltage QRS amplitude in limb leads <5 mm
- R/S ratio <1 in leads V5 or V6.

None of these is very sensitive or specific for COPD but it has been shown that the more severe the COPD, the more likely a person is to have an ECG change or dysrhythmia.[62]

Supraventricular dysrhythmias, such as atrial fibrillation or flutter, ventricular ectopic beats, and nonsustained ventricular tachycardia, are most commonly associated with AECOPD. They are precipitated by hypoxia, cor pulmonale, acidosis, or the adrenergic stimulation of bronchodilators. Multifocal atrial tachycardia is considered more specific to COPD but it is uncommon. ST-segment or T-wave changes as well as Q waves may indicate an ischemic precipitant to the AECOPD. But poor R-wave progression, ST-segment, and T-wave abnormalities in the right precordial leads may be seen in persons with COPD without ischemia owing to repolarization abnormalities secondary to right ventricular hypertrophy.[60]

Imaging

The chest radiograph of patients with COPD can present with findings, such as flattened diaphragms (the most reliable finding and best seen on the lateral view), an increased anteroposterior diameter with an enlarged retrosternal space greater than 2.5 cm in front of the ascending aorta on the lateral view, oligemia, and bullae.[63] None of these findings is diagnostic and can be seen in other conditions. A chest radiograph, however, should always be performed in AECOPD[46] to look for cause, an alternative diagnosis, or a complication, such as a pneumothorax. A retrospective review of 685 episodes of AECOPD showed 16% of patients had a clinically significant abnormality on chest radiograph, of which most were new infiltrates or pulmonary edema.[64] Another study showed that 21% of admissions had their management altered by initial chest radiograph.[65] The incidence of pulmonary embolus is 3% in the ED AECOPD population and up to 25% in those hospitalized with AECOPD.[66] CT scan with pulmonary angiography should be considered when there is significant suspicion that the cause of the AECOPD is a pulmonary embolus.

Spirometry

The initial assessment and diagnosis of AECOPD is based on clinical evaluation, and spirometry is both difficult and inaccurate in patients with exacerbations. Thus, spirometry is not recommended in the diagnosis of AECOPD.[46]

TREATMENT
Prehospital

Most prehospital emergency medical services in North America are staffed by nonphysician providers with various levels of training that follow physician-developed protocols for patient care and treatment. The accurate diagnosis of acutely dyspneic patients can be difficult in the prehospital setting and there is only moderate agreement between paramedics and emergency physicians as to etiology in the dyspneic patient population.[67,68] Many prehospital protocols are not COPD specific but have been developed to treat the broader diagnoses of bronchospasm and dyspnea.

Paramedics with advanced life support training use a greater diversity of medications and have been shown to improve outcomes in patients with respiratory distress compared with paramedics with basic life support training.[69] Interventions used to treat AECOPD in the prehospital setting include oxygen, bronchodilators, noninvasive positive pressure ventilation, and intubation. There is ongoing debate as to whether high-flow oxygen in the prehospital setting may cause hypercapnic respiratory failure in patients with AECOPD and this is addressed in the following section on oxygen therapy. Given the challenge of diagnosing AECOPD in the prehospital setting, oxygen should not be withheld from hypoxic patients and the standard remains to provide oxygen to saturations at or above 92%.[70,71] Bronchodilators, including β_2-agonists and anticholinergics, are commonly used by paramedics when bronchospasm is suspected and have been shown to improve patient dynpnea subjectively and objectively.[72,73] Continuous positive airway pressure (CPAP) ventilation is becoming more popular and readily available in prehospital medicine and in many cities it is a standard of care for patients with severe dyspnea. There is mounting evidence that prehospital NIPPV is feasible, improves symptoms, prevents intubation, shortens ICU stay, and may decrease mortality.[74–76] The use of prehospital endotracheal intubation remains controversial and is fraught with potential complications.[77] In the setting of agonal respirations, obtundation, and respiratory arrest, however, paramedics with advanced airway management training should secure the airway with the most effective method at their disposal.

Oxygen

Supplemental oxygen should be administered to improve the hypoxemia of patients with AECOPD. The goals of arterial oxygen saturation (Sao_2) greater than 90% and Pao_2 greater than 60 mm Hg are recommended by consensus guidelines as is blood gas verification 30 to 60 minutes after supplemental oxygen has been started.[5,46] It is hypothesized that increases in administered fraction of inspired oxygen (Fio_2) cause V/Q mismatch in the lungs, which leads to worsening carbon dioxide retention, hypercapnea, and a respiratory acidosis that is associated with neurologic and cardiorespiratory depression in patients with COPD.[78] Judicious use of oxygen and titration to a Sao_2 of only 88% to 92% is accepted practice to prevent carbon dioxide retention, hypercapnea, and respiratory acidosis. There is evidence to support the assertion that increased oxygen is associated with hypercapnea, respiratory acidosis, and ICU admission but this does not occur in every patient given increased Fio_2.[79] One randomized trial suggests that prehospital high-flow oxygen increases mortality in patients with respiratory distress and suspected AECOPD but the issue still remains controversial.[80]

Bronchodilators

Bronchodilators are considered first-line therapy for patients with AECOPD and are central to symptomatic control.[4–8] Although the airflow obstruction in COPD is generally irreversible, a reversible component often exists. Bronchodilators improve the reversible component of airflow obstruction that contributes to hyperinflation and resulting dyspnea by widening the airways. The 2 first-line classes of bronchodilators used in AECOPD are inhaled short-acting β_2-agonists, such as albuterol (salbutamol), and inhaled anitcholinergic agents, such as ipatropium bromide.[5–7,46]

β_2-Agonists relax airway smooth muscle by stimulating airway β_2-adrenergic receptors that increase intracellular cyclic AMP, which antagonizes smooth muscle bronchoconstriction. Their onset is within minutes, peak effect is at 30 minutes, and their effect lasts 4 to 6 hours. Common side effects include tachycardia, tremor, hypokalemia, and a transient hypoxia from V/Q mismatch.[81] The parasympathetic nervous system and its cholinergic signaling to muscarinic pulmonary acetylcholine receptors cause bronchoconstriction and mucus secretion. Inhaled anticholinergics competitively inhibit the muscarinic pulmonary acetylcholine receptors. These agents have a slower onset than β_2-agonists, with their effects starting at 15 minutes, peak effect at 60 to 90 minutes, and duration of 6 to 8 hours. Common anticholinergic side effects include dry mouth, tremor, and urinary retention and, if exposed to the eye during nebulization, anticholinergics can precipitate acute angle closure glaucoma in those at risk.[81]

There is some thought that anticholinergic agents may be superior to β_2-agonists to treat the reversible component of COPD based on disease pathophysiology and on anticholinergic mechanism of action. This may be the case in stable COPD.[82] In AECOPD, the evidence does not favor one over the other. A well-done systematic review showed no significant difference in changes in FEV_1 between β_2-agonists and the anticholinergic ipratropium bromide–treated patients at 90 minutes (weighted mean difference [WMD] 0.0 L; 95% CI, −0.19 to 0.19) and 24 hours (WMD 0.05 L; 95% CI, −0.14 to 0.05) and no advantage to adding ipratropium to β_2-agonist treatment (WMD 0.02 L; 95% CI, −0.08 to 0.12). The side effects described in the review were minor and no significant differences in hemodynamics were observed.[83] Consensus guidelines favor a short-acting β_2-agonist as the first-line bronchodilator owing to its quicker onset of action. If a prompt response to these drugs does not occur, the addition of an anticholinergic is recommended.[46]

The optimal dosing of bronchodilators in an AECOPD has yet to be established. There is little evidence to support the dose amount or frequency of dosing. One study in admitted patients with AECOPD did not show a significant difference in clinical outcomes in patients treated every 4 hours with either 2.5 mg or 5 mg of nebulized albuterol.[84] Another ED-based study of 86 patients with AECOPD compared hourly and every 20-minute dosing of albuterol. It showed a nonsignificant trend toward FEV_1 improvement at 2 hours in those with every 20-minute dosing and post hoc analysis showed significant improvement in those with the most severe obstruction (FEV_1 <20%) given the every 20-minute albuterol.[85] Although far from conclusive, this evidence falls in line with the empiric practice of many emergency physicians: with worsening severity of AECOPD, the frequency of bronchodilators is increased. The method of delivery is by metered dose inhaler (MDI) or by nebulization. There does not seem to be a difference in outcomes based on method of administration.[86] The decision to administer bronchodilators by nebulizer or MDI, therefore, is based on several factors. In severe exacerbations, an altered mental status favors the use of nebulized bronchodilators. Infection control and costs favor the use of MDIs.

Methylxanthines, such as aminophylline and theophylline, have fallen out of favor and are rarely used in EDs.[87] Current evidence does not support the use of methylxanthines in AECOPD and the authors of a Cochrane review[88] conclude that methylxanthines have no early beneficial effects in lung function, the late clinical improvements are modest and inconsistent, and adverse effects are significant. These agents should be avoided.

Intravenous magnesium sulfate ($MgSO_4$) is a smooth muscle relaxant and has been shown to improve airflow and decrease hospitalizations in severe asthma exacerbations.[89] Current guidelines, however, make no mention of its use in AECOPD. There are 2 randomized controlled trials comparing $MgSO_4$ to placebo in patients with AECOPD. In the first study, ED patients were randomized to receive 1.5 g intravenous $MgSO_4$ or placebo after receiving a dose of albuterol, which resulted in a significant improvement in peak expiratory flow in those given $MgSO_4$.[90] The second crossover randomized controlled trial comparing 1.2 g $MgSO_4$ and placebo showed significantly improved

FEV_1 when $MgSO_4$ was given after salbutamol.[91] Intravenous $MgSO_4$ has few side effects if dosed properly it can be considered in combination with β_2-agonists.

Steroids

The inflammatory response that is believed to underlie much of the pathophysiology of AECOPD has generated interest in the use of systemic corticosteroids for managing the condition. Several randomized controlled trials have looked at the benefits and risks of systemic steroid administration in AECOPD with an emphasis on the outcomes of treatment failures, duration of hospitalization, relapse, mortality, and surrogate outcomes directed at indices of lung function. The study of inhaled cortico-steroids has been restricted largely to its role as chronic therapy for the prevention of exacerbations.[92]

A Cochrane review published in 2009 represents the most comprehensive work on this subject.[93] Ten studies (n = 1051) were included in the analysis. Steroid use resulted in significantly fewer treatment failures, defined as the need to seek additional medical therapy within 30 days (odds ratio [OR] 0.50; 95% CI, 0.36–0.69). In other words, the number of patients needed to treat (NNT) with corticosteroids to avoid one treatment failure in this time period was 10 (95% CI, 7–16). Duration of hospital-ization was significantly shorter with corticosteroid treatment (mean difference −1.22 days; 95% CI, −2.26 to −0.18). FEV_1 also demonstrated significant improve-ments both at the early time point and at end of treatment. There was a significant improvement in breathlessness but no significant effect on mortality. There was an increased likelihood of an adverse event (hyperglycemia, weight gain, or insomnia) associated with corticosteroid treatment (OR 2.33; 95% CI, 1.60–3.40) with a number needed to harm of 5 (95% CI, 4–9). The risk of hyperglycemia specifically, was signif-icantly increased (OR 4.95; 95% CI, 2.47–9.91). A study of approximately 80,000 hospitalizations for COPD suggests that there is no advantage to high-dose cortico-steroids over low-dose regimens and that lower-dose regimens may actually improve outcomes.[94]

Antibiotics

In contrast to the role of corticosteroids in improving outcomes, the benefits of antimi-crobial therapy for the treatment of AECOPD are less certain. The primary problem is that there is significant heterogeneity in the many studies that have looked at this question. The evidence includes both hospitalized and discharged patients, myriad antibiotic regimens, and many studies conducted in eras and settings with variable bacteriologic susceptibility to therapy.

The most recent and up-to-date systematic review of the comparison of antibiotics to placebo does provide some useful guidance as to their optimal use.[95] Thirteen trials with 1557 patients were included, which were deemed moderate to good quality. Regarding the primary outcome of antibiotics on treatment failure, there was much heterogeneity across all trials explained by the severity of exacerbations in the studies examined. The investigators found that antibiotics did not reduce treatment failures in outpatients with mild to moderate exacerbations (pooled OR 1.09; 95% CI, 0.75–1.59; I^2 = 18%). In admitted patients with severe exacerbations, however, antibiotics had a substantial benefit on treatment failure rates (pooled OR 0.25; 95% CI, 0.16–0.39; I^2 = 0%; NNT 4; 95% CI, 3–5) and on mortality (pooled OR 0.20; 95% CI, 0.06–0.62; NNT 14; 95% CI, 12–30). Not surprisingly, antibiotics were associated with a higher rate of adverse events than placebo, namely diarrhea.

Understanding of which antibiotics to select and the duration of therapy is some-what more limited due to a paucity of studies powered to measure rates of treatment failure. A comparison of the major clinical practice guidelines on the topic is instructive. When choosing an antibiotic, GOLD[46] and Department of Veterans Affairs and Department of Defense (VA/DoD)[8] recommend stratifying patients according to the severity of their exacerbation. For mild exacerbations with no risk factors for poor outcomes, GOLD recommends oral treatment with a β-lactam, a tetracycline, or trimethoprim/sulfamethoxazole. For moderate exacerbations with risk factors for poor outcome, they recommend a β-lactam/β-lactamase inhibitor, and for severe exacerbations with risk factors for *Pseudomonas aeruginosa* infection, a fluoroquinolone. VA/DoD recommends considering doxycycline, trimethoprim/sulfamethoxazole, or a second-generation cephalosporin for uncomplicated exacerbations of COPD. For complicated exacerbations, the VA/DoD recommends a β-lactam/β-lactamase inhibitor or a fluoroquinolone. According to VA/DoD, choice of antibiotic agents may be determined based on the frequency of exacerbations in the past 12 months, severity of underlying COPD, presence of cardiac disease, and recent (within 3 months) antibiotic exposure for each patient. Comparative effectiveness research published recently suggests that macrolides are equivalent to fluoroquinolones for AECOPD and carry slightly lower rates of diarrhea[96] whereas a systematic review indicated that 5-day regimens or shorter are as effective as longer courses of antimicrobials in COPD.[97]

Noninvasive Positive Pressure Ventilation

NIPPV refers to a respiratory assist device that reduces the work of breathing by supplying pressurized air through a mask by continuous positive airway pressure (CPAP) or bilevel positive airway pressure (BiPAP). NIPPV is an extremely important component of the emergency physician's armamentarium and is indicated for moderate to severe dyspnea, tachypnea, acidosis (pH <7.35) and hypercapnic respiratory failure (PaCO$_2$ >45 mm Hg) in AECOPD.[43] The intervention has been studied extensively in several randomized trials that have been synthesized in a Cochrane review.[98] Fourteen studies were included in the review with 622 and 541 patients contributing to the outcomes of treatment failure (intubation) and mortality, respectively. NIPPV resulted in decreased mortality (NNT 10 [95% CI, 7–20]; relative risk [RR] 0.52 [95% CI, 0.35–0.76]), decreased need for intubation (NNT 4 [95% CI, 4–5]; RR 0.41 [95% CI, 0.33–0.53]), and reduction in treatment failure (NNT 5 [95% CI, 4–6]; RR 0.48 [95% CI, 0.37–0.63]). Rapid improvement of pH within the first hour (WMD 0.03; 95% CI, 0.02–0.04), Paco$_2$ (WMD −0.40 kPa; 95% CI −0.78 to −0.03), and respiratory rate (WMD −3.08 breaths per minute; 95% CI, −4.26 to −1.89) correlated with the reported benefits. In addition, complications associated with treatment (RR 0.38; 95% CI, 0.24–0.60) and length of hospital stay (WMD −3.24 days; 95% CI, −4.42 to −2.06) were also reduced in the NIPPV group. NIPPV may not be tolerated by some patients due to altered mental status, discomfort, or a constricting sense of panic. Appropriate timing is an important consideration as well because its value is probably limited in the agonal and preterminal phases of respiratory failure.

Intubation and Mechanical Ventilation

Despite the clinical benefits of NIPPV in patients with moderate to severe AECOPD, 20% to 30% require intubation and mechanical ventilation.[99–101] Patients with severe AECOPD can present to an ED in extremis where there is an immediate indication for intubation and mechanical ventilation (**Box 3**).[46]

Patients with AECOPD who require intubation and mechanical ventilation have a poorer prognosis, with mortality rates between 20% and 73% and a mean life expectancy of 1 year.[102] Before a decision is made to intubate these patients, clinicians must

---

Box 3
Indications for intubation and mechanical ventilation

- Unable to tolerate NIPPV or NIPPV failure
- Severe dyspnea with use of accessory muscles and paradoxic abdominal motion
- Respiratory frequency >35 breaths per minute
- Life-threatening hypoxemia
- Severe acidosis (pH <7.25) and/or hypercapnia ($Paco_2$ >8.0 kPa, 60 mm Hg)
- Respiratory arrest
- Somnolence, impaired mental status
- Cardiovascular complications (hypotension, shock)
- Other complications (metabolic abnormalities, sepsis, pneumonia, pulmonary embolism, barotrauma, massive pleural effusion)

Data from the Global Strategy for the Diagnosis, Management and Prevention of COPD, Global Initiative for Chronic Obstructive Lung Disease (GOLD) 2011. Available from: http://www. goldcopd.org/.

---

ensure whether a patient is a candidate for invasive ventilation. There are several factors that influence the decision. First and foremost are the patient's wishes. Discussion regarding advance directives and do-not-intubate/do-not-resuscitate wishes should take place with patients or appropriate representatives. The pros of mechanical ventilation (prolonging survival) as well as the cons (barotrauma, infection, and failure to wean from the ventilator) should be clearly explained.

Considerations before laryngoscopy and intubation

Patients with AECOPD who require intubation present unique challenges. These patients are often very hypoxic. Although standard preoxygenation via bag valve mask or nonrebreather mask is indicated before rapid sequence intubation, these methods can fail to get patients above an oxygen saturation of 90%. Even if preoxygenation does successfully increase the oxygen saturation above 90%, due to extremely small reserves and significant V/Q mismatch, desaturation occurs precipitously once a patient is sedated and paralyzed. As a possible solution, preoxygenation with NIPPV has been proposed to remedy high-risk hypoxic patients with significant V/Q mismatch and shunt. Applying NIPPV with increased CPAP settings, a patient's oxygenation can significantly improve. Starting with a CPAP setting of 5 and titrating up to a maximum of 15 cm H_2O, 100% saturation can be achieved in patients in whom nonrebreather mask or bag valve mask preoxygenation does not result in adequate saturations.[103]

Furthermore, these patients can have a significantly altered level of consciousness, be combative, and may fight the efforts of preoxygenation. Therefore, delayed sequence intubation (DSI) can be used. DSI is essentially procedural sedation to allow for preoxygenation. Ketamine, if not contraindicated, is administered to produce a dissociative state where breathing and airway reflexes are maintained, thus allowing for unresisted preoxygenation.[103]

The application of high-flow oxygen to a patient via nasal prongs before sedation and paralysis and continuing its use through laryngoscopy can extend the time before hypoxia occurs.[103-106]

Finally, because these patients can be volume depleted from their work of breathing and have exhausted most of their catecholamine stores by the time they require intubation, these patients should be given 500 mL to 1 L of fluid to prevent significant drops in blood pressure from the induction agent and mechanical positive pressure ventilation.[107,108]

Mechanical ventilation and postintubation management

The goals of intubation and mechanical ventilation in patients with AECOPD are to improve and maintain oxygenation, provide rest to the muscles of respiration, continue inhaled bronchodilator therapy, and prevent dynamic hyperinflation and ventilator-induced lung injury.[107,108] Initial ventilator settings for intubated patients with AECOPD are listed in **Box 4**.[109]

The ventilator is initially set to an Fio_2 of 1.0. The mode of ventilation chosen is often based on institutional culture and the physician. In general, however, assist control ventilation is recommended because it allows less work for a patient's muscles of respiration.

Patients with obstructive pulmonary disease require prolonged time for expiration owing to the airway obstruction. When a patient with AECOPD is put on a mechanical ventilator, a standard set exhalation time may be too short to fully evacuate the lungs before the next breath is initialized (also known as breath stacking), which results in gas trapping and the phenomenon known as dynamic hyperinflation (DHI). The consequences of DHI are significant because it can result in poor perfusion of inspiratory muscles, reduce the pressure-generating capacity of the respiratory muscles, increase the work of breathing, and raise mean intrathoracic pressure.[110–113] Ultimately DHI can cause hypoxia and severely elevated intrathoracic pressures, which can result in hypotension, obstructive shock, and pulseless electrical activity (PEA) arrest. Moreover, barotrauma, such as pneumothorax, pneumomediastinum, and pneumoperitoneum, correlate with the degree of DHI. Thus, the ventilator is set to minimize DHI, by setting a low tidal volume (6–8 mL/kg ideal body weight) and a low respiratory rate (8–10 breaths per minute), and to maximize time for complete expiration (I:E ratio of 1:4–1:5).[109]

The consequence of these ventilator settings is a decrease in minute ventilation and subsequent elevation in $Paco_2$ and respiratory acidosis. This resulting respiratory acidosis should be tolerated to a serum pH as low as 7.15 to prevent DHI and its consequences. This ventilation strategy is known as permissive hypercapnea. Allowing patients to develop severe respiratory acidosis below pH 7.15 from permissive

---

Box 4
Initial ventilator settings

Mode: assist control

Fio_2: 1.0

Tidal volume: 6–8 mL/kg

Inspiration/expiration (I:E) ratio: 1:4–1:5

Positive end-expiratory pressure (PEEP): 0 cm H_2O

Respiratory rate: 8–10 breaths/min

Inspiratory flow: 80–100 L/min

Data from Jain S, Hanania N, Guntupalli K. Ventilation of patients with asthma and obstructive lung disease. Crit Care Clin 1998;14:685–705.

hypercapnia can result in cardiac arrhythmias and death so a sodium bicarbonate infusion or the administration of tris-hydroxymethyl aminomethane (THAM) may be considered to maintain pH. Moreover, patients can become agitated by the elevations in $Paco_2$ so good sedation and occasional paralysis are required.[108] Prolonged neuromuscular paralysis, however, should not be used unless necessary because the myopathy resulting from the combination of steroids and paralytics can be devastating.[114,115]

Predicting DHI can be achieved by observing for auto-PEEP or an elevated plateau pressure on the mechanical ventilator. The first indicator of DHI that can be seen on a mechanical ventilator is auto-PEEP, which represents an elevated alveolar pressure at the end of expiration.[109] It can be seen on the ventilator flow-time tracing demonstrated in **Fig. 1**.

The presence of auto-PEEP represents the presence of DHI. The degree of auto-PEEP, however, does not correlate to the degree of DHI[110] and it may be falsely

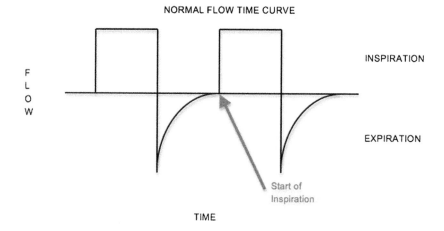

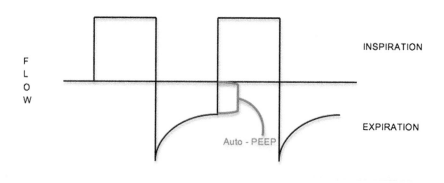

Fig. 1. Flow-time ventilator curves showing normal inspiration-expiration (*upper*) and auto-PEEP (*lower*).

low in severe obstruction. The second and more accurate indicator of DHI is via plateau pressure, which is the airway pressure measured during an inspiratory pause on the ventilator. A plateau pressure above 30 cm H_2O is considered significantly elevated and correlates with complications of DHI.[109]

If auto-PEEP or an elevated plateau pressure occur, this can be treated with further bronchodilator therapy, optimizing sedation, decreasing the respiratory rate, and decreasing the tidal volume. Furthermore, the emergency physician should remain vigilant for the most dramatic complication of DHI, which is significant hypotension or PEA arrest. If this occurs, it is likely that increased intrathoracic pressure has become high enough to produce an obstructive shock or arrest. Disconnection from the ventilator and resultant decrease in intrathoracic pressures can improve vital signs and cause return of spontaneous circulation.[116] In addition, manually squeezing the chest to decrease the hyperinflation may help. If a tension pneumothorax is suspected, immediate needle decompression followed by tube thoracostomy is required.

Peak pressures on the ventilator do not correlate well with DHI and its consequences but should be kept under 50 cm H_2O. A sudden rise in peak pressure is useful because it predicts endotracheal tube blockage, mucus plugging, and pneumothorax. A sudden drop in peak pressure may indicate extubation or endotracheal tube disconnection.[113]

It is theorized that in severe airway obstruction, uses of low-density gases, such as helium-oxygen mixtures (heliox), can help reduce patient inspiratory work and facilitate ventilation. Although a few trials exist comparing heliox to standard air-oxygen mixtures, definitive evidence of benefit is lacking.[117,118]

Palliative and End-of-Life Care

Providing palliative care to seriously ill patients with COPD can be as important as resuscitating these patients. The goals of palliative care are to control pain and other distressing symptoms, reduce suffering, improve the quality of seriously ill patients' lives, and support those patients and their families.[119] Many patients with severe or end-stage COPD do not want to be resuscitated or intubated or have ICU care, and their preference is for comfort care. Emergency physicians should have some familiarity with basic palliative care assessments and treatments as well as knowledge of local and institutional palliative care resources.

One useful tool for emergency physicians to evaluate the palliative needs of patients with advanced COPD is rapid palliative care assessment.[120] This can be performed after or concurrently with the initial ABCs in critically ill patients and consists of an ABCD approach:

A. Does the patient have any **advance directives** in place regarding life-sustaining measures? If so, what are they? All efforts should be made by the emergency physician to honor advance directives, including do-not-resuscitate or do-not-intubate orders as well as other end-of-life care preferences. Involve the patient's treating physician if possible.

B. How can you make the patient **feel better**? This is the symptom-management phase of the acute resuscitation. In end-stage COPD, dyspnea is the most distressing symptom. If a patient does not want intubation and ventilation, there are several therapies that can provide patient comfort. NIPPV is effective in patients with do-not-intubate orders[121] and when used solely as a palliative treatment, because it has been shown to reduce dyspnea shortly after initiation during an episode of hypercapnic respiratory failure[122] and in terminally ill patients.[123] Opioids can reduce the uncomfortable sensations associated with labored breathing. A systematic review and meta-analysis found evidence in favor of using oral or inject-able opioid drugs for the palliative treatment of breathlessness when compared with placebo.[124]

C. Are there **caregivers** at the bedside or who can be reached by phone? Family and caregiver involvement is important to clarify any issues or advance directives in a patient with altered mental status. As a patient nears death, the family should be considered an extension of the patient because the comfort and communica-tion provided by a physician can help the family grieving process.

D. Does the patient have **decision-making capacity**? If advance directives do not exist, the patient's wishes should be elucidated. But patients must have the capacity to make decisions to go forward with their wishes. This involves 3 elements. First, do patients have knowledge of the choices? Do patients under-stand the consequences of their decision? Can they weigh their options against a stable set of values? In the absence of directives, family or caregiver input, and patient decision-making capacity, the emergency physician should proceed with full resuscitative treatment until further information is available.

Treatments Beyond the ED

Emergency physicians can have a significant impact on the quality of life of a person with COPD not only by treating the exacerbation but also by providing referral to specialists and outpatient programs that offer assessments and therapies that improve morbidity and mortality.

The single most cost-effective way to improve quality of life and decrease mortality for patients with COPD is smoking cessation.[125,126] An AECOPD may represent a teachable moment for patients and providing resources for smoking cessation or referral to a smoking cessation program can have significant impact.

Long-term oxygen therapy (>15 hours per day) in patients with severe COPD and Pao_2 less than 55 mm Hg has been shown to increase survival and can also have a beneficial impact on hemodynamics, hematologic characteristics, exercise capacity, lung mechanics, and mental state.[127–129] Further drug therapy with long-acting anticholinergics, inhaled steroids, or combination of an inhaled steroid and a long-acting β_2-agonist has been shown to reduce exacerbations and improve lung function and health status in those with moderate to severe disease.[130–132]

Lung volume reduction surgery is used to treat select patients with severe emphysema in the upper lobes by removing the most damaged areas of the lung, thus reducing hyper-inflation. Improvements in mortality and decreases in AECOPD are reported for these procedures.[133] Because of the high risk of the procedure for patients with the most severe disease, alternatives have been studied, including bronchoscopic lung volume reduction.[134,135] Finally, in appropriately selected patients with advanced COPD, lung transplantation has been shown to improve quality of life and functional capacity.[129]

Pulmonary rehabilitation programs involving exercise training, nutrition counseling, and education about COPD have been shown to improve survival, improve exercise capacity, decrease dyspnea, reduce hospitalizations, improve anxiety and depres-sion, and improve quality of life.[129,136]

Hospital at-home programs are an emerging entity in the care of patients with COPD and AECOPD. They involve having specially trained respiratory care nurses visiting patients at home to assess patients, monitor their disease status, and aid with the management of their disease. These programs have been shown no different than standard inpatient hospital care with respect to hospital readmission rates and mortality. Furthermore, patients prefer to be treated at home.[137]

DISPOSITION
Hospital Admission

Factors associated with increased admission rates in AECOPD include older age and female gender, more pack-years of smoking, recent use of inhaled corticosteroid, self-reported activity limitation in the past 24 hours, tachypnea, and a concomitant diagnosis of pneumonia.[138] Respiratory failure, organ dysfunction, or hemodynamic instability are all reasons for ICU admission. Hospitalization is also necessary for any patient with persistent shortness of breath that does not improve with medications, hypoxia, worsening hypercapnea, altered mental status, and symptoms that interrupt activities of daily living, such as sleeping and eating. Admission should also be strongly considered for patients with significant comorbid illness or a poorly supportive home environment or one in which they cannot cope.[139] Referral for admission to hospital by emergency physicians mirrors recommendations of consensus guidelines.[137]

Home

The judgment to send a patient home from an ED after an AECOPD is based on several factors. Patient symptoms and hemodynamics should have returned to baseline. The level of function and ability to perform activities of daily living should be close to their pre-exacerbation levels. Therapy with bronchodilators should be required less than every 4 hours. It is important that patients understand their treatment regimen and they should be observed using and taught how to properly use bronchodilators. Patients should be returning to supportive living conditions where help can be accessed if it is needed.[46,138]

When a decision is made to discharge a patient from an ED, prescriptions may include steroids, antibiotics, and bronchodilators, if needed. Moreover, influenza[140] and pneumococcal vaccines should be given to unimmunized patients to reduce future exacerbations. Follow-up should be made with appropriate primary care and specialists if patients do not already have adequate follow-up. Referral to programs that aid in smoking cessation and assessment of patients for pulmonary rehabilitation and hospital at home should also be considered. Finally, instructions should be given to return to an ED if the symptoms of exacerbation reoccur.

REFERENCES

1. World Health Statistics 2008. Geneva (Switzerland): World Health Organization; 2008. p. 30. Available at: http://www.who.int/whosis/whostat/EN_WHS08_Full.pdf. Accessed January 4, 2011.
2. Mannino DM, Homa DM, Akinbami LJ, et al. Chronic pulmonary disease surveillance—United States, 1971-2000. MMWR Surveill Summ 2002;51(SS-6):1–16.
3. Brown DW, Croft JB, Greenlund KJ, et al. Deaths from chronic obstructive pulmonary disease—United States, 2000-2005. MMWR Morb Mortal Wkly Rep 2008;57:1229–32.
4. Global strategy for the diagnosis, management, and prevention of COPD, updated 2010. Global Initiative for Chronic Obstructive Lung Disease (GOLD). Available at: http://www.goldcopd.org. Accessed January 4, 2011.
5. American Thoracic Society/European Respiratory Society Task Force. Standards for the diagnosis and management of patients with COPD. Version 1.2. New York: American Thoracic Society; 2004 [updated 2005 September 8]. Available at: http://www.thoracic.org/go/copd. Accessed January 4, 2011.

6. O'Donnell DE, Hernandez P, Kaplan A, et al. Canadian Thoracic Society recommendations for management of chronic obstructive pulmonary disease—2008 update—highlights for primary care. Can Respir J 2008;15(Suppl A):1A–8A.

7. National Institute for Clinical Excellence (NICE). Chronic obstructive pulmonary disease. National clinical guideline on management of chronic obstructive pulmonary disease in adults in primary and secondary care. Thorax 2004; 59(Suppl 1):1–232.

8. VA/DoD clinical practice guideline for management of outpatient chronic obstructive pulmonary disease. Department of Veterans Affairs and Department of Defense. Available at: http://www.healthquality.va.gov/chronic_obstructive_pulmonary_disease_copd.asp. Accessed April 17, 2011.

9. Chapter 1 Definition. In: Global strategy for the diagnosis, management and prevention of COPD, Global Initiative for Chronic Obstructive Lung Disease (GOLD) 2010. p. 1–6. Avialable at: http://www.goldcopd.org. Accessed April 17, 2011.

10. Snider G. The definition of emphysema: report of the National Heart, Lung and Blood Institute, Division of Lung Diseases Workshop. Am Rev Respir Dis 1985; 132:182.

11. Husain AN. The lung. In: Kumar V, Abbas A, Faustos N, et al, editors. Robbins and cotran pathologic basis of disease. 8th edition. Philidelphia: Saunders Elsevier; 2010. Available at: http://www.mdconsult.com/books/about.do?about=true&eid=4–u1.0-B978-1-4377-0792-2.X5001-9–TOP&isbn=978-1-4377-0792-2&uniqId=239435368-2. Accessed January 15, 2011.

12. Kanner RE, Anthonisen NR, Connett JE. Lower respiratory illnesses promote FEV1 decline in current smokers but not ex-smokers with mild chronic obstructive pulmonary disease: results from the lung health study. Am J Respir Crit Care Med 2001;164:358–64.

13. Pelkonen M, Notkola IL, Nissinen A, et al. Thirty-year cumulative incidence of chronic bronchitis and COPD in relation to 30-year pulmonary function and 40-year mortality: a follow-up in middle-aged rural men. Chest 2006;130:1129–37.

14. US Surgeon General. The health consequences of smoking: chronic obstructive pulmonary disease. Washington, DC: US Department of Health and Human Services; 1984.

15. Berglund DJ, Abbey DE, Lebowitz MD, et al. Respiratory symptoms and pulmonary function in elderly non-smoking population. Chest 1999;115:49–59.

16. Trupin L, Earnest G, San Pedro M, et al. The occupational burden of chronic obstructive pulmonary disease. Eur Respir J 2003;22:462–9.

17. Matheson MC, Benke G, Raven J, et al. Biological dust exposure in the workplace is a risk factor for chronic obstructive pulmonary disease. Thorax 2005; 60:645–51.

18. OroczoLevi M, Garcia Aymerich J, Villar J, et al. Wood smoke exposure and risk of chronic obstructive pulmonary disease. Eur Respir J 2006;27:5426.

19. Smith KR. Inaugural article: national burden of disease in India from indoor air pollution. Proc Natl Acad Sci U S A 2000;97:13286–93.

20. Sezer H, Akkurt I, Guler N, et al. A case control study on the effect of exposure to different substances on the development of COPD. Ann Epidemiol 2006;16: 59–62.

21. Smith KR, Mehta S. The burden of disease from indoor air pollution in developing countries: comparison of estimates [abstract]. Int J Hyg Environ Health 2003;206: 279–89. Available at: http://www.ncbi.nlm.nih.gov/pubmed/12971683. Accessed January 16, 2011. PMID 12971683.

22. Celli BR, Halbert RJ, Nordyke RJ, et al. Airway obstruction in never smokers: results from the third national health and nutrition examination survey. Am J Med 2005;118:1364–72.
23. Prescott E, Lange P, Vestbo J. Socioeconomic status, lung function and admission to hospital for COPD: results from the Copenhagen City Heart Study. Eur Respir J 1999;13:1109–14.
24. Postma DS, Kerkhof M, Boezem HM, et al. Asthma and COPD: common genes common environments? Am J Respir Crit Care Med [abstract] 2011;183(12): 1588–94. Available at: http://www.ncbi.nlm.nih.gov/pubmed/21297068. Accessed February 16, 2011. PMID 21297068.
25. Stoller JK, Aboussouan LS. Alpha1 antitrypsin deficiency. Lancet 2005;365: 2225–36.
26. McCloskey SC, Patel BD, Hinchliffe SJ, et al. Siblings of patients with severe chronic obstructive pulmonary disease have a significant risk of airflow obstruction. Am J Respir Crit Care Med 2001;164(8 Pt 1):1419–24.
27. Hurst JR, Vestbo J, Anzueto A, et al. Susceptibility to exacerbation in chronic obstructive pulmonary disease. N Engl J Med 2010;363:1128–38.
28. Lawlor DA, Ebrahim S, Davey Smith G. Association of birth weight with adult lung function: findings from the British Women's Heart and Health Study and a metaanalysis. Thorax 2005;60:851–8.
29. Xu X, Weiss ST, Rijcken B, et al. Smoking, changes in smoking habits, and rate of decline in FEV1: new insight into gender differences. Eur Respir J 1994;7: 1056–61.
30. Silverman EK, Weiss ST, Drazen JM, et al. Gender related differences in severe, early onset chronic obstructive pulmonary disease. Am J Respir Crit Care Med 2000;162:215–28.
31. Sethi S, Maloney J, Grove L, et al. Airway inflammation and bronchial bacterial colonization in chronic obstructive pulmonary disease. Am J Respir Crit Care Med 2006;173:991–8.
32. Retamales I, Elliott WM, Meshi B, et al. Amplification of inflammation in emphysema and its association with latent adenoviral infection. Am J Respir Crit Care Med 2001;164:469–73.
33. Diaz PT, King MA, Pacht ER, et al. Increased susceptibility to pulmonary emphysema among HIV seropositive smokers. Ann Intern Med 2000;132:369–72.
34. MacNee W. Pathogenesis of chronic obstructive pulmonary disease. Clin Chest Med 2007;28:479–513.
35. Kim V, Rogers TJ, Criner GJ. New concepts in the pathobiology of chronic obstructive pulmonary disease. Proc Am Thorac Soc 2008;5:478–85.
36. Hogg JC, Timens W. The pathology of chronic obstructive pulmonary disease. Annu Rev Pathol 2009;4:435–59.
37. Scichilone N, Battaglia S, La Sala A, et al. Clinical implications of airway hyperresponsiveness in COPD. Int J Chron Obstruct Pulmon Dis 2006;1:49–60.
38. Postma DS, Kerstjens HA. Characteristics of airway hyperresponsiveness in asthma and chronic obstructive pulmonary disease. Am J Respir Crit Care Med 1998;158:S187–92.
39. Tashkin DP, Altose JE, Connett RE, et al. Methacholine reactivity predicts changes in lung function over time in smokers with early chronic obstructive pulmonary disease. Am J Respir Crit Care Med 1996;153:1802–11.
40. Hospers JJ, Postma DS, Rijcken B, et al. Histamine airway hyper-responsiveness and mortality from chronic obstructive pulmonary disease: a cohort study. Lancet 2000;356:1313–7.

41. Reilly JJ, Silverman EK, Shapiro SD. Chronic obstructive pulmonary disease. In: Fauci AS, Kasper DL, Longo DL, et al, editors. Harrison's principles of internal medicine. 17th edition. New York: McGraw Hill Medical; 2008.

42. O'Donnell DE, Revill SM, Webb KA. Dynamic hyperinflation and exercise intolerance in chronic obstructive pulmonary disease. Am J Respir Crit Care Med 2001;164:770–7.

43. Chapter 4 Pathology, pathogenesis, and pathophysiology. In: Global strategy for the diagnosis, management and prevention of COPD, Global Initiative for Chronic Obstructive Lung Disease (GOLD) 2010. p. 24–9. Available at: http://www.goldcopd.org. Accessed April 17, 2011.

44. Chaouat A, Naeije R, Wetitzenblum E. Pulmonary hypertension in COPD. Eur Respir J 2008;32:1371–85.

45. Stone AC, Nici L. Other systemic manifestations of chronic obstructive pulmonary disease. Clin Chest Med 2007;28:553–7.

46. Chapter 5 Management of COPD, component 4 manage exacerbations. In: Global strategy for the diagnosis, management and prevention of COPD, Global Initiative for Chronic Obstructive Lung Disease (GOLD) 2010. p. 64–72. Available at: http://www.goldcopd.org. Accessed April 17, 2011.

47. Rosychuk RJ, Voaklander DC, Senthilselvan A, et al. Presentations to emergency departments for chronic obstructive pulmonary disease in Alberta: a population-based study. CJEM 2010;12:500–8.

48. Donaldson GC, Seemungal TA, Bhowmik A, et al. Relationship between exacerbation frequency and lung function decline in chronic obstructive pulmonary disease. Thorax 2002;57:847–52.

49. Makris D, Moschandreas J, Damianaki A, et al. Exacerbations and lung function decline in COPD: new insights in current and ex-smokers. Respir Med 2007; 101:1305–12.

50. Seemungal TA, Donaldson GC, Bhowmik A, et al. Time course and recovery of exacerbations in patients with chronic obstructive pulmonary disease. Am J Respir Crit Care Med 2000;161:1608–13.

51. Patil SP, Krishnan JA, Lechtzin N, et al. In-hospital mortality following acute exacerbations of chronic obstructive pulmonary disease. Arch Intern Med 2003;163:1180–6.

52. MacDonald M, Beasley RW, Irving L, et al. A hypothesis to phenotype COPD exacerbations by aetiology. Respirology 2011;16:264–8.

53. Salpeter SR, Ormiston TM, Salpeter EE. Cardioselective beta-blockers for chronic obstructive pulmonary disease (Updated January 2011). Cochrane Database Syst Rev 2005;4:CD003566.

54. Chapter 5 Management of COPD, component 1 assess and monitor disease. In: Global strategy for the diagnosis, management and prevention of COPD, Global Initiative for Chronic Obstructive Lung Disease (GOLD) 2010. p. 33–41. Available at: http://www.goldcopd.org. Accessed April 17, 2011.

55. Garcia-Pachon E, Padilla-Navas I. Frequency of Hoover's sign in stable patients with chronic obstructive pulmonary disease. Int J Clin Pract 2006; 60:514–7.

56. Straus SE, McAlister FA, Sackett DL, et al. The accuracy of patient history, wheezing, and laryngeal measurements in diagnosing obstructive airway disease. CARE-COAD1 Group. Clinical Assessment of the Reliability of the Examination-Chronic Obstructive Airways Disease. JAMA 2000;283:1853–7.

57. Palm KH, Decker WW. Acute exacerbations of chronic obstructive pulmonary disease. Emerg Med Clin North Am 2003;21:331–52.

58. Kelly AM. Can venous blood gas analysis replace arterial in emergency medical care? Emerg Med Australas 2010;22:493–8.
59. Lim BL, Kelly AM. A meta-analysis on the utility of peripheral venous blood gas analyses in exacerbations of chronic obstructive pulmonary disease in the emergency department. Eur J Emerg Med 2010;17:246–8.
60. Rodman DM, Lowenstein SR, Rodman T. The electrocardiogram in chronic obstructive pulmonary disease. J Emerg Med 1990;8:607–15.
61. Thomas AJ, Apiyasawat S, Spodick DH. Electrocardiographic detection of emphysema. Am J Cardiol 2011;107:1090–2.
62. Holtzman D, Aronow WS, Mellana WM, et al. Electrocardiographic abnormalities in patients with severe versus mild or moderate chronic obstructive pulmonary disease followed in an academic outpatient pulmonary clinic. Ann Noninvasive Electrocardiol 2011;16:30–2.
63. Friedman PJ. Imaging studies in emphysema. Proc Am Thorac Soc 2008;5:494–500.
64. Emerman C, Cydulka R. Evaluation of high-yield criteria for chest radiography in acute exacerbation of chronic obstructive pulmonary disease. Ann Emerg Med 1993;22:680–4.
65. Tsai T, Gallagher E, Lombardi G, et al. Guidelines for the selective ordering of admission chest radiography in adult obstructive airway disease. Ann Emerg Med 1993;22:1854–8.
66. Rizkallah J, Man SF, Sin DD. Prevalence of pulmonary embolism in acute exacerbations of COPD: a systematic review and metaanalysis. Chest 2009;135:786–93.
67. Ackerman R, Waldron RL. Difficulty breathing: agreement of paramedic and emergency physician diagnoses. Prehosp Emerg Care 2006;10:77–80.
68. MacLeod BA, Lorei J, Wolfson AB. The accuracy of prehospital diagnosis in patients with dyspnea. Ann Emerg Med 1990;19:459.
69. Stiell IG, Spaite DW, Field B, et al. Advanced life support for out-of-hospital respiratory distress. N Engl J Med 2007;356:2156–64.
70. Moore SW. Respiratory emergencies. In: MacDonald RD, Burgess RJ, editors. Nancy Caroline's Emergency care in the streets. 6th edition (Canadian Edition). Mississauga (Canada): Jones and Bartlett Publishers; 2010. p. 26.5–26.45.
71. Fleischman R, Daya M, Sahni R. Respiratory distress. In: Krohmer JR, Sahni R, Schwartz B, et al, editors. Emergency Medical services: clinical practice and systems oversight. USA: Kendall/Hunt Publishing; 2009. p. 211–22.
72. Zehner WJ Jr, Scott JM, Iannolo PM, et al. Terbutaline vs albuterol for out-of-hospital respiratory distress: randomized, double-blind trial. Acad Emerg Med 1995;2:686–91.
73. Rodenberg H. Effect of levalbuterol on prehospital patient parameters. Am J Emerg Med 2002;20:481–3.
74. Warner GS. Evaluation of the effect of prehospital application of continuous positive airway pressure therapy in acute respiratory distress [abstract]. Prehospital Disaster Med 2010;25:87–91.
75. Thompson J, Petrie DA, Ackroyd-Stolarz S, et al. Out-of-hospital continuous positive airway pressure ventilation versus usual care in acute respiratory failure: a randomized controlled trial. Ann Emerg Med 2008;52:232–41.
76. Schmidbauer W, Ahlers O, Spies C, et al. Early prehospital use of non-invasive ventilation improves acute respiratory failure in acute exacerbation of chronic obstructive pulmonary disease. Emerg Med J 2011;28(7):626–7. Available at: http://emj.bmj.com/. Accessed March 1, 2011.

77. Wang HE, Thomson DP. Airway management. In: Krohmer JR, Sahni R, Schwartz B, et al, editors. Emergency medical services: clinical practice and systems oversight. USA: Kendall/Hunt Publishing; 2009. p. 383–403.

78. Murphy R, Driscoll P, O'Driscoll R. Emergency oxygen therapy for COPD patients. Emerg Med J 2001;18:333–9.

79. Plant PK, Owen JL, Elliot MW. One year period prevalence study of respiratory acidosis in acute exacerbations of COPD: implications for the provision of non-invasive ventilation and oxygen administration. Thorax 2000;55:550–4.

80. Austin MA, Wills KE, Blizzard L, et al. Effect of high flow oxygen on mortality in chronic obstructive pulmonary disease patients in prehospital setting: randomised controlled trial. BMJ 2010;341:c5462.

81. Rennard SI. Treatment of stable chronic obstructive pulmonary disease. Lancet 2004;364(9436):791–802.

82. Tashkin DP, Ashutosh K, Bleecker ER, et al. Comparison of the anticholinergic bronchodilator ipratropium bromide with metaproterenol in chronic obstructive pulmonary disease. A 90-day multi-center study. Am J Med 1986;81:81–90.

83. McCrory DC, Brown CD. Anticholinergic bronchodilators versus beta2-sympathomimetic agents for acute exacerbations of chronic obstructive pulmonary disease (Updated 2008). Cochrane Database Syst Rev 2003;1:CD003900.

84. Nair S, Thomas E, Pearson SB, et al. A randomized controlled trial to assess the optimal dose and effect of nebulized albuterol in acute exacerbations of COPD. Chest 2005;128:48–54.

85. Emerman CL, Cydulka RK. Effect of different albuterol dosing regimens in the treatment of acute exacerbation of chronic obstructive pulmonary disease. Ann Emerg Med 1997;29:474–8.

86. Turner MO, Gafni A, Swan D, et al. A review and economic evaluation of bronchodilator delivery methods in hospitalized patients. Arch Intern Med 1996;156:2113–8.

87. Cydulka RK, Rowe BH, Clark S, et al. Emergency department management of acute exacerbations of chronic obstructive pulmonary disease in the elderly: the Multicenter Airway Research Collaboration. J Am Geriatr Soc 2003;51:908–16.

88. Barr RG, Rowe BH, Camargo CA. Methylxanthines for exacerbations of chronic obstructive pulmonary disease (Updated 2008). Cochrane Database Syst Rev 2003;2:CD002168.

89. Rowe BH, Bretzlaff J, Bourdon C, et al. Magnesium sulfate for treating exacerbations of acute asthma in the emergency department. Cochrane Database Syst Rev 2000;1:CD001490.

90. Skorodin MS, Tenholder MF, Yetter B, et al. Magnesium sulphate in exacerbations of chronic obstructive pulmonary disease. Arch Intern Med 1995;155:496–501.

91. Abreu González J, Hernández García C, Abreu González P, et al. Effect of intravenous magnesium sulphate on chronic obstructive pulmonary disease exacerbations requiring hospitalization: a randomized placebo-controlled trial. Arch Bronconeumol 2006;42:384–7.

92. Agarwal R, Aggarwal AN, Gupta D, et al. Inhaled corticosteroids vs placebo for preventing COPD exacerbations: a systematic review and metaregression of randomized controlled trials. Chest 2010;137:318–25.

93. Walters JAE, Gibson PG, Wood-Baker R, et al. Systemic corticosteroids for acute exacerbations of chronic obstructive pulmonary disease. Cochrane Database Syst Rev 2009;1:CD001288.

94. Lindenauer PK, Pekow PS, Lahti MC, et al. Association of corticosteroid dose and route of administration with risk of treatment failure in acute exacerbation of chronic obstructive pulmonary disease. JAMA 2010;303:2359–67.
95. Puhan MA, Vollenweider D, Latshang T, et al. Exacerbations of chronic obstructive pulmonary disease: when are antibiotics indicated? A systematic review. Respir Res 2007;8:30.
96. Rothberg MB, Pekow PS, Lahti M, et al. Comparative effectiveness of macrolides and quinolones for patients hospitalized with acute exacerbations of chronic obstructive pulmonary disease (AECOPD). J Hosp Med 2010;5: 261–7.
97. El Moussaoui R, Roede BM, Speelman P, et al. Short-course antibiotic treatment in acute exacerbations of chronic bronchitis and COPD: a meta-analysis of double-blind studies. Thorax 2008;63:415–22.
98. Ram FSF, Picot J, Lightowler J, et al. Non-invasive positive pressure ventilation for treatment of respiratory failure due to exacerbations of chronic obstructive pulmonary disease (updated with no changes in 2009). Cochrane Database Syst Rev 2004;3:CD004104.
99. Carratù P, Bonfitto P, Dragonieri S, et al. Early and late failure of noninvasive ventilation in chronic obstructive pulmonary disease with acute exacerbation. Eur J Clin Invest 2005;35:404–9.
100. Merlani PG, Pasquina P, Granier JM, et al. Factors associated with failure of noninvasive positive pressure ventilation in the emergency department. Acad Emerg Med 2005;12:1206–15.
101. Confalonieri M, Garuti G, Cattaruzza MS, et al. A chart of failure risk for noninvasive ventilation in patients with COPD exacerbation. Eur Respir J 2005;25:348–55.
102. Dales RE, O'Connor A, Hebert P, et al. Intubation and mechanical ventilation for COPD: development of an instrument to elicit patient preferences. Chest 1999; 116:792–800.
103. Weingart SD. Preoxygenation, reoxygenation, and delayed sequence intubation in the emergency department. J Emerg Med 2011;40(6):661–7. Available at: http://www.sciencedirect.com/science/journal/07364679. Accessed March 18, 2011.
104. Teller LE, Alexander CM, Frumin MJ, et al. Pharyngeal insufflation of oxygen prevents arterial desaturation during apnea. Anesthesiology 1988;69:980–2.
105. Taha SK, Siddik-Sayyid SM, El-Khatib MF, et al. Nasopharyngeal oxygen insufflation following pre-oxygenation using the four deep breath technique. Anaesthesia 2006;61:427–30.
106. Ramachandran SK, Cosnowski A, Shanks A, et al. Apneic oxygenation during prolonged laryngoscopy in obese patients: a randomized, controlled trial of nasal oxygen administration. J Clin Anesth 2010;22:164–8.
107. Nelson BP, Jagoda AS. Reactive airways disease. In: Walls RM, Murphy MF, editors. Manual of emergency airway management. 3rd edition. Philadelphia: Lippincott, Williams, and Wilkins; 2008. p. 351–6.
108. Santanilla JI, Daniel B, Yeow M. Mechanical ventilation. Emerg Med Clin North Am 2008;26:849–62.
109. Jain S, Hanania N, Guntupalli K. Ventilation of patients with asthma and obstructive lung disease. Crit Care Clin 1998;14:685–705.
110. Koh Y. Ventilatory management in patients with chronic airflow obstruction. Crit Care Clin 2007;23:169–81.
111. Kawagoe Y, Permutt S, Fessler HE. Hyperinflation with intrinsic PEEP and respiratory muscle blood flow. J Appl Physiol 1994;77:2440–8.

112. Fleury B, Murciano D, Talamo C, et al. Work of breathing in patients with chronic obstructive pulmonary disease in acute respiratory failure. Am Rev Respir Dis 1985;131:822-7.

113. Roussos C, Macklem PT. The respiratory muscles. N Engl J Med 1982;307:786-97.

114. Douglass JA, Tuxen DV, Horne M, et al. Myopathy in severe asthma. Am Rev Respir Dis 1992;146:517-9.

115. Kupfer Y, Namba T, Kaldawi E, et al. Prolonged weakness after long-term infusion of vecuronium bromide. Ann Intern Med 1992;117:484-6.

116. Gladwin MT, Pierson DJ. Mechanican ventilation of the patient with severe chronic obstructive pulmonary disease. Intensive Care Med 1998;24:898-910.

117. Rodrigo GJ, Pollack CV, Rodrigo C, et al. Heliox for treatment of exacerbations of chronic obstructive pulmonary disease. Cochrane Database Syst Rev 2001;1: CD003571.

118. Andrews R, Lynch M. Heliox in the treatment of chronic obstructive pulmonary disease. Emerg Med J 2004;21:670-5.

119. American Academy of Hospice and Palliative Medicine (AAHPM). Available at: http://www.aahpm.org/about/default/overview.html#Definition. Accessed March 26, 2011.

120. Devader TE, Albrecht R, Reiter M. Initiating palliative care in the emergency department. J Emerg Med 2011. Available at: http://www.sciencedirect.com/science/journal/07364679. Accessed April 1, 2011.

121. Levy M, Tanios MA, Nelson D, et al. Outcomes of patients with do-not-intubate orders treated with noninvasive ventilation. Crit Care Med 2004;32: 2002-7.

122. Bott J, Carrol MP, Conway JH, et al. Randomised controlled trial of nasal ventilation in acute ventilatory failure due to chronic obstructive airways disease. Lancet 1993;341:1555-7.

123. Cuomo A, Conti G, Delmastro M, et al. Noninvasive mechanical ventilation as a palliative treatment of acute respiratory failure in patients with end-stage solid cancer. Palliat Med 2004;18:602-10.

124. Jennings AL, Davies AN, Higgins JPT, et al. Opioids for the palliation of breathlessness in advanced disease and terminal illness (updated 2011). Cochrane Database Syst Rev 2001;3:CD002066.

125. Anthonisen NR, Connett JE, Kiley JP, et al. Effects of smoking intervention and the use of an inhaled anticholinergic bronchodilator on the rate of decline of FEV1. The Lung Health Study. JAMA 1994;272:1497-505.

126. Anthonisen NR, Skeans MA, Wise RA, et al. The effects of smoking cessation intervention on 14.5 year mortality: a randomized clinical trial. Ann Intern Med 2005;142:233-9.

127. Cranston JM, Crockett A, Moss J, et al. Domiciliary oxygen for chronic obstructive pulmonary disease. Cochrane Database Syst Rev 2005;4:CD001744.

128. Tarpy SP, Celli BR. Long-term oxygen therapy. N Engl J Med 1995;333:710-4.

129. Chapter 5 Management of COPD, component 3 manage stable COPD. In: Global strategy for the diagnosis, management and prevention of COPD, Global Initiative for Chronic Obstructive Lung Disease (GOLD) 2010. p. 48-63. Available at: http://www.goldcopd.org. Accessed April 17, 2011.

130. Barr RG, Bourbeau J, Camargo CA. Tiotropium for stable chronic obstructive pulmonary disease. Cochrane Database Syst Rev 2005;2:CD002876.

131. Nannini LJ, Cates CJ, Lasserson TJ, et al. Combined corticosteroid and long-acting beta-agonist in one inhaler versus placebo for chronic obstructive pulmonary disease. Cochrane Database Syst Rev 2007;4:CD003794.

132. Nannini LJ, Cates CJ, Lasserson TJ, et al. Combined corticosteroid and long-acting beta-agonist in one inhaler versus long-acting beta-agonists for chronic obstructive pulmonary disease. Cochrane Database Syst Rev 2007;4:CD006829.

133. National Emphysema Treatment Trial Research Group. A randomized trial comparing lung-volume-reduction surgery with medical therapy for severe emphysema. N Engl J Med 2003;348:2059–73.

134. Hopkinson NS, Toma TP, Hansell DM, et al. Effect of bronchoscopic lung volume reduction on dynamic hyperinflation and exercise in emphysema. Am J Respir Crit Care Med 2005;171:453–60.

135. Ernst A, Anantham D. Endoscopic management of emphysema. Clin Chest Med 2010;31:117–26.

136. Puhan MA, Gimeno-Santos E, Scharplatz M, et al. Pulmonary rehabilitation following exacerbations of chronic obstructive pulmonary disease. Cochrane Database Syst Rev 2009;1:CD005305.

137. Ram FSF, Wedzicha JA, Wright JJ, et al. Hospital at home for acute exacerbations of chronic obstructive pulmonary disease. Cochrane Database Syst Rev 2003;4:CD003573.

138. Tsai CL, Clark S, Cydulka RK, et al. Factors associated with hospital admission among emergency department patients with chronic obstructive pulmonary disease exacerbation. Acad Emerg Med 2007;14:6–14.

139. American Thoracic Society/European Respiratory Society Task Force. Standards for the diagnosis and management of patients with COPD. Version 1.2. New York: American Thoracic Society; 2004 [updated 2005 September 8]. Available at: http://www.thoracic.org/go/copd. p. 170–5. Accessed April 3, 2011.

140. Poole P, Chacko EE, Wood-Baker R, et al. Influenza vaccine for patients with chronic obstructive pulmonary disease. Cochrane Database Syst Rev 2006;1: CD002733.

Pneumonia in Adults: the Practical Emergency Department Perspective

Karen G.H. Woolfrey, MD, FRCP(C)[a,b,c],*

KEYWORDS

- Pneumonia • Community-acquired • Classification • Treatment
- Adult • Pneumococcus

INTRODUCTION AND PERSPECTIVE

Pneumonia is an inflammation of the lung most commonly caused by infection with bacteria, viruses, and other organisms. It is both a common and a potentially serious disease. It is estimated that there were more than 500,000 hospital admissions in the United States in 2009 from pneumonia. Whereas pneumonia managed as an outpatient is a less severe disease, pneumonia requiring hospitalization is associated with approximately 15% mortality. Pneumonia is often a complication of a preexisting condition or infection such as influenza. The 2009 national vital statistics identified pneumonia and influenza as the eighth leading cause of death.[1] Pneumonia consistently accounts for most of these deaths. Close to 90% of the deaths attributed to pneumonia occur in the population older than 65 years. In this cohort, pneumonia and influenza combine as the seventh leading cause of death.[2,3]

The Center for Disease Control's Advisory Committee on Immunization Practices recommends annual influenza vaccination for everyone older than 6 months.[4] (The emergence of serious drug-resistant pneumococci also accentuates the urgent need for pneumococcal immunization. Together, pneumonia and influenza represented a cost to the US economy in 2005 of $40.2 billion. In 2010, the economic costs of all lung diseases were projected to be approximately $173.4 billion.[5])

The challenge for emergency department (ED) care is to recognize the diagnosis, initiate early and appropriate empiric antibiotic therapy, risk stratify patients with respect to severity of illness, and recognize indications for admission. This challenge

No funding support received.

The author has nothing to disclose.

[a] Department of Medicine, University of Toronto, Toronto, Ontario, Canada

[b] Royal College Emergency Medicine Residency Training Program, University of Toronto, Toronto, Ontario, Canada

[c] Postgraduate Education, Department of Emergency Medicine, Sunnybrook Health Sciences Centre, Toronto, Ontario, Canada

* 2075 Bayview Avenue, Room C7-53, Toronto, Ontario M4N 3M5, Canada.

E-mail address: karen.woolfrey@sunnybrook.ca

emed.theclinics.com

must be balanced with an emphasis on cost-effective management, recognizing the changing spectrum of pathogenesis and a cognizance toward variable and less common presentations.

PATHOGENESIS

Infectious transmission in pneumonia occurs most commonly either by microaspiration or by direct droplet inhalation. However, the development of clinical pneumonia requires either a defect in host defense mechanisms or inoculation with virulent organisms. Several pneumonic pathogens are spread by droplets. This mode of transmission bypasses the upper tract defenses and deposits directly in the lower respiratory tract. **Fig. 1** shows the 2 most common modes of transmission and the infectious organisms most commonly associated with each.

Host defenses can be impaired in many ways. **Fig. 2** shows some common conditions that are associated with an increased risk of the development of pneumonia and the manner in which these conditions impair host defenses.

Pneumonia can also be transmitted through less common mechanisms. These mechanisms may include: hematogenous spread; invasion from infection in contiguous structures (pleura or subdiaphragmatic structures); direct inoculation (as a result of surgery or bronchoscopy); and reactivation, most commonly in immunocompromised hosts. The most common organisms that are implicated in reactivation, even after many years, include *Pneumocystis jiroveci*, *Mycobacterium tuberculosis*, and cytomegalovirus.

CAUSE AND CLASSIFICATION

The challenge in the ED is not in making the diagnosis of pneumonia but rather in identifying the cause of the infection such that the appropriate antibiotic treatment can be instituted in a timely manner. This strategy is of particular importance in those patients with higher risk of mortality (ie, hospitalized inpatients). Because microbiological testing results are not available at the time of the ED assessment, the initial therapy with antibiotics is empiric.

To facilitate the decision-making process with regard to the institution of empiric antibiotics, it is helpful to classify pneumonia. The traditional classification was based on the terminology of typical or atypical pneumonia. The traditional clinical

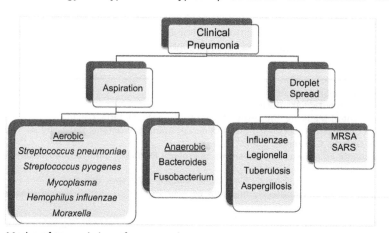

Fig. 1. Modes of transmission of pneumonia.

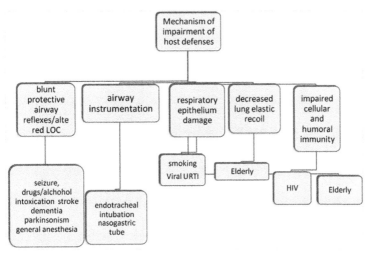

Fig. 2. Host conditions that predispose to pneumonia. URTI, upper respiratory tract infection.

presentation of typical pneumonia, most commonly caused by *Streptococcus pneumoniae*, included high fever, rigors, cough with rust-colored sputum, and laboratory findings of leukocytosis. Microbiology revealed gram-positive encapsulated diplococci. The classic chest radiograph (CXR) appearance in this setting was lobar consolidation. *Streptococcus pneumoniae* accounts for approximately 60% of community-acquired pneumonia (CAP). **Fig. 3** shows a CXR with this typical appearance.

The clinical presentation of atypical pneumonia was a more gradual onset, dry cough, in patients who often look well and are ambulatory. Microbiology often did not identify any organisms on Gram stain because most commonly they did not have cell walls. The CXR appearance was more often an interstitial pattern. **Fig. 4** shows a CXR with this atypical interstitial appearance. The most commonly described atypical organisms are *Mycoplasma*, *Legionella*, and *Chlamydophila*. The challenge with this traditional classification is that in clinical practice the presentations of these infections have considerable overlap whereby a pneumococcal infection may present with an interstitial pattern on CXR and atypical clinical symptoms and vice versa.

A more practical classification for the ED is to consider the environmental contact combined with host factors, because this can provide guidance with respect to the

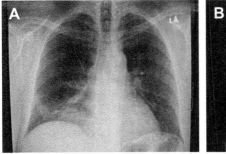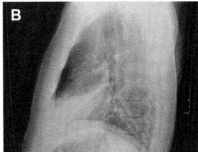

Fig. 3. (A) CXR, posteroanterior, lobar consolidation. (B) CXR, lateral, lobar consolidation.

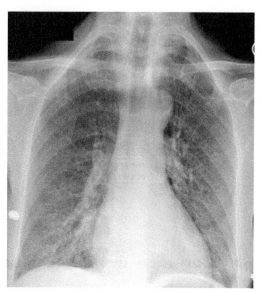

Fig. 4. CXR, posteroanterior, interstitial pattern.

likely offending agent. This practical classification is important for the ED in guiding treatment. Hence, the history in the ED should focus not only on the pattern of symptoms but also on the setting in which the pneumonia is acquired, any geographic travel or animal exposures in conjunction with any host risk factors that could predispose to certain types of infection and also predict patient outcome. The classification can be broadly divided into 4 categories: CAP; hospital-acquired pneumonia (HAP); health care-associated pneumonia (HCAP); and ventilator-associated pneumonia (VAP).

Community-acquired pneumonia (CAP) is defined as an acute infection of the pulmonary parenchyma, occurring outside the hospital, with clinical symptoms accompanied by the presence of an infiltrate on CXR[6] The diagnosis of CAP requires that a patient has not been hospitalized or in a nursing home in the previous 14 days. The most common pathogens implicated in the development of CAP are *Streptococcus pneumoniae, Mycoplasma pneumoniae, Hemophilus influenzae, Clamydophilia* sp, and viruses.

Two classifications of pneumonia are associated with exposure to the health care environment. HAP is a new respiratory infection that presents more than 48 hours after hospital admission. HCAP is infection in patients hospitalized for 2 or more days in the previous 90 days. This group includes patients undergoing dialysis or chemotherapy, chronic wound care, or home intravenous antibiotics care, the immunocompromised patient population, and patients from nursing home facilities.

VAP is pneumonia that is diagnosed more than 48 hours after a patient has been intubated and placed on a ventilator in the intensive care unit (ICU).

Fig. 5 provides a schematic view of this classification of pneumonia and the pathogenic organisms most commonly associated with infection. The latter 3 classes (HAP, VAP, and HCAP) are predominately associated with gram-negative bacteria. *Acinetobacter* is a pathogen associated with VAP specifically, and the 3 encapsulated bacteria (*Streptococcus pneumoniae, Klebsiella,* and *H influenzae*) are all associated with particularly higher morbidity and mortality.[7]

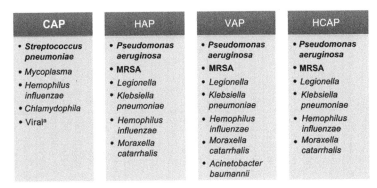

Fig. 5. Classification of pneumonia. [a]Viral, includes influenza A and B, adenovirus, respiratory syncytial virus, and parainfluenza.

Mortality from pneumonia varies depending on the causative organism, but *Streptococcus pneumoniae* has the highest mortality. The incidence of *Streptococcus pneumoniae* in 2008 was 100/100,000 adults/y. The mortality statistics for pneumococcal pneumonia in 2005 published by the World Health Organization were 1.6 million deaths worldwide. Even in developed countries the statistics indicate 10% to 20% mortality. The greatest risk of pneumococcal pneumonia is usually among people who have chronic illness such as lung, heart, or kidney disease, sickle cell anemia, or diabetes. But high rates are also noted in patients recovering from severe illness, those residing in nursing homes or chronic care facilities, and those patients older than 65 years.[8] Other high mortality causes include *Klebsiella*, *Legionella*, and methicillin-resistant *Staphylococcus aureus* (MRSA).

The clinical symptoms that characterize pneumonia caused by various agents often overlap, and the interobserver variability of physical findings has been shown to be high. This finding has led to an approach of antibiotic treatment of pneumonia in the ED, which is mostly empiric. However, to facilitate diagnostic decision making, various epidemiologic conditions have been shown to be related to specific pathogens in patients with pneumonia.[9] These classic associations are shown in **Table 1**.

The typical cardiovascular reaction to fever is tachycardia. However, certain pneumonias may be associated with fever and relative bradycardia (Faget sign). These pneumonias include *Legionella*, *Mycoplasma*, and tularemia. Other infections associated with this clinical sign include yellow fever, typhoid fever, brucellosis, and Colorado tick fever.

It is also often useful to consider the pathogenic organisms in pneumonia with respect to age of the host. **Table 2** shows the most typical organisms based on age classification.

DIAGNOSTIC TESTS
Laboratory Tests

Complete blood count
The white blood cell count (WBC) is neither sensitive nor specific to identify the likely causative agent of pneumonia (ie, bacterial or viral), but may be correlated with the severity of illness.[10,11] However, the WBC count may be useful in 2 scenarios: first, neutropenia, which may indicate immunosuppression; and second, lymphopenia, which may indicate immunosuppression from AIDS.

Table 1
Epidemiologic conditions, risk factors, and classic presentations of pneumonia associated with specific pathogens

Pathogen	Symptoms	Associated Condition	Radiographic/Laboratory Findings
Streptococcus pneumoniae	Rapid onset, rust sputum, chills, rigors	Alcoholism; COPD/smoking; HIV (early); postinfluenza; IVDU; endobronchial obstruction	Leukocytosis; gram-positive encapsulated diplococci; lobar infiltrate
Staphylococcus aureus	Gradual onset; postviral illness	IVDU; postinfluenza; structural lung disease[a]; endobronchial obstruction	Gram-positive cocci in clusters; associated with abscess, pleural effusion
Klebsiella	Fever, rigors; current-jelly sputum	Alcoholism; COPD; diabetes; elderly;	Bulging minor fissure; gram-negative encapsulated bacillus
Pseudomonas		HAP; VAP; HCAP; cystic fibrosis; hot tub use; COPD/smoking	Patchy infiltrates; gram-negative bacillus
Hemophilus influenzae	Gradual onset	Elderly; HIV (early); COPD/ smoking; postinfluenza; endobronchial obstruction	Patchy infiltrates; pleural effusion; gram-negative encapsulated coccobacillus
Moraxella catarrhalis		COPD/smoking	Gram-negative diplococcus
Chlamydophila pneumoniae	Gradual onset; dry cough; staccato cough (neonates)	COPD/smoking	Patchy infiltrates; Gram stain negative
Mycoplasma	Insidious onset; young adults		Gram stain negative; CXR, intestinal and perihilar; pleural effusion; extrapulmonary manifestations: bullous myringitis, cold agglutinins, morbilliform rash, hemolytic anemia, Guillain-Barré
Legionella	High mortality; relative bradycardia (Faget sign); GI symptoms; no person-to-person spread	Elderly, COPD/smoking; hotel/ cruise ship[b]	Gram stain negative; patchy infiltrates; hyponatremia; nonspecific LFT abnormalities

Anaerobes	Aspiration: oral pathogens or gram-negative enteric pathogens	Alcoholics; edentulous, neuromuscular disease, recent intubation; endobronchial obstruction	CXR: right middle lobe or right upper lobe infiltrates lung abscess
Hantavirus	Acute lung injury and shock; rodent urine/feces	Rodent urine/feces; travel to southwestern United States	
CA-MRSA			CXR: lung abscess
Bordetella pertussis	Cough more than 2 weeks; posttussive vomiting		
Yersinia pestis	Buboes; high person-to-person transmission	Fleas from rodents; hematogenous spread	
Bacillus anthracis	No person-to-person transmission; also GI and skin infection	Inhaled spores	Wide mediastinum
Francisella tularensis	Tularemia; lymphadenopathy; ulcerated skin lesions	Infected rabbits	
Coxiella burnetii	Q fever	Cattle and sheep exposure	Spirochete
Chlamydophila psittaci	Psittacosis	Infected birds	
Histoplasma capsulatum; *Coccidioides immitis;* *Blastomyces dermatitidis*	Histoplasmosis (bat/bird droppings); coccidiomycosis (southwestern United States); blastomycosis (erythema nodosum); slow gradual onset	Dirt/construction exposure	Patchy infiltrate
SARS	Coronavirus; acute lung injury; shock; young adults; travelers (Southeast Asia); highly contagious and lethal		
Mycobacterium tuberculosis		Alcoholics; lung abscess; HIV (early); IVDU	

(continued on next page)

Table 1
(continued)

Pathogen	Symptoms	Associated Condition	Radiographic/Laboratory Findings
Acinetobacter		Alcoholics; VAP	
HIV (early)			
Streptococcus pneumoniae; H influenzae; M tuberculosis			
HIV (late) *Pneumocystis jiroveci; Cryptococcus; Histoplasma; Aspergillus; Mycobacterium kansasii; Pseudomonas aeruginosa; H influenzae*	Opportunistic infection; progressive SOB		CD4 <200; increased LDH; low oxygen saturation

Abbreviations: CA-MRSA, community-acquired MRSA; COPD, chronic obstructive pulmonary disease; GI, gastrointestinal; HIV, human immunodeficiency virus; IVDU, intravenous drug use; LDH, lactate dehydrogenase; LFT, liver function test; SARS, severe acute respiratory syndrome; SOB, shortness of breath.

^a Structural lung disease: bronchiectasis.

^b Hotel or cruise ship stay within the previous 2 weeks.

Table 2
Age related pneumonia pathogens

Age Range	Suspected Organism
0–3 weeks	Group B streptococcus, *Listeria*, *E coli*
3 weeks–3 months	*Streptococcus pneumoniae*, *Chlamydia*, *Bordetella pertussis*, viral (respiratory syncytial virus, parainfluenzae)
4 months–4 years	Viral, *Streptococcus pneumoniae*, *Mycoplasma*
4 years–15 years	*Mycoplasma*, *Streptococcus pneumoniae*
Adults: CAP, HAP, VAP, HCAP	See **Table 1**

Blood cultures and sputum cultures

The laboratory detection of pneumonia can be difficult because of problems in obtaining an optimal specimen for diagnosis.[12] Blood cultures from pneumococcal pneumonia cases are often negative, and respiratory specimens such as sputum or nasopharyngeal samples can be confounded by the presence of normal flora.

The 2003 guidelines from the Infectious Diseases Society of America (IDSA) and the American Thoracic Society (ATS) recommend 2 blood cultures for patients hospitalized with pneumonia.[6,13] However, low rates of secondary bacteremia have led many to question the usefulness and cost-effectiveness of routine blood cultures. Studies have repeatedly shown sensitivity of blood cultures in patients admitted to the hospital with CAP to be between 7% and 10%. Patients with CAP who had blood cultures performed had a less than 2% chance of having a change in therapy directed by blood culture results. Severity of pneumonia, as measured by the Pneumonia Severity Index (PSI), also poorly correlates with the yield of blood cultures.[14] Blood cultures should be considered in patients who have a host defect in the ability to clear bacteremia. These patient groups include those with asplenia, complement deficiencies, chronic liver disease, and leucopenia.[15,16]

The Agency for Healthcare Research and Quality (AHRQ) has made recommendations regarding the use of blood cultures in adult patients with CAP.[17] The AHRQ states that routine blood cultures are not recommended in patients admitted with CAP. Consideration should be given to obtaining blood cultures in higher-risk patients admitted with CAP (ie, those with severe disease, immunocompromise, significant comorbidities, or other risk factors for infection with resistant organisms).

The benefits of sputum culture are also controversial. A meta-analysis has shown the use of sputum Gram stain to have low yield.[18] The initial limitation is that less than 50% of patients do not produce an adequate sample. Despite this finding, when a sputum sample has more than 25 polymorphonuclear cells per low-power field and there is a predominant organism, the causative organism is identified in more than 80% of cases. The interpretation of the sputum culture is also problematic. For properly handled samples the sensitivity is approximately 75%. This sensitivity is lower if antibiotics therapy has been started before the sample is taken. In addition, because of the possibility of culturing bacteria that colonize the oropharynx, false-positive results may occur. This finding is especially true for debilitated patients, who are more likely to be colonized with pathogens. However, certain organisms are always pathogenic and can be assumed to be causing disease if they are identified. These organisms include *Legionella* species, *Mycobacterium tuberculosis,* and the endemic fungi.[19]

The current IDSA/ATS guidelines for CAP in adults published in 2007[7] state that sputum cultures should be considered in patients when it is expected that the findings will result in a change in antibiotic management or that the test is likely to have high yield. The specific guidelines recommend therefore the use of sputum cultures in the following 8 circumstances: ICU admission; failure of outpatient antibiotic management; cavitary infiltrates; active alcohol abuse; severe obstructive or structural lung disease; positive *Legionella* urinary antigen test (UAT); positive pneumococcal UAT; or pleural effusion.

Serologic testing

Serologic testing is available for *Chlamydia* sp, *Legionella*, and some fungi. In the ED these investigations are useful only from a retrospective perspective because they usually require both acute and convalescent serum titers. Rapid antigen tests are also available for influenza and respiratory syncytial virus (RSV). These tests may be useful as an adjunctive ED test for infection control purposes for hospital inpatients and as an aid in decision making regarding family and contact prophylaxis.

UATs are commercially available for *Streptococcus pneumoniae* and *Legionella pneumophilia*. These tests have the highest diagnostic yield in patients with more severe illness. These antigen tests are rapid, simple to use, have high specificity in adults (<90%), and, most importantly, have the ability to detect the organism after antibiotics have been started.[20,21]

Serologic testing can be useful as an aid to tailoring antibiotic management. This finding is of particular importance for the identification of *Mycobacterium* or the identification of antibiotic-resistant strains. The latter have been implicated in increased mortality[22] and in increased risk of clinical failure.[23] The identification of certain pathogens may have important epidemiologic implications. These implications include severe acute respiratory syndrome (SARS), influenza, legionnaire disease, and agents of bioterrorism. Cost is the greatest impedance to testing in all patients. The cost/benefit ratio must be considered.[24]

Microbiological testing in severe CAP in patients admitted to the ICU has been shown to both identify the causative agent and lead to changes in antibiotic therapy, both of which, in this setting, have had a positive impact on patient outcome.[25]

Imaging Modalities

CXR

The diagnosis of CAP is based on the presence of select clinical features (cough, fever, sputum production, or pleuritic chest pain) and is supported by imaging of the lung. The CXR remains the reference standard for the diagnosis of pneumonia. It has been shown to have greater sensitivity and specificity than the physical examination of the chest for diagnosis of pneumonia.[26] The CXR is not only useful in making the diagnosis of pneumonia but also in aiding in differentiating pneumonia from other common causes of cough and fever, or in identifying an alternative diagnosis.

There is considerable overlap in the classic CXR appearances associated with specific pathogens. However, CXR has low sensitivity for the diagnosis of pneumonia in the very elderly population and in the neutropenic population.

Computed tomography scan/magnetic resonance imaging

Computed tomography (CT) of the chest has been shown to have greater sensitivity than CXR for the diagnosis of pneumonia. However, the clinical significance of these findings when the CXR is negative is unclear.[27] For patients who are hospitalized with suspected pneumonia but have a negative CXR, it is recommended to treat the condition empirically and repeat the CXR in 24 to 48 hours.

CT scanning has been shown to be beneficial for the diagnosis of pneumonia in the neutropenic patient.[27,28] CT scanning can be useful in those patients who do not respond to initial therapy. In addition to ruling out other diagnoses such as pulmonary emboli, a CT scan can disclose other reasons for antibiotic failure, including pleural effusions, lung abscess, or central airway obstruction. Magnetic resonance imaging has been shown to have similar sensitivity compared with CT and has been recommended for follow-up examinations in this patient population to minimize repeated radiograph exposure.[29]

Ultrasonography
Recently the use of bedside ultrasonography has been studied in the ED diagnosis of pulmonary conditions including pneumonia. Bedside lung ultrasonography has been shown to be 96% sensitive and 96% specific in the diagnosis of radio-occult (negative CXR) pleural-pulmonary lesions.[30] A recent systematic review[31] has also shown bedside lung ultrasonography to be an ideal tool for the diagnosis of emergency pulmonary conditions, with the benefit of the absence of radiation.

HOSPITAL ADMISSION DECISIONS

Diagnostic and treatment decisions for pneumonia are based on assessing the severity of illness. These assessments also affect the decision between inpatient and outpatient treatment and ICU admission versus admission to a general ward.

Scoring Systems

Two scoring systems have been developed that can assist in the identification of patients who may be candidates for outpatient treatment: CURB-65 is a severity of illness score,[32] and the PSI[33] is a prognostic model (**Table 3**).

The use of these objective criteria must be supplemented by physician judgment. Factors such as patient compliance to oral medication and outpatient social support

Table 3
Comparison of CURB-65 and PSI scores

CURB - 65	PSI
Confusion +1	Age
Blood urea nitrogen >7 mmol/L +1	Female −10
Respiratory rate >30 +1	Nursing home resident +10
Systolic blood pressure <90 mm Hg or diastolic blood pressure <60 mm Hg +1	Neoplastic disease history +30
Age >65 y +1	Liver disease +20
	Congestive heart failure +10
	Cerebrovascular disease +10
	Renal disease +10
	Altered mental status +20
	Respiratory rate >29 +20
	Systolic blood pressure <90 +20
	Temperature <35°C or >39.9°C +15
	Pulse >124 +10
	pH <7.35 +30
	Blood urea nitrogen <29 +20
	Sodium <130 +20
	Glucose >13.8 +10
	Hematocrit <30% +10
	Partial pressure oxygen <60 +10
	Pleural effusion on radiograph +10

systems should be taken into account. The ATS has also developed criteria to assist in the decision making regarding which patients require higher-level monitoring or an ICU admission directly from the ED.[7]

The PSI uses a 2-step approach to risk assessment. Patients are first identified as low-risk and recommended for outpatient management. The low-risk patients are those less than 50 years, who do not have significant comorbid conditions, and who have no concerning features on physical examination. Patients who do not meet these low-risk criteria are then classified into categories based on age, comorbid illness, abnormal physical examination findings, and laboratory abnormalities. Scoring is divided into 5 classes and each class is associated with a predicted mortality: class 1, points 0, mortality 0.1%; class 2, points less than 70, mortality 0.6%; class 3, points 71–90, mortality 2.8%; class 4, points 91–130, mortality 8.2%; class 5, points greater than 130, mortality 29.2%. Classes 1, 2, and 3 are considered low-risk patients, class 4, moderate-risk, and class 5, high-risk. Hospital admission is recommended for those patients who score more than 91 (class 4). This score has been shown to decrease overall admission rates and decrease health care costs.[34] However, the scoring system does not consider dynamic observation of patients over time, the ability to take oral medications, home supports, and access to follow-up.

CURB-65 is a more simplified tool that uses 5 criteria to determine patients at lower risk for adverse events. These criteria are confusion; uremia (blood urea nitrogen [BUN] >7 mmol/L); respiratory rate (>30); blood pressure (<90 systolic, or >60 diastolic); age 65 years or greater. Each criterion is rated equally for a total score of 5. The risk of 30-day mortality increases with increasing score. A score of 1 point is the lowest-risk group, with an estimated 2.7% 30-day mortality; outpatient treatment is recommended. Two points is the moderate-risk group, with a 6.8% 30-day mortality; either outpatient treatment with close follow-up or inpatient treatment is recommended in this group. Three points is the severe group, with an estimated 14% mortality; inpatient treatment is recommended in this group with consideration for an ICU admission. Four and 5 points are the highest-risk groups. There is an estimated 27.8% mortality in these groups and an ICU admission is recommended.

Comparison of the PSI and CURB-65 scores reveals that they are equivalent in predicting mortality.[35] Both the 28-day mortality and the inhospital mortality for PSI level V and CURB >/- 3 were equivalent.[36] Both scoring indices have also been shown to accurately predict outcomes in patients with HCAP.[37] However, there are no randomized trials of hospital admission strategies that directly compare the 2 scoring systems. In addition, no prospective criteria have been validated for the decision-making process for an ICU admission.[38] PSI also underperforms in the elderly population.[39] This finding is suspected secondary to the inappropriate weight given to the age variable in the scoring system. This situation is of concern because elderly patients often have atypical presentations and worse outcomes.

The ATS has developed criteria to assist with inhospital disposition decision making. These criteria are divided into major and minor criteria. Direct admission to an ICU or high-level monitoring unit is recommended for patients with either of the major criteria or with 3 of the minor criteria. Major criteria are invasive mechanical ventilation or septic shock with the need for vasopressors. **Table 4** shows the minor criteria for severe CAP.

MANAGEMENT

The goal of therapy is eradication of the infecting microorganism, with resultant resolution of clinical disease. Antimicrobials are the mainstay of treatment. The ATS

Table 4
Minor criteria for severe CAP

Physical Examination	CXR	Laboratory
Respiratory rate >30/min	Multilobar infiltrates	Leukopenia: WBC <4000 cells/mm^3
Blood pressure: requires aggressive intravenous fluids		Thrombocytopenia: platelet count <100,000 cells/mm^3
Hypoxemia: Pao$_2$/Fio$_2$ ratio <250		
Mental status: confusion		
Hypothermia: temperature <36°C		

advocates an empiric approach to treatment based on clinical presentation. This approach also incorporates the presence of risk factors for *Pseudomonas* species, gram-negative organisms, and drug-resistant *Streptococcus pneumoniae* (DRSP).[7]

Table 5 provides a schematic view of the current recommended treatments for various patient populations with pneumonia.

The most common pathogens in this mild (ambulatory) group are all adequately covered by macrolide antibiotics (see **Fig. 5**). Macrolide antibiotics are recommended as monotherapy in this patient population. The use of fluoroquinolones to treat

Table 5
Recommended antibiotic treatment

Outpatient	Inpatient Hospital Ward[a]	Inpatient ICU
Healthy/no risk factors for DRSP Macrolide[b] or Doxycycline	Respiratory fluoroquinolone or β-lactam plus macrolide	Minimum treatment β-lactam plus macrolide
Comorbidity[c] Respiratory fluoroquinolone[d] or β-lactam[e] plus macrolide		Antipseudomonal coverage Imipenen; meropenem plus ciprofloxacin or levofloxacin or β-lactam plus aminoglycoside plus azithromycin or β-lactam plus aminoglycoside plus antipseudomonal fluoroquinolone
		CA-MRSA Vancomycin or linezolid

[a] Increasing resistance rates suggest that empiric therapy with a macrolide alone is not recommended in this population.
[b] Macrolide antibiotics include azithromycin, clarithromycin, and erythromycin; doxycycline can be used as a macrolide alternative.
[c] Cardiovascular: coronary artery disease or congestive heart failure, valvular heart disease; Pulmonary: asthma, chronic obstructive pulmonary, interstitial lung disorders; Renal: preexisting renal disease with a documented abnormal serum creatinine level outside the period of the pneumonia episode; Hepatic: preexisting viral or toxic hepatopathy; Central nervous system: vascular or nonvascular encephalopathy, diabetes mellitus and treatment with oral anti-diabetics or insulin; Neoplastic illness: any solid tumor active at the time of presentation or requiring antineoplastic treatment within the preceding year.
[d] Respiratory fluoroquinolones included moxifloxacin and levofloxacin.
[e] β-Lactams include high-dose amoxicillin (1 g 3 times a day) or amoxicillin clavulanate (750 mg twice a day) or ceftriaxone or cefuroxime.

ambulatory patients with pneumonia without comorbid conditions, risk factors for DRSP, or recent antibiotic use is not recommended because of the concern for the development of fluoroquinolone resistance.[40] Comorbidity or recent antimicrobial therapy increased the likelihood of infection with DRSP, and enteric gram-negative bacteria. In these patients, therapeutic options include either a respiratory fluoroquinolone or a combination therapy with a β-lactam antibiotic effective against *Streptococcus pneumoniae* plus a macrolide. Recommended β-lactams include: high-dose amoxicillin or amoxicillin clavulanate. Oral cephalosporins can also be used as alternatives. Agents in the same class as the patient has been receiving previously should not be used to treat patients with recent antibiotic exposure.

For patients who are admitted to a hospital ward, the combination treatment of a β-lactam plus a macrolide or monotherapy with a fluoroquinolone has been shown to be associated with a significant reduction in mortality compared with that of the administration of a cephalosporin alone.[41] The choice between dual or monotherapy should be based on the patient's previous 3-month antibiotic exposure. Initial therapy for admitted patients is usually intravenous, but oral therapy can be considered for patients without risk factors for severe pneumonia, especially with highly bioavailable agents such as fluoroquinolones.[42]

Patients admitted to the ICU with pneumonia are those who are usually diagnosed with severe pneumonia initially from the ED. The antimicrobial treatment in this patient population must be broader. The minimum recommended treatment of these patients is a β-lactam plus either azithromycin or a fluoroquinolone. For all patients admitted to the ICU, antimicrobial coverage should include that for *Streptococcus pneumoniae* and *Legionella*. This combination therapy is recommended for at least 48 hours or until results of diagnostic tests are known. In the mechanically ventilated ICU patient, treatment with a fluoroquinolone alone has been associated with inferior outcome.[43]

In the critically ill ICU patient with severe pneumonia, many microorganisms other than *Streptococcus pneumoniae* and *Legionella* sp must be considered. Of particular importance is *Pseudomonas* sp and gram-negative bacteria.[44] Therefore, standard empiric treatment regimes in this population should include coverage for *Streptococcus pneumoniae*, *Legionella* sp, and *H influenzae*, all of the atypical organisms, Enterobacteriaceae sp, and Pseudomonadaceae sp (see **Table 5**). Penicillin-allergic patients should have the β-lactam substituted with azetreonam, a synthetic monocyclic β-lactam antibiotic. The excess mortality associated with MRSA indicates empiric coverage for this organism in this patient population. For suspected MRSA (end-stage renal disease, injection drug abuse, previous influenza, and previous recent antibiotic use) vancomycin or linezolid should be added.

SPECIAL TREATMENT CONSIDERATIONS
Timing of Antibiotics

There seems to be a causal relationship between antibiotic timing and improved outcomes, especially in the elderly population.[45] Early antibiotic treatment does not seem to shorten the time to clinical stability but has been shown to decrease length of hospital stay.[46] However, there is insufficient evidence to establish an overall benefit in mortality or morbidity from antibiotics administered in less than 8 hours from ED arrival in patients with CAP without severe sepsis. For patients admitted through the ED, the first antibiotic dose should be administered while the patient is still in the ED.

Transition from Parenteral Antibiotics to Oral Antibiotics

Most hospitalized patients are initially treated with parenteral antibiotics. The transition to oral antibiotics can occur when the patient has become clinically stable and has shown clinical improvement. Criteria for clinical stability include temperature less than 37.8°C, heart rate less than 100/min, respiratory rate less than 24/min, systolic blood pressure greater than 90 mm Hg; room air oxygen saturation of greater than 90%; and normal mental status.[47] This transition should be balanced with an assessment of the ability to ingest oral medications in patients with normal functioning gastrointestinal tracts.

Duration of Treatment

It is recommended that the duration of treatment be a minimum of 5 days and that the patient be afebrile for 48 to 72 hours before discontinuation of treatment. The patient should not possess any signs of clinical instability at the time of discontinuation of treatment.[47] Few controlled trials have evaluated the optimum duration of antibiotic therapy in either inpatients or outpatients. However, most patients with CAP are treated for 7 to 10 days or longer.

Noninvasive Positive Pressure Ventilation

In patients with pneumonia, noninvasive positive pressure ventilation (NPPV) has been shown to be well tolerated, safe, and associated with a significant reduction in respiratory rate, need for endotracheal intubation, and duration of ICU stay. NPPV does not decrease overall duration of overall hospitalization or inhospital mortality, except in the subgroup of patients with pneumonia and underlying chronic obstructive pulmonary disease (COPD).[48] However, other studies of patients with hypoxic respiratory failure have failed to show a benefit of NPPV, with many patients eventually requiring intubation.[49] Hence, these conflicting data do not support the routine use of NPPV in patients with severe pneumonia, with the exception of patients with underlying COPD. The ATS and the IDSA currently recommend a cautious trial of NPPV for refractory hypoxemia in patients with severe pneumonia.[7]

Hypotensive, Fluid-resuscitated Patients with Severe Pneumonia

Corticosteroids have been studied in patients with septic shock and have yielded no benefit. A recent 2010 Cochrane review of 20 randomized trials revealed that corticosteroids did not change 28-day mortality. Furthermore, corticosteroids did show a statistically significant increase in adverse events such as hyperglycemia and hypernatremia.[50,51]

Recombinant human activated protein C (APC) has also been studied in patients with severe sepsis. A Cochrane Review of 4434 adult patients yielded no benefit. There was no difference in mortality between the control group and those who received APC, regardless of the severity of the sepsis. However, use of APC was associated with a higher risk of serious bleeding.[52]

Diffuse Bilateral Pneumonia and Acute Respiratory Distress Syndrome

Mortality for patients with severe diffuse bilateral pneumonia or acute respiratory distress syndrome (ARDS) is extremely high. The ARDSnet trial revealed a significant reduction in mortality with the use of low tidal volume ventilation (6 mL/kg ideal body weight) or what has become known as a lung protective ventilation strategy. With this intervention, the number needed to treat (NNT) to avoid 1 death is 9 (NNT = 9).[53,54] The ATS therefore has made a level 1 recommendation that patients with diffuse bilateral pneumonia or ARDS should be mechanically ventilated with low tidal volumes.

DRSP

Antibiotic resistance patterns vary considerable among countries/regions and evolve over time. Globally, 1.6 million people die of invasive pneumococcal disease annually.

This incidence is highest in extremes of age, in patients with comorbidity, and in those with defects in immunity. The development of drug-resistant strains of microorganisms has placed a challenge on effective treatment options.[55,56]

Emergency physicians should be aware that the patients at the highest risk of infection with DRSP include those who take antibiotics frequently, patients who are exposed to others who commonly receive antibiotics, children younger than 6 years (especially those in daycare facilities and their immediate family members), adults older than 70 years, and those with underlying immunosuppression.

Penicillin resistance occurs in a stepwise fashion with irreversible mutations of the penicillin binding proteins. In the United States, penicillin resistance decreased from 1999 to 2005. This decrease was reported in both the pediatric and the adult population. This decline is a reflection of the introduction of the 7-valent pneumococcal conjugate vaccine.[57,58]

During this same period, resistance rates to macrolides did not change, but resistance to fluoroquinolones increased, likely reflecting an increase in use. The resistance of fluoroquinolone is highest in adults older than 64 years and in patients with underlying COPD.

The impact of antimicrobial resistance on clinical outcome remains controversial. Host factors such as extremes of age, immunosuppression, and comorbidity likely also influence mortality.[59]

Prescribing antibiotics for respiratory infection contributes to the development of resistance to that antibiotic. The effect seems to be greatest in the month immediately after treatment but may persist for up to 12 months. Reduction in antibiotic use may reduce the potential for antimicrobial resistance.[60]

Antibiotic resistance is a problem that can be combated at the ED level through a combination of appropriate antibiotic selection, prescribing patterns, use of antibiotic resistance profiles, surveillance protocols, and an understanding of new antibiotic treatment options.

Nonresponding Pneumonia

Nonresolving pneumonia is a clinical syndrome in which clinical symptoms of pneumonia do not improve or worsen despite an initial 10 days of antibiotic therapy or in which radiographic opacities fail to resolve within 12 weeks. Mortality among nonresponding patients is greatly increased compared with patients who initially respond to treatment. Overall mortality as high as 49% has been reported for nonresponding hospitalized patients with pneumonia.[61] Nonresponse mandates either a transfer to a higher level of care, further diagnostic testing, or a change in treatment. Inadequate host response is the most common cause of apparent treatment failure. Patients older than 65 years, those with COPD, diabetes, alcoholism, or those who are undergoing immunosuppressive therapy are the most likely to be nonresponders.

Emergency physicians should be aware that as many as 10% of patients with CAP and up to 60% of patients with HAP have inadequate responses to initial empiric therapy. As many as 20% of these patients are diagnosed with diseases other than pneumonia.[62]

SPECIAL PATIENT POPULATIONS
MRSA

There are 2 patterns of MRSA: the hospital-acquired strain (HA-MRSA) and those more recently identified strains that are phenotypically distinct and have become known as community-acquired MRSA (CA-MRSA).[63] The latter are resistant to fewer antimicrobials than are the hospital-acquired MRSA strains. However, most of these strains do contain a toxin associated with the clinical features of necrotizing pneumonia, shock, respiratory failure, and the formation of abscesses and empyema. This strain should be suspected in patients with cavitary infiltrates on CXR. It is estimated that 2% of CA-MRSA infections result in pneumonia.[64]

CA-MRSA pneumonia is associated with an influenzalike illness, occurs most commonly in young healthy individuals, and has high mortality. The recommended parenteral antibiotic treatment is vancomycin or linezolid. The addition of rifampicin may also be considered. The management of CA-MRSA should also include culture of blood, sputum, and pleural specimens in the case of pleural effusion. Empyema is an associated complication and should be drained. It is recommended that patients with this diagnosis be admitted to an ICU. Respiratory infection control measures are important for the prevention of nosocomial spread of MRSA.[65]

VIRAL PNEUMONIAS
Influenza

In the ambulatory setting, in uncomplicated cases of viral pneumonia caused by influenza, treatment within 48 hours of symptoms with oseltamivir or zanamivir is recommended. These neuraminidase inhibitors have been shown to reduce median time to resolution of symptoms by 0.5 to 2.5 days. In this patient population, both oral oseltamivir and inhaled zanamivir reduce the likelihood of complications of the lower respiratory tract.[66]

In the hospitalized patient population, it is postulated that oseltamivir may reduce viral shedding and therefore treatment even greater than 48 hours of symptom onset may confer some benefit. Oseltamivir has been shown to have a broad influenza spectrum (both influenza A and B) and a low risk of resistance.

Amantadine is effective against influenza A only. Recent circulating influenza viruses in North America have been resistant to amantadine. Hence, treatment or chemoprophylaxis with amantadine is not currently recommended.[67]

Pandemic Influenza

Influenza A from H5N1 (Avian) and H1N1 (pandemic influenza A) have a greater severity of infection than routine seasonal influenza. Both strains possess pandemic potential. These strains have been associated with acute respiratory failure and mortality greater than70%. The usual clinical presentation is fever, cough, and respiratory distress progressive over 3 to 5 days. Exposure to dead or dying poultry in an area with known or suspected H5N1 activity has been reported by most patients with avian influenza A.[68]

Rapid bedside tests to detect influenza A have been used as screening tools. It is recommended that confirmed cases be treated with oseltamivir. The current recommendation is for a 5-day course of treatment at the standard dosage of 75 mg 2 times daily. Oseltamivir has been shown to have a significant mortality reduction, especially when started within 6 to 8 days after symptom onset. The mortality benefit seems to affect all age groups.[69] All such patients should also be placed in respiratory isolation and droplet precautions used.

The cause of viral pneumonia is most likely unknown to the emergency physician at initial presentation. No universal empiric therapy for viral pneumonia can be recommended. Causes of viral pneumonia other than influenza A and B include RSV, adenovirus, rhinovirus, enteroviruses, human metapneumovirus, hantavirus, and varicella zoster virus. Evidence for antiviral treatment of CAP caused by viruses other than influenza comes mainly from case reports and treatment of immunocompromised patients. Ribavirin has been shown to be efficacious against RSV, human metapneumovirus, and parainfluenza. It can be used in intravenous form for the treatment of severe pneumonia caused by these viruses, from experience with immunocompromised patients.[70] Ribavirin aerosol treatment has been shown to be less efficacious.

Human Immunodeficiency Virus and Tuberculosis

The use of HAART (highly active antiretroviral therapy) has decreased the incidence of opportunistic infection in patients infected with the human immunodeficiency virus (HIV). Respiratory infections are the most common type of opportunistic infection in the population with HIV. Pneumonia is associated with high mortality in the immunocompromised patient population. *Pneumocystis jiroveci* is the most common opportunistic infection in the HIV population. Traditionally, such infection in a patient with HIV is believed to represent reactivation of latent colonization. Those with CD4 counts less than 200 cells/mm^3 are at the greatest risk. Among patients with HIV and Pneumocystis pneumonia (PCP), mortality is 10% to 20%. This mortality increases substantially with the need for mechanical ventilation. The addition of corticosteroids to the standard treatment of PCP has been shown to decrease both mortality and the need for mechanical ventilation. Corticosteroids are indicated in patients with PCP and substantial hypoxemia (Pao$_2$ <70 mm Hg; A-a gradient >35 mm Hg on room air).[71–73]

However, the most common cause of bacterial pneumonia in the population with HIV remains *Streptococcus pneumoniae*. Patients infected with this microorganism develop pneumonia more frequently than do patients who do not have HIV and they have a more severe clinical course when infected.[74] Pneumococcal infections occur in patients with HIV with CD4 counts less than 500 cells/mm^3.

In 2010, 11,181 tuberculosis (TB) cases were reported in the United States for a rate of 3.6 cases per 100,000 population.[75] HIV is considered the greatest risk factor for TB infection. TB can occur in the early stage of HIV with CD4 cell counts less than 300 cells/mm^3. Patients with HIV are more likely to develop active TB once infected and they have a higher risk of death. It is estimated that in 2009, there were 1.1 million HIV-positive patients with TB worldwide and 380,000 deaths from TB in the population with HIV. HIV is also the most important risk factor for progression from latent to active TB. Early diagnosis of TB can be difficult because of a lack of specific clinical findings, such as abnormal CXR or positive skin test result. In patients with more advanced HIV disease, extrapulmonary disease is more common.[76] Treatment of latent TB infection has been shown to reduce the risk of active TB in HIV-positive patients, especially those with a positive skin test.[77]

SUMMARY

Pneumonia is a common disease presentation to the ED. The challenge for the emergency physician is to recognize the diagnosis, initiate early and appropriate empiric antibiotic therapy, risk stratify patients with respect to severity of illness, and recognize indications for admission. Treatment should consider not only empiric therapy guidelines but also the environment in which the pneumonia was contracted and the host factors that may implicate risk for a particular microorganism.

The emergency physician should initiate antibiotic treatment in the ED for all patients who are diagnosed with pneumonia and should be vigilant regarding respiratory isolation and droplet precautions. Disposition should be based not only on the severity of the presenting symptoms, but the underlying comorbidities of the patient, the clinical likelihood of deterioration, and the access to outpatient follow-up.

REFERENCES

1. Heron M, Hoyert D, Murphy S, et al. Deaths: final data for 2006. Natl Vital Stat Rep 2009;57(14):1–134.
2. Trends in pneumonia and influenza morbidity and mortality. Morbidity and Mortality Weekly Report 2010;59(14):425.
3. McCullers J. Insights into the interaction between influenza virus and pneumococcus. Clin Microbiol Rev 2006;19:571–82.
4. Centre for Disease Control and Prevention Advisory Committee on Immunization Practices (ACIP), Universal Annual Influenza Vaccination. February 24, 2010.
5. Chartbook on cardiovascuar, lung, and blood diseases, 2009. National Heart Lung and Blood Institute; 2009.
6. Mandell LA, Bartlett JG, Dowell SF, et al. Update of practice guidelines for the management of community-acquired pneumonia in immunocompetent adults. Clin Infect Dis 2003;37:1405–33.
7. Mandall LA. Infectious Disease Society of America/American Thoracic Society consensus guidelines for the management of community-acquired pneumonia in adults. Clin Infect Dis 2007;44:S27–72.
8. Epidemiology and Prevention of Vaccine Preventable Diseases, 2006. CDC National Immunization Program; 2006.
9. Neidermann MS, Mandell LA, Anzueto A, et al. Guidelines for the management of community-acquired pneumonia in adults, diagnosis, assessment of severity, antimicrobial therapy and prevention. Clin Infect Dis 2007;44(Suppl 2):527–72.
10. Vernet G. Laboratory based diagnosis of pneumococcal pneumonia–state of the art and unmet needs. Clin Microbiol Infect 2011;17(Suppl 3):1–13.
11. Kruger S, Pletz MW, Rohde G. Biomarkers in community acquired pneumonia–what did we learn from the CAPNETZ study? Pneumologie 2011;65(2):110–3.
12. Craven DE. Blood cultures for community acquired pneumonia–piecing together a mosaic for doing less. Am J Respir Crit Care Med 2004;169:327–8.
13. Niederman MS, Mandell LA, Anzueto A, et al. Guidelines for the management of adults with community-acquired pneumonia. Diagnosis, assessment of severity, antimicrobial therapy, and prevention. Am J Respir Crit Care Med 2001;163(7): 1730–54.
14. Campbell SG, Marrie TJ, Ansey R, et al. The contribution of blood cultures to the clinical management of adult patients admitted to the hospital with community-acquired pneumonia: a prospective observational study. Chest 2003;123:571–82.
15. Metersky MA, Ma A, Bratzler DW, et al. Predicting bacteremia in patients with community acquired pneumonia. Am J Respir Crit Care Med 2004;169:342–7.
16. Paganin F, Lilienthal F, Bourdin A, et al. Severe community-acquired pneumonia: assessment of microbial activity as mortality factor. Eur Respir J 2004;24:779–85.
17. Nazarian DJ, Eddy OL, Lukens TW, et al. American College of Emergency Physician Clinical policy: critical issue in the management of adult patients presenting to the emergency department with community-acquired pneumonia. Ann Emerg Med 2009;54(3):704–31.
18. Reed WW, Byrd GS, Gates RH Jr, et al. Sputum gram stain in community acquired pneumococcal pneumonia: a meta-analysis. West J Med 1996;165:197–204.
19. Metersky M. When to obtain cultures from patients with community-acquired pneumonia. J Respir Dis 2005;26(4):143–8.

20. Yzerman EP, den Boer JW, Lettinga KD, et al. Sensitivity of three urine antigen tests associated with clinical severity in a large outbreak of Legionnaires' disease in the Netherlands. J Clin Microbiol 2002;40(9):3232–6.
21. Strålin K, Kaltoft MS, Konradsen HB, et al. Comparison of two urinary antigen tests for establishment of pneumococcal etiology of adult CAP. J Clin Microbiol 2004;42:3620–5.
22. Kollef MH, Sherman G, Ward S, et al. Inadequate antimicrobial treatment of infections: a risk factor for hospital mortality among critically ill patients. Chest 1999; 115(46):72–4.
23. Arancibia F, Ewig S, Martinez JA, et al. Antimicrobial treatment failure in patient with CAP. Am J Respir Crit Care Med 2000;162:154–60.
24. Sepsis and CAP: partnerships for diagnostic development. RFA no: RFA-AI-04–043. US Department of Health and Human Service; 2004.
25. Rello J, Bodi M, Mariscal D. Microbiological testing and outcome in patients with severe community acquired pneumonia. Chest 2003;123:174–80.
26. Wipf JE, Lipsky BA, Hirschmann HV, et al. Diagnosing pneumonia by physical examination: relevant or relic? Arch Intern Med 1996;165:197–204.
27. Syrjala H, Broas M, Suramo I, et al. High resolution computed tomography for the diagnosis of community-acquired pneumonia. Clin Infect Dis 1998;27:358–63.
28. Huessel CP, Kauczor HU, Ullmann AJ. Pneumonia in the neutropenic patient. Eur Radiol 2004;14(2):256–71.
29. Reiger C, Herzog P, Fiegl M, et al. Pulmonary MRI–a new approach to the evaluation of the febrile neutropenic patient with malignancy. Support Care Cancer 2008;16(6):599–606.
30. Volpicelli G, Cardinale L, Berchialla P, et al. A comparison of different diagnostic tests in the bedside evaluation of pleuritic pain in the ED. Am J Emerg Med 2012; 30(2):317–24.
31. Reissig A, Copetti R, Kroegel C. Current role of emergency ultrasound of the chest. Crit Care Med 2011;39(4):839–45.
32. Lim WS, van der Eerden MM, Liang R, et al. Defining community acquired pneumonia severity on presentation to hospital: an international derivation and validation study. Thorax 2003;58:377.
33. Fine MJ, Auble TE, Yealy DM, et al. A prediction rule to identify low-risk patients with community-acquired pneumonia. N Engl J Med 1997;336(4):243–50.
34. Marrie TJ, Lau CY, Wheeler SL, et al. A controlled trial of a critical pathway for treatment of community-acquired pneumonia. CAPITAL Study Investigators. Community-Acquired Pneumonia Intervention Trial Assessing Levofloxacin. JAMA 2000;283(6):749–55.
35. Aujesky D, Auble TE, Yealy DM, et al. Prospective comparison of three validated prediction rule for prognosis in CAP. Am J Med 2005;118:384.
36. Richard G, Levy H, Laterre PF, et al. CURB-65, PSI, APACHE II to assess mortality rate in patients with severe sepsis and community acquired pneumonia in PROWESS. J Intensive Care Med 2011;26(1):34–40.
37. Fang WF, Yang KY, Wu CL, et al. Application and comparison of scoring indices to predict outcomes in patients with healthcare-associated pneumonia. Crit Care 2011;15(1):R32.
38. Moran GJ, Talan DA, Abrahamian FM. Diagnosis of pneumonia in the ED. Infect Dis Clin North Am 2008;22:53.
39. Chen JH, Chang SS, Liu JJ, et al. Comparison of clinical characteristics and performance of pneumonia severity score and CURB-65 among younger adults, elderly and very old subjects. Thorax 2010;65(11):971–7.

40. Heffelfinger JD, Dowell SF, Jorgensen JH, et al. Management of community-acquired pneumonia in the era of pneumococcal resistance: a report from the Drug-Resistant Streptococcus pneumoniae Therapeutic Working Group. Arch Intern Med 2000;160:1399–408.

41. Gleason PP, Meehan TP, Fine JM, et al. Associations between initial antimicrobial therapy and medial outcomes for hospitalized elderly patients with pneumonia. Arch Intern Med 1999;159:2562–72.

42. Marras TK, Nopmaneejumruslers C, Chan CK. Efficacy of exclusively oral antibiotic therapy in patients hospitalized with non-severe community acquired pneumonia: a retrospective study and meta-analysis. Am J Med 2004;116: 385–93.

43. Levoy O, Saux P, Bedos JP, et al. Comparison of levofloxacin and cefotaxime combined with ofloxacin for ICU patients with community-acquired pneumonia who do not require vasopressors. Chest 2005;128:172–83.

44. File TM. Community acquired pneumonia. Lancet 2003;362:1991–2001.

45. Houck PM, Batzler DW. Administration of first hospital antibiotics for community-acquired pneumonia: does timeliness affect outcomes? Curr Opin Infect Dis 2005;18(2):151–6.

46. Siber SH, Garrett C, Singh R, et al. Early administration of antibiotics does not shorten time to clinical stability in patients with moderate to severe community acquired pneumonia. Chest 2003;124:1798–804.

47. Menendez R, Torres A, Rodriguez de Castro F, et al. Reaching stability in community acquired pneumonia: the effects of the severity of disease, treatment, and the characteristics of patients. Clin Infect Dis 2004;39:1783–90.

48. Confalonieri M, Potena A, Carbone G, et al. Acute respiratory failure in patients with severe community acquired pneumonia. A prospective randomized evaluation of non-invasive ventilation. Am J Respir Crit Care Med 1999;160:1585–91.

49. Antonelli M, Conti G, Moro ML, et al. Predictors of failures of non-invasive positive pressure ventilation in patients with acute hypoxemic respiratory failure: a multicenter study. Intensive Care Med 2001;27:1718–28.

50. Annane D, Bellissant E, Bollaert PE, et al. Corticosteroids for treating severe sepsis and septic shock. Cochrane Database Syst Rev 2010;12. DOI: 10.1002/14651858.CD002243.pub2.

51. Sprung CL, Annane D, Keh D, et al. CORITCUS Study Group. Hydrocortisone therapy for patients with septic shock. N Engl J Med 2008;358(2):111–24.

52. Marti-Carcajal AJ, Salanti G, Cardina-Zorrila AF, et al. Human recombinant activated Protein C for severe sepsis. Cochrane Database Syst Rev 2000;1:CD004388.

53. Eisner MD, Thompson T, Hudson LD, et al. Efficacy of low tidal volume ventilation in patients with different clinical risk factors for acute lung injury and acute respiratory distress syndrome. Am J Respir Crit Care Med 2001;164:231–6.

54. Petrucci N, Lacovelli W. Lung protective ventilation strategy for the acute respiratory syndrome. Cochrane Database Syst Rev 2007;3:CD003844.

55. Van Bembeke F, Reinert RR, Appelbaum PC, et al. Multidrug-resistant Streptococcus pneumoniae infections: current and future therapeutic option. Drugs 2007;67(16):2355–82.

56. Johnson DM, Stilwell MG, Fritsche TR, et al. Emergence of multidrug-resistant Streptococcus pneumoniae: report from the SENTRY Antimicrobial Surveillance Program (1999-2003). Diagn Microbiol Infect Dis 2006;56(1):69–74.

57. Lynch J III, Zhanel George G. Streptococcus pneumoniae: epidemiology and risk factors, evolution of antimicrobial resistance, and impact of vaccine. Curr Opin Pulm Med 2010;16:217–25.

58. Centers for Disease Control and Prevention (CDC). Pneumonia hospitalizations among young children before and after introduction of pneumococcal conjugate vaccine–Unites States 1997-2006. MMWR Morb Mortal Wkly Rep 2009;58:1–4.
59. Lynch JP, Zhanel GG. Streptococcus pneumoniae: does antimicrobial resistance matter? Semin Respir Crit Care Med 2009;30:210–38.
60. Costelloe C, Metcalfe C, Lovering A, et al. Effect of antibiotic prescribing in primary care on antimicrobial resistance in individual patients: systematic review and meta-analysis. BMJ 2010;340:c2096.
61. Menendez R, Torres A, Zalacain R, et al. Risk factors of treatment failure in community acquired pneumonia: implications for disease outcome. Thorax 2004;59:960–5.
62. Almirall J, Bolibar I, Vidal J, et al. Epidemiology of community acquired pneumonia in adults: a population based study. Eur Respir J 2000;15:757–63.
63. Deresinski S. Methicillin-resistant Staphylococcus aureus: an evolutionary, epidemiologic, and therapeutic odyssey. Clin Infect Dis 2005;40:562–73.
64. Fridkin SK, Hageman JC, Morrison M, et al. Methicillin-resistant Staphylococcus aureus disease in three communities. N Engl J Med 2005;352:1436–44.
65. Barton-Forbes M, Hawkes M, Moore D, et al. Guidelines for the prevention and management of CA-MRSA: a perspective for Canadian health care practitioners. Can J Infect Dis Med Microbiol 2006;17(Suppl C):1B–24B.
66. Treanor JJ, Hayden FG, Vrooman PS, et al. Efficacy and safety of the oral neuraminidase inhibitor oseltamivir in treating acute influenza: a randomized controlled trial. US Neuramidase Study Group. JAMA 2000;283:1016–24.
67. Jefferson T, Demicheli V, Rivetti D, et al. Antivirals for influenza in healthy adults: systematic review. Lancet 2006;367:303–13.
68. Rothberg MB, Haessler SD. Complications of seasonal and pandemic influenza. Crit Care Med 2010;38(Suppl 4):e91–7.
69. Adisasmito W, Chan PK, Lee N, et al. Effectiveness of antiviral treatment in human influenza A(H5N1) infections: analysis of a Global Patient Registry. J Infect Dis 2010;202(8):1154–60.
70. Hopkins P, McNeil K, Kermeen F, et al. Human metapneumovirus in lung transplant recipients and comparison to respiratory syncytial virus. Am J Respir Crit Care Med 2008;178:876–81.
71. Bozette SA, Sattler FR, Chiu J, et al. A controlled trial of early adjunctive treatment with corticosteroids for Pneumocystis carinii pneumonia in the acquired immunodeficiency syndrome. N Engl J Med 1990;323:1451–7.
72. Gagnon S, Boota AM, Fischl MA, et al. Corticosteroids as adjunctive therapy for severe Pneumocystis carinii pneumonia in the acquired immunodeficiency syndrome. N Engl J Med 1990;323:1444–50.
73. Briel M, Bucher H, Boscacci R, et al. Adjunctive corticosteroids for Pneumocystis jiroveci pneumonia. Cochrane Database Syst Rev 2006;3:CD006150.
74. Hirsehick RE, Glassroth J, Jordan MC, et al. Bacterial pneumonia in person infected with HIV. N Engl J Med 1995;333(13):845–51.
75. Centers for Disease Control and Prevention (CDC). Trends in TB–US 2010. MMWR Morb Mortal Wkly Rep 2011;60(11):333–7.
76. Centers for Disease Control and Prevention (CDC). Trends in tuberculosis incidence–United States, 2006. MMWR Morb Mortal Wkly Rep 2007;56(11):245–50.
77. Akolo C, Adetifa I, Shepperd S, et al. Treatment of latent TB in HIV infected patients. Cochrane Database Syst Rev 2010;1:CD000171.

Evaluation and Management of Seasonal Influenza in the Emergency Department

Marc Afilalo, MD, MCFP(EM), CSPQ, FRCP(C)[a],*,
Errol Stern, MD, CSPQ, FRCP(C)[b], Matthew Oughton, MD, FRCP(C)[c]

KEYWORDS

- Influenza - Seasonal - Emergency department

Influenza is an acute infectious respiratory disease of viral cause that occurs annually in outbreaks, epidemics, and occasionally pandemics of varying severity and attack rates depending on the influenza virus subtype involved. Although most seasonal flu cases do not produce long-term sequelae, influenza continues to cause substantial morbidity and mortality despite multiple landmark discoveries in infectious diseases during the previous century.[1,2] In the past 2 decades, influenza mortality has even risen, in large part because of an aging population.[3] Worldwide, flu epidemics account for an estimated 3 to 5 million cases leading to approximately 245,000 to 500,000 deaths annually.[4] The Centers for Disease Control and Prevention (CDC) estimates there are about 36,000 influenza-related deaths each year in the United States, and between 1972 and 1992, influenza accounted for an estimated 426,000 deaths.[1,5] In Canada, the Laboratory Center for Disease Control estimates that 70,000 to 75,000 influenza-associated hospitalizations and 6000 to 7000 deaths occur from influenza each year.[6] In Europe, between 40,000 and 220,000 deaths are estimated to be caused by influenza in a moderate flu season and during a severe epidemic respectively.[7]

Influenza also imposes a huge financial burden on health care systems and society overall. Data from the United States reveal that influenza accounts for more than

The authors have nothing to disclose.

[a] Emergency Department, Jewish General Hospital, 3755 Côte Ste-Catherine Road, Room D-012, Montreal, Quebec, Canada, H3T 1E2

[b] Emergency Department, Jewish General Hospital, 3755 Côte Ste-Catherine Road, Room D-010, Montreal, Quebec, Canada, H3T 1E2

[c] Department of Medicine, Division of Infectious Diseases, Jewish General Hospital, 3755 Côte Ste-Catherine Road, Pavilion A/Room A-923, Montreal, Quebec, Canada, H3T 1E2

* Corresponding author.

E-mail address: marc.afilalo@mcgill.ca

Emerg Med Clin N Am 30 (2012) 271–305

doi:10.1016/j.emc.2011.10.011

0733-8627/12/$ – see front matter © 2012 Elsevier Inc. All rights reserved.

emed.theclinics.com

226,000 hospitalizations, an estimated 3.1 million hospitalization days, with costs of more than $5 billion annually.[3,8] Costs related to influenza epidemics surpass $12 billion and cause millions of lost work hours each year.[9]

Timely diagnosis of influenza and early recognition of an influenza outbreak or epidemic are key components in preventing influenza-related complications, hospitalizations, and deaths. As the primary gateway to the health care system, emergency departments (EDs) are the most frequent points of entry for patients with influenza who seek medical attention. As a result, emergency physicians are well positioned to play a pivotal role in promptly identifying and adequately managing influenza community outbreaks and epidemics.

This article provides an updated overview of influenza to enhance the clinical judgment of emergency physicians and facilitate accurate decision making and diagnosis of seasonal influenza, thereby minimizing influenza's potential morbidity and mortality.

EPIDEMIOLOGY
Seasonality of Influenza

The epidemiology of influenza differs globally. Influenza outbreaks can occur during a specific season, referred to as seasonal influenza, or influenza activity can be present throughout the year. In northern and southern hemisphere temperate zones, influenza is highly seasonal and attacks predominantly occur during the winter months. For northern hemisphere countries like the United States and Canada, seasonal influenza usually starts in November, peaks from December to March, and abates in May,[10] whereas for southern hemisphere countries like Australia, the flu starts in May, peaks in June to September, and ends in November. Substantial fluctuations in influenza viral transmission patterns may occur with peaks occurring much earlier or later than anticipated.[11] In contrast, tropical regions lacking a distinct winter season exhibit different patterns of activity, in which influenza viruses may be isolated year round[12] with biannual influenza outbreaks.[13]

Onset and Time Course of Influenza Outbreaks

Typical outbreaks usually begin suddenly, spread in the community peaking during a period of 2 to 3 weeks, and continue for an average duration of 3 months.[14] In terms of clinical signs important for the emergency physician, the first indication of onset of a flu outbreak in a community is a surge in pediatric febrile respiratory illnesses, followed by increases in adult influenza-like illnesses (ILI).[15]

As the predominant front line of health care systems, EDs including emergency physicians are well positioned to detect local outbreaks of the flu in their early stages and notify appropriate public health authorities to take proper measures to contain the outbreak. Similarly, emergency physicians can play a pivotal role in containing emerging flu pandemics by keeping abreast of global influenza epidemics.

CLASSIFICATION AND DESCRIPTION OF INFLUENZA VIRUSES

Influenza viruses belong to the Orthomyxoviridae class of viruses and structurally consist of an inner core and outer membrane. The core contains a nucleoprotein antigen that determines the classification of the influenza virus into its 3 basic types: A, B, or C.[16] The outer membrane contains a coat of proteins including glycoproteins. Influenza A viruses are categorized based on 2 immunologically important glycoproteins: hemagglutinin (H) with 16 different subtypes (H1–H16) and neuraminidase (N) with 9 different subtypes (N1–N9).[17] For instance, the influenza A (H1N1) virus responsible for the 2009 flu pandemic expresses hemagglutinin 1 (H1) and neuraminidase 1

(N1) subtypes, whereas influenza A (H2N2) virus, which caused the influenza pandemic of 1957 to 1958, expresses hemagglutinin 2 (H2) and neuraminidase 2 (N2) subtypes. Influenza B and C viruses are not subcategorized.

Influenza A, B, and C viruses have similar structural and biologic characteristics but differ antigenically with varying prevalence and virulence. Influenza A is the most prevalent of the 3, frequently causes seasonal outbreaks and epidemics in humans, and infection with this subtype leads to more severe morbidity than influenza B and C. In addition, influenza A is the only subtype that causes pandemics. Influenza A H1N1 and H3N2 are currently the predominant virus subtypes causing influenza infection in humans. Since 1977, these 2 flu viruses have been circulating, causing seasonal influenza worldwide, whereas influenza A H2N2 subtype has not circulated in humans since 1968.[10]

Influenza B viruses circulate less widely than influenza A, causing fewer seasonal outbreaks and epidemics, whereas influenza C viruses cause only sporadic cases or minor outbreaks but not epidemics. In both cases, humans develop antibodies to these influenza viruses during childhood that provide some protection later against severe disease.[18] However, in children less than 6 years of age who have not yet acquired antibodies to influenza C, this virus can cause serious respiratory infections.[19]

Antigenic Drift and Antigenic Shift

Influenza A viruses, more than influenza B and C viruses, have a natural tendency to periodically undergo hemagglutinin and neuraminidase antigenic changes. Small point mutations in the RNA gene segments that code for these 2 glycoproteins lead to minor hemagglutinin and neuraminidase antigenic changes called **antigenic drifts** that result in localized outbreaks. Large mutations with viral gene reassortment that result in major hemagglutinin and neuraminidase antigenic changes referred to as **antigenic shifts** are associated with more widespread epidemics and pandemics. Influenza A, because of their greater propensity for antigenic variation, is the only influenza virus type able to undergo antigenic shifts, whereas all 3 virus types (influenza A, B, and C) have the ability to undergo antigenic drifts.

PATHOGENESIS AND PATHOPHYSIOLOGY
Cellular Pathogenesis

Influenza viral infection starts with transfer of virus-laden respiratory secretions from an infected person to an immunologically susceptible host. The virus initially attaches to the epithelial cells of the upper respiratory tract and, if not neutralized by the host's immune system, the virus can continue to invade more and more cells as the virus descends the respiratory tract. After adsorption and binding of viral hemagglutinin to host cell sialic acid–conjugated glycoproteins, the virus enters the host cell. This adsorption and binding is deemed necessary for virus cell entry,[20] and is epidemiologically significant because the configuration of sialic acid–conjugated glycoproteins differs from one species to another, which may exert a crucial role in limiting transfer of influenza viruses across species.[21] Once the virus has entered the host cell, it immediately disrupts normal cell function and starts replicating and releasing its viral progeny. Neuraminidase is essential for viral release and propagation.[22] Viral replication leads to host cell degradation and death via several mechanisms that shut off protein synthesis and release potent cytokines.[23,24] Cytokines, such as type I interferons, interleukins, tumor necrosis factor, as well as other inflammatory mediators, are thought to cause coughing and other systemic symptoms of flu.

Virus replication starts within 4 to 6 hours of host cell infection, and continues until about 24 hours before symptom onset.[25] The duration between incubation period, symptom onset, and virus shedding can range from 18 to 72 hours depending, in part, on inoculum dose.[26]

Virus Shedding

The quantities of shed virus measured in specimens exhibit a distinct pattern and temporally correlate with symptom onset and severity of illness. Virus shedding is observed starting within 24 hours before the onset of symptoms, peaks in 1 to 2 days after the onset of symptoms develop, remains high for another 1 to 2 days correlating with when the illness is most severe, and then rapidly declines, coming to an end approximately 7 to 10 days after infection. However, in certain circumstances, virus shedding can continue for weeks. Two key factors that influence the duration of viral shedding are age and severity of illness.[27–29] Young children, because of their relative lack of immunity, can shed virus for 10 days or more.[29,30] Patients with chronic diseases and more severe, complicated influenza shed the virus for an average of 2 days longer than uncomplicated influenza.[27,31,32] In elderly[31] and immunocompromised patients,[33–37] viral shedding and potential infectivity can persist for weeks, even months.

Pathophysiology

Multiple pathologic changes and pulmonary function abnormalities are observed during active uncomplicated acute influenza infection. Bronchoscopy often shows inflammation and edema of the bronchial mucosa, most notably in the lower respiratory tract, that lead to decreased forced flow rates and increased pulmonary resistance, which may persist for weeks after clinical recovery. In patients with asthma and chronic obstructive pulmonary disease, influenza can cause acute decreases in forced expiratory vital capacity (FVC) and forced expiratory volume in 1 second (FEV1).[38,39] Virus infection can advance into the lung parenchyma either via inhalation or contiguous spread from the upper respiratory tract causing primary viral pneumonia. Tracheitis, bronchitis, and bronchiolitis are seen, characterized by submucosal hyperemia, edema, focal hemorrhage with bloody fluid, and loss of normal ciliated epithelium.[40]

Disruption of the normal epithelial barrier to infection, and abnormalities in ciliary clearance mechanisms, along with increased adherence of bacteria to virus-infected epithelial cells, predispose to bacterial superinfection. The most common pathogens responsible for bacterial infection are *Staphylococcus aureus*, *Streptococcus pneumoniae*, and *Haemophilus influenzae*.

CLINICAL PRESENTATION
Clinical Signs and Symptoms

The signs and symptoms of seasonal influenza are variable in severity, and dependent on the age of the patients. In adults, influenza is usually characterized by respiratory symptoms with other constitutional symptoms such as fever, myalgia, malaise, and headache. An abrupt onset is common, such that patients are often able to report the time of onset. Respiratory symptoms and cough may initially be mild, but can progress causing dyspnea and pleuritic chest pain. Degree of fever is variable; fever in the elderly is usually not as severe as in young patients. During the flu season, patients with influenza-like symptoms and proven influenza infection were more likely to have cough (93% vs 80%), fever (68% vs 40%), cough and fever together (64% vs 33%), and/or nasal congestion (91% vs 81%) compared to those without influenza.[41] For decreasing the likelihood of influenza, the absence of fever (likelihood ratio [LR], 0.40; 95% confidence interval [CI], 0.25–0.66), cough (LR, 0.42; 95% CI, 0.31–0.57), or nasal congestion (LR, 0.49; 95% CI, 0.42–0.59) were the only findings that had summary LRs less than 0.5.[42] Patients may also present with isolated gastrointestinal or central nervous system (CNS) involvement.

Children with influenza often do not present with the classic symptoms. They often cannot describe their symptoms, and tend to have more gastrointestinal symptoms. Symptoms can mimic bacterial sepsis with high fevers, and children with influenza may present with febrile seizures.[43]

In uncomplicated influenza, there are a few physical findings. There may be evidence of hyperemia of the pharynx, even with severe sore throat complaints. Mild cervical lymphadenopathy and otitis media may be present, especially in younger patients. A dry cough is usually noted on chest examination with clear lungs or rhonchi, unless complicated by pneumonia. If there are no complications, fever and body aches can last 3 to 5 days, and the cough and lack of energy may last for 2 or more weeks.[44]

Complications Contributing to Clinical Presentation (Symptomatology)

Pneumonia is the major complication of influenza and occurs especially in high-risk patients:

- Children aged less than 5 years (especially those aged <2 years)
- Adults aged 65 years or more
- Persons with chronic diseases
- Persons with immunosuppression
- Women who are pregnant or postpartum (within 2 weeks after delivery)
- Persons aged 18 years or younger who are receiving long-term aspirin therapy
- First Nations/Alaska Natives
- Persons who are morbidly obese (ie, body mass index [BMI] greater than or equal to 40)
- Residents of nursing homes and other chronic-care facilities.[45]

Pneumonia can either be of viral or secondary bacterial cause. Primary viral pneumonias are uncommon but tend to have increased symptom severity. However, during influenza outbreaks, influenza virus types A and B are responsible for more than half of all community-acquired viral pneumonia cases. Secondary bacterial pneumonia is a significant complication of influenza, accounting for 25% of all influenza deaths.[46] Children hospitalized with influenza-associated pneumonia have a higher risk for intensive care admission, respiratory failure, and death compared to those hospitalized with influenza without pneumonia. Classically, influenza patients complicated with pneumonia have an exacerbation of fever and respiratory symptoms after an initial improvement. The most common bacterium is *S pneumonia*, accounting for approximately 50% of cases. *Staphylococcus aureus* and *Haemophilus influenza* are also important common organisms. During the 2006 to 2007 influenza season, 51 cases of community-acquired *S aureus* pneumonia were reported to the CDC. Almost 50% of these cases had antecedent or concomitant viral illness, and just under 80% of the *S aureus* cultures were MRSA. The median age was 16 years, 44% had no known pertinent medical history, and approximately half of patients, for whom final disposition was known, died a median of 4 days after symptom onset. Despite the selection bias in the cases reported, *community-associated S aureus* (CA-MRSA) pneumonia accounts for severe pneumonia with high mortality in young otherwise healthy patients with influenza. Therefore, empiric therapy for severe community-acquired pneumonia should include treatment against S aureus, including MRSA.[47]

Neurologic complications include encephalitis, transverse myelitis, and Guillain-Barré syndrome. Reye syndrome has been reported in patients using aspirin after influenza infections. Myositis is rare, but has been reported more commonly in children than adults. It presents in early convalescence with acute onset of pain and tenderness in the lower leg muscles severe enough to limit walking. Serum creatine kinase (CK) levels transiently increase, with complete recovery generally occurring in 3 to 4 days; renal failure is rare.[48]

Cardiovascular involvement occurs by directly affecting the myocardium or exacerbating existing cardiovascular conditions. The frequency of myocardial involvement in influenza infection is variable, with rates of up to 10% having been reported in the literature, although this depends on the methods used to detect myocardial involvement. Although many patients are asymptomatic, a significant proportion of these have electrocardiogram changes. Fulminant myocarditis resulting in cardiogenic shock and death may occur. When a patient's condition deteriorates with hemodynamic compromise, cardiac involvement should be considered. The mainstay of treatment of influenza myocarditis is supportive. Cardiovascular deaths also increase during influenza epidemics by increased deaths from coronary artery disease. These deaths have been shown to be reduced by influenza vaccination, which should be offered to all patients with cardiovascular disease.[49]

Other rare complications encountered include toxic shock syndrome in conjunction with secondary S aureus infection and parotitis.[50]

ED EVALUATION

Influenza can be difficult to diagnose based on clinical symptoms alone because the initial symptoms of influenza can be similar to those caused by other infectious agents including Mycoplasma pneumoniae, adenovirus, respiratory syncytial virus, rhinovirus, parainfluenza viruses, and Legionella.

It is important for the ED to develop clinical pathways to identify ILI so that contagious patients can be segregated and treated effectively. The CDC defines ILI as patients with temperature greater than 37.8°C (100°F) plus either cough or sore throat in the absence of a known cause other than influenza. As described, patients with influenza may have atypical presentations. Fever is not always present, especially in premature infants, young infants, elderly patients, or immunosuppressed patients, and patients may present with only myalgias, headache, fatigue, or other complications.[51] The ED needs to consider the variability of clinical presentations and the prevalence of influenza in the community regarding investigation and treatment, and infection control isolation protocol.

Patients with suspected influenza should have standard laboratory investigations such as a complete blood count and electrolytes; the results are usually nonspecific, but leukopenia is typical and thrombocytopenia may be present. Patients with physical signs that suggest meningitis should undergo a lumbar puncture. In patients with hypoxemia, the elderly, or high-risk patients with pulmonary symptoms, a chest radiograph should be performed to exclude pneumonia. Dyspnea and chest pain are typically used as indicators for obtaining a chest radiograph. Shortness of breath may be a useful indicator of pneumonia-complicating influenza.[52] Radiological findings include bilateral interstitial infiltrates, and focal infiltrates may indicate superimposed bacterial pneumonia.

Diagnostic Workup (Who to Test)

Diagnostic testing does not have to be performed on every patient who presents to the ED with ILI, especially when there is a circulating influenza outbreak or epidemic. Confirmation of influenza virus infection is not required for clinical decisions to prescribe antiviral medication. The decision to administer influenza treatment or chemoprophylaxis should be based on clinical illness and epidemiologic factors, and the start of therapy should not be delayed pending results, especially during an influenza outbreak.[51] Influenza diagnostic testing is not clinically indicated when test results will not alter a patient's clinical care or influence clinical practice for other patients (**Fig. 1**). A positive influenza test may be used to confirm influenza virus in the community, which may affect clinical practice related to home care guidance, hospital infection control practices, future testing practices, and so forth. Neither the rapid influenza test nor clinical prediction rules were superior to clinical judgment alone in the diagnosis of influenza. In one study of 258 patients with 21% confirmed influenza, the overall clinical judgment had a sensitivity of 29% (95% CI, 18%–43%) and specificity 92% (95% CI, 87%–95%), which improved to a sensitivity of 67% (95% CI, 39%–86%) and specificity of 96% (95% CI, 81%–99%) when patients presented within 48 hours. Rapid influenza tests only had a sensitivity of 33% (95% CI, 22%–47%) and specificity of 98% (95% CI, 96%–99%), and a clinical prediction rule showed a sensitivity of 40% (95% CI, 27%–54%) and specificity of 92% (95% CI, 87%–95%).[53] Thus, in times of high disease prevalence such as during influenza outbreaks or epidemics, most patients exhibiting ILI symptoms can be diagnosed clinically as having influenza, without performing any diagnostic tests. Clinicians should consult the CDC's Global Flu Activity Update (http://www.cdc.gov/flu/international/activity.htm) for the latest updates on the international flu situation, and FluView (http://www.cdc.gov/flu/weekly/) for a summary of flu activity in the United States.

Diagnostic testing is ideally indicated in 2 circumstances: (1) for sporadic cases of ILI, during periods of low disease prevalence, and (2) for severely ill patients. Influenza should be confirmed in sporadic cases of ILI to rule out another viral diagnosis, for example severe acute respiratory syndrome (SARS) or coronavirus. Diagnostic testing is recommended in severely ill patients because there is a greater urgency to make the correct diagnosis to provide appropriate medical management. In these 2 cases, rapid influenza diagnostic tests (RIDTs) and reverse transcriptase polymerase chain reaction (RT-PCR) are appropriate.

The 2009 evidence-based clinical practice guidelines for the diagnosis, management, and chemoprophylaxis of seasonal influenza developed by the Infectious Diseases Society of America recommend that the following patient populations undergo diagnostic testing for influenza if testing results will influence medical management (**Box 1**).[54]

Types of Specimens and Detection of Influenza Virus

Influenza virus can be isolated from different types of specimens, including nasal, throat, or nasopharyngeal swabs, aspirates or washes, and sputum samples. Nasopharyngeal specimens (swabs and aspirates) are more sensitive for detecting the virus than throat swabs or sputum specimens[54,55]; in one comparison of 3 rapid assays and immunofluorescence for influenza detection, sensitivity for all of these methods increased by approximately 40% when nasopharyngeal swabs instead of throat swabs were used.[56] Acceptable specimens also vary depending on the specific diagnostic test (**Table 1**). The optimal time frame for collecting diagnostic specimens

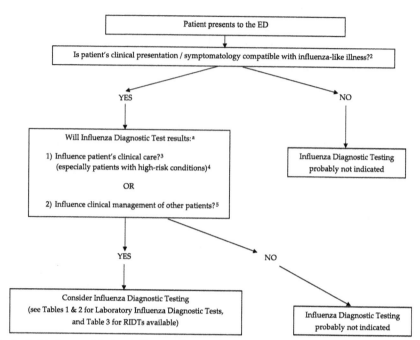

Fig. 1. Guide for considering influenza diagnostic testing (IDT) for patients presenting to the ED with influenza-like illness symptoms when influenza activity is high in the community.[1] [1]Confirmation of influenza virus infection by diagnostic testing is not required for clinical decisions to prescribe antiviral medications. Decisions to administer antiviral medications for influenza treatment or chemoprophylaxis, if indicated, should be based upon clinical illness and epidemiologic factors, and start of therapy should not be delayed pending testing results (http://www.cdc.gov/flu/professionals/diagnosis/clinician_guidance_ridt.htm). **Respiratory specimens should be collected from an ill patient as early as possible after onset of symptoms (ideally <48–72 hours after onset) to help maximize influenza testing sensitivity.** [2]Influenza like-illness (history of feverishness or documented fever with either cough or sore throat), fever with other respiratory symptoms, etc. Note that some persons may have atypical presentations (eg, elderly, very young infants, immunosuppressed, and patients with certain chronic medical conditions). Fever is not always present (eg, premature infants, young infants, elderly, immunosuppressed). Other symptoms associated with influenza include myalgias, headache, and fatigue. Complications include exacerbation of underlying chronic disease, (eg, congestive cardiac failure, asthma), pneumonia, bacterial co-infection, bronchiolitis, croup, encephalopathy, seizures, myositis, and others. [3]eg, Decisions on use of antibiotics or antiviral medications, on conducting further diagnostic tests, on recommendations for home care, or on recommendations for ill persons living with persons with high-risk conditions. Consult Infectious Disease Society of America, American Thoracic Society, Association of American Physicians, and Advisory Committee on Immunization Practices for antibiotic guidance. [4]Persons ≥65 years or <2 years; pregnant women; persons with chronic lung disease (including asthma), heart disease, renal, metabolic, hematologic and neurologic disease; immunosuppression; and morbid obesity. [5]eg, Decisions on changing infection control practices (such as in hospitalized patients); if a positive influenza test result is used for confirming influenza virus circulation in the community which might inform clinical practices related to home care guidance, hospital infection control practices, future testing practices, etc. RIDT, rapid influenza diagnostic testing. [a]*Initiation of antiviral treatment, if clinically indicated, should not be delayed pending influenza diagnostic test results.* (*Adapted from* the Centers for Disease Control and Prevention (CDC) website: Guidance for Clinicians on the Use of Rapid Influenza Diagnostic Tests for the 2010-2011 Influenza Season. Available at: http://www.cdc.gov/flu/professionals/diagnosis/clinician_guidance_ridt.htm. Accessed September 30, 2011.)

Box 1
Indications for testing for influenza

During influenza season (testing should be done in the following persons if the result will influence clinical management)

- Outpatient immunocompetent persons of any age at high risk of developing influenza complications (eg, hospitalization or death) presenting with acute febrile respiratory symptoms 5 days or less after illness onset (when virus is usually being shed)
- Outpatient immunocompromised persons of any age presenting with febrile respiratory symptoms, irrespective of time since illness onset (because immunocompromised persons can shed influenza viruses for weeks to months)
- Hospitalized persons of any age (immunocompetent or immunocompromised) with fever and respiratory symptoms, including those with a diagnosis of community-acquired pneumonia, irrespective of time since illness onset
- Elderly persons and infants presenting with suspected sepsis or fever of unknown origin, irrespective of time since illness onset
- Children with fever and respiratory symptoms presenting for medical evaluation, irrespective of time since illness onset
- Persons of any age who develop fever and respiratory symptoms after hospital admission, irrespective of time since illness onset
- Immunocompetent persons with acute febrile respiratory symptoms who are not at high risk of developing complications secondary to influenza infection may be tested for purposes of obtaining local surveillance data

Throughout the year (testing should be done for the following persons)

- Health care personnel, residents, or visitors in an institution experiencing an influenza outbreak who present with febrile respiratory symptoms within 5 days after illness onset
- Persons who are epidemiologically linked to an influenza outbreak (eg, household and close contacts of persons with suspected influenza, returned travelers from countries where influenza viruses may be circulating, participants in international mass gatherings, and cruise ship passengers) who present within 5 days after illness onset

From Harper SA, Bradley JS, Englund JA, et al. Seasonal influenza in adults and children – diagnosis, treatment, chemoprophylaxis, and institutional outbreak management: clinical practice guidelines of the Infectious Diseases Society of America. Clin Infect Dis 2009;48(8):1003–32; with permission.

---

largely depends on the amount of viral shedding at the time of testing. In immunocompetent children and adults, in whom viral shedding is brief, specimen samples yield the best results during the first 1 to 5 days of illness.[54,57] Low viral titers in the first 12 to 24 hours following onset of clinical illness have been suggested as a cause of false-negative results in patients tested early[58]; similarly, specimens obtained after 5 days of illness have an increased likelihood of false-negative results because of decreased virus shedding. Immunocompetent infants and young children spread virus for longer ($\geq$1 week), which ideally permits the collection of specimens after 5 days of illness.[54] Irrespective of age, specimen collection in immunocompromised persons can also exceed 5 days of illness because virus shedding in this patient population can last for weeks, even months.[54]

In the ED, collection of serum specimens is not recommended for diagnostic purposes because results are not readily available and therefore cannot guide clinical decision making and management.[54]

Table 1
Laboratory diagnostic testing methods for influenza currently available in the United States

Diagnostic Testing Method(s)	Acceptable Specimens	Influenza Virus Types Detected	Time to Final Result
Immunofluorescence microscopy Direct fluorescent antibody staining Indirect fluorescent antibody staining	1. NP swab/aspirate 2. Nasal swab/aspirate/wash 3. Throat swab	A and B	≈1–4 h
Viral culture Conventional culture Rapid shell vial culture	1. NP swab/aspirate 2. Nasal swab/aspirate/wash 3. Throat swab 4. Bronchioalveolar lavage	A and B	Conventional culture ≈3–10 d Rapid shell vial culture ≈1–3 d
RT-PCR	1. NP swab/aspirate 2. Nasal swab/aspirate/wash 3. Throat swab 4. Bronchioalveolar lavage 5. Sputum	A and B	≈1–6 h
RIDTs	Depends on specific RIDT (see **Table 3**)	A and B[a]	≈10–15 min
Serologic testing[b]	Paired acute and convalescent serum samples[c]	A and B	≥2 wk

Abbreviation: NP, nasopharyngeal.
[a] Most RIDTs detect A and B, some detect A or B, others only A (see **Table 3**).
[b] Serologic testing is not recommended for routine patient diagnosis.
[c] A fourfold or greater increase in antibody titer from the acute (collected within the first week of illness) to the convalescent phase (collected 2–4 weeks after the acute sample) indicates recent infection.
Data from Refs.[55,59,64]

Table 2
Laboratory diagnostic testing methods for influenza currently available in Canada

Test	Method	Influenza Virus Types Detected	Turnaround Time[a]
RT-PCR (nucleic acid testing)	RNA detection	A and B	24–96 h (6–8 h to perform test)
Viral culture	Virus isolation	A and B	2–10 d
Direct immunofluorescence tests Indirect immunofluorescence tests	Antigen detection	A and B	2–4 h
Point-of-care tests	Antigen detection	A and B	0.5 h

[a] Length of time needed from specimen collection until results are available.
From Canadian Public Health Laboratory Network. Guidance for laboratory testing for detection and characterization of human influenza virus for the 2010-2011 respiratory virus season. Available at: http://www.cphln.ca/documents/EN_Influenza_Seasonal_Best_Practices_2010-2011.pdf. Accessed September 30, 2011; with permission.

Influenza Laboratory Testing Methods

Several different laboratory testing methods for detecting influenza virus are available in the United States (**Table 1**) and Canada (**Table 2**). These methods include immunofluorescence microscopy (direct or indirect antibody staining), viral culture (conventional and rapid), RT-PCR, RIDTs, and serologic testing. Among these testing methods, RIDTs with rapid processing yielding timely results that can influence clinical decision making and patient management are most pertinent for the needs of the ED.

Based on which type(s) of influenza virus (A and/or B) can be detected, diagnostic tests can be categorized into 3 types: (1) those that detect only influenza A; (2) those that detect either influenza A or B, but cannot discriminate between the two; and (3) tests that both detect and distinguish between influenza A or B viruses. Only RT-PCR and viral culture can identify influenza strains.

RIDTs

RIDTs are rapid antigen point-of-care tests capable of identifying influenza A and B viral types in respiratory specimens in approximately 10 to 15 minutes.[59] RIDTs are immunoassays that come in user-friendly, diagnostic kits with varying complexity that either: (1) only detect influenza A virus, (2) detect but cannot distinguish between influenza A and B viruses, or (3) both detect and distinguish between influenza A and B viruses. Commercial RIDTs currently available in the United States and Canada are listed in **Table 3**, and general RIDT characteristics, including advantages and disadvantages, are described in **Box 2**. RIDTs are valuable in the ED because they produce results in a timely and clinically relevant manner that facilitate on-site point-of-care diagnosis of influenza that, according to limited research, has led to a decrease in demand for further diagnostic tests (eg, chest radiography, blood cultures) and the use of antibiotics, thus resulting in decreased patient costs.[61]

Recommendations for the use of RIDTs were developed and promulgated by the World Health Organization (WHO) (**Box 3**). The CDC has recently issued guidelines for clinicians on the use of RIDTs for the 2010 to 2011 influenza season.[59]

A major drawback of RIDTs is their limited reliability in accurately detecting influenza virus, which depends on a wide variety of factors, including RIDT sensitivity, specificity, positive and negative predictive values, type of specimen collected, and time of collection with respect to onset of symptoms. Although RIDTs exhibit high specificities ranging between 90% and 95%, RIDTs have substantially lower sensitivities, ranging from about 70% to 90% in children, decreasing even further to approximately 40% to 60% or lower in adults, compared with viral culture and RT-PCR.[54,62,63] Thus, if RIDTs are the only diagnostic assay used in a center, positive results can be trusted but a negative result cannot reliably exclude disease. **Table 4** displays specifically selected commercially available RIDTs and corresponding test sensitivities, specificities, and positive and negative predictive values, which also vary according to the study.

Time of specimen collection also influences the accuracy of RIDT results: the closer within the period of viral shedding and illness the specimen sample is obtained, the more accurate the result.[60,64] In an effort to minimize false interpretation of RIDTs, the CDC has published the following guidance statements that emergency physicians and other health care professionals must keep in mind when performing and interpreting RIDTs[59,65]:

1. The reliability of a positive RIDT result increases in patients with clinical signs and symptoms consistent with influenza.
2. Collection of specimens within 48 to 72 hours of illness onset increases the likelihood of producing a positive RIDT result.

Table 3
Examples of commercial rapid influenza diagnostic tests (RIDTs) currently available in the United States and Canada

Rapid Influenza Diagnostic Test (RIDT) Name	Manufacturer	Influenza Virus Type Detected	Distinguishes Between A and B?	Acceptable Specimens	Time to Final Results	Approved in the United States	Approved in Canada
BinaxNOW® Flu A and Flu B	Binax Inc., www.binax.com	A and B	Yes	NP swab nasal wash/aspirate	15 min	Yes	Yes
BinaxNOW® Influenza A and B	Binax Inc., www.binax.com	A and B	Yes	NP swab nasal wash/aspirate/swab	15 min	Yes	Yes
BioSign® Flu A + B	Princeton BioMeditech Corp. www.pbmc.com	A and B	Yes	NP swab/wash/aspirate	15 min	Yes	No
Clearview Exact® Influenza A and B	Alere www.alere.com	A and B	Yes	Nasal swab	15 min	Yes	No
Clearview Exact® II Influenza A and B	Alere www.alere.com	A and B	Yes	Nasal swab	15 min	Yes	No
Directigen™ EZ Flu A + B	Becton-Dickinson, www.bd.com	A and B	Yes	NP swab/wash/aspirate throat swab	15 min	Yes	No
Directigen™ Flu A	Becton-Dickinson, www.bd.com	A	Detects A only	NP swab/wash/aspirate pharyngeal swab	15 min	Yes	Yes
Directigen™ Flu A + B	Becton-Dickinson, www.bd.com	A and B	Yes	NP swab/wash/aspirate lower nasal swab, throat swab, bronchioalveolar lavage	15 min	Yes	Yes
Flu OIA	Thermo Biostar, Inc., www.biostar.com	A and B	No	NP swab, throat swab nasal aspirate, sputum	20 min	Yes	Yes
ImmunoCard STAT! Flu A and B	Meridian Bioscience, Inc., www.meridianbioscience.com	A and B	Yes	NP swab/aspirate nasal swab/wash	15–20 min	Yes	Yes
Influ-A Respi-Strip	Coris BioConcept, www.corisbio.com	A	No	NP swab	5–15 min	No	Yes
Influ-A and B Respi-Strip	Coris BioConcept, www.corisbio.com	A and B	Yes	NP swab/wash/aspirate	5–15 min	No	Yes

3M™ Rapid Detection Flu A + B Test	3M www.3m.com	A and B	Yes	NP swab/aspirate nasal wash/aspirate	15 min	Yes	No
OSOM® Influenza A and B	Genzyme www.genzyme.com	A and B	Yes	Nasal swab	10 min	Yes	No
SAS™ FluAlert A	SA Scientific Inc., www.sascientific.com	A only	No	Nasal wash/aspirate	15 min	Yes	No
SAS™ FluAlert B	SA Scientific Inc., www.sascientific.com	B only	No	Nasal wash/aspirate	15 min	Yes	No
SAS™ FluAlert A and B	SA Scientific Inc., www.sascientific.com	A and B	Yes	Nasal wash/aspirate	15 min	Yes	No
QuickVue® Influenza Test	Quidel Corporation www.quidel.com	A or B	No	Nasal swab/wash/aspirate	10 min	Yes	No
QuickVue® Influenza A + B Test	Quidel Corporation www.quidel.com	A and B	Yes	NP swab nasal swab/wash/aspirate	10 min	Yes	Yes
Quick S-INFLU A/B Seiken	Denka Seiken Co., Ltd. www.denkaseiken.co.jp	A and B	Yes	Nasal swab/aspirate	25 min	Yes	Yes
TRU FLU®	Meridian Bioscience Inc., www.meridianbioscience.com	A and B	Yes	NP swab/aspirate nasal wash	15 min	Yes	No
XPECT™ Flu A and B	Remel Inc., www.remelinc.com Thermofisher	A and B	Yes	Nasal swab/wash throat swab, (sputum, NP Swab, tracheal aspirates, bronchoalveolar wash)	15 min	Yes	Yes
ZstatFlu-II test	Zyme Tx, Inc., www.zymetx.com	A and B	No	Throat swab	30 min	Yes	No

Abbreviation: NP, nasopharyngeal.

Adapted from World Health Organization: WHO recommendations on the use of rapid testing for influenza diagnosis. July 2005. Available at: http://www.who.int/influenza/resources/documents/rapid_testing/en/index.html. Accessed September 30, 2011; with permission, and Centers for Disease Control and Prevention (CDC) website: Guidance for Clinicians on the Use of Rapid Influenza Diagnostic Tests for the 2010-2011 Influenza Season. Available at: http://www.cdc.gov/flu/professionals/diagnosis/clinician_guidance_ridt.htm. Accessed September 30, 2011.

Box 2
Advantages and disadvantages of RIDTs

Advantages

1. Simple to perform

2. Results available within 15 minutes

3. Produce results in a timely and clinically pertinent manner

4. Selective RIDTs are waived from CLIA requirements in the United States, permitting their use in any medical facility (including doctor's office)

Disadvantages

1. No uniformity in distinguishing between influenza A or B virus

2. Do not identify virus strains

3. Do not identity influenza A virus subtypes

4. Frequently yield false-negative results because of reduced test sensitivity (40%–70%), particularly during increased influenza activity

5. False-positive results can be produced, particularly during months of low influenza activity

Abbreviation: CLIA, Clinical Laboratory Improvement Amendment of 1988.

Data from Centers for Disease Control and Prevention. Guidance for clinicians on the use of rapid influenza diagnostic tests for the 2010-2011 influenza season. Available at: http://www.cdc.gov/flu/professionals/diagnosis/clinician_guidance_ridt.htm. Accessed September 30, 2011.

---

3. Different RIDTs have different acceptable specimens and test specifications. Accuracy of RIDT results depends on collecting a good quality, acceptable specimen; following test procedures according to RIDT package instructions; and using appropriate viral transport media, consistent with specifications (if testing is to be performed at another location than the specimen collection).

Box 3
WHO recommendations on the use of RIDTs for influenza diagnosis in countries with influenza surveillance

WHO RIDT recommendations

1. Influenza surveillance should be used to guide the optimal use of rapid tests.

2. At the beginning of the influenza season or an influenza outbreak, rapid tests may influence clinical decisions and contribute to clinical awareness.

3. During periods of high influenza activity, it is impractical to test every individual meeting an influenza case definition. Clinical judgment and local influenza surveillance data should be used for case management in the first instance. Rapid tests are recommended to be used only when they can influence timely patient management.

4. During periods of low influenza activity, if rapid tests are used, positive results must be interpreted with caution and confirmed by immunofluorescence assay, viral culture, or RT-PCR.

5. Because of the differing complexity of rapid tests, education of laboratory personnel about methods and limitations before their use is essential.

Data from World Health Organization. WHO recommendations on the use of rapid testing for influenza diagnosis. July 2005. Available at: http://www.who.int/influenza/resources/documents/rapid_testing/en/index.html. Accessed September 30, 2011; with permission.

4. Use RIDTs with high sensitivity and specificity (see **Table 4**):
   a. RIDT sensitivities are generally low to moderate, ranging between 10% and 70% (most are approximately 50%–70%) compared with the gold standard viral culture or RT-PCR. An RIDT with low sensitivity yields false-negative results.
   b. RIDT specificities are generally high, approximately 90% to 95%, compared with the gold standard viral culture or RT-PCR. An RIDT with high specificity yields few false-positives.
5. Disease prevalence (level of influenza activity) in the community affects the accuracy of RIDT results:
   a. During periods of high disease prevalence (high influenza activity) at the height of the influenza season:
      i. Likelihood of true-positive RIDT results increases (positive predictive value [PPV] is high)
      ii. Likelihood of false-negative RIDT results increases (negative predictive value [NPV] is low)
   b. During periods of low disease prevalence (low influenza activity) usually at the start and end of the influenza season:
      i. Likelihood of false-positive RIDT results increases (PPV is low)
      ii. Likelihood of true-negative RIDT results increases (NPV is high).

RT-PCR

RT-PCR is replacing viral culture as a reference standard because it is currently the most sensitive, specific, and versatile diagnostic test available for diagnosing influenza.[66] Based on nucleic acid amplification, RT-PCR can detect the influenza virus but also differentiate between virus types, subtypes, and even determine viral strain, all in approximately 4 to 6 hours. As a result, RT-PCR has become the recommended test of choice for accurately diagnosing influenza in a timely fashion.[54] During the recent pandemic, the CDC released a method through the WHO for RT-PCR detection of influenza A that allowed clinical and reference laboratories to standardize methodology and thus produce data that could be compared between laboratories.[67] However, the major advantage of RT-PCR lies in its ability to more readily detect influenza viruses in people with chronic lung diseases and immunosuppressed persons, who may exhibit lower levels of the virus.[68] In these susceptible patients, RT-PCR can efficiently and accurately confirm the diagnosis of influenza to support therapeutic and infection control decisions.

Immunofluorescence

Immunofluorescence yields timely results within 2 to 4 hours, and this can be used as a screening test. However, immunofluorescence has several disadvantages, including lower sensitivity (47%–93%)[69,70] and specificity compared with viral culture, and is labor intensive, requiring specially trained laboratory personnel who may not be available 24/7, even in large hospitals. In addition, test performance depends on an adequate specimen sample that must include respiratory epithelium cells.[54]

Viral Culture

Influenza virus can be cultured either by isolation of virus in cell culture (conventional tube culture), which provides results in 3 to 10 days, or by shell vial culture, which offers the advantage of a faster turnaround time of 48 to 72 hours.[54] Because of the lengthy turnaround times of either method, viral culture is not a useful diagnostic test in the ED for aiding initial clinical decision making and management. However,

Table 4
Ease of use, sensitivity, specificity, and positive and negative predictive values of selective RIDTs

RIDT Name	General Ease of Use	Ease of Interpretation	Sensitivity[a]	Specificity[a]	Positive Predictive Value[a]	Negative Predictive Value[a]
BinaxNOW Flu A and Flu B	Easy	Easy	(1) A, 78%–82%; B, 58%–71%; (2) A, 52%; B, 54%; (3) A, 73%; B, 100%	(1) A, 92%–94%; B, 58%–71%; (2) 93% combined; (3) A, 95%; B, 100%	(3) 93% combined	(3) 89% combined
BinaxNOW Influenza A and B	Easy	Easy	(1) A, 100%; B, 92%–100%	(1) A, 92%–93%; B, 94%–99%	—	—
Directigen Flu A	Moderate	Easy	(1) 67%–96%; (4–8) 75%–100%	(1) 88%–100%; (4–8) 92%–100%	(4–8) 92%–100%	(4–8) 89%–100%
Directigen Flu A+B	Moderate	Easy	(1) A, 96%; B, 88% (3,11,14,16) A, 55%–100%; B, 62%–88%; (3) 29% (11–15) 55%–88%	(1) A, 99.6%; B, 96.8%; (3,11,14,15) A, 99%; B, 93%–100% (3,11–15) 93%–100%	(1) A, 96%; B, 80% (11–14) 74%–89%; (14,15) A, 81%; B, 90%–100% (3) 93% combined	(1) Flu A, 99.6%; Flu B, 98% (11–14) 93%–98% (14,15) A, 99%; B, 97% (3) 85% combined
Flu OIA	Moderate	Moderate	(1,17) 62%–88% (18,20,22) 46%–64% (21) 48%–100%	(1,17) 52%–80% (18–20,22) 74%–97% (22) 93%–97%	(18–19) 73%–91%	(18–19) 56%–77%
QuickVue Influenza Test	Easy	Easy	(1) AB, 73%–81% (13–14,24–28) AB, 55%–91%	(1) AB, 96%–99% (13–14,24–28) AB, 83%–99%	(1) AB, 92%–96% (13–14,24–25,28) AB, 55%–93%	(1) AB, 85%–93% (13–14,25–25,28) AB, 77%–99%
QuickVue Influenza A+B Test	Easy	Easy	(1) A,72%–77%; B, 73%–82%	(1) A, 96%–99%; B, 96%–99%	(1) A, 87%–91%; B, 80%–90%	(1) A, 90%–96%; B, 94%–97%
Influ AB Quick	Easy	Easy	(1) A, 90%–93%; B, 92%–93%; (15) A, 55%–58%; B, 63%–67%	(1) A, 98%–99%; B, 98%–99% (15) A, 100%; B, 99.6%	(15) 91%	(15) 98%

			Sensitivity	Specificity	PPV	NPV
Quick S-Influ A/B Seiken	Easy	Easy	(1) A, 90%–93%; B, 92%–93% (29) A, 81%; B, 88%	(1) A, 98%–99%; B, 98%–99% (29) A, 96%; B, 99%	—	—
XPECT Flu A and B	Moderate	Easy	(1) A, 89%–100%; B, 93%–100% (30) A, 92%–94%; B, 98%	(1) A, 100%; B, 100% (30) A, 100%; B, 100%	(28) A, 100%; B, 100%	(30) A, 98%–99%; B, 99.7%
Wampole Clearview Flu A/B	—	Easy	(1) A, 92% B, 98%	(1) A, 100%; B, 100%	—	—
ZstatFlu-II test	Easy	Easy	(4–7,12,23,31–32) 65%–96% A, 76%; B, 41%	(4–5,31–32) 77%–98%	(4–5,31) 59%–76%	(4–5,31) 90%–98%
Influ A Respi-Strip	Easy	Easy	(1) A, 91%	(1) A, 86%	(1) A, 94%	(1) A, 80%
Influ A and B Respi-Strip	Easy	Easy	(1) A, 99% B, 72.2%	(1) A, 88%; B, 100%	(1) A, 78%; B, 100%	(1) A, 99%; B, 98%
Espline Influenza A and B-N	—	—	(33–34) A, 85%–100%; B, 72%–91%	(33–34) A/B, 98%–100%	—	—
Capila FluA,B	Easy	Easy	(1) A,69%–94%; B, 81%–96% (35) A/B, 75%–82%	(1) A, 93%–95%; B, 96%–99% (35) A/B, 94%–100%	—	—
RapidTesta FLU AB	—	—	(36) A, 82%–83%; B, 80%–83%	(36) A, 98%–99%; B, 98%	—	—
ImmunoCard STAT! Flu A and B	Easy	Easy	(1) A, 83%; B, 100%	(1) A, 98%; B, 100%	—	—

[a] See Appendix 1 for sensitivity, specificity, positive predictive value, and negative predictive value references.
Data from World Health Organization. WHO recommendations on the use of rapid testing for influenza diagnosis. July 2005. Available at: http://www.who.int/influenza/resources/documents/rapid_testing/en/index.html. Accessed September 30, 2011; with permission.

viral culture allows for subsequent analyses, including sensitivity testing and subtyping performed by reference laboratories.

During the influenza season, viral culture is indicated primarily for confirming negative RIDT and immunofluorescence results, as well as for influenza virus surveillance because it provides key information regarding influenza virus strains and subtypes.[54] During the off-season, viral culture is indicated in patients who present to the ED within 5 days of symptom onset with suspected ILI, especially if the person is epidemiologically linked to an influenza outbreak.[54]

Serologic Testing

Serologic testing is not useful or recommended in the ED because results are not readily available and therefore cannot facilitate clinical judgment, diagnosis, or management of influenza.[57] Serologic tests that include hemagglutinin inhibition, neutralization, complement-fixation, and enzyme-linked immunosorbent assay (ELISA) are mainly used to establish a diagnosis retrospectively and for research purposes.[57] Because most individuals have previously been infected with influenza viruses, to reliably determine antibody titers, a single serum sample collected in the ED is inadequate, but paired specimen samples (acute and convalescent sera) are needed.

Interpretation of Laboratory Test Results

Whenever interpreting any influenza diagnostic test, the emergency physician or other health care professional must keep in mind the limitations of these tests, especially for RIDTs. In addition, the clinician should be aware of the disease prevalence in the community at any given time, because the level of influenza activity is known to affect the accuracy and reliability of test results. With respect to patient management, a positive influenza test result does not necessarily rule out any overlying coinfection by additional pathogens, and in the case of initial negative influenza test results from less sensitive diagnostic methods like RIDTs, the clinician should contemplate additional diagnostic testing (such as RT-PCR or culture) and decide whether antiviral treatment should be initiated empirically.

ED MANAGEMENT
Antiviral Medications

Currently, 4 antiviral medications from 2 drug classes have been approved and are available for the treatment and prevention of influenza in the United States, Canada, and most other countries. These medications include amantadine and rimantadine, which belong to the drug class adamantanes, and oseltamivir (Tamiflu; Roche) and zanamivir (Relenza; GlaxoSmithKline), which belong to the class neuraminidase (NA) inhibitors. Adamantanes are active only against influenza A virus, whereas NA inhibitors are active against both influenza A and B viruses. Other antiviral pharmacologic properties are compared in **Table 5**. In the last several years, adamantines have become less clinically useful because of their widespread resistance to influenza A (H3N2) and 2009 (H1N1) virus strains.[71] As a result, amantadine and rimantadine are currently not recommended for the treatment or chemoprophylaxis of influenza A virus.[45]

Guideline Indications for Antiviral Treatment

The goals of influenza pharmacotherapy are to decrease symptoms, prevent associated complications, and reduce functional disability, hospitalizations, and mortality. Treatment decisions on administering antiviral therapy should take into account factors such as time since symptom onset, underlying conditions, and severity of disease.

Table 5
Comparison of antiviral medication pharmacologic properties

	Amantadine	Rimantadine	Zanamivir	Oseltamivir
Protein target	M2	M2	Neuraminidase	Neuraminidase
Activity	A only	A only	A and B	A and B
Side effects	CNS (13%) GI (3%)	GI (6%) GI (3%)	? Bronchospasm	GI (9%)
Metabolism	None	Multiple (hepatic)	None	Hepatic
Excretion	Renal	Renal and other	Renal	Renal (tubular secretion)
Drug interactions	Antihistamines Anticholinergics	None	None	Probenecid (increased levels of oseltamivir)
Dose adjustments needed	≥65 y old CCl <50 mL/min	≥65 y old CrCl <10 mL/min	None	CrCl <30 mL/min Severe liver dysfunction
Contraindications	Acute-angle glaucoma	Severe liver dysfunction	Underlying airway disease	None
FDA-approved Indications				
Therapy	Adults and children ≥1 y of age	Adults only	Adults and children ≥7 y of age	Adults and children ≥1 y of age[a]
Prophylaxis	Yes	Yes	No	Adults and children ≥13 y of age[b]

Abbreviations: CrCl, creatinine clearance; FDA, US Food and Drug Administration; GI, gastrointestinal.
[a] FDA has authorized treatment of S-OIV with oseltamivir in children greater than or equal to 3 months of age.
[b] FDA has authorized prophylaxis for S-OIV with oseltamivir in children greater than or equal to 1 year of age.
Data from Treanor J. Influenza viruses, including avian influenza and swine influenza. In: Mandell GL, Bennett JE, Dolin R, editors. Mandell, Douglas, and Bennett's principles and practice of infectious diseases. 7th edition. Philadelphia: Churchill Livingston Elsevier; 2010. p. 2265–88.

According to the CDC[45] and other published guidelines,[54] antiviral treatment is recommended for patients infected by the influenza virus who meet the following criteria:

1. Patients with laboratory-confirmed or highly suspected influenza virus infection considered high risk for developing influenza complications (**Box 4**). Treatment is recommended irrespective of illness severity or vaccination status;

Box 4
Persons at high risk for influenza complications recommended for antiviral therapy

1. Infants aged less than 2 years[a]
2. Adults aged 65 years or more
3. Women who are pregnant or postpartum (within 2 weeks after delivery)
4. Persons with asthma or other chronic pulmonary diseases, such as cystic fibrosis in children or chronic obstructive pulmonary disease in adults
5. Persons with hemodynamically significant cardiovascular disease (except hypertension alone)
6. Persons with chronic renal dysfunction
7. Persons with hepatic disorders
8. Persons with hematological conditions (including sickle cell anemia and other hemoglobinopathies)
9. Persons with chronic metabolic disease (including diabetes mellitus)
10. Persons with neurologic and neuromuscular disorders (including cerebral palsy, epilepsy [seizure disorders], stroke, intellectual disability [mental retardation], muscular dystrophy, and spinal cord injury)
11. Persons with immunosuppressive disorders (including those caused by immunosuppressive therapy)
12. Persons with cancer
13. Persons with human immunodeficiency virus infection
14. Persons aged less than 19 years receiving long-term aspirin therapy (eg, for conditions such as rheumatoid arthritis or Kawasaki disease)
15. American Indians/Alaska Natives
16. Persons morbidly obese (ie, BMI$\geq$40)
17. Residents of any age of nursing homes or other long-term care institutions

[a] Although all children aged less than 5 years are considered at higher risk for complications from influenza, the highest risk is for those aged less than 2 years, with the highest hospitalization and death rates among infants aged less than 6 months. Because many children with mild febrile respiratory illness might have other viral infections (eg, respiratory syncytial virus, rhinovirus, parainfluenza virus, or human metapneumovirus), knowledge about other respiratory viruses as well as influenza virus strains circulating in the community is important for treatment decisions.

Data from Centers for Disease Control and Prevention. Antiviral agents for the treatment and chemoprophylaxis of influenza - Recommendations of the Advisory Committee on Immunization Practices (ACIP). MMWR Recomm Rep 2011;60(No. RR-1):1–28; and Harper SA, Bradley JS, Englund JA, et al. Seasonal influenza in adults and children – diagnosis, treatment, chemoprophylaxis, and institutional outbreak management: clinical practice guidelines of the Infectious Diseases Society of America. Clin Infect Dis 2009;48(8):1003–32.

2. Patients with laboratory-confirmed or highly suspected influenza virus infection requiring hospitalization, irrespective of underlying illness or vaccination status;
3. Patients with laboratory-confirmed or highly suspected influenza virus infection who have severe, complicated, or progressive illness;

Antiviral treatment should be considered for adults and children with influenza virus infection who meet the following criteria:

1. Outpatients at high risk of complications (see **Box 4**) with illness that is not improving and who have a positive influenza test result from a specimen obtained more than 48 hours after onset of symptoms;
2. Outpatients with laboratory-confirmed or highly suspected influenza virus infection who are not at increased risk of complications, whose onset of symptoms is less than 48 hours before ED presentation, and who would like to shorten the duration of illness and further reduce their risk of complications;
3. Outpatients with laboratory-confirmed or highly suspected influenza virus infection who are in close contact with persons at high risk of complications secondary to influenza infection;
4. Patients whose onset of symptoms occurred more than 48 hours before ED presentation with persisting moderate to severe illness may also benefit from treatment.

Benefits of Early Initiation Antiviral Treatment (≤48 Hours After Symptom Onset)

Because viral titers rapidly decrease by day 3 to 4 of illness in untreated, previously healthy persons, efficacy of antiviral therapy is directly related to time of treatment initiation.[72] Studies have found that early treatment, especially initiated within the first 6 hours of symptom onset, provides the greatest benefit in reducing symptoms.[72] Antiviral treatment initiated within 48 hours of onset of influenza illness can lead to shorter duration of symptoms and decreased illness severity. Studies administering NA inhibitor antiviral medications in previously healthy patients with uncomplicated influenza resulted in a shorter duration of illness by 1 to 2 days.[28,29,73–79] In addition, research has shown that early initiation of treatment with antivirals can also decrease the rate of serious influenza-related complications (eg, pneumonia, respiratory failure, and death) in high risk patients.[80] In contrast, slight or no benefit has been observed in healthy people when antiviral treatment is started more than 48 hours after the onset of uncomplicated influenza.[45] As a result, influenza antiviral treatment, when clinically indicated, should be initiated in a timely fashion, preferably within 48 hours of symptom onset, and not after laboratory confirmation of influenza.

Benefits of Antiviral Treatment Administered More Than 48 Hours After Symptom Onset

In certain patient populations, antiviral treatment may still be beneficial even if given more than 48 hours after symptom onset. These patients include pregnant women, patients with severe or progressive illness requiring hospitalization, and patients at high risk for suffering influenza complications. A study by Siston and colleagues[81] found that, in pregnant women, treatment with antiviral medications decreased respiratory complications and death even when initiated 3 to 4 days after symptom onset compared with 5 days or more. Based on observational studies, oseltamivir decreases severe clinical outcomes in hospitalized patients with influenza. In a multivariate analysis, treatment with oseltamivir led to a significantly decreased risk of death within 15 days of hospitalization (odds ratio [OR], 0.2; 95% CI, 0.1–0.8).[82] Benefits were detected even in patients whose treatment was initiated more than 48 hours after the onset of symptoms. A study by Lee and colleagues[83] found that among 99 hospitalized patients (median age, 70 years) with laboratory-confirmed influenza who received oseltamivir, benefits were observed even when oseltamivir was started up to 96 hours after illness onset.

Choice of Antiviral Medication

Influenza virus vulnerability to antiviral drugs is continuously evolving. As a result, emergency physicians need to be familiar with the most recently updated information available on antiviral resistance and recommendations on antiviral use. As of January 2011, the CDC recommends the following antiviral drugs for treatment and chemoprophylaxis of seasonal influenza (**Table 6**).[45]

ISOLATION AND PREVENTION OF NOSOCOMIAL SPREAD OF INFLUENZA

The most effective way to prevent and control seasonal influenza is through immunization of both health care workers and patients.[84] Procedures should be institutionalized, which ensures that patients and visitors with respiratory infection symptoms follow triage procedures in the ED that effectively isolate them as rapidly as possible.

In hospital entrances and the ED triage, there should be clear signage with instructions regarding respiratory hygiene and cough etiquette. Face masks should be available to cover the nose and mouth when coughing or sneezing, and waste receptacles are needed to dispose of contaminated tissues. There should also be instructions on how and when to perform hand hygiene. Passive signage asks patients to self-identify; the triage health care team should actively ask patients about possible symptoms while maintaining a distance of at least 1 m from them. Waiting times should be minimized and closely monitored, with staffing adjustments made accordingly. During periods of increased influenza activity, facilities should consider setting up pretriage stations that facilitate rapid screening of patients for symptoms of influenza to separate those patients from others. Registration can identify the charts of patients with potential influenza to expedite care. Waiting rooms should be segregated into 2 areas; patients with and without respiratory symptoms. When possible, physical barriers should separate the patients.

In the ED, patients should be evaluated in single treatment areas.[85] The health care worker should use personal protection equipment (PPE), including a surgical mask, and a face-shield or mask with visor attachment, if there is a high chance of splash or spray of respiratory secretions. Gloves and a long-sleeved gown should be worn when entering the room of a patient with suspected or confirmed influenza.[85] The health care worker should remove all PPE just before leaving the patient's room and discard it in the hands-free waste and linen receptacle within the room. Hand hygiene should be performed after removing gloves and gown, before removing mask and protection, and again after leaving the room.[86]

If a patient with droplet precautions in the ED needs to be moved for investigation, the patient should wear a face mask and continue to follow cough etiquette and hand hygiene. There should be appropriate communication to other personnel about patients with suspected or confirmed influenza before transferring them to other departments (eg, radiology) and admitting units in the facility.

Some procedures performed on patients with suspected or confirmed influenza infection may be more likely to generate higher concentrations of infectious respiratory aerosols. These procedures include intubation and related procedures (eg, manual ventilation, open endotracheal suctioning, cardiopulmonary resuscitation, sputum induction, nebulized therapy, and noninvasive positive pressure ventilation such as continuous positive airway pressure [CPAP] or biphasic positive airway pressure [BiPAP]). Although there are limited data available on influenza transmission related to such aerosols, many authorities recommend the additional precautions to be used when such procedures are performed.[87] The number of health care workers present should be limited to only those essential for patient care and support. Those present should have received influenza vaccine. There should be a low threshold for intubation rather than using prolonged aerosol-generating procedures such as BiPAP and CPAP. The health care worker should wear respiratory protection including a fitted N95 respirator during aerosol–generating procedures. N95 respirators should be used in the context of a comprehensive respiratory protection program that includes fit testing and training as required under the respiratory protection standard (29 CFR 1910.134) of the Occupational Safety and Health Administration (OHSA).[88] The procedures should be conducted in an airborne infection isolation room (AIIR), when feasible. AIIRs reduce the concentration of infectious aerosols and prevent spread into adjacent areas using controlled air exchanges and directional airflow. AIIR are negative-pressure rooms relative to the surrounding areas, with a minimum of 6 air exchanges per hour. The air should be exhausted directly to the outside or filtered through a high-efficiency particulate air (HEPA) filter before recirculation. There should be environmental surface cleaning following the procedure.

Visitors should not be present during aerosol-generating procedures. Visits to patients with suspected or confirmed influenza should be controlled such that visitors should be instructed to limit their movement within the facility. Facilities should provide instruction before visitors enter a patient's room on hand hygiene, limiting surfaces touch, and use of PPE.[89] Visitors should be advised to contact their health care provider for information on influenza vaccination, if this has not been received; if they are high-risk patients (as described earlier),[45] chemoprophylaxis may be offered if they are in close contact with the patient.

Health care workers in the ED presumably receive education and training programs on preventing transmission of all infectious agents, including influenza. These programs should be updated periodically and competency should be documented. Health care workers who develop fever and respiratory symptoms should be instructed not to report to work, or, if working, they should put on a face mask and promptly notify their supervisor and/or infection control personnel. Health care workers should be excluded from work for at least 24 hours after they no longer have fever. Those with ongoing respiratory symptoms should be evaluated to determine appropriateness of contact with patients. Health care workers caring for immunocompromised patients should be considered for temporary assignment or exclusion from work for 7 days from symptom onset or until the resolution of symptoms, whichever is longer.[85] Administration of antiviral treatment and chemoprophylaxis of health care workers should be considered when appropriate. Early treatment with antiviral agents and vaccination are especially important for health care workers at higher risk for influenza complications, including pregnant women and women up to 2 weeks after giving birth; persons 65 years and older; and persons with chronic diseases such as asthma, heart disease, diabetes, diseases that suppress the immune system, and morbid obesity.[45] Work reassignment should be considered

Table 6
Recommended dosage and schedule of influenza antiviral medications[a] for treatment[b] and chemoprophylaxis[c]

Antiviral Agent	Treatment/ Chemoprophylaxis	Age Groups (y)				
		1–6	7–9	10–12	13–64	≥65
Zanamivir	**Treatment**					
	Influenza A	Not approved	10 mg twice a day	10 mg twice a day	10 mg twice a day	10 mg twice a day
	Influenza B	Not approved	10 mg twice a day	10 mg twice a day	10 mg twice a day	10 mg twice a day
	Chemoprophylaxis					
	Influenza A	Not approved for ages 1–4 y	Children aged 5–9 y 10 mg every day	10 mg every day	10 mg every day	10 mg every day
	Influenza B	Not approved for ages 1–4 y	Children aged 5–9 y 10 mg every day	10 mg every day	10 mg every day	10 mg every day
Oseltamivir[d]	**Treatment**					
	Influenza A					
	Weight of Child (kg)	≤15 / >15–23 / >23–40 / >40	≤15 / >15–23 / >23–40 / >40	≤40 / >40		
	Dose	30 mg twice a day / 45 mg twice a day / 60 mg twice a day / 75 mg twice a day	30 mg twice a day / 45 mg twice a day / 60 mg twice a day / 75 mg twice a day	Dose varies[e] / 75 mg twice a day	75 mg twice a day	75 mg twice a day
	Influenza B					
	Weight of Child (kg)	≤15 / 15–23 / 23–40 / >40	≤15 / 15–23 / 23–40 / >40	≤40 / >40		
	Dose	30 mg twice a day / 45 mg twice a day / 60 mg twice a day / 75 mg twice a day	30 mg twice a day / 45 mg twice a day / 60 mg twice a day / 75 mg twice a day	dose varies[e] / 75 mg twice a day	75 mg twice a day	75 mg twice a day

Chemoprophylaxis

Influenza A

Weight of Child (kg)	≤15	>15-23	>23-40	>40	≤15	>15-23	>23-40	>40	≤40	>40
Dose	30 mg every day	45 mg every day	60 mg every day	75 mg every day	30 mg every day	45 mg every day	60 mg every day	75 mg every day	dose varies[e]	75 mg every day

Influenza B

Weight of Child (kg)	≤15	>15-23	>23-40	>40	≤15	>15-23	>23-40	>40	≤40	>40
Dose	30 mg every day	45 mg every day	60 mg every day	75 mg every day	30 mg every day	45 mg every day	60 mg every day	75 mg every day	dose varies[e]	75 mg every day

[a] Zanamivir is manufactured by GlaxoSmithKline (Relenza, an inhaled powder). Zanamivir is approved for treatment of persons aged greater than or equal to 7 years and approved for chemoprophylaxis of persons aged greater than or equal to 5 years. Zanamivir is administered through oral inhalation by using a plastic device included in the medication package. Patients benefit from instruction and demonstration of the correct use of the device. Zanamivir is not recommended for those persons with underlying airway disease. Oseltamivir is manufactured by Roche Pharmaceuticals (Tamiflu, a tablet). Oseltamivir is approved for treatment or chemoprophylaxis of persons aged greater than or equal to 1 year. Oseltamivir is available for oral administration in 30 mg, 45 mg, and 75 mg capsules and liquid suspension. No antiviral medications are approved for treatment or chemoprophylaxis of influenza among children less than 1 year old. This information is based on data published by the FDA (Available at: http://www.fda.gov/Drugs/DrugSafety/informationbyDrugClass/ucm100228.htm).

[b] Recommended duration for antiviral treatment is 5 days. Longer treatment courses can be considered for patients who remain severely ill after 5 days of treatment.

[c] Recommended duration is 10 days when administered after a household exposure and 7 days after the most recent known exposure in other situations. For control of outbreaks in long-term care facilities and hospitals, CDC recommends antiviral chemoprophylaxis for a minimum of 2 weeks and up to 1 week after the most recent case was identified.

[d] A reduction in the dose of oseltamivir is recommended for persons with creatinine clearance less than 30 mL/min.

[e] For the recommended treatment dose for oseltamivir for children aged 10 to 12 years who weigh 40 kg or less, please see weight of child and dose for age groups 7 to 9 years.

Data from Centers for Disease Control and Prevention. Antiviral agents for the treatment and chemoprophylaxis of influenza - recommendations of the Advisory Committee on Immunization Practices (ACIP). MMWR 2011;60(No. RR-1):1–28.

for those at higher risk to avoid potentially high-risk exposure such as performing or assisting aerosol-generating procedures in patients with suspected or confirmed influenza.

The ED should have adequate isolation facilities and clear protocols of rapid admission to the wards to prevent boarding. Lastly, discharge instructions should be developed and given to every patient with influenza discharged home from the ED.

Discharge instructions for adult patients with suspected or confirmed influenza

The Emergency Department team feels that you have the seasonal flu or influenza and your symptoms are mild enough to send you home for observation and recovery of your illness.

Influenza is contagious, and you should use proper precautions so that you do not pass your infection on to others.

When you leave the Emergency Department, please wear a mask and keep it on until you arrive home if you cannot keep a distance of 2 m from others. You may also wear it at home, as necessary.

Do not use public transportation (bus, subway) to go home. Go straight home; do not make any stops on the way (eg, drug store, grocery store). If you were given a prescription, make arrangements for a family member or friend to pick it up.

You should isolate yourself in your home until 7 days after the onset of illness or at least 24 hours after symptoms have resolved, whichever is longer. Do not go to work, school, or public places. Do not share personal items, such as towels, drinking cups, cutlery, thermometers, and toothbrushes.

Always use hygiene and prevention measures to avoid contamination:

- Wash your hands frequently.
- Cough or sneeze into the crook of your elbow rather than into your hands.
- Use tissues and dispose in waste basket.
- Keep your surroundings clean.

While at home, it is important that you monitor your own health to be sure that your illness does not worsen. You should consult your doctor or return to the Emergency Department if you develop one of these symptoms: shortness of breath, difficulty breathing, chest pain, recurrent vomiting, or high fever 38.5°C (101.3°F).

Household contacts should:

- Pay attention to the onset of any illness
- Stay home if mild flulike symptoms occur
- Go to a doctor with a fever more than 38°C (100.4°F) and belong to a group at risk of developing influenza complications (children less than 2 years of age, pregnant women, person 65 years old and older, and persons with chronic diseases such as asthma, heart disease, diabetes, and diseases that suppress the immune system)
- Go to a doctor with a fever more than 38°C (100.4°F) and one of these symptoms:
  - Shortness of breath
  - Difficulty breathing
  - Chest pain
  - Recurrent vomiting
  - Child who is too quiet and less active than normal, or refuses to play, or is agitated

SEASONAL VERSUS PANDEMIC INFLUENZA

The symptoms of an influenza pandemic can be similar to those of seasonal flu (ie, fever, headache, myalgia, coryza, gastrointestinal symptoms, sore throat, or cough). In the last century, 4 influenza pandemics were caused by novel influenza viruses. The most significant was in 1918, when the so-called Spanish flu killed 40 to 50 million people worldwide.[90] In 2009, there was the emergence of a novel H1N1 virus, a genetic combination of human and swine influenza viruses. Because many persons have little or no immunity to a new pandemic virus, the disease can spread quickly. With the H1N1 pandemic, the rate of infection was highest among young individuals; infections were less common in persons older than 65 years, perhaps secondary to preexisting immunity against antigenically similar viruses.[91–93] There are several differences between seasonal and pandemic influenza[94]:

Seasonal and pandemic influenza	
Seasonal Influenza	**Pandemic Influenza**
Seasonal flu happens every year	An influenza pandemic happens only 2 or 3 times a century
Seasonal flu is usually around from November to April, and then stops	An influenza pandemic usually comes in 2 or even 3 waves several months apart. Each wave lasts about 2 months
About 10% of the population gets ordinary seasonal flu each year	About 35% of the population may get the influenza during the course of the full outbreak
Seasonal flu is hardest on people who do not have a strong immune system: the very young and old, and those with certain chronic illnesses	People of any age may become seriously ill with influenza during a pandemic. Often it affects a younger population
In a normal flu season, a minority die of complications from the flu, such as pneumonia	During an influenza pandemic, many more persons are infected and there may be many more deaths (see FluAid 2.0 regarding estimates based on attack rates)
Annual flu shots are protective from seasonal flu	There is no existing vaccine for an influenza pandemic. It takes 4 to 6 months after the pandemic starts to develop a vaccine
Antivirals should help the seasonal flu	Antivirals may help but the effectiveness is unknown until the virus is identified

Adapted from Ontario Ministry of Health and Long-Term Care. What you should know about a flu pandemic. http://www.healthgov.on.ca/en/public/programs/emu/pan_flu/#4. Accessed May 2011.

The WHO is responsible for monitoring the spread of influenza worldwide, declaring a pandemic, and coordinating the global response. However, the local health care systems need to develop surveillance to detect and monitor for a pandemic strain. It is important for the emergency physician to be cognizant that patients presenting with severe ILI, with epidemiologic links to southeast Asia, in particular China, with no diagnosis within the first 72 hours of hospitalization may represent the patient with an emerging respiratory infection.[95] Patients with severe respiratory infections are those with fever and new onset of cough or shortness of breath with radiographic evidence of acute respiratory distress syndrome or other life-threatening complications such as encephalitis. The emergency physician should enquire about the patient's travel history or any close contact with persons who have traveled (especially from southeast Asia) or contact with any health care provider.[95] Such patients require isolation and consultation with the infection control team. During a pandemic, a comprehensive screening process is needed at triage to limit the exposure to other patients and health care workers. Further elaboration of pandemics is beyond the scope of this article.

REFERENCES

1. Simonsen L, Clarke MJ, Williamson GD, et al. The impact of influenza epidemics on mortality: introducing a severity index. Am J Public Health 1997;87(12): 1944–50.
2. Simonsen L, Clarke MJ, Schonberger LB, et al. Pandemic versus epidemic influenza mortality: a pattern of changing age distribution. J Infect Dis 1998;178(1): 53–60.
3. Thompson WW, Shay DK, Weintraub E, et al. Mortality associated with influenza and respiratory syncytial virus in the United States. JAMA 2003;289(2): 179–86.
4. World Health Organization. Influenza. Available at: http://www.who.int/mediacentre/factsheets/2003/fs211/en/.htm. Accessed September 30, 2011.
5. Centers for Disease Control and Prevention. Key facts about the flu. Available at: http://www.cdc.gov/flu/keyfacts.htm. Accessed September 30, 2011.
6. Molinari NM, Ortega-Sanchez IR, Messonnier ML, et al. The annual impact of seasonal influenza in the US: measuring disease burden and costs. Vaccine 2007;25(27):5086–96.
7. Neuzil KM, Reed GW, Mitchel EF, et al. Influenza-associated morbidity and mortality in young and middle-aged women. JAMA 1999;281(10):901–7.
8. Canadian Consensus Conference on Influenza. Can Commun Dis Rep 1993; 19(17):136–42, 145–7.
9. Nichol KL, Margolis KL, Wuorenma J, et al. The efficacy and cost effectiveness of vaccination against influenza among elderly persons living in the community. N Engl J Med 1994;331:778–84.
10. Centers for Disease Control and Prevention. Recommendations of the Advisory Committee on Immunization Practices (ACIP), 2006. MMWR Recomm Rep 2006;55(RR10):1–42.
11. Dowdle WR, Coleman MT, Gregg MB. Natural history of influenza type A in the United States, 1957-1972. Prog Med Virol 1974;17:91–135.
12. Ng TP, Pwee KH, Niti M, et al. Influenza in Singapore: assessing the burden of illness in the community. Ann Acad Med Singapore 2002;31:182–8.
13. Monto AS. Epidemiology of influenza. Vaccine 2008;26(Suppl 4):D45–8.
14. Glezen WP, Couch RB. Interpandemic influenza in the Houston area, 1974-76. N Engl J Med 1978;298(11):587–92.
15. Dolin Raphael. Epidemiology of influenza. UpToDate; 2010. Available at: http://www.uptodate.com/contents/epidemiology-ofinfluenza?source=search_result&search=Epidemiology+of+Influenza&selectedTitle=1%7E150. Accessed September 30, 2011.
16. Pons MW. Isolation of influenza virus ribonucleoprotein from infected cells. Demonstration of the presence of negative-stranded RNA in viral RNP. Virology 1971;46(1):149–60.
17. Beigel JH. Influenza. Crit Care Med 2008;36(9):2660–6.
18. Homma M, Ohyama S, Katagiri S. Age distribution of the antibody to type C influenza virus. Microbiol Immunol 1982;26:639–42.
19. Matsuzaki Y, Katsushima N, Nagai Y. Clinical features of influenza C virus infection in children. J Infect Dis 2006;193(9):1229–35.

20. Springer GF, Schwick HG, Fletcher MA. The relationship of the influenza virus inhibitory activity of glycoproteins to their molecular size and sialic acid content. Proc Natl Acad Sci U S A 1969;64:634–41.
21. Suzuki Y, Ito T, Suzuki T, et al. Sialic acid species as a determinant of the host range of influenza A viruses. J Virol 2000;74:11825–31.
22. Gottschalk A. The influenza virus neuraminidase. Nature 1958;181:377–8.
23. Adachi M, Matsukura S, Tokunaga H, et al. Expression of cytokines on human bronchial epithelial cells induced by influenza virus A. Int Arch Allergy Immunol 1997;113:307–11.
24. Ottolini MG, Blanco JCG, Eichelberger MC, et al. The cotton rat provides a useful small animal model for the study of influenza virus pathogenesis. J Gen Virol 2005;86:2823–30.
25. Couch RB, Douglas RG Jr, Fedson DS, et al. Correlated studies of a recombinant influenza-virus vaccine. III. Protection against experimental influenza in man. J Infect Dis 1971;124(5):473–80.
26. Jordan WS, Badger GF, Dingle JH. A study of illness in a group of Cleveland families. XVI. The epidemiology of influenza 1948-1953. Am J Hyg 1958;68: 169–89.
27. Ison MG, Gnann JW Jr, Nagy-Agren S, et al. Safety and efficacy of nebulized zanamivir in hospitalized patients with serious influenza. Antivir Ther 2003;8: 183–90.
28. Treanor JJ, Hayden FG, Vrooman PS, et al. Efficacy and safety of the oral neuraminidase inhibitor oseltamivir in treating acute influenza: a randomized controlled trial. JAMA 2000;283(8):1016–24.
29. Whitley RJ, Hayden FG, Reisinger KS, et al. Oral oseltamivir treatment of influenza in children. Pediatr Infect Dis J 2001;20(2):127–33.
30. Sato M, Hosoya M, Kato K, et al. Viral shedding in children with influenza virus infections treated with neuraminidase inhibitors. Pediatr Infect Dis J 2005; 24(10):931–2.
31. Leekha S, Zitterkopf NL, Espy MJ, et al. Duration of influenza A virus shedding in hospitalized patients and implications for infection control. Infect Control Hosp Epidemiol 2007;28(9):1071–6.
32. Lee N, Chan PK, Hui DS, et al. Viral loads and duration of viral shedding in adult patients hospitalized with influenza. J Infect Dis 2009;200(4):492–500.
33. Klimov A, Rocha E, Hayden FG, et al. Prolonged shedding of amantadine-resistant influenzae A viruses by immunodeficient patients: detection by polymerase chain reaction-restriction analysis. J Infect Dis 1995;172(5):1352–5.
34. Englund JA, Champlin RE, Wyde PR, et al. Common emergence of amantadine- and rimantadine-resistant influenza A viruses in symptomatic immunocompromised adults. Clin Infect Dis 1998;26(6):1418–24.
35. Boivin G, Goyette N, Bernatchez H. Prolonged excretion of amantadine-resistant influenza A virus quasi species after cessation of antiviral therapy in an immunocompromised patient. Clin Infect Dis 2002;34(5):e23–5.
36. Nichols WG, Guthrie KA, Corey L, et al. Influenza infections after hematopoietic stem cell transplantation: risk factors, mortality, and the effect of antiviral therapy. Clin Infect Dis 2004;39(9):1300–6.
37. Weinstock DM, Gubareva LV, Zuccotti G. Prolonged shedding of multidrug-resistant influenza A virus in an immunocompromised patient. N Engl J Med 2003;348(9):867–8.
38. Kondo S, Abe K. The effects of influenza virus infection on FEV1 in asthmatic children. The time-course study. Chest 1991;100(5):1235–8.

39. Smith CB, Kanner RE, Goldern CA, et al. Effect of viral infections on pulmonary function in patients with chronic obstructive pulmonary diseases. J Infect Dis 1980;141(3):271–80.
40. Louria DB, Blumenfeld HL, Ellis JT, et al. Studies on influenza in the pandemic of 1957-1958. II. Pulmonary complications of influenza. J Clin Invest 1959;38: 213–65.
41. Monto AS, Gravenstein S, Elliott M, et al. Clinical signs and symptoms predicting influenza infection. Arch Intern Med 2000;160(21):3243–7.
42. Call SA, Vollenweider MA, Hornung CA, et al. Does this patient have influenza? JAMA 2005;293(8):987–97.
43. Chiu SS, Tse CY, Lau YL, et al. Influenza A infection is an important cause of febrile seizures. Pediatrics 2001;108(4):E63.
44. Influenza symptoms and laboratory diagnostic procedures. Centers for Disease Control and Prevention; 2010. Available at: http://www.cdc.gov/flu/professionals/diagnosis/labprocedures.htm. Accessed September 30, 2011.
45. Centers for Disease Control and Prevention. Antiviral agents for the treatment and chemoprophylaxis of influenza - Recommendations of the Advisory Committee on Immunization Practices (ACIP). MMWR Recomm Rep 2011; 60(No. RR-1):1–28.
46. Simonsen L. The global impact of influenza on morbidity and mortality. Vaccine 1999;17(Suppl 1):S3.
47. Kallen AJ, Brunkard J, Moore Z, et al. Staphylococcus aureus community-acquired pneumonia during the 2006 to 2007 influenza season. Ann Emerg Med 2009;53(3):358–65.
48. Cox NJ, Subbarao K. Influenza. Lancet 1999;354(9186):1277–82.
49. Mamas MA, Fraser D, Neyses L. Cardiovascular manifestations associated with influenza virus infection. Int J Cardiol 2008;130(3):304–9.
50. British Infection Society, British Thoracic Society, Health Protection Agency. Pandemic flu: clinical management of patients with an influenza-like illness during an influenza pandemic. Provisional guidelines from the British Infection Society, British Thoracic Society, and Health Protection Agency in collaboration with the Department of Health. Thorax 2007;62(Suppl 1):1–46.
51. Influenza diagnostic testing algorithm. Centers for Disease Control and Prevention; 2010. Available at: http://www.cdc.gov/flu/professionals/diagnosis/testing_algorithm.htm. Accessed September 30, 2011.
52. Oliveira EC, Lee B, Colice GL. Influenza in the intensive care unit. J Intensive Care Med 2003;18(2):80–91.
53. Stein J, Louie J, Flanders S, et al. Performance characteristics of clinical diagnosis, a clinical decision rule, and a rapid influenza test in the detection of influenza infection in a community sample of adults. Ann Emerg Med 2005;46(5):412–9.
54. Harper SA, Bradley JS, Englund JA, et al. Seasonal influenza in adults and children – diagnosis, treatment, chemoprophylaxis, and institutional outbreak management: clinical practice guidelines of the Infectious Diseases Society of America. Clin Infect Dis 2009;48(8):1003–32.
55. Centers for Disease Control and Prevention. Role of laboratory diagnosis of influenza. Available at: http://www.cdc.gov/flu/professionals/diagnosis/labrole.htm. Accessed September 30, 2011.
56. Smit M, Beynon KA, Murdoch DR, et al. Comparison of the NOW Influenza A & B, NOW Flu A, NOW Flu B, and Directigen Flu A & B assays, and immunofluorescence with viral culture for the detection of influenza A and B viruses. Diagn Microbiol Infect Dis 2007;57(1):67–70.

57. Centers for Disease Control and Prevention. Influenza Symptoms and laboratory diagnostic procedures. Available at: http://www.cdc.gov/flu/professionals/diagnosis/labprocedures.htm. Accessed September 30, 2011.
58. Landry ML. Diagnostic tests for influenza infection. Curr Opin Pediatr 2011;23(1): 91–7.
59. Centers for Disease Control and Prevention. Guidance for clinicians on the use of rapid influenza diagnostic tests for the 2010-2011 influenza season. Available at: http://www.cdc.gov/flu/professionals/diagnosis/clinician_guidance_ridt.htm. Accessed September 30, 2011.
60. WHO recommendations on the use of rapid testing for influenza diagnosis. World Health Organization; 2005. Available at: http://www.who.int/influenza/resources/documents/rapid_testing/en/index.html. Accessed September 30, 2011.
61. Bonner AB, Monroe KW, Talley LI, et al. Impact of the rapid diagnosis of influenza on physician decision-making and patient management in the pediatric emergency department: results of a randomized, prospective, controlled trial. Pediatrics 2003;112(2):363–7.
62. Hurt AC, Alexander R, Hibbert J, et al. Performance of six influenza rapid tests in detecting human influenza in clinical specimens. J Clin Virol 2007;39(2):132–5.
63. Raphael D. Clinical manifestations of seasonal influenza in adults. UpToDate; 2010. Available at: http://www.uptodate.com/contents/clinical-manifestations-of-seasonal-influenza-in-adults?view. Accessed September 30, 2011.
64. Petric M, Comanor L, Petti CA. Role of the laboratory in diagnosis of influenza during seasonal epidemics and potential pandemics. J Infect Dis 2006;194(Suppl 2): S98–110.
65. Centers for Disease Control and Prevention. Rapid Diagnostic testing for influenza. Available at: http://www.cdc.gov/flu/professionals/diagnosis/rapidclin.htm. Accessed September 30, 2011.
66. Cox NJ, Zeigler T. Influenza viruses. In: Murray PR, Benson EJ, Jorgemson H, et al, editors. Manual of clinical microbiology. 8th edition. Washington, DC: American Society for Microbiology Press; 2003. p. 1360–7.
67. CDC protocol of realtime RTPCR for influenza A (H1N1). World Health Organization; 2009. Available at: http://www.who.int/csr/resources/publications/swineflu/CDC RealtimeRTPCR_SwineH1Assay-2009_20090430.pdf. Accessed September 30, 2011.
68. van Elden LJR, van Kraaij MGJ, Nijhuis M, et al. Polymerase chain reaction is more sensitive than viral culture and antigen testing for the detection of respiratory viruses in adults with haematological cancer and pneumonia. Clin Infect Dis 2002;34(2):177–83.
69. Pollock NR, Duong S, Cheng A, et al. Ruling out novel H1N1 influenza virus infection with direct fluorescent antigen testing. Clin Infect Dis 2009;49:66–8.
70. Ginocchio CC, Zhang F, Manji R, et al. Evaluation of multiple test methods for the detection of the novel 2009 influenza A (H1N1) during the New York City outbreak. J Clin Virol 2009;45(3):191–5.
71. Centers for Disease Control and Prevention. FluView: 2009-2010 influenza season week 20 ending May 22, 2010. Available at: http://www.cdc.gov/flu/weekly/weeklyarchives2009-2010/weekly20.htm. Accessed September 30, 2011.
72. Aoki FY, Macleod MD, Paggiaro P, et al. Early administration of oral oseltamivir increases the benefits of influenza treatment. J Antimicrob Chemother 2003; 51(1):123–9.
73. Hayden FG, Osterhaus AD, Treanor JJ, et al. Efficacy and safety of the neuraminidase inhibitor zanamivir in the treatment of influenza virus infections. GG167 Influenza Study Group. N Engl J Med 1997;337(13):874–80.

74. Monto AS, Fleming DM, Henry D, et al. Efficacy and safety of the neuraminidase inhibitor zanamivir in the treatment of influenza A and B virus infections. J Infect Dis 1999;180(2):254–61.

75. Nicholson KG, Aoki FY, Osterhaus AD, et al. Efficacy and safety of oseltamivir in treatment of acute influenza: a randomized controlled trial. Neuraminidase Inhibitor Flu Treatment Investigator Group. Lancet 2000;355(9218):1845–50.

76. Hedrick JA, Barzilai A, Behre U, et al. Zanamivir for treatment of symptomatic influenza A and B infection in children five to twelve years of age: a randomized controlled trial. Pediatr Infect Dis J 2000;19(5):410–7.

77. Lalezari J, Campion K, Keene O, et al. Zanamivir for the treatment of influenza A and B infection in high-risk patients: a pooled analysis of randomized controlled trials. Arch Intern Med 2001;161(2):212–7.

78. Monto AS, Webster A, Keene O. Randomized, placebo-controlled studies of inhaled zanamivir in the treatment of influenza A and B: pooled efficacy analysis. J Antimicrob Chemother 1999;44(Suppl 2):23–9.

79. The MIST (Management of Influenza in the Southern Hemisphere Trialists) Study Group. Randomized trial of efficacy and safety of inhaled zanamivir in treatment of influenza A and B virus infections. Lancet 1998;352(9144):1877–81.

80. Piedra PA, Schulman KL, Blumentals WA. Effects of oseltamivir on influenza-related complications in children with chronic medical conditions. Pediatrics 2009;124(1):170–8.

81. Siston AM, Rasmussen SA, Honein MA, et al. Pandemic 2009 influenza A (H1N1) virus illness among pregnant women in the United States. JAMA 2010;303(15):1517–25.

82. McGeer A, Green KA, Plevneshi A, et al. Antiviral therapy and outcomes of influenza requiring hospitalization in Ontario, Canada. Clin Infect Dis 2007;45(12):1568–75.

83. Lee N, Cockram CS, Chan PKS, et al. Antiviral treatment for patients hospitalized with severe influenza infection may affect clinical outcomes. Clin Infect Dis 2008;46(8):1323–4.

84. Public Health Agency of Canada. National Advisory Committee on Immunization Statement on Seasonal Trivalent Inactivated Influenza vaccine (TIV) for 2010-2011. An Advisory Committee Statement (ACS). Canadian Communicable Disease Report 2010;36:ACS-6.

85. Siegel JD, Rhinehart E, Jackson M, et al, and the Healthcare Infection Control Practices Advisory Committee. 2007 Guideline for isolation precautions: preventing transmission of infectious agents in healthcare settings. Available at: http://www.cdc.gov/hicpac/pdf/isolation/Isolation2007.pdf. Accessed September 30, 2011.

86. Public Health Agency of Canada. Guidance: infection prevention and control measures for healthcare workers in acute care and long-term care settings — seasonal influenza. Available at: http://www.phac-aspc.gc.ca/nois-sinp/guide/ac-sa-eng.php. Accessed September 30, 2011.

87. Epidemic- and pandemic-prone acute respiratory diseases: infection prevention and control in health care. Epidemic and pandemic alert and response. World Health Organization; 2008. Available at: http://www.who.int/csr/resources/publications/EPR_AM3_E3.pdf. Accessed September 30, 2011.

88. United States Department of Labor, Occupational Safety and Health Administration (OSHA). Respiratory Protection 1910.134. Personal protective equipment. Available at: http://www.osha.gov/pls/oshaweb/owadisp.show_document?p_table=STANDARDS&p_id=12716. Accessed September 30, 2011.

89. Centers for Disease Control and Prevention. Guidelines and recommendations prevention strategies for seasonal influenza in healthcare settings. Available at: http://www.cdc.gov/flu/professionals/infectioncontrol/healthcaresettings.htm. Accessed September 30, 2011.

90. The Ontario health plan for an influenza pandemic in brief. Ontario Ministry of Health and Long-Term Care; 2009. Available at: http://www.health.gov.on.ca/english/providers/program/emu/pan_flu/ohpip2/brief_08.pdf. Accessed September 30, 2011.

91. Novel Swine-Origin Influenza A (H1N1) Virus Investigation Team. Emergence of a novel swine-origin influenza A (H1N1) virus in humans. N Engl J Med 2009; 360(25):2605–15.

92. Belshe RB. Implications of the emergence of a novel H1 influenza virus. N Engl J Med 2009;360(25):2667–8.

93. Fisman DN, Savage R, Gubbay J, et al. Older age and a reduced likelihood of 2009 H1N1 virus infection. N Engl J Med 2009;361(20):2000–1.

94. Ontario Ministry of Health and Long-Term Care. What you should know about a flu pandemic. What is the difference between the ordinary/seasonal influenza – or "flu" – and an influenza pandemic? Available at: http://www.health.gov.on.ca/en/public/programs/emu/pan_flu/#4. Accessed September 30, 2011.

95. Early detection of severe emerging or re-emerging respiratory infections through severe respiratory illness (SRI) surveillance. Public Health Agency of Canada; 2006. Available at: http://www.phac-aspc.gc.ca/eri-ire/pdf/02-SRI-Surveillance-Protocol_e.pdf. Accessed September 30, 2011.

APPENDIX 1: REFERENCES FOR TABLE 4 (SENSITIVITY, SPECIFICITY, PPV, AND NPV OF SELECTIVE RIDTS)

1. Manufacturer's product information or product insert.

2. Landry ML, Cohen S, Ferguson D. Comparison of Binax NOW and Directigen for rapid detection of influenza A and B. J Clin Virol 2004;31:113–5.

3. Weinberg A, Walker M. Evaluation of three immunoassay kits for rapid detection of influenza A and B. Clin Diagn Lab Immunol 2005;12:367–70.

4. Dominguez EA, Taber LH, Couch RB. Comparison of rapid diagnostic techniques for respiratory syncytial virus and influenza A virus respiratory infections in young children. J Clin Microbiol 1993;31:2286–90.

5. Noyla DE, Clark B, O'Donnell FT, et al. Comparison of a new neuraminidase detection assay with an enzyme immunoassay, immunofluorescence, and culture for rapid detection of influenza A and B viruses in nasal wash specimens. J Clin Microbiol 2000;38:1161–5.

6. Ryan-Poirier KA, Katz JM, Webster RG, et al. Application of Directigen FLU-A for the detection of influenza A virus in human and nonhuman specimens. J Clin Microbiol 1992;30:1072–5.

7. Waner JL, Todd SJ, Shalaby H, et al. Comparison of Directigen FLU-A with viral isolation and direct immunofluorescence for the rapid detection and identification of influenza A virus. J Clin Microbiol 1991;29:479–82.

8. Leonardi GP, Leib H, Birkhead GS, et al. Comparison of rapid detection methods for influenza A and their value in health care management of institutionalized geriatric patients. J Clin Microbiol 1994;32:70–4.

9. Johnston SL, Bloy H. Evaluation of a rapid enzyme immunoassay for detection of influenza A virus. J Clin Microbiol 1993;31:142–3.

10. Yuen KY, Chan PK, Peiris M, et al. Clinical features and rapid viral diagnosis of human disease associated with avian influenza A H5N1 virus. Lancet 1998;351: 467–71.

11. Chan KH, Maildis N, Pope W, et al. Evaluation of the Directigen FluA+B test for rapid diagnosis of influenza virus type A and B infections. J Clin Microbiol 2002;40:1675–80.

12. Hamilton MS, Abel DM, Ballam YJ, et al. Clinical evaluation of the ZstatFlu-II test: a chemiluminescence rapid diagnostic test for influenza virus. J Clin Microbiol 2002;40:2331–4.

13. Ruest A, Michaud S, Deslandes S, et al. Comparison of the Directigen Flu A+B test, the QuickVue Influenza test, and clinical case definition to viral culture and reverse transcription-PCR for rapid diagnosis of influenza virus infection. J Clin Microbiol 2003;41:3487–93.

14. Cazacu AC, Greer J, Taherivand M, et al. Comparison of lateral-flow immunoassay and enzyme immunoassay with viral culture for rapid detection of influenza virus in nasal wash specimens from children. J Clin Microbiol 2003; 41:2132–4.

15. Dunn JD, Gordon GL, Kelley C, et al. Comparison of the Denka Seiken INFLU A-B Quick and BD Directigen Flu A+B kits with fluorescent-antibody staining and shell vial culture methods for rapid detection of influenza viruses. J Clin Microbiol 2003;41:2180–3.

16. Landry ML, Ferguson D. Suboptimal detection of influenza virus in adults by the Directigen Flu A+B enzyme immunoassay and correlation of results with the number of antigen-positive cells detected by cytospin immunofluorescence. J Clin Microbiol 2003;41:3407–9.

17. Covalciuc KA, Webb KH, Carlson CA. Comparison of four clinical specimen types for detection of influenza A and B viruses by optical immunoassay (FLU OIA test) and cell culture methods. J Clin Microbiol 1999;37:3971–4.

18. Boivin G, Hardy I, Kress A. Evaluation of a rapid optical immunoassay for influenza viruses (FLU OIA test) in comparison with cell culture and reverse transcription-PCR. J Clin Microbiol 2001;39:730–2.

19. Hindiyeh M, Goulding C, Morgan H, et al. Evaluation of Biostar FLU OIA assay for rapid detection of influenza A and B viruses in respiratory specimens. J Clin Virol 2000;17:119–26.

20. Schultze D, Thomas Y, Wunderli W. Evaluation of an optical immunoassay for the rapid detection of influenza A and B viral antigens. Eur J Clin Microbiol Infect Dis 2001;20:280–3.

21. Tucker SP, Cox C, Steaffens J. A flu optical immunoassay (ThermoBioStar's FLU OIA): a diagnostic tool for improved influenza management. Philos Trans R Soc London B Biol Sci 2001;356:1915–24.

22. Herrmann B, Larsson C, Zweygberg BW. Simultaneous detection and typing of influenza viruses A and B by a nested reverse transcription-PCR: comparison to virus isolation and antigen detection by immunofluorescence and optical immunoassay (FLU OIA). J Clin Microbiol 2001;39:134–8.

23. Rodriguez WJ, Schwartz RH, Thorne MM. Evaluation of diagnostic tests for influenza in a pediatric practice. Pediatr Infect Dis J 2002;21:193–6.

24. Bellei N, Benfica D, Perosa AH, et al. Evaluation of a rapid test (QuickVue) compared with the shell vial assay for detection of influenza virus clearance after antiviral treatment. J Virol Methods 2003;109:85–8.

25. Pregliasco F, Puzelli S, Mensi C, et al. Influenza virological surveillance in children: the use of the QuickVue rapid diagnostic test. J Med Virol 2004;73:269–73.

26. Quach C, Newby D, Daoust G, et al. QuickVue influenza test for rapid detection of influenza A and B viruses in a pediatric population. Clin Diagn Lab Immunol 2002;9:925–6.

27. Yamazaki M, Mitamura K, Kimura K, et al. Clinical evaluation of an immunochromatography test for rapid diagnosis of influenza. Kansenshogaku Zasshi 2001;75:1047–53.

28. Kawakami C, Shimizu H, Watanabe S, et al. Evaluation of immunochromatography method for rapid detection of influenza A and B viruses. Kansenshogaku Zasshi 2001;75:792–9.

29. Fujieta T. Evaluation of new rapid influenza virus detection kit- QUICK S-INFLU A/B "SEIKEN." Jpn J Med Pharmacol Sci 2004;51:127–30.

30. Cazacu AC, Demmler GJ, Neuman MA, et al. Comparison of a new lateral-flow chromatographic membrane immunoassay to viral culture for rapid detection and differentiation of influenza A and B viruses in respiratory specimens. J Clin Microbiol 2004;42:3661–4.

31. Noyola DE, Paredes AJ, Clark B, et al. Evaluation of a neuraminidase detection assay for the rapid detection of influenza A and B virus in children. Pediatr Dev Pathol 2000;3:162–7.

32. Rawlinson WD, Waliuzzaman ZM, Fennell M, et al. New point of care test is highly specific but less sensitive for influenza A and B in children and adults. J Med Virol 2004;74:127–31.

33. Mitamura K, Yamazaki M, Ichikawa M, et al. Evaluation of an immunochromatography test using enzyme immunoassay for rapid detection influenza A and B viruses. Kansenshogaku Zasshi 2004;78:597–603.

34. Hara M, Takao S, Fukuda S, et al. Comparison of three rapid diagnostic kits using immunochromatography for detection of influenza A viruses. J Jpn Assoc Infect Dis 2004;78:935–42.

35. Kubo N, Ikematsu H, Nabeshima S, et al. Evaluation of an immunochromatography test kit for rapid diagnosis of influenza. Kansenshogaku Zasshi 2003;77:1007–14.

36. Yamazaki M, Mitamura K, Ichikawa M, et al. Evaluation of flow-through immunoassay for rapid detection of influenza A and B viruses. Kansenshogaku Zasshi 2004;78:865–71.

Acute Aortic Dissection in the Emergency Department: Diagnostic Challenges and Evidence-Based Management

Suneel Upadhye, MD, MSc, FRCPC*, Karen Schiff, MD, FRCPC

KEYWORDS

- Aortic dissection • Emergency department
- Evidence-based medicine

ACUTE AORTIC DISSECTION

Acute aortic dissection (AAD) is a rare but potentially catastrophic disease that remains difficult to diagnose in the emergency department (ED). It carries a significant in-hospital mortality of 27%, even when properly diagnosed.[1] In a recently published guideline from the American College of Cardiology (ACC)/American Heart Association (AHA), mortality estimates for AAD were placed at 40% for immediate death, 1% per hour for incremental death thereafter if initially surviving the acute dissection event, and 20% for perioperative death.[2] There is a 50% to 70% reported survival rate after initial surgery depending on patient age and cause. This article focuses on the epidemiology, clinical assessments, diagnostic challenges, and management strategies for AAD in the ED.

AAD: EPIDEMIOLOGY

The International Registry of Acute Aortic Dissection (IRAD) was created in 2000 to follow patterns and outcomes in AAD.[3] This registry of 464 cases (mean age 63 years, men 65%), found an overall mortality of 27.4%, with a surgical versus nonsurgical

Funding support: None. Neither of the authors has any direct financial interests, professional relationships, or other conflicts of interest relevant to this article.

Division of Emergency Medicine, McMaster University, Room 254, Second Floor, McMaster Building, 237 Barton Street East, Hamilton, Ontario, L8L 2X2, Canada

* Corresponding author.

E-mail address: upadhyes@mcmaster.ca

Emerg Med Clin N Am 30 (2012) 307–327

doi:10.1016/j.emc.2011.12.001

0733-8627/12/$ – see front matter © 2012 Published by Elsevier Inc.

emed.theclinics.com

mortality of 26% versus 58% respectively for proximal (type A) dissections. Mortalities for distal (type B) dissections were 10.7% for medical management and 31% for surgical management (performed in 20% of type B candidates).

The true incidence of aortic dissection is difficult to define because acute AAD can be instantly fatal in the prehospital setting (and death may be attributed to other causes). In addition, AAD may be missed on initial presentation, leading to early mortality as a result of misclassification.[2] Population-based prevalence studies suggest that the incidence of AAD may range from 2.5 to 3 cases per 100,000 person years in the United States (6000–10,000 new cases annually), to 16 cases per 100,000 annually in Sweden.[2] There is a higher incidence of AAD in men (65%) and with increasing age.[1,2]

Left untreated, patients with a proximal (type A) acute dissection have a mortality of approximately 75% within 2 weeks.[4] With successful initial therapy, the 5-year survival rate is 75%. The 10-year survival rate for surgically repaired dissections is 40% to 60%.

The medicolegal issues surrounding missed diagnosis of AAD remain significant. There is no central repository of pooled medicolegal cases/outcomes in the United States available to physicians for quality assurance purposes. However, the Risk Factor Study conducted by the Sullivan Group in the United States in 2006 examined the documentation of risk factors for acute diagnoses in 91,286 ED records analyzed, and found that risk factors for AAD were poorly documented (26%) compared with 86% documentation for coronary artery disease risk factors.[5] In this study, although medical physicians performed most patient assessments (83.6%), it was noted that nurse practitioners (48.9%) and template users (50.2%) were the best at documenting the relevant risk factors. In Canada, the Canadian Medical Protection Agency (CMPA) has issued 2 recent bulletins concerning AAD cases and outcomes.[6,7] In the first bulletin, 2 cases of atypical chest pain with nonclassic features were reviewed.[6] In the first case, the findings of experts suggested that a detected large blood pressure differential between patient arms should have alerted the treating physicians to the possible diagnosis of AAD. In the second, there was a complete lack of typical and atypical findings. The second bulletin reviewed 32 cases that generated 34 medico-legal cases; 56% of these were either dismissed or judged in favor of the physician.[7] Common misdiagnoses included acute coronary syndrome (19%), musculoskeletal pain (20%), pneumonia/pulmonary embolism (20%), pericarditis (12%), gastrointestinal (GI) pain (9%), and other causes (20%). The bulletin cautioned physicians to consider the diagnosis of AAD in situations of sudden severe chest pain, accompanying visceral symptoms (nausea, vomiting, pallor, diaphoretic), normal/minimally abnormal electrocardiography (ECG) findings, and inappropriate reliance on classic features such as tearing chest pain, blood pressure/pulse discrepancies, new cardiac murmurs, and chest radiograph mediastinal widening as potentially misleading.

AAD: PATHOPHYSIOLOGY

Normal cardiac contractions involve swinging movements of the heart in the pericardium resulting in small flexions of the ascending and descending aorta; the latter is tethered just distal to the left subclavian artery.[1] This repetitive swinging (37 million beats per year) creates repetitive stresses on the layers of the aortic wall. The aortic wall is composed of 3 layers: the innermost intima, the media (composed of elastic connective tissue and smooth muscle), and the outermost adventitia.

Hemodynamic stressors to the aortic inner walls can be the result of prolonged hypertension, inherently weakened connective tissue walls (eg, Ehlers-Danlos syndrome), or a bicuspid aortic valve that alters the laminar flow of ejected blood toward the aortic wall rather than the central vascular lumen.[1]

Dissection occurs when the medial layers have degenerated through normal aging or other pathologic processes, and pulsatile blood flow tears through the intimal layer into the media. The resulting false lumen can then extend distally or proximally. This distention can lead to obstruction of other arterial origins from the aortic trunk, rupture back into the true vascular lumen, or into the pericardial sac or pleural cavity. External rupture can be more common because the adventitial layers are thin walled. The most important predictors of continuing dissection are the degree of sustained hypertension, and the upstroke surge pressure (slope) of the pulse wave during contraction (upstroke pattern on apex cardiogram; change in pressure [dP]/change in time [dt]).[1] False lumens can also be the result of spontaneous hemorrhage of the vasa vasorum into the aortic wall; this occurs in 8% to 15% of cases and explains the absence of an intimal tear in certain cases.[1,8] Intramural hematomas seem to be more common in the descending aortas of elderly hypertensive patients.[8]

CLASSIFICATION OF AAD

The anatomic distribution as well as the acuity of the dissection have important prognostic and therapeutic implications. Consequently, dissections are classified according to anatomic location as well as acuity.

There are 2 different anatomic classification systems for aortic dissection that are commonly used, the Stanford and DeBakey classifications. The Stanford classification divides dissections into types A and B.[9] Specifically, any dissection involving the ascending aorta (proximal to the brachiocephalic artery) is classified as type A, whereas type B dissections involve only the descending aorta (distal to the subclavian artery). The DeBakey system describes dissection according to the origin of the intimal tear and the extent of the dissection using type I, II, and III classifications.[10] In DeBakey type I dissections, the intimal tear originates in the ascending aorta and extends to the arch and often beyond to the descending aorta. DeBakey type II dissections originate in, and are confined to, only the ascending aorta. DeBakey type III dissections originate in and propagate to the descending aorta. DeBakey type III dissections were then further subdivided into IIIa and IIIb classifications by Larson and Edwards,[11] in which the former involves only the thoracic descending aorta and the latter extends below the diaphragm (**Fig. 1**, **Table 1**). Although vascular surgeons may debate the relative usefulness of either classification system for surgical management planning, for emergency physicians, it is not as important which classification system is used, so long as an accurate assessment of ascending versus descending aorta involvement can be made to differentiate management strategies. The Stanford system, with an A versus B dichotomy, is easier to use than the 3-level DeBakey system (with subdivisions).

For temporal classification purposes, AAD can be categorized as acute if diagnosis occurs within 2 weeks of pain onset, subacute if within 2 to 6 weeks, and chronic if more than 6 weeks after onset of pain.[1,2]

According to the IRAD, 62% of dissections are type A, whereas the remaining 38% are type B.[3] Although more common, type A dissections are also associated with a higher mortality. The overall mortality for patients with type A dissection in IRAD was 27.4% (26.6% mortality for those who underwent surgery compared with 58% for those who were treated medically).[3] Conversely, with appropriate medical antihypertensive management, 90% of patients with uncomplicated type B dissections survived to hospital discharge.[12]

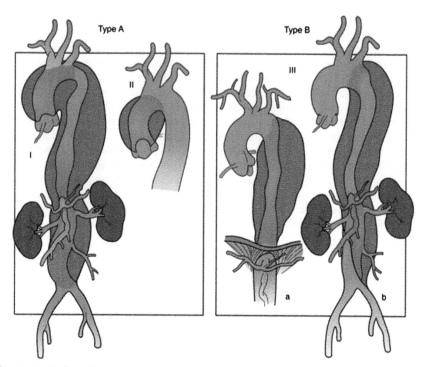

Fig. 1. Aortic dissections.

AAD: CLINICAL ASSESSMENT IN THE ED
Risk Factors for AAD

Aortic dissection occurs most frequently in men and with advancing age.[1] However, in the IRAD database, female patients with AAD were older than their male counterparts (mean age onset, 63 years), less likely to present within 6 hours of onset, less likely to endorse abrupt onset or have pulse deficits, and more likely to have mental status changes or congestive heart failure.[2] Women were also less likely to be properly diagnosed within 24 hours of symptom onset, and subsequently had higher in-hospital mortality (30% vs 21%, $P = .001$) than men.

Table 1 Classifications of AADs	
Classification of Aortic Dissection	
Stanford	
Type A	Involving the ascending aorta
Type B	Not involving the ascending aorta
DeBakey	
Type I	Originates in ascending aorta and extends to arch and often beyond into the descending aorta
Type II	Originates and localized to the ascending aorta
Type III	Originates and is localized to the descending aorta only Type IIIa: involves thoracic descending aorta only Type IIIb: extends beyond the diaphragm

There are several known/reported risk factors for AAD (**Table 2**). Common medical risk factors include a history of hypertension (70%–90%), prior cardiac surgery/catheterization (18%), a bicuspid aortic valve (14%), or a history of connective tissue disorders (eg, Marfan syndrome, Ehler-Danlos syndrome). Inflammatory vascular disorders also hold a higher risk of AAD.[2,13] IRAD data show that for patients less than 40 years old with AAD, 50% had a history of Marfan syndrome.[2] Patients may also be at risk of acquired AAD with significant exertion or trauma.[1] A positive family history in first-degree relatives has been associated in 13% to 19% of patients with AAD without an identified genetic syndrome.[2]

There are specific populations that deserve special mention when considering the diagnosis of AAD in the ED. Cocaine, methylenedioxymethamphetamine (MDMA; known as ecstasy), and other stimulant use have been associated with an increased risk of AAD.[1,14–18] Acute β-blocker withdrawal and fluctuations in circadian cortisol levels have also been implicated in AAD.[8] There are case reports of spontaneous AAD in recreational weight lifters.[19–21] Certain infectious diseases have also been associated with AAD, including tuberculous aortitis, and insidious *Salmonella* aortitis causing type B dissection.[22,23] An increasing incidence of AAD in pregnancy has been reported,[2,4,24–28] including cases associated with cocaine use, inflammatory arteritis, and otherwise previously healthy women with no prior aortic disease.[29] Half of dissections of women younger than 40 years occur in pregnancy.[4] Pregnancy has been associated with altered hemodynamic states (increased heart rate and stroke volume), and increased estrogen and progesterone changes, which may induce

Table 2	
Risk factors for aortic dissection	
Risk Category	**Associated Disorders**
Increased aortic wall stress	Hypertension (especially uncontrolled) Pheochromocytoma Cocaine/stimulant use Weight lifting/other Valsalva situations Deceleration injury/blunt trauma Aortic coarctation
Medical conditions affecting aortic medial layers	Genetic disorders/syndromes: Ehler-Danlos, Marfan, Turner, Loeys-Dietz, Noonan, congenital bicuspid aortic valve, familial dissections/aneurysms Inflammatory vasculitides: syphilis, granulomatous arteritis, tuberculous, salmonella, Takayasu, giant cell, systemic lupus erythematosus, Behçet
Iatrogenic wall injury	Cardiac/valvular surgery, intra-aortic balloon pump use, aortic cannulation, cross-clamping sites, catheterization
Other	Male sex Age >50 y Pregnancy Polycystic kidney disease Chronic corticosteroid use or immunocompromised states

Data from Hiratazka LF, Bakris GL, Beckman JA, et al. 2010 ACCF/AHA/AATS/ACR/ASA/SCA/SCAI/SIR/STS/SVM Guidelines for the diagnosis and management of patients with thoracic aortic disease. Circulation 2010;121:e266–369. doi:10.1161/CIR.0b013e33181d4739e; and Chen K, Varon J, Wenker OC, et al. Acute thoracic aortic dissection: the basics. J Emerg Med 1997;15:859–67.

histologic changes in arterial walls that predispose to dissection.[18] In addition, it is possible to present to ED with AAD with no known risk factors[30]; there is no clear reported evidence on the incidence of risk factor–free AAD.

Presentations of Acute Thoracic Aortic Dissection

Historical features

The diagnosis of acute thoracic aortic dissection (TAD) in the ED is complicated by it being a rare clinical condition with potentially catastrophic outcomes, and does not necessarily present with classic findings. Typical features include sudden acute chest pain (90%) that is excruciating, severe at onset, and of a sharp/ripping/tearing quality.[1,2,4] It may be possible to localize the dissection origin based on location of pain: anterior (ascending aorta), neck/jaw (arch), interscapular (descending aorta), and lumbar/abdominal (subdiaphragmatic). Migratory pain may be rare (17%). Of concern, pain may ease or abate over time, or change as the dissection extends and begins to involve other organ systems.[2] For example, type A dissections typically present with chest pain (71% anterior), and, less commonly, with back pain (47%) or abdominal pain (21%). Type B dissections are more likely to present as back pain (64%), followed by chest or abdominal pain (63% and 43% respectively).[2] Visceral symptoms including nausea, vomiting, diaphoresis, apprehension, and lightheadedness may accompany the onset of dissection.

In the CMPA case review series of missed AAD (n = 32 patients), the symptom distribution was as follows: sudden-onset severe chest pain (91%), visceral symptoms (pallor, vomiting, diaphoresis 78%), intermittent pain (75%), radiation to back/neck/arms/jaw (69%), pleuritic/positional pain (44%), pyrexia (22%), syncope (9%), and tearing quality (3%).[8] The author concluded that, although there may be some classic findings of TAD that should prompt the inclusion of TAD in a differential diagnosis of acute chest pain in the ED, the reliance on the presence of these features, or the absence thereof, may not be sufficient to include or exclude the diagnosis.

The most comprehensive systematic review to date by Klompas,[30] and the subsequent abstract,[31] summarize the difficulty of relying on certain clinical features for the diagnosis of TAD. The likelihood ratios (LRs) for various clinical findings are summarized in **Table 3**.

The studies suggest that there is poor reliability in the symptomatic descriptions of pain quality when determining the likelihood of TAD in a patient with chest pain in the

Table 3 Summary of LRs for symptoms/signs of TAD		
Symptom	**+ LR (95% CI)**	**− LR (95% CI)**
Sudden onset of pain	1.6 (1.0–2.4)	0.3 (0.2–0.5)
Tearing/ripping pain[a]	1.2 (0.2–8.1) 10.8 (5.2–22.0)	0.99 (0.9–1.1) 0.4 (0.3–0.5)
Migrating pain[a]	1.1 (0.5–2.4) 7.6 (3.6–16.0)	0.97 (0.6–1.6) 0.6 (0.5–0.7)
History of hypertension	1.6 (1.2–2.0)	0.5 (0.3–0.7)
Focal neurologic deficit	6.6–33.0	0.71–0.87
Diastolic murmur	0.9–1.7	0.79–1.1
Pulse deficits	2.4–47.0	0.62–0.93

[a] Unpooled data from 2 studies.

Data from Klompas M. Does this patient have an acute thoracic aortic dissection? JAMA 2002;287:2262–72.

ED. However, the 2000 study by von Koloditsch and colleagues[32] merits some attention. This work was a prospective study of patients in the ED with chest pain (n = 250, 128 confirmed TAD cases) presenting to a German university hospital center, with a mean age of 53 years, 78% men, and 61% type A dissection. The outcomes of this specific study suggest that the positive and negative LRs for tearing/ripping pain (10.8 and 0.4 respectively), and for migrating pain (7.6 and 0.6 respectively) approach clinically significant levels for ED physician decision making.[33]

A final precaution remains, in that up to 12% of TAD cases may be painless, and present only with complications involving other body systems.[4] These patients tended to be older, possible steroid users or patients with Marfan, or presenting with syncope, stroke, or congestive heart failure.[2]

Physical findings of AAD

The physical examination findings associated with AAD are unreliable and frequently absent in patients with AAD, based on the location of the dissection and the extent of involvement of surrounding structures or organ systems. An examination of the peripheral pulses in the upper extremities or assessment of blood pressure differentials can reveal some important clues for the diagnosis. Historically, a blood pressure differential of 20 to 30 mm Hg was reported to be significant for TAD,[18] and a differential greater than 20 mm Hg was confirmed in a prospective study by von Koloditsch and colleagues[32] as a significant predictor of AAD. However, other studies have shown that up to 20% of normal patients may have a pulse differential of 20 mm Hg without AAD,[18] and 53% of normal patients have difference of 10 mm Hg.[21] The Klompas[30] meta-analysis of clinical findings with AAD suggested that the pooled sensitivity of pulse deficits is 31% (95% confidence interval [CI] 24–39) but a positive LR of 5.7 (95% CI 1.4–23.0). New aortic regurgitation murmurs arise in 32% to 76% of patients with AAD,[1,2] but have a pooled sensitivity of 28% (95% CI 21–36) and a disappointing positive LR of 1.4 (95% CI 1.0–2.0).

Complications of acute aortic regurgitation may range from nonexistent to life-threatening congestive heart failure or cardiogenic shock, depending on the extent and magnitude of dissection into the aortic valve root. Other clues to significant aortic regurgitation complicated by pericardial tamponade may include jugular venous distension, muffled heart sounds, tachycardia, and hypotension.[1] Acute aortic dissection into the pericardium with subsequent tamponade is reported to be the second most common cause of death in AAD.[18]

AAD can be complicated by mass compression effects on adjacent structures, leading to superior vena cava syndrome, Horner syndrome (sympathetic chain), hoarseness (recurrent laryngeal nerve), dyspnea (tracheobronchial tree), and dysphagia (esophagus).[4] A pulsatile sternoclavicular joint, although rare, may provide a diagnostic clue to the diagnosis with compression manifestations of upper chest/lower neck phenomena.[4]

End-organ presentations of AAD

Cardiovascular complications These can include aortic regurgitation and related disorders (discussed earlier), pulse deficits, blood pressure differentials, syncope, myocardial infarction, congestive heart failure, and cardiogenic shock.[1,2,4,8] Low sensitivity findings from the Klompas[30] review include pericardial rubs (sensitivity 6%, 95% CI 3%–13%), congestive heart failure (sensitivity 15%, 95% CI 4%–33%), shock (sensitivity 19%, 95% CI 15%–26%), and new myocardial infarction on ECG (sensitivity 7%, 95% CI 4%–14%). It is important to recognize an ST-elevation myocardial infarction (STEMI) in the setting of potential proximal AAD (incidence

3%), because thrombolytic therapy is contraindicated in these situations; this reportedly occurs in 0.1% to 0.2% of STEMI cases.[1] STEMI is most common in the right coronary circulation, leading to posteroinferior infarctions caused by dissection into the right coronary ostium.[18] Evidence of myocardial ischemia on ECG is reported in up to 19% of AAD cases.[2] There are also reports of proximal dissections extending into the atrial septa leading to conduction abnormalities.[4] Both atrial fibrillation[34] and intractable supraventricular tachycardia[35] cases have been reported. Painless acute congestive heart failure has been reported in the setting of a type B dissection.[36] In addition, AAD as a cause of cardiac arrest should be suspected in patients of older age, known aortic aneurysms, male gender, and initial pulseless electrical activity rhythm,[37] as well as those with polycystic kidney disease.[38]

Syncope Syncope complicates approximately 13% of cases of AAD.[2] This syncope can be the result of acute cardiac dysfunction (described earlier), vascular outflow obstruction in the arch/carotid arteries, neurologic vasovagal pain responses, or from acute hypovolemia caused by hemorrhage into third spaces. Syncope inappropriately attributed to heat-related illness in a young healthy male patient with a painless AAD has been reported.[39] Painless syncope is also reported elsewhere in the emergency literature.[40]

Neurologic complications Focal neurologic deficits can complicate AAD with a pooled sensitivity of 17% (95% CI 12%–23%).[30] Neurologic deficits can result from hypotension, malperfusion, distal thromboembolism, or nerve compression from mass effects.[2] Proximal arch dissections are more likely to cause intracranial and brainstem deficits, whereas distal arch dissections may involve the spinal cord and lower extremities.[1] Cerebral ischemia and stroke syndromes are the most common central nervous system effects of proximal AAD, occurring 5% to 15% of the time[8]; chest pain in the setting of new focal neurologic deficit is highly predictive of proximal AAD involving the cerebral circulation.[8] It is critical for ED physicians to consider AAD in the setting of acute stroke syndromes, because contraindicated thrombolytic therapy in this setting can lead to catastrophic outcomes.[1] Sudden coma from basilar artery occlusion[41] and transient locked-in syndrome[42] have both been described in the setting of painless AAD, as has acute vertigo.[43] Focal central findings may be localized from vaso-occlusive or thromboembolic causes, or diffuse if resulting from systemic hypotension. The spinal cord may be susceptible to injury if AAD involves the origins of the intercostal spinal arteries, the artery of Adamkiewicz, or the thoracic radicular artery, resulting in clinical syndromes of transverse myelitis, anterior cord syndromes, and paraplegia or quadraplegia.[8] This may be particularly true in watershed areas of the cord. Multiple cases exist of painless neurologic deficits of the legs of variable onset and duration (incidence 10%); the common theme is that the index of suspicion for ED physicians should be high for AAD in the setting of sudden paralysis of the lower extremities even in the absence of chest symptoms.[9,44–49] Of interest, 50% of neurologic symptoms may be transient, and one-third may not present with chest pain, complicating the potential AAD diagnosis.[2]

Ears/nose/throat complications As stated previously, several structures in the throat and upper thorax can be compressed by mass effect of proximal/arch dissection, including the trachea (dyspnea, stridor), esophagus (dysphagia), recurrent laryngeal nerve (hoarseness), and sympathetic chain (ipsilateral Horner syndrome). Serious comorbidities have resulted from initial benign presentations including sore throat,[50] hoarseness,[51] and hoarseness with collapse and neck bruising.[52] The recurrent theme is of benign and potentially misleading complications in the face of painless AAD.

Respiratory complications Respiratory effects of AAD can include mass effects on the tracheobronchial tree (dyspnea), hemorrhage into the lung tissues (hemoptysis 3%) and pleural space, pleural effusions, and death.[2,53]

GI complications Mesenteric ischemia is the most common GI complication of AAD, and the most common cause of death in type B dissection.[2] By the time unreliable serum markers become positive, it is often too late to salvage the dead bowel. Rare but catastrophic GI bleeding can also result from mesenteric ischemia or from aortoenteric fistula.[54,55]

Other atypical presentations Chronic aortic dissection has been reported in the literature as presenting with fever of unknown origin,[56] renal colic, and mesenteric ischemia.

Other diagnoses mimicking AAD There are sparse case reports of thymic diseases presenting as an AAD, including a 49-year-old hypertensive woman with marfanoid features presenting with tearing chest pain and a para-aortic bulge on chest radiograph but normal aortogram, ultimately diagnosed as an invasive thymoma.[57] Another case involved an 80-year-old hypertensive man presenting with sudden severe chest and back pain, but investigations ultimately revealed an thymic carcinoid tumor.[58] A case of Takayasu arteritis presenting with AAD to the ED has also been described.[59]

The value of combined clinical findings in arriving at a diagnosis of AAD has been examined.[32] The findings examined in combination included severe sudden-onset tearing pain, blood pressure or pulse differentials between the arms, and/or mediastinal widening on chest radiograph. The positive LRs for diagnosing AAD with 0, 1, 2, or 3 combined findings increased exponentially through 0.1 (95% CI 0.0–0.2), 0.5 (95% CI 0.3–0.8), 5.3 (95% CI 3.0–9.4), and 66.0 (95% CI 4.1–1062.0) respectively. However, these 3 findings were only present in 27% of the 128 patients included in this study.

The overarching themes in the diverse literature regarding AAD assessment in the ED become readily apparent. The classic features of AAD are rarely present in combination to suggest an obvious diagnosis in the ED. The clinical manifestations of AAD may be a result of the dissection process itself, the location and extension of the dissection, and the subsequent end organs affected by the compromised blood flow or mass effects caused by the dissection. Seemingly unrelated clinical features more consistent with other, more common diagnostic entities may delay or confound the ultimate diagnosis of AAD, with potentially serious sequelae. In addition, there are many AAD mimics that may initially suggest AAD, but ultimately are diagnosed as something else. The lesson for all ED physicians is one of awareness and vigilance of common and atypical presentations of this dangerous condition, and of investigating them appropriately to make a proper and safe diagnosis.

AAD: DIAGNOSTIC STRATEGIES IN THE ED

Once the possibility of AAD has been considered, the emergency physician must make the proper diagnosis. Routine initial tests readily available in the ED (ECG, chest radiograph, laboratory markers) all have variable reliability in making a diagnosis of AAD.

Electrocardiography

The ECG is often normal or may show nonspecific changes in the setting of aortic dissection. Data collected from the IRAD revealed that the ECG was normal in 31% of cases, whereas 26% showed left ventricular hypertrophy reflecting long-standing hypertension.[3] The Klompas[30] review also noted a poor LR+ (0.2–3.2) and LR− (0.84–1.2) for left ventricular hypertrophy findings on ECG in the setting of AAD. The primary usefulness of the ECG in this clinical setting is to consider or exclude alternative diagnoses.

It is imperative to consider the possibility of aortic dissection in the setting of ischemia, especially inferior ischemia, because proximal dissections may extend to involve the right coronary artery.[60] In the review by Klompas,[30] 7% of patients with aortic dissection showed evidence of acute ischemia (either ST elevation or new Q waves) on the ECG. In this setting, the AHA 2010 guidelines on thoracic aortic disease recommended that, because of the uncommon event of dissection-associated coronary disorder, ST elevation should be treated as a primary cardiac event unless the patient is considered to be at high risk for aortic dissection.[2]

Laboratory Markers: D-Dimer and Other Serum Biomarkers

The use of a screening D-dimer in the diagnosis of TAD has been shown to be a highly useful marker, with reported sensitivities ranging from 94%[61] to 99%.[62] Despite this high sensitivity, a 2008 review by Sutherland and colleagues[63] commented that, because of the wide CIs quoted in the studies, the poorly defined eligibility criteria for study inclusion, and the possibility of false-negatives in patients with thrombosed false lumens, D-dimers should not be used as the sole screening tool in this clinical setting. This conclusion was echoed in the 2010 AHA guidelines for diagnosis and management of patients with thoracic aortic disease in which D-dimer screening was not recommended at this time because of the lack of large prospective evaluation, limitations in accurately assessing posttest probability of a negative D-dimer, and the potential for a negative D-dimer result in patients with a thrombosed false lumen or ascending aortic intramural hematoma.[2] A recently published meta-analysis of 7 studies (298 patients with AAD, 436 without) suggests that using a D-dimer cutoff of 500 ng/mL had an excellent negative LR (LR− 0.06, 95% CI 0.03–0.12) to exclude AAD, but not a good positive LR to include an AAD diagnosis (LR+ 2.43, 95% CI 1.89–3.12).[64] These investigators concluded that using a cutoff of less than 500 ng/mL may be useful to exclude the diagnosis of AAD and avoid the need for advanced imaging. However, there was significant heterogeneity in the included studies, and this information has not yet been prospectively validated in the ED. With further investigation and large prospective evaluation, D-dimer assays may show diagnostic promise and become part of a useful screening strategy or clinical decision rule for diagnosis of AAD.

Serum biomarkers reflecting smooth muscle damage have also been investigated in the setting of AAD. Specifically, serum smooth muscle myosin heavy chain (released with arterial wall smooth muscle damage) and calponin (a smooth muscle troponinlike protein) have been evaluated by Suzuki and colleagues.[65,66] Although further investigation is required, both biomarkers show promise and, in the future, may assist in the diagnosis of aortic dissection.

Although not helpful in the screening or diagnosis of aortic dissection, C-reactive protein levels have been shown to have prognostic value and predict adverse long-term outcomes. In a small cohort study of 255 Austrian patients with symptomatic aortic disease, cumulative mortality from 1 to 6 months was 32% to 40%, and there was a near-linear increase in hazard ratio from 0.7 to 2.6 through increasing C-reactive protein level quartiles.[67]

Chest Radiography

Approximately 90% of patients with aortic dissection have abnormalities on the chest radiograph,[4] and therefore the presence of a normal chest radiograph may help to decrease the likelihood of aortic dissection. In the review by Klompas,[30] a pooled analysis of 1337 chest radiographs also reported abnormalities in 90% of patients with aortic dissection. Furthermore, Klompas[30] showed that, in the absence of an abnormal aortic contour or mediastinal widening, the likelihood of AAD is significantly decreased (negative LR 0.3; 95% CI 0.2–0.4). The most common radiographic changes associated with dissection were abnormal aortic contour (pooled sensitivity 71%) and widening of the mediastinum (pooled sensitivity 64%). Other radiographic findings may include pleural effusion, displacement of intimal calcification, abnormalities of the aortic knob, and displacement of trachea or nasogastric tube deviation to the right.[68] Because of the lack of sensitivity and nonspecific chest radiography findings present in aortic dissection, it is imperative to proceed with additional imaging techniques.

Advanced Imaging Modalities

In the clinical setting, where a rapid diagnosis is crucial because of the critical nature of AAD, several factors are considered when deciding how to proceed with advanced diagnostic imaging.[69–71] Specifically, variables such as testing risks and benefits, access and availability to imaging modalities, accuracy of technique, and individual patient variables are carefully considered.[69] Historically, aortic dissection was evaluated with aortography, a modality that has now largely been replaced with noninvasive diagnostic strategies, including helical computed tomography (CT), magnetic resonance imaging (MRI), and transesophageal echocardiography (TEE). Although transthoracic echocardiography (TTE) may provide useful bedside information in the setting of aortic dissection, it does not have sufficient sensitivity or specificity to be the solitary diagnostic modality used. Specifically, TTE has shown a sensitivity of only 59.3% in the detection of AAD.[71] Further limiting the use of TTE is the inability to visualize the entire aorta.[69] As bedside ED ultrasound continues to grow and develop, findings consistent with aortic dissection may be observed at the bedside by the ED physician.[70] A case report study recently described 5 cases in which ED physicians used bedside ED ultrasound to aid in the diagnosis of TAD.[70]

Transesophageal echocardiography

Transesophageal echocardiography (TEE) may play an important role in the diagnosis of aortic dissection. This imaging modality may be of particular usefulness in the hemodynamically unstable patient, in which a timely diagnosis is imperative and transfer out of an acute care setting to the radiology department is not possible. TEE has been shown to have a high sensitivity with reported values of 98%.[71] In the systematic review of different imaging modalities, TEE was shown to have comparable sensitivity (98%) and sensitivity (95%) with CT and MRI.[72] TEE also offers the advantages that it is able to show aortic regurgitation and pericardial effusion. Although visualization of the branches of the aortic arch and distal ascending aorta historically limited the usefulness of TEE, probe technologic advancements have improved the visualization of these anatomic regions.[73]

CT

According to the IRAD, the most common diagnostic modality initially used is CT, with 61% of patients undergoing CT.[3] With technological advancements, helical CT offers many advantages and shows in a pooled analysis a high sensitivity and specificity of 100% and 98%, respectively.[72] In this study, Shiga and colleagues[72] concluded that helical CT was the optimal imaging modality for ruling out aortic dissection in patients with a low clinical pretest probability for aortic dissection. The limitations of CT include use of ionizing radiation and contrast media, need for patient transfer out of the acute care setting, and limited ability to assess the aortic valve. Conversely, CT is generally readily available, quick to complete, delineates anatomy of the entire aorta well, and may show alternative disorders considered in the differential diagnosis for aortic dissection.

In the meta-analysis of 16 studies conducted by Shiga and colleagues,[72] CT, MRI, and TEE were found to be equally effective in ruling out or confirming the diagnosis of TAD (**Table 4**). Accordingly, in the recent 2010 AHA guidelines for the diagnosis and management of patients with thoracic aortic disease, a class I recommendation was made that either urgent TEE, MRI, or CT imaging be used to determine a definitive diagnosis in patients with high clinical suspicion for aortic dissection. Furthermore, the AHA recommends that, if the initial diagnostic test is negative in a patient with high clinical suspicion for aortic dissection, a second imaging modality should be completed.[2]

In summary, TEE, CT, and MRI all show acceptable diagnostic abilities and the initial imaging modality should be dictated by patient characteristics and availability of resources. If the initial imaging test is negative in the context of a high clinical suspicion, the clinician should proceed with a second diagnostic imaging modality. The algorithm (**Fig. 2**) from the 2010 ACC/AHA guidelines summarizes a diagnostic approach to diagnostic decision making for AAD in the ED.

AAD: MANAGEMENT ISSUES

Once the diagnosis of AAD has been confirmed, the management decisions in the ED are straightforward. Patients with evidence of hypotension need to be urgently resuscitated with intravenous (IV) fluids, blood products, and immediately transported to the operating room to optimize survival chances.[1] Although there may be some advocacy for permissive hypotension in the management of ruptured abdominal aortic aneurysms to limit the use of blood products and to suppress exsanguination, there is no literature to support this strategy in the hypertensive patient with AAD.[73] The only contemporary report of minimal benefit with permissive hypotension in AAD management was in a small case series of endovascular patients who had endovascular stent grafts placed and observed for leaks[74]; no comments were provided regarding permissive hypotension in medical management alone, and this is not addressed in the ACC/AHA 2010 guidelines.[2] Conversely, in the hypotensive patient, use of vasopressors to support blood pressure must be cautious given the risk of propagating the dissection.[2] Similarly, inotropic agents may increase ventricular contraction rate and force, which will increase shear forces on the aortic wall. Blood pressures in 4 limbs should be constantly monitored to follow potential evolution of intimal flaps obstructing flow into an extremity and causing pseudohypotension. In cases of severe hypotension/shock or pulseless electrical activity with presumed pericardial tamponade, emergency pericardiocentesis may be warranted. For patients being transported to a regional vascular center for definitive care, all appropriate measures to optimize hemodynamic stability and safe transfer should be achieved before transportation of the patient.

Medical Management of AAD

In patients with hemodynamically stable dissections, the goals of ED management include pain control, heart rate and blood pressure control to avoid excessive shear forces on the intimal layers of the arterial walls (dP/dt = speed at which blood is ejected into the aorta with each ventricular contraction).[8] Analgesia can usually be achieved with titratable opioids, which relieve pain, decrease sympathetic tone, and augment the effects of rate control and vasodilation.[1,2] Target systolic blood pressures of 100 to 120 mm Hg and heart rates less than 60 beats/min can be achieved using β-adrenergic blockers (esmolol, labetalol) or vasodilators such as sodium nitroprusside, nitroglycerin, or fenoldopam. However, the use of vasodilators as a single agent is discouraged because of the associated reflex tachycardia and resulting increased shear forces across arterial intimal walls (dP/dt). As a result, a concomitant β-blocker (eg, esmolol) should be used (assuming no contraindications such as

Table 4
Summary of performance characteristics for advanced AAD imaging

Imaging Technique	Including Studies No.	Meta-Analysis Results				
		Sensitivity	Specificity	Positive LR	Negative LR	Diagnostic Odds Ratio
TEE	10	98 (95–99)	95 (92–97)	14.1 (6.0–33.2)	0.04 (0.02–0.08)	6.1 (5.0–7.2)
Helical CT	3	100 (96–100)	98 (87–99)	13.9 (4.2–46.0)	0.02 (0.01–0.11)	6.5 (4.4–8.7)
MRI	7	98 (95–99)	98 (95–100)	25.3 (11.1–57.1)	0.05 (0.03–0.10)	6.8 (5.5–8.0)

Data from Shiga T, Wajima Z, Apfel C, et al. Diagnostic accuracy of transesophageal echocardiography, helical computed tomography, and magnetic resonance imaging for suspected thoracic aortic dissection. Systematic review and meta-analysis. Arch Intern Med 2006;166:1350–6; and Greenberg RK, Haulon S, Khwaja J, et al. Contemporary management of acute aortic dissection. J Endovasc Ther 2003;10:476–85.

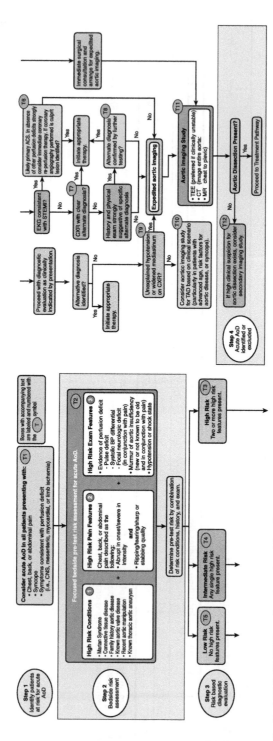

Fig. 2. AHA/ACC 2010 evaluation algorithm for AAD. ACS, acute coronary syndrome; AoD, aortic dissection; BP, blood pressure; CNS, central nervous system; CXR, chest radiograph; MR, magnetic resonance. (*Reproduced from* Hiratazka LF, Bakris GL, Beckman JA, et al. 2010 ACCF/AHA/AATS/ACR/ASA/SCA/SCAI/SIR/STS/SVM Guidelines for the diagnosis and management of patients with thoracic aortic disease. Circulation 2010;121:e266–369. doi:10.1161/CIR.0b013e33181d4739e; with permission.)

chronic obstructive pulmonary disease (COPD) or high-risk bronchospastic disease). Labetolol may be an attractive single-agent choice because it has both α_1-specific and nonspecific β-adrenergic properties (7:1 ratio of β vs α blockade for IV labetalol). Another advantage of these titratable IV agents is rapid onset and short duration of action, which can be turned off quickly as needed.[4] Trimethaphan (a ganglionic blocker and vasodilator) has both dP/dt and systolic blood pressure reduction properties, making it an acceptable alternative to esmolol/nitroprusside combination or labetalol, especially in the context of contraindications to either agent; side effects include tachyphylaxis, significant hypotension, respiratory depression, urinary retention, and ileus.[8] These blood pressure targets should be cautiously maintained without causing end-organ ischemia. Calcium channel blockers are less desirable agents for blood pressure and heart rate control, particularly nifedipine (and all dihydropyridines), which has negligible inotropic and chronotropic activities and may increase reflex sympathetic tone and arterial wall stress.[1,2]

The starting doses of various agents are listed in **Table 5**.

Surgical Management of AAD

Type A acute dissections require prompt surgical treatment in a qualified vascular or cardiac surgery center. Expeditious surgery can reduce in-hospital mortality to 27% compared with medically treated type A dissections (mortality 56%).[1] Autopsy studies have suggested that untreated type A dissections can increase mortality by 1% per hour up to a cumulative 50% mortality within the first 48 hours of diagnosis.[9]

The definitive management of type B dissections is less clear. Appropriate medical management can limit mortality to 10%.[1] Surgery may be reserved for patients with ongoing pain, refractory hypertension, occlusion of major arterial trunk origins, frank leaking or rupture, or development of local aneurysms. Patients with local aneurysms have been reported to have in-hospital 30-day mortalities of 32%[1]; the triad of hypotension, branch vessel involvement, and absence of chest pain is an independent predictor of in-hospital death.

Longer Term Follow-Up

After the acute phase of management, long-term β-blockade is warranted regardless of medical versus surgical management.[4] Repeat surgery is required in 10% to 20% of cases because of redissection, compression of mediastinal structures, blood leakage, or aneurysm formation. Type B dissections initially managed medically often go on to elective surgery because of aneurismal dilatation or limb ischemia.[4]

Routine follow-up examinations are recommended on a schedule of 3 to 6 months.[4]

Table 5 Initial medications for blood pressure control in aortic dissection			
Medication Class (Agent)	**Starting Dose**	**Infusion Regimen**	**Cautions for Use**
β-Blockers			
1. Esmolol	Bolus 500 μg/kg	50–200 μg/kg/min	COPD or high-risk bronchospasm; consider selective β-blocker such as metoprolol or atenolol
2. Labetalol	Bolus 20 mg every 5–10 min to 80–300 mg total	1–2 mg/min	
Sodium Nitroprusside		0.5–3.0 μg/kg/min	Concomitant use of β-blocker to avoid reflex tachycardia, possible cyanide toxicity with prolonged use

Pitfalls in AAD Management

Because the incidence of AAD is rare compared with other important causes of acute chest pain in the ED (eg, acute coronary syndrome [ACS], pulmonary embolism, pneumothorax, esophageal rupture), a rapid and reliable approach to ruling out AAD is important, especially in the context of a time-dependent emergency such as STEMI, when medical and reperfusion treatments must be implemented as soon as possible.[21] The incidence of STEMI is nearly 800 times that of AAD, but proximal dissection rarely can lead to STEMI.[21] Use of antiplatelet agents, anticoagulants, and fibrinolytics can be disastrous in the patient with STEMI who has a proximal AAD with coronary involvement as opposed to the more common atherosclerotic plaque rupture causes. Fatality rates of 71% have been reported in patients misdiagnosed with AAD-STEMI due to catastrophic hemorrhage.[21] Recognition of key risk factors, clinical features, or lack of response to conventional ACS treatments should prompt ED physicians to at least consider an AAD diagnosis before embarking on potentially irreversible fibrinolysis decisions.

Other barriers to expeditious diagnosis of AAD in the context of ED chest pain may include lack of awareness of AAD incidence/risk factors, lack of readily available screening tests for AAD, and institutional care pathways for more common chest pain presentations (eg, ACS, pulmonary embolism), which steer clinicians away from the rare, but equally dangerous, diagnosis of AAD.[2]

Prognosis for AAD

There has been little progress in developing prognostic methods to accurately predict outcomes for patients with AAD. The most common determinant of outcomes seems to be the maximal aortic diameter measurement,[75] but this is not universally reliable depending on different dissection types (A vs B). For type A dissections, observational data from the IRAD data registry (n = 591 patients) suggest that a diameter cutoff of 5.5 cm may be useful to guide elective surgery decisions, but there was no difference in mortality.[76] For type B dissections, an incremental increase of 5 mm in maximal aortic diameter on CT scan had an odds ratio of 1.41 (95% CI 1.04–1.92) of in-hospital death, rupture, or organ malperfusion in one retrospective series of 220 patients,[77] and a diameter of 40 mm or more was predictive of needing elective surgery in another series of 180 patients.[78] In a recent review of the IRAD database (n = 1480 type B patients), increasing ascending aortic dimensions were associated with higher surgical incidence, but no difference in mortality or cause of death at different width cutoffs (<40 mm, 41–45 mm, >46 mm).[79] However, it was noted that higher ascending aorta widths were associated with more open procedures involving root/aortic valve/ascending aorta/arch repairs, and those with widths less than 40 mm were more likely to undergo conservative endovascular repairs.

Recent ACC/AHA Guideline 2010 Recommendations

The recently published ACC/AHA guideline describes the following recommendations for management of AAD[2]:

1. Initial management (level of evidence)
   a. Class I recommendations
      i. IV β-blockade titrated to heart rate of 60 beats per minute or less in the absence of contraindications (C).
      ii. If β-blockade is contraindicated, consider nondihydropyridine calcium channel blockers for same goal as described earlier (C).

iii. After target heart rate is achieved, if persistent systolic blood pressure still is greater than 120 mm Hg then consider vasodilators (nitroprusside, angiotensin-converting enzyme inhibitors) administered intravenously to further reduce blood pressure without compromising end-organ perfusion (C).

iv. Beware β-blockade or calcium channel blockade if there is evidence of acute aortic regurgitation caused by loss of compensatory tachycardia (C).

b. Class III recommendations

i. Initiate rate control before using vasodilators to avoid reflex tachycardia causing increased aortic wall stresses and propagation of dissection (C).

2. Definitive management (level of evidence)

a. Urgent surgical consultation should be obtained for all patients diagnosed with AAD, regardless of anatomic location, once the diagnosis is made or highly suspected (C).

b. Ascending AAD should be urgently evaluated for immediate surgery to avoid life-threatening complications (B).

c. Descending AAD should be managed medically unless life-threatening complications arise (eg, malperfusion of end organs, dissection progression, enlarging aneurysm, worsening symptoms, or inability to control blood pressure [level B]).

Most of these recommendations are in keeping with other evidence sources reviewed in this article. These suggestions are manageable in the ED, provided that there is adequate access to resources for advanced diagnosis and critical care.

Acute Dissection in Pregnancy

Pregnant women with potential AAD present unique diagnostic problems for emergency physicians. Pregnancy is associated with several important hemodynamic and physiologic stresses for women.[28] These stresses include large changes in intravascular volume, compensatory cardiac output demands (heart rate, inotropism), and intimal wall connective tissue changes due to hormonal influences. Patients are most at risk of AAD expansion and rupture in the third trimester, especially during the peripartum and postpartum periods (up to 3 months after birth). The unique circumstances of preeclampsia can raise the risk of missed type A dissection due to overlap with type B symptoms.[28] Urgent surgical repair by specialized vascular and obstetric teams may be warranted because of unique considerations of aortic repair coupled to maintaining fetal viability. If the timing is appropriate for fetal development, urgent AAD repair may coincide with emergency delivery by cesarean section, with strict monitoring of maternal and fetal hemodynamics.[26,28,80] Placental malperfusion is the leading cause of fetal death if the advancing dissection involves occlusion of the internal iliac artery and uterine arterial insufficiency. There are case reports of AAD in pregnancy managed surgically with concomitant operative delivery, with the presence of previously discussed risk factors including cocaine use,[25] Ehlers-Danlos syndrome,[24] and Takayasu arteritis.[27] In pregnant women with acute undifferentiated chest pain or dyspnea presentations, AAD should be high on the differential diagnosis for evaluation and management in the ED.

AAD: SUMMARY

For emergency physicians assessing acute undifferentiated chest pain, the diagnosis of AAD remains one of the most sinister challenges. The key clinical features and initial diagnostic tests do not always lead to this diagnosis, and the potential mimics involving cardiovascular, abdominal, neurologic, and other systems are numerous and easily misleading. Astute physicians should always have an awareness of potential risk factors for AAD, classic versus atypical presentations, careful physical examination findings, and a high index of suspicion/low threshold for moving on to advanced imaging techniques to reliably include or exclude this diagnosis. An ongoing awareness of new diagnostic modalities to facilitate the AAD diagnosis should be maintained. Once properly diagnosed, initial management steps targeting pain, heart rate, and blood pressure control can be undertaken to optimize hemodynamic stability, and subsequent definitive surgical consultation can then be undertaken. Failure to consider AAD in these situations (and document risk assessments accordingly) can lead to clinically adverse outcomes for patients and medicolegal liability for physicians.

REFERENCES

1. Ankel F. Aortic dissection. In: Marx JA, Hockberger RS, Walls RM, et al, editors. Rosen's emergency medicine: concepts and clinical practice. 7th edition. Philadelphia: Mosby Elsevier Publishing; 2010. p. 1088–92. Chapter 83.
2. Hiratazka LF, Bakris GL, Beckman JA, et al. 2010 ACCF/AHA/AATS/ACR/ASA/SCA/SCAI/SIR/STS/SVM guidelines for the diagnosis and management of patients with thoracic aortic disease. Circulation 2010;121:e266–369.
3. Hagan PG, Neinaber CA, Isselbacher EM, et al. The International Registry of Acute Aortic Dissection (IRAD) – new insights into an old disease. JAMA 2000;283:897–903.
4. Chen K, Varon J, Wenker OC, et al. Acute thoracic aortic dissection: the basics. J Emerg Med 1997;15:859–67.
5. Haffner JW, Parrish SE, Hubler JR, et al. Risk factor documentation for life-threatening disease in US emergency department patients [abstract 209]. Ann Emerg Med 2006;48:S65.
6. Thoracic aortic dissection: Medicolegal difficulties. CMPA Bulletin IS0768-E 2008. Available at: https://www.cmpa-acpm.ca/cmpapd04/docs/resource_files/infosheets/2007/com_is0768-e.cfm. Accessed March 11, 2011.
7. Risk identification for all physicians – thoracic aortic dissections: "tearing" apart the data. CMPA bulletin R10812E 2008. Available at: https://www.cmpa-acpm.ca/cmpapd04/docs/resource_files/risk_id/2008/com_ri0812-e.cfm. Accessed October 8, 2008.
8. Knaut AL, Cleveland JC. Aortic emergencies. Emerg Med Clin North Am 2003;21:817–45.
9. Daily PO, Trueblood HW, Stinson EB, et al. Management of acute aortic dissections. Ann Thorac Surg 1970;10(3):237–47.
10. DeBakey ME, McCollum CH, Crawford ES, et al. Dissection and dissecting aneurysms of the aorta: 20 year follow-up of 527 patients treated surgically. Surgery 1982;92:1118.
11. Larson EW, Edwards WD. Risk factors for aortic dissection: a necropsy study of 161 patients. Am J Cardiol 1984;53:849–55.
12. Suzuki T, Mehta RH, Ince H, et al. Clinical profiles and outcomes of acute type B aortic dissection in the current era: lessons from the International Registry of Acute Aortic Dissection (IRAD). Circulation 2003;108(Suppl 1):11312–7.
13. Ando M, Okita Y, Tagusari O, et al. A surgically treated case of Takayasu's arteritis complicated by aortic dissections localized in the ascending and abdominal aorta. J Vasc Surg 2000;31:1042–5.
14. Fisher A, Holroyd BR. Cocaine-associated dissection of the thoracic aorta. J Emerg Med 1992;10:723–7.
15. McDermott JC, Schuster MR, Crummy AB, et al. Crack and aortic dissection. Wis Med J 1993;92:453–5.

16. Perron AD, Gibbs M. Thoracic aortic dissection secondary to crack cocaine ingestion. Am J Emerg Med 1997;15:507–9.
17. Palmiere C, Burkhardt S, Staub C, et al. Thoracic aortic dissection associated with cocaine abuse. Forensic Sci Int 2004;141:137–42.
18. Rogers RL, McCormack R. Aortic disasters. Emerg Med Clin North Am 2004;22: 887–908.
19. Schorr JS, Horowitz MD, Livingstone AS. Recreational weight lifting and aortic dissection: case report. J Vasc Surg 1993;17:774–6.
20. Ragucci MV, Thistle HG. Weight lifting and type II aortic dissection. A case report. J Sports Med Phys Fitness 2004;44:424–7.
21. Woo K, Schneider JI. High-risk chief complaints I: chest pain – the big three. Emerg Med Clin North Am 2009;27:685–712.
22. Kimura N, Yamaguchi A, Noguchi K, et al. Type B aortic dissection associated with *Salmonella* infection. Gen Thorac Cardiovasc Surg 2007;55:212–6.
23. Choi JB, Yang HW, Oh SK, et al. Rupture of ascending aorta secondary to tuberculous aortitis. Ann Thorac Surg 2003;75:1965–7.
24. Babatasi G, Massetti M, Bhoyroo S, et al. Pregnancy with aortic dissection in Ehler-Danlos syndrome. Staged replacement of the total aorta (10 year follow up). Eur J Cardiothorac Surg 1997;12:671–4.
25. Madu EC, Shala B, Baugh D. Crack-cocaine-associated aortic dissection in early pregnancy-a case report. Angiology 1999;50:163–8.
26. Shihata M, Preforius V, MacArthur R. Repair of an acute type A aortic dissection combined with an emergency cesarean section in a pregnant woman. Interact Cardiovasc Thorac Surg 2008;7:938–40.
27. Lakhi NA, Jones J. Takayasu's arteritis in pregnancy complicated by peripartum aortic dissection. Arch Gynecol Obstet 2010;282:103–6.
28. Stout CL, Scott EC, Stokes GK, et al. Successful repair of a ruptured Stanford type B aortic dissection during pregnancy. J Vasc Surg 2010;51:990–2.
29. Kim TE, Smith DD. Thoracic aortic dissection in an 18-year-old woman with no risk factors. J Emerg Med 2010;38:e14–44.
30. Klompas M. Does this patient have an acute thoracic aortic dissection? JAMA 2002;287:2262–72.
31. Bushnell J, Brown J. Clinical assessment for acute thoracic aortic dissection. Ann Emerg Med 2005;46:90–2.
32. Von Koloditsch Y, Schwartz AG, Nienaber CA. Clinical prediction of acute aortic dissection. Arch Intern Med 2000;160:2977–82.
33. Gallagher EJ. Clinical utility of likelihood ratios. Ann Emerg Med 1998;31:391–7.
34. Chew HC, Lim SH. Aortic dissection presenting with atrial fibrillation. Am J Emerg Med 2006;24:379–80.
35. Den Uil CA, Caliskan K, Bekkers JA. Intractable supraventricular tachycardia as first presentation of thoracic aortic dissection: case report. Int J Cardiol 2010;144:e5–7.
36. Liu JF, Ge QM, Chen M, et al. Painless type B aortic dissection presenting as acute congestive heart failure. Am J Emerg Med 2010;28:646.e5–7.
37. Meron G, Kurkciyan I, Sterz F, et al. Non-traumatic aortic dissection or rupture as a cause of cardiac arrest: presentation and outcome. Resuscitation 2004;60: 143–50.
38. Lee CC, Chang WT, Fang CC, et al. Sudden death caused by dissecting thoracic aortic aneurysm in a patient with autosomal dominant polycystic kidney disease. Resuscitation 2004;63:93–6.
39. Vuckovic SA. An usual presentation of ascending aortic arch dissection. J Emerg Med 2000;19:149–52.

40. Young J, Herd AM. Painless acute aortic dissection and rupture presenting as syncope. J Emerg Med 2002;22:171–4.

41. Sung PS, Fang CW, Chen CH. Acute aortic dissection mimicking basilar artery occlusion in a patient presenting with sudden coma. J Clin Neurosci 2010;17: 952–3.

42. Nadour W, Goldwasser B, Beiderman RW, et al. Silent aortic dissection presenting as transient locked-in syndrome. Tex Heart Inst J 2008;35:359–61.

43. Demiroyoguran NS, Karcioglu O, Topacoglu H, et al. Painless aortic dissection with bilateral carotid involvement presenting with vertigo as the chief complaint. Emerg Med J 2006;23:e15.

44. Greenwood WR, Robinson MD. Painless dissection of the thoracic aorta. Am J Emerg Med 1986;4:330–3.

45. Beach C, Manthey D. Painless acute aortic dissection presenting as left lower extremity numbness. Am J Emerg Med 1998;16:49–51.

46. Joo JB, Cummings AJ. Acute thoracoabdominal aortic dissection presenting as painless, transient paralysis of the lower extremities: a case report. J Emerg Med 2000;19:333–7.

47. Hsu YC, Lin CC. Paraparesis as the major initial presentation of aortic dissection: report of four cases. Acta Neurol Taiwan 2004;13:192–7.

48. Karascostas D, Anthomelides G, Ioannides P, et al. Acute paraplegia in painless aortic dissection. Rich imaging with poor outcomes. Spinal Cord 2010;48:87–9.

49. Huang SM, Du F, Wang CY, et al. Aortic dissection presenting as isolated lower extremity pain in a young man. Am J Emerg Med 2010;28:1061.e1–3.

50. Liu WP, Ng KC. Acute thoracic aortic dissection presenting as sore throat: report of a case. Yale J Biol Med 2004;77:53–8.

51. Chen HC, Lin CJ, Tzeng YS, et al. Hoarseness as an unusual initial presentation of aortic dissection. Eur Arch Otorhinolaryngol 2005;262:189–91.

52. Al-Hity W, Playforth MJ. Collapse, hoarseness of the voice and swelling and bruising of the neck: an unusual presentation of thoracic aortic dissection. Emerg Med J 2001;18:508–9.

53. Tristano AG, Tairouz Y. Painless right hemorrhagic pleural effusions as presentation sign of aortic dissecting aneurysm. Am J Med 2005;188:794–5.

54. O'Dell KB, Hakim SN. Dissecting thoracic aortic aneurysm in a 22-year-old man. Ann Emerg Med 1990;19:316–8.

55. Firstenberg MS, Sai-Sudhakar CB, Sirak JH, et al. Intestinal ischemia complicating ascending aortic dissection: first things first. Ann Thorac Surg 2007;84:e8–9.

56. Gorospe L, Sendino A, Pacheco R, et al. Chronic aortic dissection as a cause of fever of unknown origin. South Med J 2002;95:1067–70.

57. Jolin SW, Steinkeler S, Yeh C. Invasive thymoma presenting as aortic dissection. Ann Emerg Med 1991;20:1233–5.

58. Vohra HA, Alzetani A, Guha T, et al. A thymic carcinoid mimicking acute aortic dissection. Cardiovasc Surg 2003;11:96–8.

59. Reichman EF, Weber JM. Undiagnosed Takayasu's arteritis mimicking an acute aortic dissection. J Emerg Med 2004;27:139–42.

60. Hirata K, Kyushima M, Asato H. Electrocardiographic abnormalities in patients with acute aortic dissection. Am J Cardiol 1995;76:1207.

61. Marill KA. Serum D-dimer is a sensitive test for the detection of acute aortic dissection: a pooled meta-analysis. J Emerg Med 2008;34(4):367–76.

62. Ohlmann P, Faure A, Morel O, et al. Diagnostic and prognostic value of circulating D-dimers in patients with acute aortic dissection. Crit Care Med 2006;34: 1358–64.

63. Sutherland A, Escano J, Coon TP. D-Dimer as the sole screening test for acute aortic dissection: a review of the literature. Ann Emerg Med 2008;52(4):339–43.

64. Shimony A, Filion KB, Mottillo S, et al. Meta-analysis of usefulness of d-dimer to diagnose acute aortic dissection. Am J Cardiol 2011;107(8):1227–34.

65. Suzuki T, Katoh H, Tsuchio Y, et al. Diagnostic implications of elevated levels of smooth-muscle myosin heavy-chain protein in acute aortic dissection. The Smooth Muscle Myosin Heavy Chain Study. Ann Intern Med 2000;133(7):537–41.

66. Suzuki T, Distante A, Zizza A, et al. Preliminary experience with the smooth muscle troponin-like protein, calponin, as a novel biomarker for diagnosing acute aortic dissection. Eur Heart J 2008;29(11):1439–45.

67. Schillinger M, Domanovits H, Bayegan K, et al. C-reactive protein and mortality in patients with acute aortic dissection. Intensive Care Med 2002;28:740–5.

68. Wheat MW. Pathogenesis of aortic dissection. In: Doroghazi RM, Slater EE, editors. Aortic dissection. New York: McGraw-Hill; 1983. p. 55–70.

69. Sarasin FP, Louis-Simonet M, Gaspoz JM, et al. Detecting acute thoracic aortic dissection in emergency department: time constraints and choice of the optimal diagnostic test. Ann Emerg Med 1996;28(3):278–88.

70. Fojtik JP, Costantino TG, Dean AJ. The diagnosis of aortic dissection by emergency medicine ultrasound. J Emerg Med 2007;32:191–6.

71. Nienaber CA, Von Kodolitsch Y, Nicolas V, et al. The diagnosis of thoracic aortic dissection by non-invasive imaging procedures. N Engl J Med 1993;328:1–9.

72. Shiga T, Wajima Z, Apfel C, et al. Diagnostic accuracy of transesophageal echocardiography, helical computed tomography, and magnetic resonance imaging for suspected thoracic aortic dissection. Systematic review and meta-analysis. Arch Intern Med 2006;166:1350–6.

73. Greenberg RK, Haulon S, Khwaja J, et al. Contemporary management of acute aortic dissection. J Endovasc Ther 2003;10:476–85.

74. Chu MW, Forbes TL, Lawlor DK, et al. Endovascular repair of thoracic aortic disease: early and midterm experience. Vasc Endovascular Surg 2007;41(3):186–91.

75. Keren A, Kim CB, Hu BS, et al. Accuracy of biplane and multiplane transesophageal echocardiography in diagnosis of typical acute aortic dissection and intramural hematoma. J Am Coll Cardiol 1996;28:627–36.

76. Pape LA, Tsai TT, Isselbacher EM, et al. Aortic diameter > or = 5.5 cm is not a good indicator of type A aortic dissection: observations from the International Registry of Acute Aortic Dissection (IRAD). Circulation 2007;116(10):1120–7.

77. Sakakura K, Kubo N, Ako J, et al. Determinants of in-hospital death and rupture in patients with a Stanford B aortic dissection. Circ J 2007;71(10):1521–4.

78. Hata M, Sezai A, Niino T, et al. Prognosis for patients with type B acute aortic dissection: risk analysis of early death and requirement for elective surgery. Circ J 2007;71(8):1279–82.

79. Booher AM, Isselbacher EM, Nienaber CA, et al. Ascending thoracic aorta dimension and outcomes in acute type B dissection (from the International Registry of Acute Aortic Dissection [IRAD]). Am J Cardiol 2011;107:315–20.

80. Papatsonis DN, Heetkamp A, van den Hombergh C, et al. Acute type A aortic dissection complicating pregnancy at 32 weeks: surgical repair after cesarean section. Am J Perinatol 2009;26(2):153–7.

Pulmonary Embolism

David W. Ouellette, MD, FRCPC[a,b,*], Catherine Patocka, MDCM[c]

KEYWORDS

- Pulmonary embolism • Diagnosis • Pregnancy • Radiation
- Venous thromboembolism • Thrombophilia • Anticoagulation
- Emergency department

Pulmonary embolism (PE) represents one of the greatest challenges in emergency medicine. It is a potentially life-threatening diagnosis that is seen in patients with chest pain and/or dyspnea, but can span the entire clinical spectrum of medical presentations from asymptomatic to cardiovascular collapse. The true incidence of PE in the general population is unknown,[1,2] but it is estimated to have an annual incidence in the United States of greater than 650,000 cases, or 0.5 to 1 per 1000.[3–6] From a patient perspective, PE has significant morbidity and mortality. It is one of the leading causes of death in the US and the third leading cause of death in hospitalized patients.[3,4] In addition, the chronic sequelae of PE, pulmonary hypertension and postthrombotic syndrome, can cause significant morbidity.[7,8] From a clinician's perspective, PE represents an entity that spans the spectrum of medical presentations from asymptomatic to cardiovascular collapse and death, and does not have any particular historical feature, physical examination finding, laboratory test, or diagnostic modality that can independently and confidently exclude its possibility.[6] Therefore, it is not surprising that PE is potentially missed more than 400,000 times per year.[9] Autopsy studies demonstrate the frequent occurrence of PE, and suggest that it is undiagnosed more often than it is diagnosed.[10,11] Further, Rodger and colleagues[5] suggest that only 30% of PE are diagnosed antemortem. Accordingly, increased efforts to diagnose PE have been globally observed, resulting in a high percentage of negative outpatient computed tomography (CT) angiograms, and subsequent concern about the radiobiological detriment of ionizing radiation.[12] It is estimated that almost 30% of suspected acute PEs may not need imaging if the proper use of clinical assessment and D-dimer were universally applied.[12]

The authors have nothing to disclose.
[a] Department of Medicine, Schulich School of Medicine and Dentistry, University of Western Ontario, London, Ontario, Canada
[b] Division of Emergency Medicine, Department of Medicine, London Health Sciences Centre, 800 Commissioners Road, London, Ontario N6A 5W9, Canada
[c] McGill Emergency Medicine Residency Program, Royal Victoria Hospital, McGill University, Room A4.62, 687 Pine Avenue West, Montreal, Quebec H3A 1A1, Canada
* Corresponding author. Division of Emergency Medicine, Department of Medicine, London Health Sciences Centre, 800 Commissioners Road, London, Ontario N6A 5W9, Canada.
E-mail address: douellettemd@gmail.com

Emerg Med Clin N Am 30 (2012) 329–375
doi:10.1016/j.emc.2011.12.004
0733-8627/12/$ – see front matter © 2012 Elsevier Inc. All rights reserved.

The role of the emergency physician (EP) is to identify potentially life-threatened patients who would benefit from early intervention and treatment, and to stabilize and treat accordingly. Although the treatment of PE is straightforward and algorithmic, the diagnostic approach is subject to significant debate and variability. It begins with an assessment of clinical probability based on the clinical presentation and risk factors, made either implicitly according to clinical judgment, or explicitly by means of clinical decision rules (CDR). Patients are classified into several categories of pretest probability (PTP), which then drives the diagnostic work-up and facilitates the interpretation of diagnostic tests.[13] The challenge, variability, and seriousness of the diagnosis has made PE an important area of research in medicine, with more than 800 to 1000 new articles published every year in the medical literature. Although numerous reviews on risk factors, diagnosis, pathophysiology, and treatment of PE have recently been published, none have addressed the topic from the point of view of the EP and the emergency department (ED) environment. This clinical review focuses on 4 main topics relevant to the EP when approaching patients with suspected or confirmed PE: (1) when to suspect the diagnosis (pathophysiology, epidemiology, risk factors, and clinical features); (2) how to make the diagnosis (diagnostic criteria, approach to investigation, and radiation risks); (3) treatment of patients with PE, including anticoagulation and thrombolysis; and (4) PE in pregnancy.

PATHOPHYSIOLOGY

PE is an obstruction of the pulmonary artery (PA) or its branches. PE most commonly occurs when a thrombus or part of a thrombus dislodges, forming an embolus, and travels through the venous system via the right ventricle (RV) into the lung. Although they may occur in any part of the venous system, most thrombi originate in the lower extremity.[14,15] Partial or total occlusion of the pulmonary circulation may also be caused by nonthrombotic agents such as cells (adipocytes, hematopoietic, amniotic, trophoblastic, or tumor cells), bacteria, fungi, parasites, foreign material (eg, central venous catheters), or gas.[16]

Thrombus formation ultimately results from the imbalance of clot formation and breakdown. Fibrin formation and deposition is increased, triggered by systemic inflammation, vascular injury, acquired hypercoagulable states, genetic thrombophilias, neoplastic abnormalities, and/or sluggish blood flow.[17] The presence of one or more elements of Virchow's triad, physiologic effects, and advancing age are important risk factors in the formation of VTE. With advancing age comes predisposition to dehydration, acquired hypercoagulable states (ie, malignancy), decreased valvular competence, venous stasis, and more cumulative effects of inflammatory damage to the vascular endothelium.[6]

Hemodynamic response to an embolus depends on its size, the individual's cardiopulmonary reserve, and many neurohumoral effects.[18] Therefore, clinical presentation may vary from asymptomatic to hemodynamic compromise and cardiogenic shock. For example, distal lung infarction results in tissue necrosis, chemokine production, and hyperinflammation. This process can produce focal, sharp, pleuritic chest pain and, over several days, lead to pleural effusion and/or consolidation. In severe cases of obstruction, hemodynamic decompensation is secondary to physical obstruction of blood flow and the resulting release of humoral factors from platelets, plasma, and tissue.[3] Acute PE may cause a progressive increase in pulmonary vascular resistance leading to increased right ventricular afterload and ultimately right ventricular dilatation and failure.[3] Right ventricular enlargement causes a leftward shift of the interventricular septum and impaired filling of the left ventricle, thereby impairing left ventricular function and cardiac output.[18] In addition to its mechanical effects, acute PE also impairs the efficient transfer of oxygen and carbon dioxide across the lung via several mechanisms. Readers are referred to the review by Goldhaber and Elliot[3] for a more in-depth discussion of the pathophysiology of PE.

EPIDEMIOLOGY AND RISK FACTORS

The overall incidence of first-time VTE is estimated to be between 70 and 113 cases/100,000/year.[19,20] Given the possibility of asymptomatic and atypical presentation, it is generally accepted that many cases of PE go unrecognized. In fact, some investigators estimate that up to 1 in 3 cases are not identified.[6,21] Early autopsy studies and pooled data suggested that over 60% of hospitalized patients had PE.[4,22] In addition, 60% to 80% of patients with DVT also have PE, but more than half are asymptomatic.[4] More recent pooled data since 1985 showed a 19% rate of PE at autopsy with 6% of patients found to have a large or fatal PE.[22] Ultimately, it may be more important to question which PEs are clinical significant and pathologic. Although there is no reliable way to measure it, PE is probably missed in the ED.[23]

The EP should be aware that PE can be a challenging diagnosis and should approach any possibility of the diagnosis seriously and systematically. PE is one of the leading causes of death in the US, and the third leading cause of death in hospitalized patients.[3,4,24–26] Mortality is estimated to be 50,000 to 200,000 patients annually, 3% to 10% if treated, and 15% to 30% if untreated.[5,6,24,27] The Prospective Investigation of Pulmonary Embolism Diagnosis (PIOPED) showed a case fatality rate of 2.5%,[28] whereas studies of low-molecular-weight heparin (LMWH) showed a rate of only 0.6% to 1.0%.[29,30] These rates are likely underestimated because patients were excluded if they were too ill to participate and most deaths from PE occur within the first 2.5 hours after the diagnosis.

The risk of VTE varies as a result of a complex interaction between multiple population risk factors. Similar to the risk factors used in the assessment of acute coronary syndrome (ACS), population risk factors provide physicians with elements that effect patient's risk of developing VTE over time. They are less useful in guiding an emergency clinician's assessment of an individual acutely symptomatic patient at the point of investigation.[31] Horlander and colleagues[32] reported a higher incidence of VTE in woman younger than 55 years, but greater among men in the older population. In the same study, an analysis of national mortality data, rates of death were 20% to 30% higher among men. Stein and colleagues[33] found that the rate of diagnosis of PE was higher in women than men (60 vs 42 per 100,000), but the age-adjusted rate was comparable.[28,33] The incidence of DVT and PE are similar in African Americans and Caucasians, whereas the mortality from PE is 50% higher in African Americans.[32–34] Asian, Pacific Islander, and American Indian patients have an even lower risk of VTE.[32,35] Young age does not exclude the diagnosis of PE, however, it is uncommon in infants and children.[36] Increasing age is accompanied by an exponential increase in PE/DVT, yet the diagnosis is missed more often in elderly patients.[19,37] In this population, a certain degree of respiratory symptoms may be inappropriately labeled as chronic.[4]

Although the definition of recognized risk factors used by individual studies varies, PIOPED II data suggests that most patients with first-time VTE have 1 or more recognized risk factors (**Box 1**).[38] However, Morgenthaler and Ryu[39] found that 12% of patients with PE lacked any known risk factor.

Box 1
Risk factors for PE[a]

Surgery within the last 3 months
Travel $\geq$4 hours in the past month
Prior pulmonary embolism
Immobilization
Trauma to lower extremity and pelvis during the past 3 months
Current or past history of thrombophilias
Malignancy
Stroke
Paresis
Paralysis
Heart failure
Chronic obstructive pulmonary disease (COPD)
Smoking
Central venous instrumentation within the past 3 months

[a] Of the patients with pulmonary embolism, 94% had $\geq$1 of the above risk factors.
Data from Stein PD, Beemath A, Matta F, et al. Clinical characteristics of patients with acute pulmonary embolism: data from PIOPED II. Am J Med 2007;120(10):871–9.

Risk factors are further categorized as inherited or acquired (transient or permanent). Inherited risk factors include major hereditary prothrombotic conditions, and they are listed in **Box 2**. The relative risk of VTE is increased by 2 to 10 times in patients with a genetic thrombophilia, but the actual risk is still low.[40] Factor V Leiden is the most common inherited risk factor and is present in about 5% of the normal population.[24,41] Antiphospholipid antibodies are associated with recurrent, unexplained fetal loss.[42] These conditions are usually only discovered after the first episode of VTE and should be suspected in any patient who presents at an early age (<40–50 years) with a PE.[42,43] **Table 1** presents the incidence of various thrombophilic disorders and associated VTE as well as the subsequent relative risk for VTE.[12]

Most first-time VTE occurs in patients with risk factors acquired over time (**Box 3**). Immobility is the most common acquired risk factor among patients with PE.[38] In addition, an association exists between atherosclerotic disease and spontaneous venous

---

Box 2
Inherited risk factors for pulmonary embolism

Factor V Leiden mutation
Antiphospholipid antibody syndrome
Antithrombin III deficiency
Protein C deficiency
Protein S deficiency
Prothrombin gene mutation
Increased factor VIII activity
Activated protein C (APC) resistance
Dysfibrinogenemia
Hyperhomocysteinemia

Table 1
Incidence of various thrombophilic disorders and associated VTE

Thrombophilic Disorders	Prevalence of Disorders in Patients with Unexplained VTE (%)	Prevalence of Disorders in General Population (%)	Frequency of VTE with Disorder (%)	Relative Risk for VTE
Inherited				
Antithrombin III deficiency	0.5–8	0.02	90	8–10
Protein C deficiency	1.5–11.5	0.3	8	4–10
Protein S deficiency	1.5–13.2	—	74–100	8–10
Factor V Leiden	20	5[a]	57	2–8
Prothrombin 20210-A mutation	6	2[a]	6	2.8
Elevated factor VIII levels	25	11[a]	—	5–6
Elevated factor XI levels	—	—	—	2.2
Heparin cofactor II deficiency	—	—	36	—
Dysfibrinogenemia	—	—	10	—
Hyperhomocysteinemia	10	5–10	—	2.5
Acquired				
Antiphospholipid syndrome	—	—	29–55	11

[a] Prevalence of disorder among whites in the general population.
Modified and reprinted from Stein PD, Matta F. Acute pulmonary embolism. Curr Probl Cardiol 2010;35(7):314–76; with permission from Elsevier.

thrombosis.[44] Thus, the most common reversible risk factors for PE include obesity, cigarette smoking, hypertension, and immobility. The degree and duration of reduced mobility or immobility that alters the risk remains unclear. A sedentary lifestyle and occupations that require prolonged ground travel or long periods of sitting increase the risk of thromboembolism. Beasley and colleagues coined the term 'eThrombosis' to describe thrombotic events secondary to prolonged periods sitting in front of the computer.[45] Air travel is a frequently quoted risk factor, but the overall incidence of severe pulmonary embolism during air travel is extremely low, only 0.4 cases per million passengers, and is primarily present in those who fly further than 5000 km (3000 miles) or for longer than 6 hours.[46] Among surgical patients, 15% of postoperative deaths may be associated with PE,[4] and the risk continues several weeks to months beyond the immediate postoperative period.[43] The most high-risk procedures are neurosurgical, oncologic, and orthopedic.[47] In patients suffering major trauma, Geerts and colleagues[48] found a 58% incidence of DVT in the lower extremity, with 18% incidence in the proximal veins. Femur, tibial, pelvic, and spinal trauma patients seem to be the most high-risk population.

Women who are pregnant or immediately postpartum are 5 to 10 times more likely to have a PE than nonpregnant patients.[24] Mechanical obstruction of blood flow leads to stasis, endothelial injury is common particularly during delivery or cesarean section, and the inherent hypercoagulable state is caused by a decrease in protein S and increase in circulating procoagulants.[49] The incidence of PE is between 1 in 20 and 1 in 1400 deliveries, with a mortality of 1 to 2 cases per 100,000 pregnancies.[24] The

---

Box 3
Acquired risk factors for pulmonary embolism

Prior history of VTE
Malignancy
Immobilization (travel, paralysis, bedridden state)
Trauma
Surgery
Pregnancy and the puerperium
Oral contraceptives/hormone replacement therapy
Central venous access devices
Advanced age
Smoking
Obesity

Medical illness

Congestive heart failure
Stroke
Sepsis/infection
Hyperviscosity syndromes: polycythemia, multiple myeloma
Nephrotic syndrome
Human immunodeficiency virus
Behçet disease

Other

Heparin-induced thrombocytopenia
Warfarin (initiation of therapy)
Chemotherapy
Plaster immobilization of injured extremity

---

highest risk time is in the immediate postpartum period which carries a 3 to 5 fold increase risk of PE.[50] A significant increase in the rate of PE also been observed with the increased rate of cesarean sections.[51]

Oral contraceptives and estrogen replacement increase the risk of VTE with a three-fold increased relative risk, and approximately 20 to 30 cases per 100,000 patients per year are reported. Originally the increased risk was attributed to the high estrogen content of the early OCP, however low estrogen plus progesterone OCP have also been associated with thrombogenicity.[52] The absolute risk remains low at 1 case per 10,000 patients per year and increases to 3 to 4 cases per 10,000 patients per year during OCP use.[52] Hormone replacement therapy increases the risk for PE by 2 to 4 times.[24]

Malignancy is identified in 17% of patients with VTE.[53] There is a well-established link between idiopathic PE and the subsequent development of cancer. Procoagulants can be produced and present in the body well before the diagnosis of cancer is made.[24,54] Pancreatic carcinoma has the highest incidence, whereas bladder tumors have the lowest incidence. Patients with lung, brain, or ovarian tumors are also particularly prone to the development of DVT and PE.[53] Many other medical conditions are associated with an increased risk of VTE.[55]

In general, EPs use population risk factors as part of their determination of the pretest probability. It can be particularly difficult for the EP to delineate which of the

Table 2
Adjusted odds ratio for PE risk factors

Historical Feature or Risk Factor	Adjusted OR (95% CI)
Patient history of VTE	2.90 (2.32–3.64)
Surgery within the previous 4 wk	2.27 (1.70–3.02)
Current estrogen use	2.31 (1.63–3.27)
Personal history of non–cancer-related thrombophilia	1.99 (1.21–3.30)
Active or metastatic cancer	1.92 (1.43–2.57)
Immobilization	1.72 (1.34–2.21)
Family history of VTE	1.51 (1.14–2.00)
Age >50 y	1.35 (1.10–1.67)
Obesity (BMI >30 kg/m²)[a]	1.13 (0.93–1.38)
Sudden onset of symptoms[a]	0.88 (0.73–1.06)
History of malignancy, now inactive[a]	0.82 (0.56–1.18)
Trauma within the previous 4 wk[a]	0.78 (0.37–1.65)
Pregnancy or postpartum state (pregnancy within past 4 wk)[a]	0.60 (0.29–1.26)
Smoking tobacco currently	0.59 (0.46–0.76)
Female sex	0.57 (0.47–0.69)

Abbreviations: BMI, body mass index; CI, confidence interval.
[a] Not statistically significant.
Adapted from Courtney DM, Kline JA, Kabrhel C, et al. Clinical features from the history and physical examination that predict the presence or absence of pulmonary embolism in symptomatic emergency department patients: results of a prospective, multicenter study. Ann Emerg Med 2010;55(4):307–15; with permission from Elsevier.

multitude of population risk factors for VTE affects the risk of PE in the individual patient presenting to the ED. A recent large prospective study of 7940 patients presenting to the ED with signs and symptoms that suggest PE attempted to delineate the predictive value of certain risk factors in PE. They calculated the adjusted odds ratios (ORs) for each of the variables (**Table 2**).[31] Factors found to be useful included prior history of VTE, surgery within the previous 4 weeks, current estrogen use, history of non–cancer-related thrombophilia, active or metastatic cancer, and immobilization.

CLINICAL FEATURES

The combination of classic findings of chest pain, dyspnea, and hemoptysis are present in fewer than 20% of patients.[56] Any complaints related to pain, shortness of breath, nonspecific malaise or functional deterioration, extremity discomfort, weakness, dizziness, or syncope could be a presentation of PE.[23] Indeed, most clinical manifestations in the diagnosis of acute PE are not sensitive, and none are specific.[12] PIOPED I and II found dyspnea, tachypnea, or pleuritic chest pain in 92% and 97% of patients, respectively.[38,57] Furthermore, 98% of patients with PE in the PIOPED study presented with one of those 3 symptoms or signs of DVT.[38,57] Most data on clinical manifestations are derived from a population already identified by the study physicians as patients with a possibility of PE and study samples generally do not include patients who were too ill or died suddenly.[12] Moreover, on physical examination, no finding is sensitive or specific for PE.[12] Physical examination may fail to reveal any clues in 28% to 58% of patients.[58]

Classically, the clinical features of PE in patients are now divided into several syndromes of presentation. These syndromes and their prevalence among patients with PE from the PIOPED II study are: (1) syndrome of pulmonary hemorrhage or infarction characterized by pleuritic chest pain or hemoptysis (41%); (2) syndrome of isolated dyspnea, in the absence of circulatory collapse, pleuritic pain, or hemoptysis (36%); and (3) syndrome of circulatory collapse defined as loss of consciousness or systolic blood pressure of 80 mm Hg or less (8%).[59,60] Hemoptysis occurs in one-third of patients with the pulmonary infarction syndrome according to the Urokinase Pulmonary Embolism Trial in 1973,[61] but more recent research does not support it as a statistically significant predictor of PE (**Tables 3** and **4**).[31,61] Pleuritic chest pain, one of the classic clinical features of PE, has been shown in many studies to be sensitive for PE, but is more common in older patients with cardiopulmonary disease.[62,63] The clinical presentation of isolated dyspnea depends mostly on the patient's cardiopulmonary reserve and the degree of pulmonary vascular obstruction. Patients may present asymptomatic with up to 50% obstruction of their pulmonary vasculature.[64] In addition, it may be challenging to clinically distinguish patients with other causes of dyspnea such as congestive heart failure (CHF), COPD, hyperventilation, and reactive airway disease. Circulatory collapse is the most severe form and may present with overt cardiac arrest, hemodynamic instability, or transient syncope. It is estimated that PE represents 4.5% of all cardiac arrests. The most common presenting rhythm was pulseless electrical activity, with 36% having a large central PE shown by transesophageal echocardiography (TEE).[65] Hemodynamic instability results from persistent right ventricular obstruction and dysfunction, decreased left ventricular filling, and thus decreased cardiac output. Although PE is thought to be

Table 3
Symptoms and signs in 500 patients with clinically suspected PE

	PE Present (n = 202)		PE Absent (n = 298)		
	No.	%	No.	%	P
Symptoms					
Dyspnea (sudden onset)	158	78	87	29	<.00001
Dyspnea (gradual onset)	12	6	59	20	.00002
Orthopnea	2	1	27	9	.00004
Chest (pleuritic)	89	44	89	30	.002
Chest pain (substernal)	33	16	29	10	.04
Fainting	53	26	38	13	.0002
Hemoptysis	19	9	16	5	.12
Cough	22	11	45	15	.22
Palpitations	36	18	46	15	.56
Signs					
Tachycardia >100/min	48	24	69	23	.96
Cyanosis	33	16	44	15	.73
Hypotension <90 mm Hg	6	3	5	2	.15
Neck vein distension	25	12	28	9	.36
Leg swelling (unilateral)	35	17	27	9	.009
Fever >38°C	14	7	63	21	.00003
Crackles	37	18	76	26	.08
Wheezes	8	4	39	13	.001
Pleural friction rub	8	4	11	4	.93

Table 4
Adjusted odds ratio of clinical symptoms of PE

Clinical Feature	Adjusted OR (95% CI)
Unilateral leg swelling	2.60 (2.05–3.30)
Hypoxemia (saturation <95%)	2.10 (1.70–2.60)
Pleuritic chest pain	1.53 (1.26–1.86)
Pulse >94 beats/min	1.52 (1.24–1.87)
Tachypnea (RR >24)	1.26 (1.02–1.56)
Dyspnea	1.26 (1.00–1.58)
Shock index >1.0[a]	1.26 (0.96–1.65)
Fever (temperature ≥38.0°C [100.4°F])[a]	1.13 (0.76–1.06)
Sudden onset of symptoms[a]	0.88 (0.73–1.06)
Hemoptysis[a]	0.78 (0.46–1.32)
Substernal chest pain	0.58 (0.46–0.72)

Abbreviation: RR, respiratory rate.
[a] Not statistically significant.
Adapted from Courtney DM, Kline JA, Kabrhel C, et al. Clinical features from the history and physical examination that predict the presence or absence of pulmonary embolism in symptomatic emergency department patients: results of a prospective, multicenter study. Ann Emerg Med 2010;55(4):307–15; with permission from Elsevier.

the cause of 1% of syncope, syncope occurs in 8% to 14% of patients with PE and it is likely a result of transient acute right ventricular outflow obstruction[66] Morgenthaler and Ryu[39] found a history of syncope in 25% of patients with PE as the cause of death.

In 1999, Miniati and colleagues[62] published a paper on the accuracy of clinical assessment in the diagnosis of PE. **Table 3** shows the prevalence of various signs and symptoms in patients with clinically suspected PE from that study.[61] Sudden-onset dyspnea, pleuritic chest pain, syncope, and unilateral leg swelling were seen more frequently in patients diagnosed with a PE. However, gradual-onset dyspnea, orthopnea, fever, and wheezing were more common in those without PEs. Recently, Courtney and colleagues[31] published a prospective, multicenter study evaluating the predictive value of many clinical features (**Table 4**). Those of particular interest to the EP include unilateral leg swelling (OR 2.60, 95% CI 2.05–3.30), hypoxemia with saturations less than 95% (OR 2.10, 95% CI 1.70–2.60), pleuritic chest pain (OR 1.53, 95% CI 1.26–1.86), and pulse greater than 94 beats/min (OR 1.52, 95% CI 1.24–1.87).[31] Tachycardia has been reported as a less sensitive clinical feature, especially in younger patients. Green and colleagues[58] found that 70% of patients less than 40 years old with a PE had heart rates less than 100 beats/min, whereas 70% of patients older than 40 years had heart rates greater than 100 beats/min. Other studies reported tachycardia occurred in only 24% to 30%.[67] Miniati and colleagues[62] found tachycardia not to be predictive of a diagnosis of PE; however, it is one of the explicit variables in the pulmonary embolism rule-out criteria (PERC) rule (**Box 4**) and has further strong validation in the recent article by Courtney and colleagues.[31]

Many studies suggest that tachypnea is the most sensitive clinical sign, being absent in only 5% to 13% of patients.[58,59] Dyspnea was the most commonly occurring symptom (73%) in patients without prior cardiopulmonary disease in both the PIOPED and PIOPED II studies, which is supported by at least 1 prospective observational study with an incidence of 92%.[68] Dyspnea may occur over seconds, minutes, hours, or days, at rest, or only with exertion.[59] Orthopnea can be a symptom of PE, but is

---

Box 4
Pulmonary embolism rule-out criteria (PERC)

A patient can be deemed very low risk and does not require any investigation for PE in the presence of[a]:

1. Low clinical suspicion (clinical gestalt <15%)

   and

2. All of the following criteria:

   Age <50 years
   Pulse <100 beats/min
   Pulse oximetry >94%
   No unilateral leg swelling[b]
   No hemoptysis[c]
   No recent surgery or trauma[d]
   No prior DVT/PE
   No hormone use[e]

---

[a] When all criteria are met, the patient is considered PERC negative.
[b] Asymmetric calf swelling viewed by raising patient's legs by the heels.
[c] In the past week.
[d] No general anesthetic in 4 weeks.
[e] Any male or female patient using hormone replacement, oral contraceptives, or estrogen.

---

neither sensitive nor specific for the diagnosis, and may be more common in patients without PE.[62]

Substernal chest pain has an OR of 0.58 and may suggest against a diagnosis of PE. Sudden onset of symptoms and hemoptysis had an OR of less than 1 but were not statistically significant,[31] which supports retrospective data that most patients who die unexpectedly from PE complain of daily pain for weeks and many had already seen a physician.[69] That is not to say that the probability of PE is reduced if a patient presents with sudden-onset symptoms, because less than half of outpatients with PE still describe their dyspnea or chest pain as sudden onset.

Cough, rales, decreased breath sounds, palpitations, lightheadedness, fever, and wheezing may result from PE but are difficult to separate from other possible concomitant illnesses.[12] Cough is usually nonproductive but may be bloody, purulent, or clear.[62] Rales and decreased breath sounds occurred in 35% of patients with PE and were the most frequently detected respiratory findings. Fever with no other source is present in 14% of patients with PE, and is usually low grade.[67,70] It was 38.3 C (101 F) or higher in only 6% of patients with a fever and greater than 38.9 C (102 F) in only 1.6%. Other atypical presentations include abdominal pain, back pain, atrial fibrillation, syncope, hiccoughs, and reactive airways disease.[56]

Occult or silent PEs likely represent many of the fatal cases of PE, because they are not routinely suspected or diagnosed, as well as most benign cases of PE, because it is probable that the lungs of healthy individuals frequently filter out these small asymptomatic emboli. The true rate of occult or silent (asymptomatic) PEs in the general population is unknown. A recent systematic review found that PE was diagnosed in 32% of patients with DVT and 15% of asymptomatic surgical patients had evidence of PE on lungs scans.[71,72] Overall, the clinical relevance of occult PEs is unknown.

DIAGNOSTIC CLINICAL ASSESSMENT AND PRETEST PROBABILITY

The clinical evaluation and diagnosis of PE is challenging, thus clinicians need a method to determine when and how to evaluate the appropriate patients. In addition, it is estimated that a considerable number of CT angiographic examinations and radiation exposure could be avoided with the proper use of a clinical history and D-dimer assay.[73] The diagnosis depends on an accurate determination of clinical pretest probability.[13,38] Determining the PTP encourages good clinical assessment and allows better interpretation of diagnostic tests. The process also identifies high-risk patients who may benefit from treatment prior to the completion of investigation, and low-risk patients in whom few, if any, investigations are required. The PTP can help the clinician to: 1) safely exclude PE, 2) determine whether to initiate investigation for PE, 3) determine how to use the diagnostic algorithm for a given patient, and 4) determine the patients who would benefit from treatment with anticoagulation prior to the completion of investigations.

Physicians may choose to make an assessment of PTP implicitly (**Fig. 1**) or explicitly (**Fig. 2**). Implicit determination of PTP, also referred to as "physician gestalt", draws on medical training, clinical experience, and clinical judgment to produce an unstructured, non-rule based estimate of PTP. Low, intermediate, and high-risk implicit PTP values have yet to be accurately determined in the literature. The influence of clinical experience on implicit PTP is unclear. Kabrhel and colleagues[74] suggest that accurate PTP determination trends with clinical experience, whereas other research suggests gestalt varies inversely with clinical experience, perhaps implying that increased clinical experience may result in reduced comfort clinically excluding PE.[74,75]

Explicit assessment of PTP relies on the use of evidence-based clinical decision rules or scoring systems to categorize the PTP.[76] Three scoring systems have been prospectively tested and validated in large clinical trials: the Geneva score, the Wells score, and the Pisa score.[13,62,77] The Pisa score is more appropriately used for hospitalized patients, whereas the Wells and Geneva scores were developed for use in the ED.[78,79]

The Geneva score was originally developed by Wicki and colleagues[77] in 2001, and later validated and revised by LeGal[80] in 2006. Klok and colleagues subsequently simplified and dichotomized the scoring system to "PE likely" and "PE unlikely" so that a patient population was selected in which a negative D-dimer assay could be used to exclude PE.[81] **Table 5** presents the simplified revised Geneva score and its clinical probabilities. No patient with a Geneva score less than or equal to 2 and a negative D-dimer test was found to have a venous thrombosis within the 3 months of follow-up.

Table 6 shows one of the more widely used CDRs, known as the Canadian (Wells) criteria. The original Wells study divided patients into low-risk, moderate-risk, and high-risk groups, based on specific signs, symptoms, and whether an alternate diagnosis was likely. The subsequent rates of PE were 3.4%, 27.8%, and 78.4%, respectively.[13] In 2000, Wells retrospectively analyzed the original data to devise a simpler scoring tool, now known as the Wells criteria. It is easy to apply and stratifies patients into low, moderate, and high risk. The study also dichotomized the patients into PE-likely and PE-unlikely cohorts to generate a patient population in which a negative D-dimer could exclude PE.[82] A patient with a negative D-dimer, in whom PE was deemed unlikely, had a 2.2% rate of PE in the derivation cohort and 1.7% rate of PE in validation cohort. **Table 6** summarizes the rates of PE with both scoring systems in the derivation and validation group. Multiple studies have validated the Wells criteria since its derivation, and the Christopher Study Investigators validated the dichotomous version, showing that only 0.5% of patients had VTE on a 3-month follow-up.[83,84]

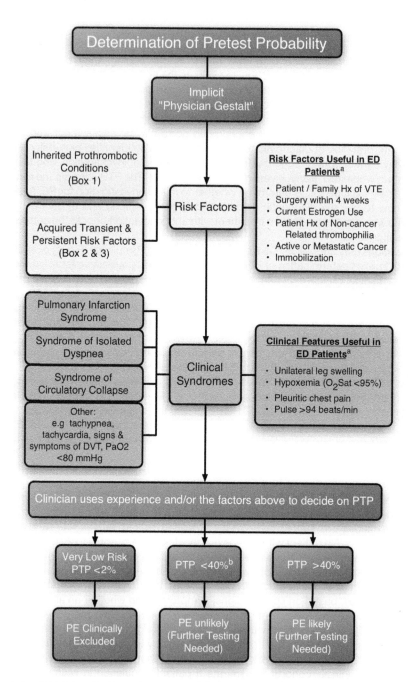

Fig. 1. Implicit determination of pretest probability. Implicit determination of PTP is a physician's gestalt judgment based on clinical experience. [a] A recent study by Courtney and colleagues[31] provided research into certain risk factors and clinical features that are useful in patients in the ED. One method, conceptualized here, illustrates how a physician determines a very-low-risk PTP, a PTP less than 40%, or a PTP greater than 40%. [b] PTP less than 40% can be further divided into PTP less than 15%, permitting application of the PERC rule, or PTP between 15% and 40%, requiring a quantitative D-dimer assay to begin the diagnostic process. Hx, history; O_2Sat, oxygen saturation; PaO_2, partial pressure of arterial oxygen.

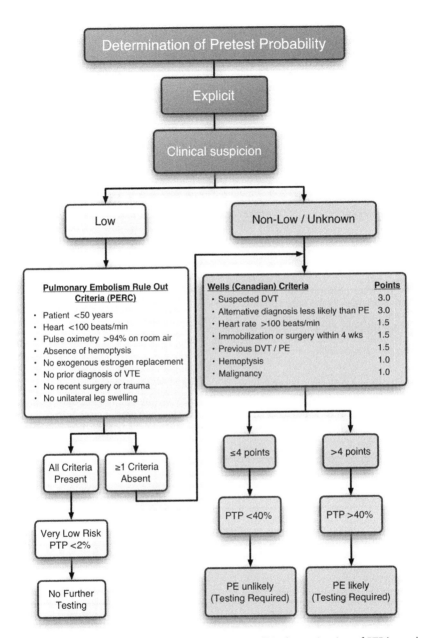

Fig. 2. Explicit determination of pretest probability. Explicit determination of PTP is an algorithmic or rule-based judgment to determine the likelihood of PE in a given patient. One method, conceptualized here, uses the PERC rule and/or the Wells criteria to place patients into very low risk, PTP less than 40%, or PTP greater than 40% risk of PE in an effort to determine how to apply a diagnostic algorithm to an individual patient. min, minutes; wks, weeks. (*Data from* Wells PS, Ginsberg JS, Anderson DR, et al. Use of a clinical model for safe management of patients with suspected pulmonary embolism. Ann Intern Med 1998;129(12): 997–1005; and Kline JA, Courtney DM, Kabrhel C, et al. Prospective multicenter evaluation of the pulmonary embolism rule-out criteria. J Thromb Haemost 2008;6(5):772–80.)

Table 5
Simplified revised Geneva score

Variable			Points
Age >65 y			1
Recent surgery/lower limb fracture (within 1 month)			1
Active malignancy (<1 year)			1
Previous DVT/PE			1
Hemoptysis			1
Unilateral lower limb pain			1
Heart rate[a]			
75–94 beats/min			1
≥95 beats/min			2
Pain on lower limb deep palpation and unilateral edema			1

Clinical Probability	PTP for PE (%)	PostTP (%)[b]	
Low	7.7	1	0–1
Moderate	29.4	3	2–4
High	64.3	12	5–7
PE unlikely	12.9	1	0–2
PE likely	64.3	5	3–7

[a] Heart rate between 75 and 94 beats/min is given a total of 1 point, while heart rate ≥95 beats/min is given a total of 2 points.
[b] Posttest probability (PostTP) of PE when combined with a high-sensitivity D-dimer assay.
Data from Klok FA, Mos IC, Nijkeuter M, et al. Simplification of the revised Geneva score for assessing clinical probability of pulmonary embolism. Arch Intern Med 2008;168(19):2131–36.

The Geneva and Wells scores have been shown in numerous studies to be comparable. The Geneva score, although calculated retrospectively, was validated prospectively in 2 independent cohorts. Both studies demonstrated consistent predictive accuracy, and a comparable accuracy with the Wells criteria.[85,86] A subsequent

Table 6
Wells criteria

Variable			Points
Hemoptysis			1.0
Malignancy (Tx within the last 6 mo, or palliative)			1.0
Previous DVT/PE			1.5
Heart rate >100 beats/min			1.5
Immobilization or surgery (within 4 wk)			1.5
Suspected DVT			3.0
An alternative diagnosis is less likely than PE			3.0

Clinical Probability	Rate of PE (%): Derivation Group		Rate of PE (%): Validation Group	
	D-dimer −ve	D-dimer +ve	D-dimer −ve	D-dimer +ve
Low	1.5	8.6	2.7	0
Moderate	7.6	36.1	2.9	37.3
High	20	79.6	20	60
PE unlikely	2.2	18.3	1.7	11.7
PE likely	16.1	57.7	10.3	60

Abbreviations: Tx, treatment, −ve, negative, +ve, positive.
Data from Wells PS, Anderson DR, Rodger M, et al. Derivation of a simple clinical model to categorize patients probability of pulmonary embolism: increasing the models utility with the SimpliRED D-dimer. Thromb Haemost 2000;83:416–20.

systemic review and meta-analysis also supports this conclusion.[87] The Wells score is validated, easy to apply, does not require any additional diagnostic studies, and is recommended by many society guidelines for patient populations with a prevalence of PE of less than 20%.[82,87–89] Its main limitation is the criterion "an alternative diagnosis is less likely," which has a moderate inter-rater reliability and represents a dichotomized implicit PTP assessment. The Geneva score does not rely on subjective criteria but was derived and validated in a cohort of patients with a prevalence of PE greater than 20%. **Fig. 2** conceptualizes an algorithm for the explicit determination of PTP. It contains a recently derived approach to the very-low-risk patient that may rule out PE before the diagnostic work-up, and one of the most commonly used objective criteria for PTP determination in PE, the Wells criteria.

Implicit Versus Explicit PTP Assessment

Evidence clearly demonstrates that physician gestalt and the 2 validated clinical decision rules show similar accuracy in discriminating between low, moderate, and high pretest probability of PE.[83,90–92] Implicit determination of PTP allows for flexibility of human judgment, and does not require spontaneous recall of the CDRs for use or documentation.[89,93] However, discordance of clinical agreement on true PTP exists, and the potential reduced accuracy of inexperienced clinicians may trend any "gestalt" PTP toward an intermediate probability and over-reliance on diagnostic tests.[94–96] In contrast, the use of CDRs provides consistent, reproducible probabilities and does not rely on clinician experience. However, the drawback lies in knowledge translation. Runyon and colleagues[93] showed that only 68% of EPs were familiar with at least 1 CDR, 18% rarely used them, 24% believed clinical gestalt was superior, and 10% even expressed medicolegal concerns. Spontaneous recall was low to moderate, and of those physicians familiar with the CDRs, only half used them in greater than 50% of the applicable cases.[93] Many clinical guidelines advocate the use of CDRs to assess clinical probability because they can be consistently applied and may trend toward increased accuracy among less experienced clinicians.[77,97] A recent policy statement published in the Annals of Emergency Medicine found insufficient evidence to support the preferential use of clinical gestalt rather than clinical decision aids.[98] Although the more recent work by Christopher and colleagues[84] has focused on simplifying the explicit algorithms from 3 categories (low, moderate, and high) to 2 categories (PE likely vs unlikely), the ability of physicians to implicitly determine PTP with only 2 categories has not been studied.

Pulmonary Embolism Rule-Out Criteria

With the widespread acceptance and use of the D-dimer, overinvestigation has been recognized as a significant problem in the process of ruling out PE.[99] The low specificity and resultant false positives of the D-dimer assay create the potential for a significant increase in pulmonary vascular imaging and radiation exposure, increased patient length of stay in overcrowded EDs, and unnecessary anticoagulation. Clinical gestalt and CDRs are both able to direct the work-up for PE, but neither can reliably identify a "very low-risk population" that requires no investigation. A "very low-risk population" is a cohort in which the PTP is below the test threshold and PE can be consistently ruled out at the bedside. The test threshold is the point at which the PTP of a disease is equal to the post-test prevalence (or false negative rate).[99] When the PTP is less than the test threshold, the probability of harm from diagnostic evaluation exceeds the potential benefit. Given the available evidence, an ideal "very low-risk population" would have PTP less than approximately 1.4% to 1.8%.[100–102] In a 2001 validation study, a Wells score less than 2 was shown to have a 1.3% probability of PE.[88] This has not been repeated to date. To address this issue, Kline and colleagues[101] derived and prospectively validated the PERC rule to identify the very-low-risk group in which PE could be safely excluded at the bedside. The result was a set of 8 criteria that, when coupled with a clinical gestalt of less than 15%, yielded a population of patients with a pretest probability less than 2% (see **Box 4**). Kline and colleagues[103] then performed a large multicenter validation study in 2008 with 8138 patients, a PE prevalence of 5.9%, and a 45-day follow-up period. In 20% of patients, the PERC rule was negative and PE was ruled out at the bedside. The PERC rule had a sensitivity of 97.4% and a specificity of 21.9%. The false-negative rate for the very-low-risk population was approximately 0.9% (95% CI 0.6%–1.6%), which is similar to negative results in quantitative D-dimer, ventilation-perfusion (V/Q) scan, CT pulmonary angiography (CTPA), and conventional pulmonary angiography. A third study by Wolf and colleagues, with a 12% prevalence of PE further supports the PERC rule.[104]

Limitations of the PERC rule include: (1) instances in which it cannot be applied (**Box 5**); (2) the main PERC studies collected patient data prospectively, but the PERC rule was applied and studied retrospectively; (3) the PERC rule was derived and validated in patient populations with a PE prevalence of 11% and 5.9% and, if used in a less restrictive fashion, particularly in populations of patients in which the prevalence of PE is greater than 20%, misdiagnosis may occur[104,105]; (4) in the PERC validation study, 23.5% of patients were either not approached, refused consent, or follow-up could not be assured.[103] Despite these problems, the PERC rule is the only tool studied to help identify very-low-risk patients.

DIAGNOSTIC TESTS
Electrocardiogram

Most routine investigations, including basic blood work, chest radiograph, electrocardiogram (ECG), cardiac troponins, brain natriuretic peptide (BNP), and arterial blood gas (ABG), are of limited value. The ECG is neither sensitive nor specific. A normal ECG can be seen in 30% of patients with PE, whereas the classic S1Q3T3 occurs in only 20% of patients with angiographically proven PE, and has a sensitivity and specificity of 54% and 62% respectively.[67,106] The most common ECG change is T-wave inversion in the precordial leads, found in 68% of patients with PE.[67] These T-wave inversions may mimic an ischemic event, which is seen in 11% of patients without prior history of cardiopulmonary disease.[103] Sinus tachycardia is the most frequent rhythm seen in patients with PE, occurring in 36%.[106] Other ECG findings include electrocardiographic manifestations of acute cor pulmonale: right bundle branch block, P-wave pulmonale, right axis deviation, and new-onset atrial fibrillation.

Box 5
Conditions in which the PERC rule cannot be used

Concurrent β-blocker use (may blunt tachycardia)

Transient tachycardia

Thrombophilia

Strong family history of thrombosis

Patients with amputations

Massively obese patients (may be difficult to clinical assess leg swelling)

Patients with baseline hypoxemia

Ultimately, an ECG is an inexpensive and rapidly available bedside test better used to suggest alternate diagnoses such as acute myocardial infarction or pericarditis.

Chest Radiograph

The chest radiography is typically nonspecific and nondiagnostic. It is reported to be normal in 12% to 24% of patients, and otherwise demonstrates a variety of nonspecific abnormalities.[67,107,108] Cardiomegaly, elevated hemidiaphragm, atelectasis, pleural effusion, consolidation, and PA enlargement are among the most common abnormalities.[109] Chest radiographs in about 65% of patients with acute PE revealed atelectasis, consolidation, elevated hemidiaphragm, or a pleural effusion.[110] Patients without cardiopulmonary disease had only blunting of the costophrenic angles, and none had an effusion more than one third of the hemithorax.[67] Hampton hump is a wedge-shaped, pleural-based, apex central pulmonary opacity that is uncommon and has a sensitivity and specificity of 22% and 82%.[111] The Westermark sign is relative oligemia usually in the presence of an ipsilateral dilated PA. It is also uncommon and has a sensitivity and specificity of 12% and 97%.[63] Ultimately, chest radiography may be more helpful in elucidating alternative diagnoses, such as pneumonia, pneumothorax, and CHF. The chest radiography may be important to the diagnostic workup because a normal chest radiograph minimizes the risk of nondiagnostic results for lung scintigraphy.

Arterial Blood Gas

In patients with normal lungs, PIOPED found that a Pco_2 greater than 36 mmHg and a normal alveolar arterial oxygen (A-a) gradient had a 98% negative predictive value (NPV) for PE.[38] In patients with no cardiopulmonary disease, 76% presented with hypoxemia, whereas 95% had an increased A-a gradient. Cvitanic and Marino[112] also found that 98% of patients had either an increased A-a gradient or hypocapnia. Generally, the ABG and A-a gradients are not sensitive or specific for PE.[113] Of those patients found not to have a PE, most had abnormally increased A-a gradients.[114] The ABG and A-a gradient may be normal in 5% to 35% of patients with PE and no prior cardiopulmonary disease.[106,115,116] Overall, despite these limitations, the unexplained presence of hypoxemia or any sudden change in the A-a gradient increases the likelihood of PE.

Troponin and Brain Natriuretic Peptide

Recently, the value of the cardiac troponin has been investigated and may be valuable to clinicians in risk stratification of those patients found to have acute PE.[117] Troponin can be increased in patients with massive acute PE and may be related to acute right ventricular strain or failure.[118] Autopsy data have shown myocardial necrosis in patients with acute PE and normal coronary arteries, which has been reproduced in animal studies.[119,120] Brain natriuretic peptide is not specific for PE and may be increased secondary to acute right ventricular strain with CHF, or other causes of pulmonary hypertension.[121]

D-dimer

D-dimer is a fibrin degradation product that indicates the presence of intravascular fibrin deposition and is usually increased in thromboembolic disease.[122] It was initially applied to patients already scheduled for imaging in an effort to reduce the number of pulmonary angiograms performed. With increasing use, the D-dimer became applied to manage patients even prior to the decision to perform diagnostic imaging. Yet an increase in the overall rate of diagnosis was not seen. D-dimer assays can be divided into 4 categories (in order of increasing sensitivity): (1) latex agglutination; (2) erythrocyte agglutination; (3) matrix screen immunoassays; and (4) enzyme-linked immunosorbent assay (ELISA) and turbidimetric techniques.[76] The first 3 categories of D-dimer assays are qualitative and have reported sensitivities of 80% to 95% and specificities of 57% to 74% in patients in the ED and therefore may not be sufficient to rule out PE.[123–125] The quantitative D-dimer assays, ELISA and turbidimetric tests, have reported sensitivities of greater than 93% and specificities of 39% to 55% (at a cutoff of 500 ng/mL; varies by institution) and are thus recommended for use to rule out the possibility of PE.[126,127] Ultimately, the use of the D-dimer measurement must be guided by clinical PTP. In patients with a high clinical suspicion for PE and a negative D-dimer, the 3-month occurrence of PE remains higher than 3%.[25] Conversely, in patients with low or intermediate PTP and a negative D-dimer (ELISA or turbidimetric assay), the NPV of PE in untreated patients is 0.14% to 0.4%.[84,128,129]

The specificity of D-dimer is low as a result of many possible false-positive cases such as trauma, cancer, pregnancy, recent surgery, and infection. **Box 6** outlines the common false-negatives and positives for the D-dimer assay. In pregnancy, the D-dimer increases with gestation, and many clinicians' think that a negative D-dimer in pregnancy (first trimester) can still be used to rule out PE. Its use in pregnancy, particularly in the second and third trimester, is controversial.[130] In the elderly, increasing age is accompanied by an increase in the false-positive rate. A D-dimer was found to only exclude 5% of patients older than 80 years, compared with 60% of those less than 40 years old.[131] An age-dependent D-dimer cutoff has been proposed, with

---

Box 6
Factors associated with an inaccurate D-dimer result in the assessment of PE

False-negative D-dimer

Symptoms of PE for >3 days

Small PE

Use of qualitative latex fixation tests

Anticoagulated patients

False-positive D-dimer

Cancer and malignancy

Recent surgery

Infection (eg, pneumonia, sepsis)

Pregnancy

Age >70 years

Disseminated intravascular coagulation

Trauma

Arterial thrombosis

Acute myocardial infarction

Vaso-occlusive sickle cell crisis

Acute cerebrovascular event

Unstable angina

Atrial fibrillation

Vasculitis

Superficial phlebitis

promising failure rates of 0.2% to 0.6%.[132] A prospective external validation study is ongoing.

Computed Tomographic Pulmonary Angiography

CTPA is thought by many to have replaced conventional pulmonary angiography as the reference standard for PE.[133] CTPA has multiple advantages compared with other lung imaging techniques (**Box 7**). CTPA is readily available, often 24 hours per day at most centers, has short acquisition times, and has a high sensitivity and specificity for the general population. One significant advantage is the ability to detect alternative diagnoses. Rates of alternative diagnoses can be as high as 67%.[134,135] One study found that 7% of the negative CTPAs showed an alternative diagnosis that required immediate action.[136] The disadvantages (see **Box 7**) include an increased nondiagnostic rate during pregnancy, nephrotoxic iodinated contrast injection, and significant breast radiation dose. Intravenous contrast injection can cause local tissue damage and anaphylactoid reactions, carries a 4% to 22% chance of contrast-induced nephropathy, and limits the use of CTPA in patients with renal insufficiency and contrast allergies.[137] The breast radiation dose may be as high as 60 mSv from a 4-slice CT, and 50–80 mSv from 64-slice CT technology, as compared with 3 mSv from a 2-view mammogram.[90,138–140]

Despite these disadvantages, CTPA is currently the dominant imaging modality in the investigation of PE and most centers use MDCT as their sole diagnostic test.[57,130] The literature has a range of sensitivities and specificities depending on CT technology, ranging from single-detector CT (SDCT) to MDCT of 16-slice to 64-slice capabilities. The current benchmark for the 3-month PE recurrence rate is 0.9% for conventional pulmonary angiography and 0.5% for a normal V/Q scan.[138,141,142] The

---

Box 7
Advantages and disadvantages of CTPA and V/Q scan

Modality	Advantages	Disadvantages
CTPA	Readily available at most centers Short acquisition time Ability to detect alternative dx Retrospective reconstructions High sensitivity/specificity Dichotomous interpretation Sole diagnostic test (MDCT) Age does not influence result	High maternal breast radiation dose Reader expertise required Expensive Nephrotoxic iodinated contrast injection Not portable Physiologic changes in pregnancy may cause nondiagnostic results Contraindicated in patients with contrast allergy and renal insufficiency
V/Q scan	Radionuclide poses minimal risk and is safe in pregnancy Safe in patients with renal insufficiency and CT contrast allergy Low maternal breast radiation Radiation dose further reduced by perfusion-only scans	Inability to provide alternative diagnoses Long acquisition time Potentially significant rate of nondiagnostic results Limited access and availability

Abbreviations: dx, diagnoses; MDCT, multidetector computed tomography; V/Q, ventilation-perfusion or lung scintigraphy.

accuracy of SDCT is controversial. The range of sensitivities and specificities of SDCT technology is 66% to 93% and 89% to 97%, respectively, limiting its effective use as the sole diagnostic test for PE.[143–145] Musset and colleagues[91] and Anderson and colleagues[146] examined the effect of bilateral compression ultrasonography (CUS) following an SDCT. In appropriately risk-stratified patients who had a negative SDCT and negative bilateral CUS, the rate of PE at 3 months was 1.8% and 0.4%.[91,146]

Newer CT technology has a sensitivity ranging between 83% and 100% and a specificity of greater than 95%.[38,57,145,147,148] PIOPED II showed a sensitivity of 83% (95% CI 76% to 92%) and a specificity of 96% (95% CI 93%–97%) with 4-slice CT technology.[57] The current MDCT has a 3-month rate of PE/DVT of less than 2% when used as a single diagnostic modality or when combined with bilateral CUS.[84] The Christopher Group Investigators found that only 1.3% (95% CT 0.7–2.0%) of patients had VTE at 3 months with a positive D-dimer (or deemed "likely for PE" by dichotomous risk stratification) and a negative MDCT.[84] Similarly a noninferiority trial by Righini and colleagues[86] compared risk-stratified patients investigated with D-dimer and MDCT versus patients investigated with D-dimer, MDCT, and bilateral CUS, and, at 3 months, showed a rate of PE of 0.3% in both groups.

Other prospective studies have raised concerns that CTPA may not reliably exclude PE, particularly in patients with high PTP. After a negative MDCT in patients with a positive D-dimer, Vigo and colleagues[149] showed a rate of PE of 19.7%. This value decreased to 1.17% (95% CI 0.24%–3.38%) in patients with a negative D-dimer. In patients with a high PTP and negative CTPA, false negatives can range from 5.3% to 40%.[57,86,91] The newest CT technology (128-slice to 256-slice) is expected to have improved sensitivity and specificity with enhanced visualization of subsegmental anatomy, but data about the performance of this generation of CT scanners and the added radiation risk are lacking.

An MDCT can be used as the sole diagnostic investigation for most low-risk patients. However, patients with a high clinical PTP and a negative MDCT may benefit from additional testing, such as bilateral CUS or lung scintigraphy, which underscores the importance of clinical context when choosing and interpreting lung imaging for the investigation of PE.

Ventilation Perfusion Lung Scan

With the advent and widespread use of CT angiography, the use of lung scintigraphy has declined precipitously over the last 15 years.[12] Given some of the disadvantages inherent to CTPA, V/Q scan still has an important role in the investigation of PE. Firm evidence exists that a V/Q scan is as accurate as CTPA. A recent study found no significant difference in the rate of PE/DVT at 3 months when comparing MDCT and V/Q.[146] PIOPED II, the largest and most significant study that evaluated the use of MDCT, showed that the sensitivity of MDCT is approximately 83%, which is similar to that of V/Q.[57] There is a growing concern about the unrestrained use of CTPA and many studies have shown that with the appropriate evaluation of clinical PTP and judicious use of lung scintigraphy, more than 30% of CTPA are potentially unnecessary.[150] Mamlouk and colleagues[73] demonstrated that CTPA was positive in only 6.4% of patients in whom PE was suspected in the ED. The major contributing factor was failure to determine accurate PTP and only 5% of patients received a D-dimer assay.

The advantages of lung scintigraphy (see **Box 7**) include low effective radiation dose of only 0.28 to 0.9 mSv and generally safe radionuclide, both in the general population and in pregnancy.[151] Disadvantages include long acquisition time, limited availability, a significant rate of nondiagnostic results, the inability to provide alternative diagnoses, and inconsistent reporting terminology and practice. V/Q is most diagnostically accurate when interpreted as normal or high probability and is concordant with clinical PTP. A normal V/Q scan essentially rules out PE with an NPV of 97%.[152–155] A high-probability scan has a positive predictive value of 85% to 90% with a sensitivity and specificity of 41% and 97%, respectively.[38] A low-probability interpretation is controversial, and many investigators advocate for additional testing, such as bilateral CUS. In contrast, 3 studies within the last 15 years have shown a 6-month PE/DVT rate of 1% without further diagnostic imaging.[38,155–157]

One of the main issues with V/Q scintigraphy is the rate of nondiagnostic interpretation, which results in further investigation and increasing costs. The rate of nondiagnostic V/Q scans ranges between 30% and 50%, and, in some studies (PIOPED I), it is as high as 70%.[38,158–160] Indeterminate rates are more common among patients with significant cardiopulmonary disease, including acute and chronic airway disease, patients with abnormal chest radiography, and the elderly.[161,162] In patients with a normal chest radiograph and without significant cardiopulmonary disease, only 11% of perfusion scans are nondiagnostic.[108] In addition, the proportion of indeterminate V/Q scans is almost twice as high in patients older than 70 years compared with patients younger than 40 years of age.[132] For lung scintigraphy to be used safely and effectively, it is important to consider and satisfy the following criteria:

1. Normal chest radiography
2. No significant cardiopulmonary disease
3. Patients less than 65 to 70 years of age
4. Women, particularly in pregnancy and those with a family history of breast cancer
5. Nuclear medicine facilities on site and available with standard consistent reporting criteria
6. The understanding that nondiagnostic results require further investigation.

Other Imaging Modalities: Ultrasound, Magnetic Resonance Imaging, Pulmonary Angiography

CUS can be used at various points in the investigation of PE: a) as an initial imaging modality; b) after a negative or inconclusive CTPA; or c) after a non-diagnostic V/Q scan. In patients with suspected PE, CUS as an initial investigation only detects 10% of DVTs.[84,163] Therefore, venous CUS should be considered as an initial imaging modality in patients with concomitant signs and symptoms of DVT, and relative or absolute contraindications to V/Q or CTPA.

Classically, CUS has been used following a nondiagnostic V/Q scan. For single negative CUS following nondiagnostic V/Q scans in patients with low PTP of PE, early studies showed a PE rate of 1.7% at 3 months.[164] However, Daniel and colleagues later showed that a single CUS had a sensitivity of only 54% and a specificity of 97% and a post-test probability of approximately 12% (95% CI 6 - 17%).[165] A single CUS should not be used to rule out PE, particularly when the test results are discordant with the PTP.[62] For these reasons, follow-up CUS examinations are obtained approximately 1 week later to assess for clot progression. Two negative CUS examinations following a nondiagnostic or indeterminate V/Q scan result in a 3-month risk of PE of less than 1%.[13,166]

Serial CUS can also be used after a negative or inconclusive CTPA. Early studies with single-slice or 4-slice multidetector CTPA showed that CUS diagnosed an additional 3.1% to 6% of DVTs in patients with negative CT.[91,167] CUS should be considered following lung imaging (lung scintigraphy, CTPA) with an indeterminate CTPA or V/Q scan, or a negative CTPA or V/Q scan in patients with an intermediate or high clinical PTP. The choice of CUS should be based on institutional ultrasound (US) proficiency, quality and type of CTPA, and expertise and consistency in lung scintigraphy.

Two echocardiography (echo) modalities can be used in the investigation of PE. Transthoracic echocardiography (TTE) is noninvasive, and rapidly available at the bedside, but lacks the sensitivity of TEE. TEE has greater sensitivity and diagnostic ability than TTE, but is invasive, of limited availability, often requires procedural sedation, and is unable to accurately detect peripheral PEs. Signs of PE on echo include increased inferior venal caval (IVC), RV and right atrial (RA) size, septal wall motion abnormalities, regional wall motion abnormalities with spared right apical function (McConnell's sign), tricuspid regurgitation, and RV thrombus.[168] Echo abnormalities are present in approximately 30% to 40% of patients with PE.[169,170] Echo is most useful in patients with contraindications to other imaging modalities, hemodynamically unstable patients who cannot be transported outside the ED, or in patients with suspected massive PE to justify thrombolytics.[171,172] TEE has a sensitivity of 5% to 20% for visualization of a clot in the RA, RV, or pulmonary artery (PA) in stable and unstable patients with submassive and massive PE.[173,174] For central PE, in patients with high clinical suspicion and evidence of RV overload, TEE has sensitivity and specificity for PE of 80% to 97% and 88% to 100%, respectively.[175,176]

Magnetic resonance angiography (MRA) has emerged as a potential alternative diagnostic imaging modality. Advantages include safer contrast material, the absence of ionizing radiation, and similar sensitivity and specificity to CTPA.[177,178] A recent study of 371 patients assessed MRA in patients with suspected PE.[179] PE was diagnosed in 28% of patients (n = 104); however, 25% of the images were technically inadequate. Of the technically adequate images, the sensitivity was 78% (95% CI 67%–86%) and the specificity was 99% (95% CI 96%–100%). In addition, sensitivity decreased significantly in segmental (64%–88%) and subsegmental (0%–40%) pulmonary arteries, whereas specificity remained greater than 92%. The combination of MRA and magnetic resonance (MR) venography had a sensitivity and specificity of 92% and 96%, respectively. However, almost 48% of the patients had inadequate imaging results.[84] MRI has several significant disadvantages. In many centers, MRI is a limited, expensive, and time-consuming resource. In addition, MRI is contraindicated in patients with implanted metallic objects and may require varying levels of patient sedation. MRI should only be considered in centres in which it is routinely performed.

Pulmonary angiography has long been considered the gold standard for the diagnosis of PE. However, CTPA has better visualization of subsegmental pulmonary arteries and greater interobserver agreement.[180,181] Pulmonary angiography is invasive, time consuming, and is not readily available at many centers. In addition, catheter PA has a higher rate of complications (6.5%) and death (0.5%), and transport out of the ED is required.[182,183] Moreover, a negative pulmonary angiogram seldom offers an alternative diagnosis.

Radiation Risks

Radiation "effective dose" is used to estimate the tissue and organ radiobiological detriment (ie, likelihood of developing cancer) from medical imaging. It is a calculated tissue weighted sum of the "Radiation Equivalent Dose" to specified organs and tissues expressed in terms of a whole body exposure. It is an estimate and is measured in Sieverts (mSv). Ionizing radiation from medical imaging now accounts for almost half of the radiation exposure to the general population, and has doubled in the past 30 years.[184] The use of CT studies has tripled since 1993.[185] At the present time, no data exists showing a causal relationship between CT scans and cancer.

However, the Biological Effects of Ionizing Radiation (BEIR) VII report has epidemiologic data from populations that received exposures from medical studies, workers with occupational exposures, Japanese atomic bomb survivors, and populations that lived near nuclear facilities during accidental release of radioactive material (eg, Chernobyl).[186] Long-term survivors of the Hiroshima and Nagasaki atomic bombs who received exposures of 10 to 100 mSv showed an increased risk of cancer.[187,188] The BEIR VII Report's LAR (lifetime attributable risk of cancer) model also predicts that 1 in 1000 persons exposed to a single dose of 10 mSv develops cancer. Although the annual natural background radiation represents an effective dose of approximately 3 mSv, which is not likely to result in a future risk of cancer, the International Commission on Radiological Protection (IRCP) confirmed that doses for CT scans approach or exceed levels associated with an increase in lifetime cancer risk. **Table 7** summarizes the average and range of effective doses for common medical imaging and the radiation-equivalent number of chest radiographs. The average effective dose of a CTPA ranges from 2–20 mSv (range: 2–40 mSv) with a radiation dose to the breast of at least 10–80 mSv.[140,151,189,190] The average effective dose from a lung ventilation perfusion scan is 0.2–1.5 mSv (range: 0.5–6.8 mSv) with an average dose of 0.28–0.9 mSv to the breast tissue.[140,151] Smith-Bindman and colleagues[191] published estimates of the radiation dose and potential cancer risk associated with common CT studies. The estimated risk of 1 radiation-induced cancer for a woman 20 years old undergoing CT for suspected PE is 1 in 330. For a woman 40 years old, the estimated risk is 1 in 620. **Table 8** provides comparisons of the radiation-induced cancer risk between common CT examinations. The threshold for CT has declined, and CT is increasingly being used among healthy individuals, in whom the risk of potential carcinogenesis could outweigh its diagnostic value. Because of the risk of radiation with CT angiography, particularly radiation of the breasts, scintigraphy may be the imaging test of choice in women less than 50 years of age. It is incumbent upon individual physicians to be aware of the institution specific radiation dose associated with their

Table 7
Effective radiation doses of selected diagnostic imaging

Diagnostic Imaging	Average Effective Dose (mSv)[a]	Range (mSv)	Chest Radiography Radiation Equivalents
Natural background radiation	1.5–3.0[b]	–	15–30
CXR (PA/Lat)	0.1	0.05–0.24	1
Pelvic radiograph	0.6	0.2–1.2	6
Abdominal radiograph	0.7	0.04–1.1	7
Lumbar spine radiograph	1.5	0.5–1.8	15
CT head	2	0.3–6	20
CT spine	6	1.5–10	60
Low dose perfusion scintigraphy	0.2	0.2–1.0	2
V/Q scan	2.2	0.5–6.8	22
CT chest	8	2–24	80
CTPA	15	2–40	150
CT abdomen	8	3.5–25	80

Abbreviations: CXR, chest radiography; Lat, lateral; mSv, milli-Sievert; PA, posteroanterior.
[a] The doses are average adult doses. The actual dose for any given patient may differ from reported average by up to ten-fold. Average doses may differ within and across institutions by 3-fold or more.
[b] Natural background radiation varies slightly by location on earth.
Data from Refs.[151,191–196]

Table 8				
Estimated odds of developing 1 radiation-induced cancer in patients undergoing CT				
	Number of Patients			
	Age 20 y		**Age 40 y**	
CT Scan	**Women**	**Men**	**Women**	**Men**
Head	4360 (3290–5110)	7350 (5540–8260)	8100 (6110–9500)	11080 (8350–12990)
Chest, no contrast	390 (290–630)	1040 (770–1670)	720 (540–1160)	1566 (1170–2520)
PE protocol	330 (230–460)	880 (610–1220)	620 (420–850)	1333 (920–1840)
Abdomen-pelvis with contrast	470 (380–700)	620 (510–930)	870 (710–1300)	942 (770–1400)

Adapted from Smith-Bindman R, Lipson F, Marcus R, et al. Radiation dose associated with common computed tomography examinations and the associated lifetime attributable risk of cancer. Arch Intern Med 2009;169(22):2078–86; with permission. Copyright © 2009 American Medical Association. All rights reserved.

diagnostic imaging, the important estimated odds of development of future radiation-induced cancer, and assess the potential risk-benefit ratio for each patient being investigated for PE.

APPROACH TO THE DIAGNOSIS OF PE

The first step is to suspect PE in the differential diagnosis, and then make an implicit or explicit determination of PTP. Physicians may find it beneficial to categorize patients as low risk (<15%), intermediate or moderate risk (15%–40%), or high risk (>40%) because these determinations may alter the diagnostic pathway at various stages of investigation (see **Figs 1** and **2**). Both the PERC rule and the Wells criteria may be used to categorize risk of PE because each is independently validated in the literature. However, even these objective criteria still contain elements of gestalt or experiential PTP determination. Once a PTP is derived, a clinician can access a multitude of suggested investigative algorithms in the literature. **Fig. 3** depicts a PTP-based algorithm for the diagnostic work-up of PE in the ED. The most important decision points include the use of the D-dimer assay, the selection of CTPA or lung scintigraphy, and the need for additional testing beyond the diagnostic algorithm. Posttest probability estimates for each pathway are also incorporated into the algorithm. In patients with inconclusive imaging tests or imaging results discordant with PTP, further investigations are generally recommended to reduce the posttest probability to less than 1% (**Fig. 4**). At this stage, the addition of the D-dimer assay, if not already completed, will be beneficial, and single or serial use of lower extremity venous ultrasonography is a reasonable low-risk investigation that reduces the rate of PE to less than 0.5% at 3 months (see **Fig. 4**).

TREATMENT OF ACUTE PE

The treatment of acute PE is systemic anticoagulation with or without thrombolysis. Anticoagulation halts clot progression and allows endogenous fibrinolysis to occur. Clot resolution occurs over weeks to months, and may be incomplete in some individuals.[64,197] Typically, an initial short-term therapy using unfractionated heparin, LMWH (eg, enoxaparin, dalteparin), or fondaparinux is used and bridges the transition to the

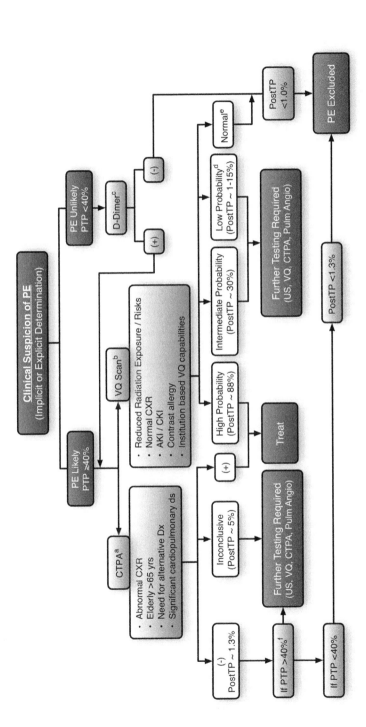

Fig. 3. A diagnostic algorithm for PE in the ED. [a] Consider the use of CTPA in patients with an abnormal CXR, those older than of 65 to 70 years, definite need of alternative diagnosis, and significant cardiopulmonary disease. [b] V/Q scans should only be used, based on the criteria described earlier, if (1) facilities are on site, (2) standardized reporting criteria are used, (3) an experienced interpretation can be obtained, (4) nondiagnostic studies are always followed by further imaging.[109] [c] Rapid ELISA or immunoturbidimetric assay. [d] In the presence of low PTP and a positive D-dimer, a low probability V/Q scan has an approximate postTP of 4%, whereas, in the presence of a moderate or high PTP, a low-probability V/Q scan has a 15% postTP. [e] The NPV of a normal V/Q scan is 97%.[76,108] [f] This algorithm includes the option to apply further testing if there is high PTP (>40%) of PE with a negative CTPA. The incidence of VTE at 3 months in patients in whom anticoagulation was withheld was 1.3%. The British Thoracic Society guidelines recommend withholding anticoagulation in the presence of a negative CTPA (level A recommendation).[84,207,208] Kline recommends further investigation in this patient population.[31] AKI, acute kidney injury; CKI, chronic kidney injury; Pulm angio, pulmonary angiogram.

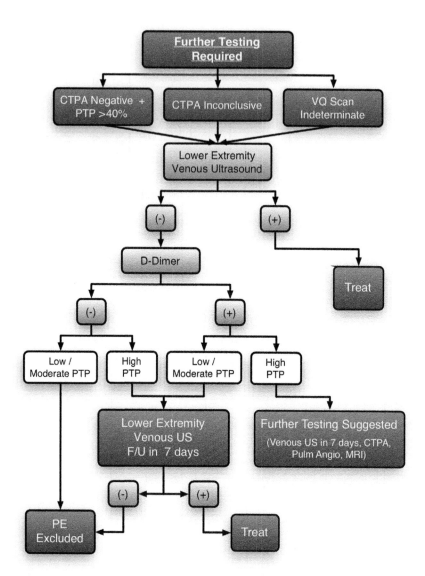

Fig. 4. A diagnostic algorithm for additional testing in patients with indeterminate imaging and the possibility of PE.

vitamin K antagonist warfarin.[198,199] Initial anticoagulation should be administered for 5 days and until the international normalized ratio (INR) is in the therapeutic range of 2.0 to 3.0 for 2 days.

In patients with a high clinical probability of PE, this treatment should begin before diagnostic imaging. In patients with low clinical PTP, it is considered safe to await confirmatory tests before initiating systemic anticoagulation.[200] In general, empiric treatment confers more benefit than harm when, PTP exceeds 30%, imaging would delay anticoagulation for greater than 24 hours, and the patient has no major contra-indications.[201] If using unfractionated heparin, it is given as a bolus dose of 5000 IU or

80 IU/kg, followed by a continuous nomogram-adjusted infusion to an activated thromboplastin time of 1.5 to 2.5 times the normal value.[202] All of the LMWHs are administered subcutaneously. Dalteparin is dosed at 200 U/kg once daily. Enoxaparin is administered at 1 mg/kg twice daily, and tinzaparin is given at 175 U/kg once daily. Fondaparinux is also delivered subcutaneously as a once-daily injection adjusted by patient weight categories. Patients weighing less than 50 kg, 50 to 100 kg, and greater than 100 kg receive doses of 5 mg, 7.5 mg, and 10 mg, respectively. The LMWHs and fondaparinux are preferable to unfractionated heparin because they are easier to administer, do not require intravenous infusions, and do not require monitoring of INR or factor Xa levels. Pregnant patients, patients with severe renal insufficiency, and those at the extremes of BMI may be eligible to have factor X levels monitored.[203,204] A 2004 meta-analysis of 12 studies showed that treatment with LMWH had an efficacy and safety profile similar to that of intravenous unfractionated heparin.[205] Similarly, a large, open-label study showed the efficacy and safety of fondaparinux to be similar to unfractionated heparin.[206]

The newer generation direct thrombin inhibitors (eg, dabigatran) are currently being studied against warfarin therapy for thromboembolic prophylaxis and the treatment of atrial fibrillation. These medications are orally administered, appear much more pharmacokinetically predictable in most patients, are easily initiated in the ED, and do not require any monitoring. Unfortunately they also lack any known reversal agent or strategy. Although off-label use for the treatment of PE is increasing, no evidence exists for their use in patients with acute PE. In patients with contraindications to anticoagulation, vena caval filters, mechanical thrombolysis and thrombectomy can be considered on an individual basis. Hemodynamically unstable patients should be treated more aggressively with pharmacologic or mechanical thrombolysis.

Thrombolysis

The use of thrombolytic agents in the treatment of PE has been studied for more than 40 years.[209] Thrombolytic agents act by promoting the conversion of endogenous plasminogen to plasmin, thereby degrading clot bound to fibrinogen and facilitating faster resolution of the clot.[197] Studies have shown that the use of thrombolytic agents in the treatment of PE results in more rapid resolution of arterial emboli, decreased PA pressure, and improvements in cardiac output and circulation.[197,210–212] A significant limitation of randomized controlled trials investigating the usefulness of thrombolytics in PE is that most studies use pulmonary perfusion parameters or hemodynamic parameters as primary endpoints.[211–214] However, these improvements in physiologic parameters have not translated into reduced mortality or recurrence risk in unselected patients with PE.[98] The use of thrombolytic agents is not without risk. The risk of major hemorrhage is 13%, twice that of heparin, and a recent meta-analysis found an intracranial hemorrhage rate of 2% with a mortality of 0.5%.[215,216] Factors associated with increased bleeding complications include increasing age, uncontrolled hypertension, recent stroke or surgery, and bleeding diathesis.[217]

Hemodynamically unstable patients should be treated more aggressively with pharmacologic or mechanical thrombolysis. In this population, mortality can be 60% or higher if untreated, and reduced to 30% or less with immediate treatment.[218] The literature provides little guidance for the EP in the administration of thrombolytic therapy. The consensus opinion among published clinical guidelines is to treat hemodynamically unstable patients with confirmed PE when the benefits outweigh the risks.[97,98] The British Thoracic Society also suggests that thrombolytic therapy may be instituted on clinical grounds alone if cardiac arrest is imminent.[97] If cardiac arrest occurs and is presumed to be due to PE, administration of fibrinolytics in patients may improve early survival, survival to discharge, and long-term neurologic function.[219,220] As a result, the 2010 American Heart Association Guidelines for Cardiopulmonary Resuscitation and Emergency Cardiovascular Care state that, if the cardiac arrest is caused by presumed PE, it is reasonable to administer fibrinolytics.[221] In the acute hemodynamically unstable patient with a massive PE, alteplase (ie, tPa) is given over 2 hours as an infusion of 100 mg, or as a 10 mg bolus, followed by a 90 mg infusion.[222,223] In patients in cardiac arrest a bolus of alteplace 50 mg or tenecteplase (tNK) 50 mg is administered over 2 min.[224,225] There are no conclusive studies comparing different thrombolytic regimens, but short infusion times of 2 hours or less are recommended in order to achieve more rapid thrombolysis and less bleeding.[198] The time frame for thrombolysis is up to 14 days after symptom onset.[226]

Given the lack of evidence showing benefit and the potential for significant bleeding complications, the use of thrombolytics in hemodynamically stable patients with PE is currently not recommended.[97,98] The use of thrombolytic therapy in subgroups of patients with PE, in particular those with right ventricular dysfunction or right heart thrombus on echocardiography, remains controversial. Patients with right ventricular dysfunction on echocardiography have more rapid return of right ventricular function and restoration of pulmonary perfusion when treated with thrombolytic agents; however, there is no evidence that these interventions decrease mortality.[197,209,211–213,227] The presence of a right heart thrombus, a rare finding, portends a worse outcome with a higher risk of recurrent PE and death.[171,228] A retrospective study of case reports and case series in patients with PE and right heart thrombus showed decreased mortality with thrombolytic therapy, although the study was limited due to selection bias.[229] Currently there are no recommendations to guide physicians in treating these subgroups of patients with PE. When faced with such cases, the physician should weigh the risks of the condition against the risks and benefits of the intervention.

PE IN THE PREGNANT PATIENT

Pregnancy is associated with an increased risk of VTE.[230] PE is the most common non-traumatic cause of death in pregnancy and the leading cause of mortality in developed countries.[43,231] Overall, the prevalence of PE in the pregnant population is quite low.[14] A meta-analysis found that more than 60% of DVTs occurred in the antepartum period, distributed equally among all trimesters, whereas 43% to 60% of PEs occurred in the postpartum period.[232,233] This increased risk is hypothesized to result from a relative hypercoagulable state in pregnancy. Fibrin and many other coagulation factors are increased, and it is common to have an acquired resistance to activated protein C.[234] In addition, free levels of protein S and general fibrinolytic activity are decreased.

The clinical pathway for the evaluation of PE in pregnant patients has been a topic of much debate and varies widely depending on institution, individual practice, and resource availability. **Fig. 5** depicts a possible algorithm for the evaluation of PE in pregnancy. The clinical diagnosis of PE in pregnant patients is fettered by the poor sensitivity and specificity of clinical findings. Leg swelling, tachypnea, tachycardia, pain, and dyspnea can be the result of normal physiologic changes in pregnancy. Physiologic dyspnea is typically mild without limiting daily activities, absent at rest, and generally does not worsen as pregnancy progresses. Dyspnea may occur by the 20th week of gestation and in up to 75% of pregnant women by 3rd trimester. Rapid-onset dyspnea or dyspnea associated with syncope, chest pain,

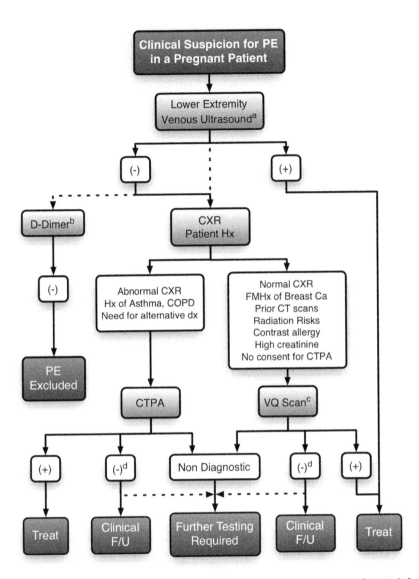

Fig. 5. A diagnostic algorithm for pregnant patients with clinical suspicion for PE. [a] If the patient has no signs and symptoms of DVT, given the low incidence of finding a lower leg DVT in all pregnant patients screened with bilateral lower leg Doppler US, some clinicians proceed straight to chest radiographs and the imaging modality of their choice (dotted line). [b] In a pregnant patient with a low PTP of PE, a negative lower leg ultrasound and a negative D-dimer may exclude the diagnosis of PE. The D-dimer may retain its NPV in pregnancy, but this is controversial given the paucity of definitive evidence (dotted line). [c] A full ventilation-perfusion scan may be used here; however, many clinicians use a perfusion-only scan to reduced radiation to the mother and fetus. Perfusion-only nuclear medicine scans yield similar results to the standard V/Q scan. [d] Few studies have examined whether additional investigation is required after a negative CTPA or V/Q scan in pregnancy. Marik and Plante[231] suggest clinical follow-up after negative diagnostic imaging. FMHx, family history; Ca, Cancer; F/U, follow-up. (*Data from* Marik PE, Plante LA. Venous thromboembolic disease and pregnancy. N Engl J Med 2008;359(19):2025–33.)

or hemoptysis, should not be attributed to physiologic dyspnea.[235] Risk factors for PE in pregnancy include heart disease, sickle cell anemia, lupus, multiple pregnancies, age greater than 35 years, obesity, smoking, African American, and cesarean section.[232,236,237]

In a patient with a high clinical suspicion for PE, a chest radiograph should be obtained to triage the patient for lung scintigraphy or CTPA, as appropriate. In patients with a low clinical suspicion, many clinicians use lower extremity venous ultrasonography and a D-dimer to initiate the work-up. The role of D-dimer in the pregnant patient is unknown. False positive results increase as the pregnancy progresses, and the inappropriate use of the D-dimer assay may result in unnecessary diagnostic examinations and radiation exposure. The NPV of a normal D-dimer in pregnancy is also controversial. It has been suggested that the quantitative high-specificity assays remain accurate regardless of trimester.[238,239] Chan and colleagues[239] showed that a negative test with a highly sensitive assay in the first and second trimesters has an NPV of 100%. However, others suggest that a negative D-dimer test may not necessarily rule out PE, but may be helpful if CUS is normal.[240] As in the non-pregnant population, a patient with a positive D-dimer and those patients with a negative D-dimer and a moderate or high PTP of PE require further investigation.

The main advantage of using lower extremity CUS is that a positive result is sufficient to initiate anticoagulation and may eliminate the need for additional imaging and radiation. The estimated prevalence of DVT in pregnant patients is between 0.06% and 8% and the prevalence among those with clinically suspected PE is uncertain.[239,241] Given only a small proportion of US studies are positive, performing a systematic US study as a first-line strategy in pregnant patients has been a matter of debate.[242] It is important to note that negative US results warrant further investigation because PE may occur in the absence of DVT, and US may fail to detect pelvic vein DVT.[243,244]

If the CUS is negative, it is reasonable to proceed with diagnostic imaging. An initial chest radiograph may be used to determine which imaging modality to use. With a normal chest radiograph, lung scintigraphy is more likely to yield an accurate result, whereas, an abnormal chest radiograph should be followed up with a CTPA.

Lung scintigraphy and CT angiography have comparable performances for diagnosis of PE during pregnancy, with no significant differences between the proportions of positive, negative, or indeterminate results.[245] Advantages of a CTPA include less radiation to the fetus during all trimesters of pregnancy and the potential to uncover alternative diagnoses.[246,247] The disadvantages include increased incidence of indeterminate results compared with the general population, fetal exposure to iodinated contrast material, and a larger dose of radiation to maternal breast tissue. Indeterminate CT results are more common in pregnant patients, mainly because of poor vascular opacification secondary to the normal physiologic increased blood volume and cardiac output that occurs during pregnancy.[248,249] The primary concern of radiation exposure during pregnancy is to the breast tissue, which is proliferating and active, and therefore more radiosensitive.[139] In addition, once imaged, patients often undergo multiple subsequent examinations for suspected recurrence.[250] Effective doses ranging from 10–80 mSv are reported in the literature which may increase the lifetime risk of breast cancer by 0.2–14% in a 30 year old woman.[91,73,151,152,251,252] The BEIR VII report estimated the lifetime attributable risk for breast cancer from a dose of 20 mGy ranges from 1/1200 for a woman aged 20 to 1/3500 for woman aged 40.[186] Studies have investigated many methods to decrease the effective radiation dose, such as bismuth shields, reduced kilovoltage, or reduced z-axis coverage, which may lower exposure by more than 50%.[253]

The advantages of V/Q scans in pregnancy include lower radiation dose to the maternal breast tissue and a decreased rate of indeterminate scans. The radiation effective dose for V/Q scans is approximately 0.5 to 2.2 mSv, and this can be reduced further to 0.2 to 0.5 mSv if perfusion-only scans are performed.[139,151] Research supports the use of perfusion-only lung scintigraphy, demonstrating that the outcome and the proportion of normal-, intermediate-, and high-probability scans is similar between perfusion-only and ventilation-perfusion scans.[254] The rate of indeterminate V/Q scans is less in pregnancy secondary to the lower frequency of cardiopulmonary disease in these younger patients.[255]

The disadvantage of lung scintigraphy is the potential fetal exposure to radiation compared with CTPA. However, the radiation effective dose of 0.64–0.8 mGy is well below the accepted limit of 50 mGy for the induction of deterministic effects in the fetus, and comparable to the natural background radiation exposure to a fetus of 1.1 to 2.5 mGy.[256–258] The combination of chest radiography, V/Q scan, CTPA, and pulmonary angiography is thought to expose the fetus to only 1.5 mGy. Perfusion-only protocols, proper hydration, and prompt emptying of the bladder after V/Q scans can further reduce the fetal radiation exposure.

In an appropriate institution, lung perfusion scans should be considered the investigation of choice for any young women. Furthermore, pregnant woman should be advised that V/Q scanning has a much lower risk of maternal breast cancer, and those with a family history of breast cancer or those who have had previous CTPA's may opt for a lung perfusion scan. Lung perfusion scans have a slightly higher theoretical risk of childhood cancer, however, exposures are well below the accepted fetal exposure limit.

MRI does not involve any radiation exposure and is not known to be harmful to the fetus. It has a high sensitivity and specificity for diagnosis of DVT. However, the PIOPED III trial recently showed a high rate of technically inadequate images when used for diagnosis of PE.[179,259] The sensitivity and specificity were 78% and 99%, respectively, when the images were considered technically accurate. However, the images were technically inadequate 25% of the time. When combined with MR venography, the sensitivity was 92% and the specificity was 96%.[179] MR pulmonary angiography should only be considered in patients for whom the standard diagnostic tests are contraindicated.

Despite the possible radiation and contract exposures, important and relevant diagnostic tests should not be withheld in pregnancy. It is important that radiation doses be kept as low as reasonably achievable ("ALARA" principle) while maintaining appropriate diagnostic quality. Ultimately, few studies exist examining whether additional investigations (eg, repeat CUS) are required after a negative CTPA or V/Q in pregnancy. Marik and Plante suggest clinical follow-up is appropriate if lower extremity US has already been performed.[247] In hemodynamically stable patients presenting early in pregnancy, anticoagulation with LMWH is recommended.[260,261] LMWH has predictable pharmacokinetics and a reduced risk of bleeding and heparin-induced thrombocytopenia. In pregnancy, the half-life of LMWH decreases because of increased renal excretion, and therefore a twice-daily regimen is often recommended.[260–262] For practical purposes, many clinicians continue to use single daily dosing. Neither heparin nor LMWH crosses the placenta and thus teratogenesis and fetal hemorrhage is not a concern.[263] Warfarin is well known to be teratogenic and is not used until the postpartum period.[260] Experience is limited with fondaparinux, danaparoid, the direct factor Xa inhibitors, and the direct thrombin inhibitors (eg, dabigatran, argatroban). In hemodynamically stable patients late in pregnancy, the challenge is the management of anticoagulation given that labor is unpredictable and delivery can be associated with significant blood loss. LMWH cannot be expeditiously reversed and thus unfractionated heparin is preferred late in pregnancy. Patients can be safely switched to subcutaneous or intravenous unfractionated heparin for the last few weeks of pregnancy, although the benefit of this approach has not been validated by clinical studies. In addition, a temporary vena caval filter can be placed before delivery as necessary.[264] After birth, anticoagulation can be resumed within 12 hours of delivery in the absence of persistent bleeding.[260] The unstable patient with massive PE and severe hemodynamic compromise should be considered for thrombolytic therapy.[265] Placental abruption after thrombolytics is a concern, but has not been reported. Successful thrombolysis has been described within 1 hour of vaginal delivery and 12 hours of cesarean section, despite being contraindicated within 10 days after cesarean section.[266]

SUMMARY

The presentation of PE ranges from incidentally discovered asymptomatic emboli to massive embolism causing an immediate threat to life. Despite an ever-expanding body of literature describing various aspects of this disease, it continues to be a challenging diagnosis to make, particularly in the ED. EPs use a combination of risk factors and clinical features to estimate a patient's PTP of having PE. Although a number CDRs are available to physicians, evidence continues to support the notion that PTP may be determined implicitly or explicitly depending on the physician's preference. Physicians should be aware of diagnostic algorithms for PE and realize that incorrect use of diagnostic tests, in particular the D-dimer, may lead to overtesting and patient harm. Furthermore, in an attempt to limit testing in patients at very low risk of having a PE the physician may choose to apply the PERC rule. In those patients who require further testing, several options are available, including CTPA, V/Q scanning, and ultrasound. Although the use and reliability of CTPA is increasing, EPs should recognize the risks of this procedure (contrast-induced nephropathy and radiation risks) and should consider alternative testing strategies when possible. In particular, alternative strategies should be considered for the investigation of pregnant patients with suspected PE. Thrombolytics are not recommended for the treatment of unselected patients with PE, despite the potential to improve physiologic parameters. The EP should risk stratify patients with known PE based on their hemodynamic stability and base the decision to thrombolyse on the known risks and benefits of the treatment.

REFERENCES

1. Dorfman GS, Cronan JJ, Tupper TB, et al. Occult pulmonary embolism: a common occurrence in deep venous thrombosis. AJR Am J Roentgenol 1987;148(2):263–6.
2. Meignan M, Rosso J, Gauthier H, et al. Systemic lung scans reveal a high frequency of silent pulmonary embolism in patients with proximal deep venous thrombosis. Arch Intern Med 2000;160(2):159–64.
3. Goldhaber SZ, Elliott CG. Acute pulmonary embolism. Part I: epidemiology, pathophysiology, and diagnosis. Circulation 2003;108(22):2726–9.
4. Ouellette DR. Pulmonary embolism. Emedicine. 2011. Available at: http://emedicine.medscape.com/article/300901-overview#a0156. Accessed May, 2011.

5. Rodger M, Wells PS. Diagnosis of pulmonary embolism. Thromb Res 2001; 103(6):V225–38.
6. White RH. The epidemiology of venous thromboembolism. Circulation 2003; 107(23 Suppl 1):I4–8.
7. Schulman S, Lindmarker P, Holmström M, et al. Post-thrombotic syndrome, recurrence, and death 10 years after the first episode of venous thromboembolism treated with warfarin for 6 weeks or 6 months. J Thromb Haemost 2006;4(4): 734–42.
8. Pengo V, Lensing AW, Prins MH, et al. Incidence of chronic thromboembolic pulmonary hypertension after pulmonary embolism. N Engl J Med 2004; 350(22):2257–64.
9. Ryu JH, Olson EJ, Pellikka PA. Clinical recognition of pulmonary embolism: problem of unrecognized and asymptomatic cases. Mayo Clin Proc 1998;73(9):873–9.
10. Lusiani L, Visona A, Bonanome A, et al. The characteristics of the thrombi of the lower limbs, as detected by ultrasonic scanning, do not predict pulmonary embolism. Chest 1996;110(4):996–1000.
11. Feied CF. Venous thrombosis and pulmonary embolism. In: Marx JA, Hockberger RS, Walls RM, et al, editors. Rosen's emergency medicine concepts and clinical practice. 5th edition, vol. 2. Atlanta (GA): Mosby; 2002. p. 1210–34.
12. Stein PD, Matta F. Acute pulmonary embolism. Curr Probl Cardiol 2010;35(7): 314–76.
13. Wells PS, Ginsberg JS, Anderson DR, et al. Use of a clinical model for safe management of patients with suspected pulmonary embolism. Ann Intern Med 1998;129(12):997–1005.
14. Nicolaides AN, Kakkar VV, Field ES, et al. The origin of deep vein thrombosis: a venographic study. Br J Radiol 1971;44(525):653–63.
15. Rollins DL, Semrow CM, Friedell ML, et al. Origin of deep vein thrombi in an ambulatory population. Am J Surg 1988;156(2):122–5.
16. Jorens PG, Van Marck E, Snoeckx A, et al. Nonthrombotic pulmonary embolism. Eur Respir J 2009;34(2):452–74.
17. Dalen JE. Pulmonary embolism: what have we learned since Virchow? Natural history, pathophysiology, and diagnosis. Chest 2002;122(4):1440–56.
18. Goldhaber SZ. Echocardiography in the management of pulmonary embolism. Ann Intern Med 2002;136(9):691–700.
19. Silverstein MD, Heit JA, Mohr DN, et al. Trends in the incidence of deep vein thrombosis and pulmonary embolism: a 25-year population-based study. Arch Intern Med 1998;158(6):585–93.
20. Anderson FA Jr, Wheeler HB, Goldberg RJ, et al. A population-based perspective of the hospital incidence and case-fatality rates of deep vein thrombosis and pulmonary embolism. The Worcester DVT Study. Arch Intern Med 1991; 151(5):933–8.
21. Goldhaber SZ. Pulmonary embolism. Lancet 2004;363(9417):1295–305.
22. Stein PD. Pulmonary embolism. 2nd edition. Oxford: Blackwell Futura; 2007.
23. Kline JA, Runyon MS. Pulmonary embolism and deep venous thrombosis. In: Marx JA, Hockenberger RS, Walls RM, editors. Rosen's emergency medicine concepts and clinical practice, vol. 1. 7th edition. Philadelphia: Mosby; 2009. p. 1124–36.
24. Martinelli I. Risk factors in venous thromboembolism. Thromb Haemost 2001; 86(91):395–403.
25. Bounameaux H. Contemporary management of pulmonary embolism: the answers to ten questions. J Intern Med 2010;268(3):218–31.

26. Tapson VF. Prophylaxis strategies for patients with acute venous thromboembolism. Am J Manag Care 2001;7(Suppl 17):S524–34.

27. Cushman M, Tsai A, Heckbert SR. Incidence rates, case fatality, and recurrence rates of deep vein thrombosis and pulmonary embolus: the Longitudinal Investigation of Thromboembolism Etiology (LITE). Thromb Haemost 2001;86.

28. Carson JL, Kelley MA, Duff A, et al. The clinical course of pulmonary embolism. N Engl J Med 1992;326(19):1240–5.

29. The Columbus Investigators. Low-molecular-weight heparin in the treatment of patients with venous thromboembolism. N Engl J Med 1997;337(10):657–62.

30. Simonneau G, Sors H, Charbonnier B, et al. A comparison of low-molecular-weight heparin with unfractionated heparin for acute pulmonary embolism. The THESEE Study Group. N Engl J Med 1997;337(10):663–9.

31. Courtney DM, Kline JA, Kabrhel C, et al. Clinical features from the history and physical examination that predict the presence or absence of pulmonary embolism in symptomatic emergency department patients: results of a prospective, multicenter study. Ann Emerg Med 2010;55(4):307–15.

32. Horlander KT, Mannino DM, Leeper KV. Pulmonary embolism mortality in the United States, 1979–1998: an analysis using multiple-cause mortality data. Arch Intern Med 2003;163(14):1711–7.

33. Stein PD, Hull RD, Patel KC, et al. Venous thromboembolic disease: comparison of the diagnostic process in men and women. Arch Intern Med 2003;163(14):1689–94.

34. Schneider D, Lilienfeld DE, Im W. The epidemiology of pulmonary embolism: racial contrasts in incidence and in-hospital case fatality. J Natl Med Assoc 2006;98(12):1967–72.

35. Meyer G, Planquette B, Sanchez O. Long-term outcome of pulmonary embolism. Curr Opin Hematol 2008;15(5):499–503.

36. Stein PD, Kayali F, Olson RE. Incidence of venous thromboembolism in infants and children: data from the National Hospital Discharge Survey. J Pediatr 2004;145(4):563–5.

37. Stein PD, Hull RD, Kayali F, et al. Venous thromboembolism according to age: the impact of an aging population. Arch Intern Med 2004;164(20):2260–5.

38. PIOPED Investigators. Value of the ventilation/perfusion scan in acute pulmonary embolism. Results of the Prospective Investigation of Pulmonary Embolism Diagnosis (PIOPED). JAMA 1990;263(20):2753–9.

39. Morgenthaler TI, Ryu JH. Clinical characteristics of fatal pulmonary embolism in a referral hospital. Mayo Clin Proc 1995;70(5):417–24.

40. Dalen JE. Should patients with venous thromboembolism be screened for thrombophilia? Am J Med 2008;121(6):458–63.

41. Rosendaal FR. Risk factors for venous thrombosis: prevalence, risk, and interaction. Semin Hematol 1997;34(3):171–87.

42. Bauer KA. The thrombophilias: well-defined risk factors with uncertain therapeutic implications. Ann Intern Med 2001;135(5):367–73.

43. Kim V, Spandorfer J. Epidemiology of venous thromboembolic disease. Emerg Med Clin North Am 2001;19(4):839–59.

44. Prandoni P, Bilora F, Marchiori A, et al. An association between atherosclerosis and venous thrombosis. N Engl J Med 2003;348(15):1435–41.

45. Beasley R, Raymond N, Hill S, et al. eThrombosis: the 21st century variant of venous thromboembolism associated with immobility. Eur Respir J 2003;21(2):374–6.

46. Lapostolle F, Surget V, Borron SW, et al. Severe pulmonary embolism associated with air travel. N Engl J Med 2001;345(11):779–83.

47. Francis CW. Prophylaxis for thromboembolism in hospitalized medical patients. N Engl J Med 2007;356(14):1438–44.

48. Geerts WH, Code KI, Jay RM, et al. A prospective study of venous thromboembolism after major trauma. N Engl J Med 1994;331(24):1601–6.

49. Danilenko-Dixon DR, Heit JA, Silverstein MD, et al. Risk factors for deep venous thrombosis and pulmonary embolism during pregnancy or post partum: a population-based, case-control study. Am J Obstet Gynecol 2001; 184(2):104–10.

50. McColl MD, Ramsay JE, Tait RC, et al. Risk factors for pregnancy associated venous thromboembolism. Thromb Haemost 1997;78(4):1183–8.

51. Kuklina EV, Meikle SF, Jamieson DJ, et al. Severe obstetric morbidity in the United States: 1998–2005. Obstet Gynecol 2009;113(2 Pt 1):293–9.

52. Vandenbroucke JP, Koster T, Briet E, et al. Increased risk of venous thrombosis in oral-contraceptive users who are carriers of factor V Leiden mutation. Lancet 1994;344(8935):1453–7.

53. Stein PD, Beemath A, Meyers FA, et al. Incidence of venous thromboembolism in patients hospitalized with cancer. Am J Med 2006;119(1):60–8.

54. Giuntini C, Di Ricco G, Marini C, et al. Pulmonary embolism: epidemiology, pathophysiology, diagnosis, and management. Chest 1995;107(Suppl 1):3S–9S.

55. Skaf E, Stein PD, Beemath A, et al. Venous thromboembolism in patients with ischemic and hemorrhagic stroke. Am J Cardiol 2005;96(12):1731–3.

56. Laack TA, Goyal DG. Pulmonary embolism: an unsuspected killer. Emerg Med Clin North Am 2004;22(4):961–83.

57. Stein PD, Fowler SE, Goodman LR, et al. PIOPED II Investigators. Multidetector computed tomography for acute pulmonary embolism. N Engl J Med 2006; 354(22):2317–27.

58. Green RM, Meyer TJ, Dunn M, et al. Pulmonary embolism in younger adults. Chest 1992;101(6):1507–11.

59. Stein PD, Beemath A, Matta F, et al. Clinical characteristics of patients with acute pulmonary embolism: data from PIOPED II. Am J Med 2007;120(10):871–9.

60. Stein PD, Henry JW. Clinical characteristics of patients with acute pulmonary embolism stratified according to their presenting syndromes. Chest 1997; 112(4):974–9.

61. Urokinase Pulmonary Embolism Trial. A national cooperative study. Circulation 1973;47(Suppl 2):II1–108.

62. Miniati M, Prediletto R, Fromichi B, et al. Accuracy of clinical assessment in the diagnosis of pulmonary embolism. Am J Respir Crit Care Med 1999;159(3):864–71.

63. Sadosty AT, Boie ET, Stead LG. Pulmonary embolism. Emerg Med Clin North Am 2003;21(2):363–84.

64. Riedel M. Acute pulmonary embolism 1: pathophysiology, clinical presentation, and diagnosis. Heart 2001;85(2):229–40.

65. Comess KA, DeRook FA, Russell ML, et al. The incidence of pulmonary embolism in unexplained sudden cardiac arrest with pulseless electrical activity. Am J Med 2000;109(5):351–6.

66. Brilakis ES, Tajik AJ. 82-year-old man with recurrent syncope. Mayo Clin Proc 1999;74(6):609–12.

67. Stein PD, Terrin ML, Hales CA, et al. Clinical, laboratory, roentgenographic and electrocardiographic findings in patients with acute pulmonary embolism and no pre-existing cardiac or pulmonary disease. Chest 1991;100(3):598–603.

68. Susec O, Boudrow D, Kline JA. The clinical features of acute pulmonary embolism in ambulatory patients. Acad Emerg Med 1997;4(9):891–7.
69. Courtney DM, Kline JA. Identification of prearrest clinical factors associated with outpatient fatal pulmonary embolism. Acad Emerg Med 2001;8(12): 1136–42.
70. Stein PD, Afzal A, Henry JW, et al. Fever in acute pulmonary embolism. Chest 2000;117(1):39–42.
71. Stein PD, Matta F, Musani MH, et al. Silent pulmonary embolism in patients with deep venous thrombosis: a systematic review. Am J Med 2010;123(5): 426–31.
72. Wolfe TR, Hartsell SC. Pulmonary embolism: making sense of the diagnostic evaluation. Ann Emerg Med 2001;37(5):504–14.
73. Mamlouk MD, vanSonnenberg E, Gosalia R, et al. Pulmonary embolism at CT angiography: implications for appropriateness, cost, and radiation exposure in 2003 patients. Radiology 2010;256(2):625–32.
74. Kabrhel C, Camargo CA Jr, Goldhaber SZ. Clinical gestalt and the diagnosis of pulmonary embolism: does experience matter? Chest 2005;127(5): 1627–30.
75. Iles S, Hodges AM, Darley JR, et al. Clinical experience and pre-test probability scores in the diagnosis of pulmonary embolism. QJM 2003;96(3):211–5.
76. Kline JA, Hernandez-Nino J, Newgard CD, et al. Use of pulse oximetry to predict in-hospital complications in normotensive patients with pulmonary embolism. Am J Med 2003;115(3):203–8.
77. Wicki J, Perneger TV, Junod AF, et al. Assessing clinical probability of pulmonary embolism in the emergency ward: a simple score. Arch Intern Med 2001;161(1):92–7.
78. Stein PD, Sostman HD, Bounameaux H, et al. Challenges in the diagnosis of acute pulmonary embolism. Am J Med 2008;121(7):565–71.
79. Einstein AJ, Henzlova MJ, Rajagopalan S. Estimating risk of cancer associated with radiation exposure from 64-slice computed tomography coronary angiography. JAMA 2007;298(3):317–23.
80. LeGal G, Righini M, Roy PM, et al. Prediction of pulmonary embolism in the emergency department: the revised Geneva score. Ann Intern Med 2006; 144(3):165–71.
81. Klok FA, Mos IC, Nijkeuter M, et al. Simplification of the revised Geneva score for assessing clinical probability of pulmonary embolism. Arch Intern Med 2008; 168(19):2131–6.
82. Wells PS, Anderson DR, Rodger M, et al. Derivation of a simple clinical model to categorize patients probability of pulmonary embolism: increasing the models utility with the SimpliRED D-dimer. Thromb Haemost 2000;83(3): 416–20.
83. Chagnon I, Bounameaux H, Aujesky D, et al. Comparison of two clinical prediction rules and implicit assessment among patients with suspected pulmonary embolism. Am J Med 2002;113(4):269–75.
84. van Belle A, Büller HR, Huisman MV, et al. Christopher Study Investigators. Effectiveness of managing suspected pulmonary embolism using an algorithm combining clinical probability, D-dimer testing, and computed tomography. JAMA 2006;295(2):172–9.
85. Klok FA, Kruisman E, Spaan J, et al. Comparison of the revised Geneva score with the Wells rule for assessing clinical probability of pulmonary embolism. J Thromb Haemost 2008;6(1):40–4.

86. Righini M, Le Gal G, Aujesky D, et al. Diagnosis of pulmonary embolism by multidetector CT alone or combined with venous ultrasonography of the leg: a randomised non-inferiority trial. Lancet 2008;371(9621):1343–52.

87. Ceriani E, Combescure C, Le Gal G, et al. Clinical prediction rules for pulmonary embolism: systematic review and meta-analysis. J Thromb Haemost 2010;8(5): 957–70.

88. Wells PS, Anderson DR, Rodger M, et al. Excluding pulmonary embolism at the bedside without diagnostic imaging: management of patients with suspected pulmonary embolism presenting to the emergency department by using a simple clinical model and D-dimer. Ann Intern Med 2001;135(2):98–107.

89. Moores LK, Collen JF, Woods KM, et al. Practical utility of clinical prediction rules for suspected acute pulmonary embolism in a large academic institution. Thromb Res 2004;113(1):1–6.

90. Kabrhel C, Courtney DM, Camargo CA Jr, et al. Potential impact of adjusting the threshold of the quantitative D-dimer based on pretest probability of acute pulmonary embolism. Acad Emerg Med 2009;16(4):325–32.

91. Musset D, Parent F, Meyer G, et al. Diagnostic strategy for patients with suspected pulmonary embolism: a prospective multicentre outcome study. Lancet 2002;360(9349):1914–20.

92. Runyon MS, Webb WB, Jones AE, et al. Comparison of the unstructured clinician estimate of pretest probability for pulmonary embolism to the Canadian score and the Charlotte rule: a prospective observational study. Acad Emerg Med 2005;12:587–93.

93. Runyon MS, Richman PB, Kline JA, et al, Pulmonary Embolism Research Consortium Study Group. Emergency medicine practitioner knowledge and use of decision rules for the evaluation of patients with suspected pulmonary embolism: variations by practice setting and training level. Acad Emerg Med 2007;14(1):53–7.

94. Rosen MP, Sands DZ, Morris J, et al. Does a physician's ability to accurately assess the likelihood of pulmonary embolism increase with training? Acad Med 2000;75(12):1199–205.

95. Richardson WS. Five uneasy pieces about pre-test probability. J Gen Intern Med 2002;17(11):882–3.

96. Jackson RE, Rudoni RR, Pascual R. Emergency physician assessment of the pre-test probability of pulmonary embolism. Acad Emerg Med 1999;6(5): 437.

97. British Thoracic Society Standards of Care Committee Pulmonary Embolism Guideline Development Group. British Thoracic Society guidelines for the management of suspected acute pulmonary embolism. Thorax 2003;58(6): 470–83.

98. American College of Emergency Physicians Clinical Policies Subcommittee. Clinical policy: critical issues in the evaluation and management of adult patients presenting to the emergency department with suspected pulmonary embolism. Ann Emerg Med 2011;57(6):628–52.

99. Robin ED. Overdiagnosis and overtreatment of pulmonary embolism: the emperor may have no clothes. Ann Intern Med 1977;87(6):775–81.

100. Pauker SG, Kassirer JP. The threshold approach to clinical decision making. N Engl J Med 1980;302(20):1109–17.

101. Kline JA, Mitchell AM, Kabrhel C, et al. Clinical criteria to prevent unnecessary diagnostic testing in emergency department patients with suspected pulmonary embolism. J Thromb Haemost 2004;2(8):1247–55.

102. Lessler AL, Isserman JA, Agarwal R, et al. Testing low-risk patients for suspected pulmonary embolism: a decision analysis. Ann Emerg Med 2010; 55(4):316–26.

103. Kline JA, Courtney DM, Kabrhel C, et al. Prospective multicenter evaluation of the pulmonary embolism rule-out criteria. J Thromb Haemost 2008;6(5): 772–80.

104. Wolf SJ, McCubbin TR, Nordenholz KE, et al. Assessment of the pulmonary embolism rule-out criteria rule for evaluation of suspected pulmonary embolism in the emergency department. Am J Emerg Med 2008;26(2): 181–5.

105. Hugli O, Righini M, Le Gal G, et al. The pulmonary embolism rule-out criteria (PERC) rule does not safely exclude pulmonary embolism. J Thromb Haemost 2011;9(2):300–4.

106. Ferrari E, Imbert A, Chevalier T, et al. The ECG in pulmonary embolism. Predictive value of negative T waves in precordial leads – 80 case reports. Chest 1997; 111(3):537–43.

107. Elliott CG, Goldhaber SZ, Visani L, et al. Chest radiographs in acute pulmonary embolism. Chest 2000;118(1):33–8.

108. Sostman HD, Miniati M, Gottschalk A, et al. Sensitivity and specificity of perfusion scintigraphy combined with chest radiography for acute pulmonary embolism in PIOPED II. J Nucl Med 2008;49(11):1741–8.

109. Edlow JA. Emergency department management of pulmonary embolism. Emerg Med Clin North Am 2001;19(4):995–1011.

110. Stein PD, Willis PW III, DeMets DL, et al. Plain chest roentgenogram in patients with acute pulmonary embolism and no pre-existing cardiac or pulmonary disease. Am J Noninvas Cardiol 1987;1:171–6.

111. Worsley DF, Alavi A. Radionuclide imaging of acute pulmonary embolism. Radiol Clin North Am 2011;39(5):1035–52.

112. Cvitanic O, Marino PL. Improved use of arterial blood gas analysis in suspected pulmonary embolism. Chest 1989;95(1):48–51.

113. Weiner SG, Burstein JL. Nonspecific tests for pulmonary embolism. Emerg Med Clin North Am 2001;19(4):943–55.

114. Kline JA, Johns KL, Coluciello SA, et al. New diagnostic tests for pulmonary embolism. Ann Emerg Med 2000;35(2):168–80.

115. Overton DT, Bocka J. The alveolar-arterial gradient in patients with documented pulmonary embolism. Arch Intern Med 1988;148(7):1617–9.

116. Stein PD, Goldhaber SZ, Henry JW. Alveolar-arterial oxygen gradient in the assessment of acute pulmonary embolism. Chest 1995;107(1):139–43.

117. Kucher N, Goldhaber SZ. Cardiac biomarkers for risk stratification of patients with acute pulmonary embolism. Circulation 2003;108(18):2191–4.

118. Pruszczyk P, Bochowicz A, Torbicki A, et al. Cardiac troponin T monitoring identifies a high-risk group of normotensive patients with acute pulmonary embolism. Chest 2003;123(6):1947–52.

119. Stein PD, Alshabkhoun S, Hatem C, et al. Coronary artery blood flow in acute pulmonary embolism. Am J Cardiol 1968;21(1):32–7.

120. Stein PD, Alshabkhoun S, Hawkins HF, et al. Right coronary blood flow in acute pulmonary embolism. Am Heart J 1969;77(3):356–62.

121. Melanson SE, Laposata M, Camargo CA Jr, et al. Combination of D-dimer and amino-terminal pro-B-type natriuretic peptide testing for the evaluation of dyspneic patients with and without acute pulmonary embolism. Arch Pathol Lab Med 2006;130(9):1326–9.

122. Farrell S, Hayes T, Shaw M. A negative SimpliRED D-dimer assay result does not exclude the diagnosis of deep vein thrombosis or pulmonary embolus in emergency department patients. Ann Emerg Med 2000;35(2):121–5.

123. Hogg K, Dawson D, Mackway-Jones K. The emergency department utility of Simplify D-dimer to exclude pulmonary embolism in patients with pleuritic chest pain. Ann Emerg Med 2005;46(4):305–10.

124. Runyon MS, Beam DM, King MC, et al. Comparison of the Simplify D-dimer assay performed at the bedside with a laboratory-based quantitative D-dimer assay for the diagnosis of pulmonary embolism in a low prevalence emergency department population. Emerg Med J 2008;25(2):70–5.

125. Kline JA, Runyon MS, Webb WB, et al. Prospective study of the diagnostic accuracy of the Simplify D-dimer assay for pulmonary embolism in emergency department patients. Chest 2006;129(6):1417–23.

126. Brown MD, Lau J, Nelson RD, et al. Turbidimetric D-dimer test in the diagnosis of pulmonary embolism: a meta-analysis. Clin Chem 2003;49(11):1846–53.

127. Brown MD, Rowe BH, Reeves MJ, et al. The accuracy of the enzyme-linked immunosorbent assay D-dimer test in the diagnosis of pulmonary embolism: a meta-analysis. Ann Emerg Med 2002;40(2):133–44.

128. Carrier M, Righini M, Djurabi RK, et al. VIDAS D-dimer in combination with clinical pre-test probability to rule out pulmonary embolism: a systematic review of management outcome studies. Thromb Haemost 2009;101(5):886–92.

129. Perrier A, Roy PM, Sanchez O, et al. Multidetector-row computed tomography in suspected pulmonary embolism. N Engl J Med 2005;28(17):1760–8.

130. Chabloz P, Reber G, Boehlen F, et al. TAFI antigen and D-dimer levels during normal pregnancy and at delivery. Br J Haematol 2001;115(1):150–2.

131. Couturaud F, Parent F, Meyer G, et al. Effect of age on the performance of a diagnostic strategy based on clinical probability, spiral computed tomography and venous compression ultrasonography: the ESSEP Study. Thromb Haemost 2005;93(3):605–9.

132. Douma RA, Le Gal G, Söhne M, et al. Potential of an age adjusted D-dimer cutoff value to improve the exclusion of pulmonary embolism in older patients: a retrospective analysis of three large cohorts. Br Med J 2010;340:c1475.

133. Remy-Jardin M, Pistolesi M, Goodman LR, et al. Management of suspected acute pulmonary embolism in the era of CT angiography: a statement from the Fleischner Society. Radiology 2007;245(2):315–29.

134. Cross JJ, Kemp PM, Walsh CG, et al. A randomized trial of spiral CT and ventilation perfusion scintigraphy for the diagnosis of pulmonary embolism. Clin Radiol 1998;53(3):177–82.

135. Kim KI, Muller NL, Mayo JR. Clinically suspected pulmonary embolism: utility of spiral CT. Radiology 1999;210(3):693–7.

136. Richman PB, Courtney DM, Friese J, et al. Prevalence and significance of nonthromboembolic findings on chest computed tomography angiography performed to rule out pulmonary embolism: a multicenter study of 1,025 emergency department patients. Acad Emerg Med 2004;11(6):642–7.

137. Mitchell AM, Kline JA. Contrast nephropathy following computed tomography angiography of the chest for pulmonary embolism in the emergency department. J Thromb Haemost 2007;5(1):50–4.

138. Task Group on Control of Radiation Dose in Computed Tomography. Managing patient dose in computed tomography. A report of the International Commission on Radiological Protection. Ann ICRP 2000;30(4):7–45.

139. Parker MS, Hui FK, Camacho MA, et al. Female breast radiation exposure during CT pulmonary angiography. AJR Am J Roentgenol 2005;185(5):1228–33.

140. Cook JV, Kyriou J. Radiation from CT and perfusion scanning in pregnancy. BMJ 2005;331(7512):350.

141. Novelline RA, Baltarowich OH, Athanasoulis CA, et al. The clinical course of patients with suspected pulmonary embolism and a negative pulmonary arteriogram. Radiology 1978;126(3):561–7.

142. Cheely R, McCartney WH, Perry JR, et al. The role of noninvasive tests versus pulmonary angiography in the diagnosis of pulmonary embolism. Am J Med 1981;70(1):17–22.

143. Perrier A, Howarth N, Didier D, et al. Performances of helical computed tomography in unselected outpatients with suspected pulmonary embolism. Ann Intern Med 2001;135(2):88–97.

144. Van Beek EJ, Brouwers EM, Song B, et al. Clinical validity of a normal pulmonary angiogram in patients with suspected pulmonary embolism – a critical review. Clin Radiol 2001;56(10):838–42.

145. Eng J, Krishnan JA, Segal JB, et al. Accuracy of CT in the diagnosis of pulmonary embolism: a systematic literature review. Am J Roentgenol 2004;183(6):1819–27.

146. Anderson DR, Kahn SR, Rodger MA, et al. Computed tomographic pulmonary angiography vs ventilation-perfusion lung scanning in patients with suspected pulmonary embolism: a randomized controlled trial. JAMA 2007;298(23):2743–53.

147. Garg K, Welsh CH, Feyerabend AJ, et al. Pulmonary embolism: diagnosis with spiral CT and ventilation-perfusion scanning – correlation with pulmonary angiographic results or clinical outcome. Radiology 1998;208(1):201–8.

148. Rufener SL, Patel S, Kazerooni EA, et al. Comparison of on-call radiology resident and faculty interpretation of 4- and 16-row multidetector CT pulmonary angiography with indirect CT venography. Acad Radiol 2008;15(1):71–6.

149. Vigo M, Pesavento R, Bova C, et al. The value of four-detector row spiral computed tomography for the diagnosis of pulmonary embolism. Semin Thromb Hemost 2006;32(8):831–7.

150. Wilson HT, Meagher TM, Williams SJ. Combined helical computed tomographic pulmonary angiography and lung perfusion scintigraphy for investigating acute pulmonary embolism. Clin Radiol 2002;57(1):33–6.

151. Radiation dose to patients from radiopharmaceuticals (addendum 2 to ICRP publication 53). Ann ICRP 1998;28(3):1–126.

152. Van Beek EJ, Brouwers EM, Song B, et al. Lung scintigraphy and helical computed tomography in the diagnosis of pulmonary embolism: a meta-analysis. Clin Appl Thromb Hemost 2001;7(2):87–92.

153. Sostman HD, Stein PD, Gottschalk A, et al. Acute pulmonary embolism: sensitivity and specificity of ventilation-perfusion scintigraphy in PIOPED II study. Radiology 2008;246(3):941–6.

154. Gray HW, Bessent RG, McKillop JH. A preliminary evaluation of diagnostic odds in lung scan reporting. Nucl Med Commun 1998;19(2):113–8.

155. Rajendran JG, Jacobson AF. Review of 6-month mortality following low-probability lung scans. Arch Intern Med 1999;159(4):349–52.

156. Tapson VF, Carroll BA, Davidson BL, et al. The diagnostic approach to acute venous thromboembolism: clinical practice guideline. American Thoracic Society. Am J Respir Crit Care Med 1999;160(3):1043–66.

157. Kahn D, Bushnell DL, Dean R, et al. Clinical outcome of patients with a 'low probability' of pulmonary embolism on ventilation-perfusion lung scan. Arch Intern Med 1989;149(2):377–9.
158. Nilsson T, Måre K, Carlsson A. Value of structured clinical and scintigraphic protocols in acute pulmonary embolism. J Intern Med 2001;250(3):213–8.
159. Prologo JD, Glauser J. Variable diagnostic approach to suspected pulmonary embolism in the ED of a major academic tertiary care center. Am J Emerg Med 2002;20(1):5–9.
160. Raskob GE, Hull RD. Diagnosis of pulmonary embolism. Curr Opin Hematol 1999;6(5):280–4.
161. Hartmann IJ, Hagen PJ, Melissant CF, et al. Diagnosing acute pulmonary embolism: effect of chronic obstructive pulmonary disease on the performance of D-dimer testing, ventilation/perfusion scintigraphy, spiral computed tomographic angiography, and conventional angiography. ANTELOPE Study Group. Advances in New Technologies Evaluating the Localization of Pulmonary Embolism. Am J Respir Crit Care Med 2000;162(6):2232–7.
162. Righini M, Goehring C, Bounameaux H, et al. Effects of age on the performance of common diagnostic tests for pulmonary embolism. Am J Med 2000;109(5):357–61.
163. Le Gal G, Righini M, Sanchez O, et al. A positive compression ultrasonography of the lower limb veins is highly predictive of pulmonary embolism on computed tomography in suspected patients. Thromb Haemost 2006;95(6):963–6.
164. Perrier A, Miron MJ, Desmarais S, et al. Using clinical evaluation and lung scan to rule out suspected pulmonary embolism: Is it a valid option in patients with normal results of lower-limb venous compression ultrasonography? Arch Intern Med 2000;160(4):512–6.
165. Daniel KR, Jackson RE, Kline JA. Utility of lower extremity venous ultrasound scanning in the diagnosis and exclusion of pulmonary embolism in outpatients. Ann Emerg Med 2000;35(6):547–54.
166. Hull RD, Raskob GE, Ginsberg JS, et al. A noninvasive strategy for the treatment of patients with suspected pulmonary embolism. Arch Intern Med 1994;154(3):289–97.
167. Anderson DR, Kovacs MJ, Dennie C, et al. Use of spiral computed tomography contrast angiography and ultrasonography to exclude the diagnosis of pulmonary embolism in the emergency department. J Emerg Med 2005;29(4):399–404.
168. Grifoni S, Olivotto I, Cecchini P, et al. Short-term clinical outcome of patients with acute pulmonary embolism, normal blood pressure, and echocardiographic right ventricular dysfunction. Circulation 2000;101(24):2817–22.
169. Gibson NS, Sohne M, Buller HR. Prognostic value of echocardiography and spiral computed tomography in patients with pulmonary embolism. Curr Opin Pulm Med 2005;11(5):380–4.
170. Kucher N, Rossi E, De Rosa M, et al. Prognostic role of echocardiography among patients with acute pulmonary embolism and a systolic arterial pressure of 90 mm Hg or higher. Arch Intern Med 2005;165(15):1777–81.
171. Kasper W, Konstantinides S, Geibel A, et al. Prognostic significance of right ventricular afterload stress detected by echocardiography in patients with clinically suspected pulmonary embolism. Heart 1997;77(4):346–9.
172. Serafini O, Bisignani G, Greco F, et al. The role of 2D-Doppler electrocardiography in the early diagnosis of massive acute pulmonary embolism and therapeutic monitoring (Italian). G Ital Cardiol 1997;27(5):462–9.

173. Cheriex EC, Sreeram N, Eussen YF, et al. Cross sectional Doppler echocardiography as the initial technique for the diagnosis of acute pulmonary embolism. Br Heart J 1994;72(1):52–7.

174. Kasper W, Meinertz T, Henkel B, et al. Echocardiographic findings in patients with proved pulmonary embolism. Am Heart J 1986;112(6):1284–90.

175. Pruszczyk P, Torbicki A, Kuch-Wocial A, et al. Transesophageal echocardiography for definitive diagnosis of haemodynamically significant pulmonary embolism. Eur Heart J 1995;16(4):534–8.

176. Pruszczyk P, Torbicki A, Pacho R, et al. Noninvasive diagnosis of suspected severe pulmonary embolism: transesophageal echocardiography vs spiral CT. Chest 1997;112(3):722–8.

177. Meaney JF, Weg JG, Chenevert TL, et al. Diagnosis of pulmonary embolism with magnetic resonance angiography. N Engl J Med 1997;336(20):1422–7.

178. Oudkerk M, van Beek EJ, Wielopolski P, et al. Comparison of contrast-enhanced magnetic resonance angiography and conventional pulmonary angiography for the diagnosis of pulmonary embolism: a prospective study. Lancet 2002; 359(9318):1643–7.

179. Stein PD, Chenevert TL, Fowler SE, et al, PIOPED III Investigators. Gadolinium-enhanced magnetic resonance angiography for acute pulmonary embolism: a multicenter prospective study (PIOPED III). Ann Intern Med 2010;152(7): 434–43.

180. Wittram C, Waltman AC, Shepard JA, et al. Discordance between CT and angiography in the PIOPED II study. Radiology 2007;244(3):883–9.

181. Diffin DC, Leyendecker JR, Johnson SP, et al. Effect of anatomic distribution of pulmonary emboli on interobserver agreement in the interpretation of pulmonary angiography. Am J Roentgenol 1998;171(4):1085–9.

182. Donato AA, Scheirer JJ, Atwell MS, et al. Clinical outcomes in patients with suspected acute pulmonary embolism and negative helical computed tomographic results in whom anticoagulation was withheld. Arch Intern Med 2003;163(17): 2033–8.

183. Stein PD, Athanasoulis C, Alavi A, et al. Complications and validity of pulmonary angiography in acute pulmonary embolism. Circulation 1992;85(2):462–8.

184. Ionizing radiation exposure of the population of the United States. National Council on Radiation Protection Report No. 160. Bethesda (MD): National Council on Radiation Protection and Measurements; 2009.

185. Berrington de González A, Mahesh M, Kim KP, et al. Projected cancer risks from computed tomographic scans performed in the United States in 2007. Arch Intern Med 2009;169(22):2071–7.

186. The National Academies. Health risks from exposure to low levels of ionizing radiation: BEIR VII phase 2. Available at: http://www.nap.edu/catalog/11340. html. Accessed January 7, 2011.

187. Pierce DA, Preston DL. Radiation-related cancer risks at low doses among atomic bomb survivors. Radiat Res 2000;154(2):178–86.

188. Preston DL, Ron E, Tokuoka S, et al. Solid cancer incidence in atomic bomb survivors: 1958–1998. Radiat Res 2007;168(1):1–64.

189. Kuiper JW, Geleijns J, Matheijssen NA, et al. Radiation exposure of multi-row detector spiral computed tomography of the pulmonary arteries: comparison with digital subtraction pulmonary angiography. Eur Radiol 2003;13(7):1496–500.

190. Huda W. When a pregnant patient has a suspected pulmonary embolism, what are the typical embryo doses from a chest CT and a ventilation/perfusion study? Pediatr Radiol 2005;35(4):452–3.

191. Smith–Bindman R, Lipson J, Marcus R, et al. Radiation dose associated with common computed tomography examinations and the associated lifetime attributable risk of cancer. Arch Intern Med 2009;169(22):2078–86.

192. Mettler FA, Huda W, Yoshizumi TT, et al. Effective doses in radiology and diagnostic nuclear medicine: a catalog. Radiology 2008;248(1):254–63.

193. Pahade FK, Litmanovich D, Pedrosa I, et al. Quality initiatives: imaging pregnant patients with suspected pulmonary embolism: what the radiologist needs to know. Radiographics 2009;29:639–54.

194. Shrimpton PC, Hillier MC, Lewis MA, et al. National survey of doses from CT in the UK: 2003. Br J Radiol 2006;79(948):968–80.

195. Diederich S, Lenzen H. Radiation exposure associated with imaging of the chest: comparison of different radiographic and computed tomography techniques. Cancer 2000;89(11 Suppl):2457–60.

196. Brenner DJ, Elliston CD. Estimated radiation risks potentially associated with full-body CT screening. Radiology 2004;232(3):735–8.

197. Arcasoy SM, Kreit JW. Thrombolytic therapy of pulmonary embolism: a comprehensive review of current evidence. Chest 1999;115(6):1695–707.

198. Kearon C, Kahn SR, Agnelli G, et al. Antithrombotic therapy for venous thromboembolic disease: American College of Chest Physicians Evidence-Based Clinical Practice Guidelines (8th edition). Chest 2008;133(Suppl 6):454S–545S.

199. Torbicki A, Perrier A, Konstantinides S, et al. Guidelines on the diagnosis and management of acute pulmonary embolism: the task force for the diagnosis and management of acute pulmonary embolism of the European Society of Cardiology (ESC). Eur Heart J 2008;29(18):2276–315.

200. Squizzato A, Galli M, Dentali F, et al. Outpatient treatment and early discharge of symptomatic pulmonary embolism: a systematic review. Eur Respir J 2009; 33(5):1148–55.

201. Hogg KE, Brown MD, Kline, et al. Estimating the pretest probability threshold to justify empiric administration of heparin prior to pulmonary vascular imaging for pulmonary embolism. Thromb Res 2006;118(5):547–53.

202. Raschke RA, Gollihare B, Peirce JC. The effectiveness of implementing the weight-based heparin nomogram as a practice guideline. Arch Intern Med 1996;156(15):1645–9.

203. Martel N, Lee J, Wells PS. Risk for heparin-induced thrombocytopenia with unfractionated and low-molecular-weight heparin thromboprophylaxis: a meta-analysis. Blood 2005;106(8):2710–5.

204. Harenberg J. Is laboratory monitoring of low-molecular-weight heparin therapy necessary? Yes. J Thromb Haemost 2004;2(4):547–50.

205. Quinlan DJ, McQuillan A, Eikelboom JW. Low-molecular-weight heparin compared with intravenous unfractionated heparin for treatment of pulmonary embolism: a meta-analysis of randomized, controlled trials. Ann Intern Med 2004;140(3):175–83.

206. Büller HR, Davidson BL, Decousus H, et al. The Matisse Investigators. Subcutaneous fondaparinux versus intravenous unfractionated heparin in the initial treatment of pulmonary embolism. N Engl J Med 2003;349(18):1695–702.

207. Goodman LR, Lipchik RJ, Kuzo RS, et al. Subsequent pulmonary embolism: risk after a negative helical CT pulmonary angiogram—prospective comparison with scintigraphy. Radiology 2000;215(5):535–42.

208. Gottsäter A, Berg A, Centergård J. Clinically suspected pulmonary embolism: is it safe to withhold anticoagulation after a negative spiral CT? Eur Radiol 2001; 11(1):65–72.

209. Ly B, Arnesen H, Eie H, et al. A controlled clinical trial of streptokinase and heparin in the treatment of major pulmonary embolism. Acta Med Scand 1978;203(6):465–70.
210. Konstantinides S, Geibel A, Kasper W, et al. Comparison of alteplase versus heparin for resolution of major pulmonary embolism. Am J Cardiol 1998;82(8): 966–70.
211. Dalla-Volta S, Palla A, Santolicandro A, et al. PAIMS 2: alteplase combined with heparin versus heparin in the treatment of acute pulmonary embolism. Plasminogen Activator Italian Multicenter Study 2. J Am Coll Cardiol 1992; 20(3):520–6.
212. A collaborative study by the PIOPED Investigators. Tissue plasminogen activator for the treatment of acute pulmonary embolism. Chest 1990;97(3): 528–33.
213. Marini C, Di Ricco G, Rossi G, et al. Fibrinolytic effects of urokinase and heparin in acute pulmonary embolism: a randomized clinical trial. Respiration 1988;54: 162–73.
214. Tibbutt DA, Davies JA, Anderson JA, et al. Comparison by controlled clinical trial of streptokinase and heparin in treatment of life-threatening pulmonary embolism. Br Med J 1974;1(5904):343–7.
215. Konstantinides S, Marder VJ. Thrombolysis in venous thromboembolism. In: Colman RW, Marder VJ, Clowes AW, et al, editors. Hemostasis and thrombosis: basic principles and clinical practice. 5th edition. Philadelphia: Lippincott Williams & Wilkins; 2006. p. 1317–29.
216. Thabut G, Thabut D, Myers RP, et al. Thrombolytic therapy of pulmonary embolism: a meta-analysis. J Am Coll Cardiol 2002;40(9):1660–7.
217. Kanter DS, Mikkola KM, Patel SR, et al. Thrombolytic therapy for pulmonary embolism. Frequency of intracranial hemorrhage and associated risk factors. Chest 1997;111(5):1241–5.
218. Wan S, Quinlan DJ, Agnelli G, et al. Thrombolysis compared with heparin for the initial treatment of pulmonary embolism: a meta-analysis of the randomized controlled trials. Circulation 2004;110(6):744–9.
219. Li X, Fu QL, Jing XL, et al. A meta-analysis of cardiopulmonary resuscitation with and without the administration of thrombolytic agents. Resuscitation 2006;70(1): 31–6.
220. Zahorec R. Rescue systemic thrombolysis during cardiopulmonary resuscitation. Bratisl Lek Listy 2002;103(7–8):266–9.
221. Vanden Hoek TL, Morrison LJ, Shuster M, et al. Part 12: cardiac arrest in special situations: 2010 American Heart Association Guidelines for Cardiopulmonary Resuscitation and Emergency Cardiovascular Care. Circulation 2010;122 (18 Suppl 3):S829–61.
222. Goldhaber SZ, Kessler CM, Heit J, et al. Randomised controlled trial of recombinant tissue plasminogen activator versus urokinase in the treatment of acute pulmonary embolism. Lancet 1988;2(8606):293–8.
223. Tebbe U, Graf A, Kamke W, et al. Hemodynamic effects of double bolus reteplase versus alteplase infusion in massive pulmonary embolism. Am Heart J 1999;138(1 Pt 1):39–44.
224. Fatovich DM, Dobb GJ, Clugston RA. A pilot randomised trial of thrombolysis in cardiac arrest (The TICA trial). Resuscitation 2004;61(3):309–13.
225. Bottiger BW, Bode C, Kern S, et al. Efficacy and safety of thrombolytic therapy after initially unsuccessful cardiopulmonary resuscitation: a prospective clinical trial. Lancet 2001;357(9268):1583–5.

226. Daniels LB, Parker JA, Patel SR, et al. Relation of duration of symptoms with response to thrombolytic therapy in pulmonary embolism. Am J Cardiol 1997; 80(2):184–8.

227. Levine M, Hirsh J, Weitz J, et al. A randomized trial of a single bolus dosage regimen of recombinant tissue plasminogen activator in patients with acute pulmonary embolism. Chest 1990;98(6):1473–9.

228. Torbicki A, Galié N, Covezzoli A, et al. Right heart thrombi in pulmonary embolism: results from the International Cooperative Pulmonary Embolism Registry. J Am Coll Cardiol 2003;41(12):2245–51.

229. Rose PS, Punjabi NM, Pearse DB. Treatment of right heart thromboemboli. Chest 2002;121(3):806–14.

230. Heit JA, Kobbervig CE, James AH, et al. Trends in the incidence of venous thromboembolism during pregnancy or postpartum: a 30-year population-based study. Ann Intern Med 2005;143(10):697–706.

231. Browse NL, Thomas ML. Source of non-lethal pulmonary emboli. Lancet 1974; 1(7851):258–9.

232. James AH, Jamison MG, Brancazio LR, et al. Venous thromboembolism during pregnancy and the postpartum period: incidence, risk factors, and mortality. Am J Obstet Gynecol 2006;194(5):1311–5.

233. Ray JG, Chan WS. Deep vein thrombosis during pregnancy and the puerperium: a meta-analysis of the period of risk and leg of presentation. Obstet Gynecol Surv 1999;54(4):265–71.

234. Brenner B. Haemostatic changes in pregnancy. Thromb Res 2004;114(5–6): 409–14.

235. Nicolaides AN, Kakkar VV, Renney JT. The soleal sinuses: origin of deep-vein thrombosis. Br J Surg 1970;57(11):860.

236. Lindqvist P, Dahlbäck B, Marsál K. Thrombotic risk during pregnancy: a population study. Obstet Gynecol 1999;94(4):595–9.

237. Larsen TB, Sørensen HT, Gislum M, et al. Maternal smoking, obesity, and risk of venous thromboembolism during pregnancy and the puerperium: a population-based nested case-control study. Thromb Res 2007;120(4): 505–9.

238. Levy MS, Spencer F, Ginsberg JS, et al. Reading between the (guidelines). Management of submassive pulmonary embolism in the first trimester of pregnancy. Thromb Res 2008;121(5):705–7.

239. Chan WS, Chunilal S, Lee A, et al. A red blood cell agglutination D-dimer test to exclude deep venous thrombosis in pregnancy. Ann Intern Med 2007;147(3): 165–70.

240. To MS, Hunt BJ, Nelson-Piercy C. A negative D-dimer does not exclude venous thromboembolism (VTE) in pregnancy. J Obstet Gynaecol 2008; 28(2):222–3.

241. Scarsbrook AF, Evans AL, Owen AR, et al. Diagnosis of suspected venous thromboembolic disease in pregnancy. Clin Radiol 2006;61(1):1–12.

242. Stone SE, Morris TA. Pulmonary embolism during and after pregnancy. Crit Care Med 2005;33(10 Suppl):S294–300.

243. Cantwell CP, Cradock A, Bruzzi J, et al. MR venography with true fast imaging with steady-state precession for suspected lower-limb deep vein thrombosis. J Vasc Interv Radiol 2006;17(11 Pt 1):1763–9.

244. Kluge A, Mueller C, Strunk J, et al. Experience in 207 combined MRI examinations for acute pulmonary embolism and deep vein thrombosis. AJR Am J Roentgenol 2006;186(6):1686–96.

245. Shahir K, Goodman LR, Tali A, et al. Pulmonary embolism in pregnancy: CT pulmonary angiography versus perfusion scanning. AJR Am J Roentgenol 2010;195(3):W214–20.

246. Scarsbrook AF, Bradley KM, Gleeson FV. Perfusion scintigraphy: diagnostic utility in pregnant women with suspected pulmonary embolic disease. Eur Radiol 2007;17(10):2554–60.

247. Marik PE, Plante LA. Venous thromboembolic disease and pregnancy. New Engl J Med 2008;359(19):2025–33.

248. U-King-Im JM, Freeman SJ, Boylan T, et al. Quality of CT pulmonary angiography for suspected pulmonary embolus in pregnancy. Eur Radiol 2008; 18(12):2709–15.

249. Andreou AK, Curtin JJ, Wilde S, et al. Does pregnancy affect vascular enhancement in patients undergoing CT pulmonary angiography? Eur Radiol 2008; 18(12):2716–22.

250. Kline JA, Courtney DM, Beam DM, et al. Incidence and predictors of repeated computed tomographic pulmonary angiography in emergency department patients. Ann Emerg Med 2009;54(1):41–8.

251. Land CE, Tokunaga M, Tokuoka S, et al. Early-onset breast cancer in A-bomb survivors. Lancet 1993;342(8865):237.

252. Allen C, Demetriades T. Radiation risk over-estimated. Radiology 2006;240(2):613–4.

253. Hurwitz LM, Yoshizumi TT, Goodman PC, et al. Radiation dose savings for adult pulmonary embolus 64-MDCT using bismuth breast shields, lower peak kilovoltage, and automatic tube current modulation. AJR Am J Roentgenol 2009; 192(1):244–53.

254. Revel MP, Cohen S, Sanchez O, et al. Pulmonary embolism during pregnancy: diagnosis with lung scintigraphy or CT angiography? Radiology 2011;258(2):590–8.

255. Cahill AG, Stout MJ, Macones GA, et al. Diagnosing pulmonary embolism in pregnancy using computed-tomographic angiography or ventilation-perfusion. Obstet Gynecol 2009;114(1):124–9.

256. Winer-Muram HT, Boone JM, Brown HL, et al. Pulmonary embolism in pregnant patients: fetal radiation dose with helical CT. Radiology 2002;224(2):487–92.

257. Patel SJ, Reede DL, Katz DS, et al. Imaging the pregnant patient for nonobstetric conditions: algorithms and radiation dose considerations. Radiographics 2007;27(6):1705–22.

258. Hurwitz LM, Yoshizumi T, Reiman RE, et al. Radiation dose to the fetus from body MDCT during early gestation. AJR Am J Roentgenol 2006;186(3):871–6.

259. Fraser DG, Moody AR, Morgan PS, et al. Diagnosis of lower-limb deep venous thrombosis: a prospective blinded study of magnetic resonance direct thrombus imaging. Ann Intern Med 2002;136:89–98.

260. Duhl AJ, Paidas MJ, Ural SH, et al. Anti-thrombotic therapy and pregnancy: consensus report and recommendations for prevention and treatment of venous thromboembolism and adverse pregnancy outcomes. Am J Obstet Gynecol 2007;197(5):457.e1–457.e21.

261. Thromboprophylaxis during pregnancy, labour and after vaginal delivery. Guideline no. 37. London: Royal College of Obstetricians and Gynaecologists; 2004.

262. Greer IA, Nelson-Piercy C. Low-molecular-weight heparins for thromboprophylaxis and treatment of venous thromboembolism in pregnancy: a systematic review of safety and efficacy. Blood 2005;106(2):401–7.

263. Forestier F, Daffos F, Capella-Pavlovsky M. Low molecular weight heparin (PK 10169) does not cross the placenta during the second trimester of pregnancy study by direct fetal blood sampling under ultrasound. Thromb Res 1984; 34(6):557–60.

264. Baglin TP, Brush J, Streff BM. Guidelines on the use of vena cava filters. Br J Haematol 2006;134(6):590–5.

265. Leonhardt G, Gaul C, Nietsch HH, et al. Thrombolytic therapy in pregnancy. J Thromb Thrombolysis 2006;21(3):271–6.

266. Stefanovic BS, Vasiljevic Z, Mitrovic P, et al. Thrombolytic therapy for massive pulmonary embolism 12 hours after cesarean delivery despite contraindication? Am J Emerg Med 2006;24(4):502–4.

Initial Management and Resuscitation of Severe Chest Trauma

Bruno Bernardin, MD[a,b,c,*], Jean-Marc Troquet, MD[c,d]

KEYWORDS

- Thoracic trauma • Severe • Management • Unstable • Blunt
- Penetrating

The chest is the site of confluence of 3 of the most important life-sustaining systems: the airway, the respiratory system, and the cardiovascular system. The potential for severe injuries by application of traumatic forces is huge. Among severely traumatized patients, 25% of deaths are thought to be secondary to chest trauma.[1] Motor vehicle crashes (MVCs), or pedestrians struck by motor vehicles, cause the majority of severe thoracic injuries.[2] In a crash, the unrestrained driver of a vehicle has about a 50% chance of sustaining a chest injury.[1] Penetrating chest trauma has the same potential for dire consequences, given the anatomic proximity and the associated harmful intent of the majority of armed assaults.

The cornerstone of care in severely injured patients consists of interventions that should be familiar to any emergency physician (EP) involved in trauma management: intubation, support of ventilation/oxygenation, and installation of thoracostomy tubes. In either blunt or penetrating injuries, 80% to 85% of chest trauma patients will respond to these maneuvers.[3–5]

The goal of this article is to provide a review of major thoracic injuries and to provide guidance in the initial management and resuscitation of victims of severe chest trauma. The authors cover injuries that are immediately or rapidly life threatening: ruptured airways, pneumothorax with or without tension, flail chest and pulmonary contusions, rupture of major blood vessels, and cardiac trauma. Bony and soft-tissue injuries, with

The authors have nothing to disclose.
[a] Department of Medicine, McGill University, Room A4.62, Royal Victoria Hospital, 687 Avenue Des Pins, Montreal, Quebec, H3A 1A1, Canada
[b] Emergency Trauma Fellowship, Montreal General Hospital, McGill University Health Center, Room B2 117-3, 1650 Avenue Cedar, Montreal, Quebec, H3G 1A4, Canada
[c] Emergency Department, Montreal General Hospital, McGill University Health Center, Room B2 117-3, 1650 Avenue Cedar, Montreal, Quebec, H3G 1A4, Canada
[d] Department of Family Medicine, McGill University, 517 Avenue des Pins, Montreal, Quebec, H2S 1S4, Canada
* Corresponding author. Emergency Department, Montreal General Hospital, McGill University Health Center, Room B2 117-3, 1650 Avenue Cedar, Montreal, Quebec, H3G 1A4, Canada.
E-mail address: bruno.bernardin@mcgill.ca

Emerg Med Clin N Am 30 (2012) 377–400
doi:10.1016/j.emc.2011.10.010
0733-8627/12/$ – see front matter © 2012 Elsevier Inc. All rights reserved.

the exception of rib fractures, are not discussed. The focus is on civilian, nonwarfare-related situations, with mechanisms of injury such as MVCs, falls, stabbings, and shootings. Blast injuries, more common in warfare situations, are not addressed directly in this article.

Each type of injury, grouped by system. is discussed separately. The authors present an approach to the resuscitation of the unstable patient presenting with undisclosed injuries following chest trauma, given that EPs are confronted with unidentified problems and must act before a final diagnosis is known. Important differences between penetrating and blunt trauma are outlined whenever necessary.

AIRWAY ISSUES: TRACHEOBRONCHIAL INJURY

Respiratory distress in trauma patients can originate from airway compromise or from a respiratory (pulmonary, chest wall) injury. Profound shock can also present as respiratory distress from circulatory insufficiency. Identification of upper airway trauma and compromise is usually straightforward and should be dealt with accordingly, usually by relief of the obstruction and by securing a definitive airway. For all patients, endotracheal intubation should be performed if any of the usual indications are met.

Identification of lower airway injury is more complex. It is a rare injury, with reported rates between 0.5% and 2% in patients arriving alive to hospital.[6–10] In a recent review of 12,187 patients seen over 15 years in a major trauma center in Toronto, Kummer and colleagues[11] found only 14 cases (0.11%). The presenting signs and symptoms vary greatly depending on the size and site of defect, pleural communication, and the ensuing air leak.[12] Many subtle presentations will manifest only as mediastinal air seen on computed tomography (CT) scan whereas the most dramatic ones are catastrophic, with respiratory distress and associated difficulties in ventilation and oxygenation.[11]

Larger defects result in dyspnea (with or without respiratory distress) and pneumothorax, possibly with tension. Intervention will be directed initially toward the pneumothorax, as the tracheobronchial injury (TBI) is often not yet suspected. Persistent pneumothorax or air leak after placement of a chest tube should alert the physician to the possibility of a TBI.[13,14] Insertion of a second chest tube is required in these cases. TBI must be suspected if a patient deteriorates rapidly following endotracheal intubation. Because of positive pressure ventilation and loss of negative intrathoracic pressure on inspiration, air leak is increased, followed by increasing difficulties with oxygenation and ventilation.

Smaller injuries initially go unnoticed, especially if the patient is breathing spontaneously. The prevalence of subcutaneous emphysema is reported to be 35% to 85%. Hemoptysis is less frequent, seen in fewer than 25% of cases.[15] TBI becomes suspected when radiological evaluation shows mediastinal air, isolated or with pneumothorax. Mediastinal air can also originate from other injuries[16]: penetrating face or neck wound with air tracking down, lung parenchyma laceration, esophageal injury, deep penetrating torso wound, or retroperitoneal injury with air tracking up the diaphragmatic hiatus. It is rare to identify the site of injury even on CT scan. Most occur within 2 cm of the carina, with predominance for the right main stem bronchus, followed by the lower trachea.[6] Left-sided defects are often better tolerated, and consequently diagnosed later (median 30 days for left side compared with 1 day for right side and 3 days for trachea).[6] This occurrence might possibly be due to the existence of greater peribronchial tissue surrounding the left main stem bronchus, which can limit air leak.[17]

Bronchoscopy is indicated in all cases of suspected TBI, with two goals in mind. With severe injury, it can be used to advance the endotracheal tube distal to the defect to decrease air leak, at times into the unaffected main stem bronchus if necessary, ensuring adequate ventilation.[15,18] Bronchoscopy also diagnoses precisely the location and size of the injury and plans possible surgical repair. Early mortality in cases of TBI results from either ventilation-oxygenation difficulties or from severe associated injuries, which frequently coexist.[6,11] Early thoracic surgery involvement is mandatory for treatment.

BREATHING

The most severe presentations resulting from thoracic trauma are respiratory distress and/or hypoxia. Injuries to consider in these cases are tension pneumothorax (TPTX), simple or open pneumothorax, and flail chest. Massive bleeding into the chest cavity can also result in respiratory impairment. Finally, pulmonary contusions usually accompany important chest injuries.

Pneumothorax and Occult Pneumothorax

A pneumothorax occurs when air accumulates between the visceral and parietal pleura. In blunt trauma this results from either lung parenchymal injury from deceleration forces, laceration by a rib fracture, or if an alveola ruptures from increased intrathoracic pressure following crush injury. In penetrating trauma, direct damage to the pleura and lung tissue allows communication between both spaces, with or without communication outside the chest wall.

The clinical manifestations of pneumothorax are proportional to many factors: its size, communication or not with the atmosphere, size of any chest wall defect, presence of associated injuries (rib fractures, flail chest, pulmonary contusions, hemothorax), as well as the premorbid condition of the patient. Physiologically, pneumothoraces can result in hampered oxygenation, ventilation, and even circulation in its more severe form with presence of associated tension, although a very important proportion is asymptomatic. Physical examination is notoriously unreliable for diagnosing the majority of traumatic pneumothoraces.

The exact incidence of traumatic pneumothorax is unknown. Various imaging modalities, namely supine chest radiography (CXR), upright CXR, ultrasonography, and CT scan, each have different sensitivities in identifying pneumothorax. With the increased use of CT scanning in trauma patients, the phenomenon of occult pneumothorax has appeared. The incidence of this phenomenon depends on the population studied and is directly proportional to the severity of the injuries. Studies in the general trauma population report an incidence of occult pneumothorax of around 2% to 7%.[19,20] Ball and colleagues[21] examined supine CXR and CT findings in 405 blunt trauma patients with an Injury Severity Score (ISS) of 12 or more. These investigators found 26% of patients with pneumothorax, of which 76% were occult when the CXR was read in the acute resuscitation setting by the trauma team.

Clinicians have also started to use an extended component of the focused assessment with sonography for trauma (E-FAST) for the detection of pneumothorax in the acute setting. Thoracic ultrasonography has shown a higher sensitivity than supine CXR for diagnosing pneumothorax. While results are promising, the exact significance of this higher diagnostic accuracy remains uncertain, as many occult pneumothoraces do not need to be drained.

Traumatologists agree that pneumothoraces in any unstable patient or those found on supine CXR should be drained, usually by insertion of a chest tube. However, there has been much debate on the most appropriate management of occult pneumothoraces in stable patients, especially for those undergoing positive pressure ventilation (PPV). The advantage of immediate drainage versus observation and insertion of chest tube only if there is clinical deterioration remains unknown. There is growing evidence and consensus that occult injuries can be safely observed even during PPV, reflected by the fact that this is now accepted by the Eastern Association for the Surgery of Trauma (EAST).[22–24]

The method of choice for drainage of traumatic pneumothorax has classically been and remains insertion of a large-caliber chest tube (size 32F and larger). Some investigators have advocated the use of a smaller chest tube, but this can only be used for stable patients with isolated pneumothorax and no other thoracoabdominal injury. Twenty percent of traumatic pneumothoraces have an associated hemothorax,[25] and smaller chest tubes can obstruct easily and become nonfunctional in the presence of even small quantities of blood in the chest cavity.

Tension Pneumothorax

Textbook and Advanced Trauma Life Support teaching focuses on a rather universal, but somewhat inaccurate, picture of the signs and symptoms of tension pneumothorax (TPTX): respiratory distress, deviated trachea, decreased breath sounds, and hypotension.[26–29] CXR findings are often described as revealing a mediastinal shift away from a large pneumothorax. This shift leads supposedly to kinking of the vena cava and decreased venous return, resulting in hypotension and, if not treated, circulatory arrest.

It must be recognized that TPTX has a different presentation, depending on whether the patient is awake and ventilating spontaneously or unconscious and on PPV.[30] These differences are well established in both animal experimental models[31–37] and human case reports.[30,38] An awake patient is able to mount a compensatory response by increasing his respiratory rate, tidal volume, negative inspiratory pressure, and chest expansion.[39] The physiologic insult is primarily hypoxic with progressive respiratory decompensation; hypotension is the terminal event of hypoxic cardiac failure or respiratory arrest. On the other hand, sedated and ventilated patients cannot compensate, and show a greater degree of impeded venous return from both the intrapleural pressure and the PPV. The deterioration is much more rapid, resulting in more rapid cardiogenic shock once the central venous pressure equals the intrapleural pressure, and causing complete obstruction of venous return.[31,40]

Reviews of case series and reports of patients with TPTX show that tracheal deviation, oxygen desaturation, and hypotension are actually inconsistent findings in (awake) spontaneously ventilating patients (<25% each).[30] By contrast, hypotension and low Sao_2 are almost universally seen in PPV patients[38,41]; deviated trachea, a late finding, is found more frequently than in awake patients but not as consistently (60%).[30,42,43]

Many investigators state that clinicians should not seek radiologic confirmation if suspecting a TPTX: "the radiograph of a tension pneumothorax is one that should never be seen".[39,44,45] Discernment should be used in most cases; this is certainly true for the patient hypoxic and hypotensive in extremis, for whom immediate chest decompression must be done. The same holds true for a patient on PPV who suddenly deteriorates with falling Sao_2, rapidly becomes hypotensive without a clear reason, becomes difficult to bag, or shows raised peak inspiratory pressures on a ventilator.[46] Identification of the affected side is not always easily done[47]; for this reason if decompression of the suspected side does not yield positive results, the other side of the chest should be drained immediately.[48] In a relatively stable patient (normal blood pressure, appropriate oxygen saturation) in whom TPTX is suspected, it is reasonable to confirm the diagnosis by immediate portable radiograph while continuously monitoring the patient. This method will exclude etiology mimicking pneumothorax, such as lobar collapse, right main stem intubation, diaphragmatic herniation, and so forth, and thus avoid unnecessary thoracostomy.

The presence of mediastinal shift on CXR does not equate with tension either. In one study of 170 pneumothoraces, there were 30 CXRs with mediastinal shift and no patient exhibited clinical features of true tension, though all were subsequently managed with thoracostomy.[49] There are also many cases of loculated pneumothoraces causing tension physiology, which had no mediastinal shift on CXR.

Needle Decompression

Indications to perform immediate decompression of a hemithorax are:

- Traumatic arrest
- Loss of blood pressure or pulse during resuscitation
- Increased difficulty to bag/raising peak ventilatory pressures combined with hypotension
- Hypotension or hypoxia/respiratory distress with decreased/absent breath sounds on one side or palpable subcutaneous emphysema.

Classic teaching recommends needle decompression of a hemithorax with placement of a large-bore intravenous catheter in the anterior second intercostal space followed by placement of a chest tube.[29] Some investigators have raised doubts about the usefulness, efficacy, and reliability of this procedure,[30] especially in the prehospital setting.[50,51] Instead, immediate open blunt dissection and thoracostomy in the mid-axillary line has been suggested. There are indeed cases reports of failed decompression of a hemithorax in the presence of a tension pneumothorax[47,50,52–54]; this can result in not recognizing the persistent presence of TPTX.[55] Needle decompression can fail for a variety of reasons.[48] The needle can be misplaced in the chest wall, outside of the pleural cavity, leading the clinician to believe there is no pneumothorax. The needle can be placed in a subcutaneous emphysema pocket or, worse, in lung tissue/bronchus; this leads the physician to believe the pneumothorax has been relieved. However, with no improvement in the patient's clinical status, as the pleural cavity remains under tension the EP may believe the pneumothorax was not responsible for the patient's condition and true thoracostomy may be delayed, with dire consequences. Finally, the needle may be placed through a vascular structure such as a subclavian or internal mammary vessel, resulting in hemorrhagic complications.[56] Marinaro and colleagues[57] demonstrated in a group of 30 patients whose chest wall thickness was measured by CT scan that insertion of the standard 5-cm cannula anteriorly would not reach the pleural space in 33% of the patients, while Lander and colleagues[58] demonstrated, by similar CT measurements, that in 18% of patients neither an anterior nor lateral approach would succeed. Another study asking physicians where they would perform a needle thoracotomy revealed that 32% incorrectly identified the second intercostal space while 95% of responders placed the needle medial to the midclavicular line,[59] resulting in a greater risk of complications.[56,60]

The minimal recommendations would be that in a context where a TPTX is suspected, if needle decompression is attempted it must be followed by immediate open blunt dissection and thoracostomy in the mid-axillary space, no matter the result of needle placement. Placement of a chest tube is secondary once the pleural space is decompressed.

Pulmonary Contusions

The incidence of pulmonary contusion in trauma populations is hard to define, as its reported occurrence depends on the population studied. Pulmonary contusions result from high-energy mechanisms of trauma with rapid deceleration, compression, shear, or inertial forces,[61] most commonly from MVCs and falls from great height.[62] Blast injuries can also result in contused lungs.[63] Damage to the lung parenchyma in the form of alveolar hemorrhage and lacerations is followed some hours later by filling of aleveoli with mucus and edema fluid.[64,65] This process leads to loss of compliance, decreased oxygen diffusion, ventilation-perfusion mismatch, and shunting. There is also experimental evidence that noncontused lung tissue will be affected some hours after injury.[66]

Clinically the patient will exhibit shortness of breath, decreased oxygenation, and increased work of breathing proportional to the degree of contused lung. One needs to remember that pulmonary contusions are dynamic processes: symptoms and signs will often progress over the next hours as pathophysiological changes evolve in the lungs.[67,68] Symptoms will typically peak at 72 hours after injury.[64]

These dynamics need to be remembered when considering CXR findings. Although the diagnosis is relatively straightforward in the context of important chest trauma with infiltrates or consolidations on plain CXR, studies have shown that up to 50% of patients with pulmonary contusions have a normal CXR on arrival whereas 92% have a positive CXR at 24 hours.[69] Another study showed that 6 hours after the injury, 21% of patients with lung contusions did not show it on CXR.[70]

CT scanning performed early is more sensitive than CXR for the diagnosis of lung contusions.[70] Many patients with normal CXR exhibit parenchymal changes on CT performed shortly after. Some investigators have found that the percentage of contused lung volume measured on CT scan is predictive of the need for mechanical ventilation or of the risk of acute respiratory distress syndrome,[71,72] the cutoff mark being somewhere between 18% and 30% of lung volume, but the patient numbers were small. It is unclear whether this is truly useful for management. These studies were done with earlier-generation scanners less sensitive than present-day machines, which are now overly sensitive for pulmonary contusions. In fact, Deunk and colleagues[73] found that patients with contusions demonstrated only on CT scan, with no contusions apparent on initial CXR, have a similar prognosis and rate of complications to patients who do not have pulmonary contusions on CT.

Treatment is supportive. Management is guided by the patient's oxygenation capabilities and secondarily by ventilation. Proper monitoring in an intensive care unit (ICU) setting, supplemental oxygen, and pulmonary toilet are the most important initial steps in the care of these patients. In the spontaneously ventilating patient, proper analgesia for coexisting rib fractures is of vital importance. In cases where oxygen demands are beyond what can be provided with face mask or when respiratory muscle fatigue is evident, consideration should be given to noninvasive positive pressure ventilation (NPPV).[74] However, the main problem remains patient selection; many patients need intubation for other injuries. In patients who are appropriate for NPPV, this modality can avoid intubation in 82% of pulmonary contusion patients with acute respiratory failure.[75] It has been demonstrated that selective intubation will have good results and will increase survival.[76,77]

If NPPV is not possible or fails, intubation becomes necessary. The goal is to optimize oxygenation while minimizing further lung tissue trauma by using lower tidal volumes (6 mL/kg) and maintaining end-inspiratory plateau pressure below 30 cm H_2O.[78] The use of positive end-expiratory pressure and other alveolar recruiting techniques such as high-frequency/inversed ratio ventilation should be considered in patients whose oxygenation is still difficult while on mechanical ventilation.[79] If a patient cannot be properly ventilated or oxygenated while on a respirator it is mandatory to exclude, and treat appropriately, other complications of severe chest trauma such as pneumothorax and hemothorax.

The topic of fluid resuscitation and its relationship to pulmonary contusions is controversial. Experimental and clinical studies on the choice and quantities of fluids show conflicting results.[64] While proper fluid and blood product resuscitation is paramount in the polytraumatized patient, overhydration of patients can contribute to worsening lung edema. Prophylactic antibiotics and steroids have no role in the management of pulmonary contusions.[64]

Rib Fractures and Flail Chest

Rib fractures are one of the most common injuries in patients with chest trauma.[80] A significant force is usually required to cause a fracture of one or more ribs. Kroell and colleagues[81] showed that a 40% deformation of the chest wall was necessary to produce multiple rib fractures or flail chest. The lateral area of the chest wall, because of its architecture and diminished muscular support, is the most susceptible.[82] Rib fractures are a marker of potentially more severe concomitant injury. There is an association between lower (9th–12th) rib fractures and abdominal injuries.[83,84] There is also an association with pneumothorax and pulmonary contusions. Children, by contrast, suffer severe underlying pulmonary/intrathoracic trauma without rib fractures,[85] because of the greater flexibility of their rib cages.

The added morbidity and mortality with each additional fracture is being more and more recognized,[86,87] especially in elderly patients in whom each additional rib fracture will accompany a relative increase in mortality rate of 19% and pneumonia rate of 27%.[88] Six or more rib fractures is associated with increased mortality from all other injuries.[89] The presence of more than 4 rib fractures increases morbidity or potential surrogate markers of such (ventilator and ICU days) in those older than 45 years, although their relatively small numbers limit the validity of these conclusions.[90,91] The pain of rib fractures will hamper proper ventilation, oxygenation, and clearing of secretions, all of which compounds associated injuries such as pulmonary contusions. Although a history of lung disease does not increase complications of rib fractures in the general population,[92] it has been recognized to result in a higher number of complications in patients older than 65 years.[93]

Patients who suffer from flail chests, the presence of 3 or more contiguous ribs fractured at 2 sites, can present in various degrees of respiratory distress. The presence of a flail segment is associated with increased mortality compared with a similar number of fractures without flail.[94] Respiratory insufficiency in flail chest results from the underlying pulmonary contusion,[76] not from the paradoxic movement of the chest. The ventilatory inefficiencies, the decreased clearing of secretions and associated atelectasis, and increased risk of pneumonia also contributes to shunting and hypoxia.[95]

Treatment of rib fractures and flail chest is supportive, aimed at pain control to allow pulmonary expansion and toilet and to provide sufficient oxygenation with supplemental oxygen as needed.[76,77] Failure of oxygenation or ventilation mandates intubation, either on presentation or later on as the symptoms of the underlying pulmonary contusions progress.

Proper analgesia can be difficult to achieve in the case of multiple rib fractures. Many modalities are available: oral or intravenous narcotics, intercostal rib blocks, paravertebral catheter analgesia, and epidural catheter analgesia. Many studies have shown the efficacy of the epidural route in controlling pain in these circumstances. It may also decrease the incidence of pneumonia according to some reports.[96,97] However, one study suggests that epidurals are associated with an increased length of stay and increased total of complications in elderly patients (mean age 77 years) who were less severely injured (ISS <9).[98] Surprisingly the EAST published guidelines recommending epidural analgesia in blunt trauma patients with multiple rib fractures.[99] The most appropriate type of pain control has not clearly been demonstrated, given the current available data.[100] Lack of superiority of epidural delivery was recently documented by Carrier and colleagues.[101] Their systematic review of 8 prospective controlled trials, totaling 232 patients, comparing epidural analgesia/anesthesia with parenteral opioids or intrapleural analgesia could not find any benefit in mortality, length of stay in ICU, or length of stay in hospital. Carrier and colleagues were able to find only that the number of days on mechanical ventilation was reduced when comparing epidural anesthesia with parenteral opioids in 73 patients. The apparent lack of benefit might well result from the small total number of patients studied so far. The authors can state that epidural anesthesia/analgesia is an effective mode of pain control for traumatized patients with multiple rib fractures, but its application is limited and has not been shown to be superior to other modes in terms of reducing morbidity or mortality.

CIRCULATION

In thoracic injuries, circulation issues can be divided into two main categories: hemorrhagic shock due to blood loss, and pump failure due to TPTX or direct cardiac injuries (blunt or penetrating).

Hemothorax

Hemorrhagic shock is the second most frequent cause of death in trauma patients and is the leading cause of early in-hospital trauma deaths.[102] In the thoracic cavity, bleeding usually comes from injuries to the chest wall (in particular intercostals or mammary arteries), the thoracic spine, the lung parenchyma, the great vessels, or the heart. Injuries to intra-abdominal organs (in particular the liver and spleen) can also cause hemorrhage in the chest cavity when the diaphragm is lacerated or ruptured. The common pathway of all such injuries is the accumulation of blood in the pleural space (a hemothorax). Its clinical presentation is variable and is not always easy to diagnose on clinical examination.

In the stable patient, the diagnosis is typically made on CXR; at least 150 to 200 mL of blood need to be present in the chest cavity for the upright CXR to identify a hemothorax.[103] As many CXRs done in trauma are performed on the supine patient, it has been shown that portable CXR on a supine patient has a sensitivity of 40% to 60% in ruling out hemothorax. E-FAST can identify as little as 20 mL of fluid in the pleural cavity, and has shown sensitivities of greater than 96% in detecting hemothorax. In addition it has been shown to be a much quicker procedure, taking about 1 minute to perform, compared with 15 minutes for a CXR. In the unstable patient with blunt trauma the diagnosis should always be suspected, and insertion of bilateral chest tube is warranted in these patients as both a diagnostic and therapeutic measure.

Because the majority of pulmonary blood supply derives from the low-pressure pulmonary vessels, expansion of the lung with apposition of the visceral and parietal pleura is usually all that is required to control these sources of bleeding.[14] Drainage of blood also prevents the formation of empyema, a common complication of retained blood in the chest cavity.

A massive hemothorax is defined as the presence of 1500 mL or more of blood in the thoracic cavity, and is the classic indication to proceed with an urgent thoracotomy. This concept, however, has been challenged for some time. It is now becoming evident that the clinical status of the patient is a more important indicator of the need for a thoracotomy. Early preparation of the patient for thoracotomy has led to better outcomes, and thresholds varying from 500 to 1000 mL of blood have been sug-gested by some investigators.[104,105]

Volume replacement remains the initial therapeutic modality for hemorrhagic shock. The use of massive transfusion protocols has been shown to be beneficial.[106] Early surgical consultation, in particular for penetrating trauma, is recommended. Angiog-raphy can be considered for the diagnosis and treatment of intercostal vessel injuries.

Aortic injury must be considered in patients who are hemodynamically unstable, or in stable patients with a significant mechanism or other confirmed thoracic injuries. For stable patients, the diagnosis can be made on contrast chest CT. For unstable patients, a transesophageal echocardiogram, performed in the emergency depart-ment (ED) or in the operating room, can assess both the heart and the aorta.

Blunt Cardiac Injury

Blunt cardiac injury (BCI) is involved in up to 20% of all deaths due to motor vehicle collision.[107] The reported incidence of BCI in all blunt thoracic trauma patients ranges from 20% to 76%.[108–111] It encompasses a wide spectrum of clinical manifestations, ranging from an asymptomatic myocardial bruise to cardiac rupture and death.[112,113] Because the right heart rests closest to the anterior chest wall, it is the most frequently involved area to be injured.[107,114] Injuries to more than one chamber occur in more than 50% of cases.[115] Common injury patterns include crush injuries, deceleration injuries, direct precordial impact, or transmitted forces from compression of the abdominal cavity. Crush injuries can sometimes cause penetrating injuries when sternal or rib fractures result in cardiac punctures or lacerations.

BCI is thought to be overdiagnosed because of the lack of an appropriate gold standard.

To address these issues and to propose an approach to the patient with BCI, the EAST published its guidelines on this topic in 1998 and classified BCI according to the sequelae of the injury[116]:

1. BCI with free wall rupture. These patients usually die at the scene. For the few who make it to the ED, the prognosis is poor even when diagnosed early (usually on echo).
2. BCI with septal rupture. These injuries are rare and often occur in combination with valvular injuries; they present with signs of valvular failure and congestive heart failure. Treatment is usually surgical.
3. BCI with coronary artery injury. Lacerations of the coronary arteries typically lead to hemopericardium and tamponade, and are usually fatal. Coronary artery dissec-tions and thrombosis can lead to myocardial infarction.
4. BCI with cardiac failure. While the aforementioned 3 entities can lead to cardiac failure, BCI can also be caused by direct injury to the cardiac muscle, leading to cardiac dysfunction and contractility.
5. BCI with complex arrhythmias. These patients often need immediate treatment because if untreated, the dysrhythmias will lead to congestive heart failure and, potentially, death.
6. BCI with minor electrocardiogram (ECG) or cardiac enzyme abnormalities. These patients are usually asymptomatic and will not require any treatment.

BCI should be suspected in patients with significant blunt trauma to the chest. In such patients the initial assessment includes an ECG[116] to assess for the presence of arrhythmia, ST abnormalities, signs of ischemia, and heart block. E-FAST should be done to assess for the presence of hemopericardium and tamponade, as well as to assess the patient's volume status. BCI can be ruled out in patients who have a normal ECG, a normal E-FAST examination, and who are hemodynamically stable.[116] In hemodynamically unstable patients BCI should be considered, but should remain a diagnosis of exclusion until all other causes of this instability have been ruled out.

Patients with hemopericardium should be resuscitated rapidly and prepared for urgent surgical treatment. ED thoracotomy might be required if their clinical status deteriorates, knowing that in such a context the survival rate is marginal. Those who remain unstable and who have dysrhythmias should be managed according to Advanced Cardiovascular Life Support protocols. Repeat E-FAST should be performed in patients who fail to improve or whose status worsens, as hemopericardium may not always be present initially.

The use of biomarkers remains a controversial topic in the assessment of patients with possible BCI. Many studies have shown that in stable patients with normal ECG, an elevated creatine kinase MB level is nonspecific for the diagnosis of BCI.[114,117–120] Troponin I and troponin T have been shown to be more specific, but still lack adequate sensitivity to have clinical utility as a screening test.[121–123] This lack of sensitivity is explained by the fact that in trauma one can often see an elevation of these biomarkers, due to catecholamine release, reperfusion injury after hypovolemic shock, microcirculatory dysfunction, or oxidative injury. Troponin can also be negative in patients with dysrhythmias, and therefore a normal troponin level does not exclude the need for cardiac monitoring and eventual need to treat the dysrhythmias. For patients who are unstable or have dysrhythmias, biomarkers should be considered if there are signs of cardiac ischemia or myocardial infarct. In such patients one has to consider that the cardiac injury might have preceded, and therefore be the cause of, the trauma.

In stable patients with a normal ECG, cardiac echocardiography does not help the clinical management and is therefore not indicated.[115,124] In all other situations (unstable patient and/or abnormal ECG), echocardiography identifies the cause(s) of the cardiac dysfunction (wall motion abnormalities, septal injuries, valvular rupture or dysfunction, thrombus), and assesses the need and response to volume resuscitation and ionotropic support. For this procedure a transesophageal echocardiogram is preferred, and can often be done intraoperatively if necessary.[125] **Fig. 1** provides a flow diagram to illustrate the assessment of possible blunt cardiac assessment.

Penetrating Cardiac Injury

Penetrating cardiac injuries are highly lethal. It is estimated that the probability of arriving alive at the hospital after suffering such an injury is between 6% and 19.3%.[126,127] Most common injuries are to the right ventricle (due to its anterior location), followed by the left ventricle.[128–130] Atrial injuries are less common and usually less severe.

Penetrating cardiac injuries typically result in hemorrhagic shock and/or cardiac tamponade. Hemorrhagic shock is responsible for the majority of deaths at the scene.[131] However, it is important to remember that because of the poor compliance of the pericardium, as little as 50 mL of blood can lead to tamponade and, therefore, lethal injuries can occur with very little amount of blood loss. Similarly to blunt trauma, clinical signs are not reliable for diagnosing tamponade in penetrating cardiac trauma.

The cardiac box, defined as the space inferior to the clavicle, superior to the costal margin, and medial to the midclavicular lines, is the area where penetrating injuries to the chest are most dangerous. However, injuries outside this area do not rule out cardiac injuries. Patients with potential cardiac injuries require immediate and rapid

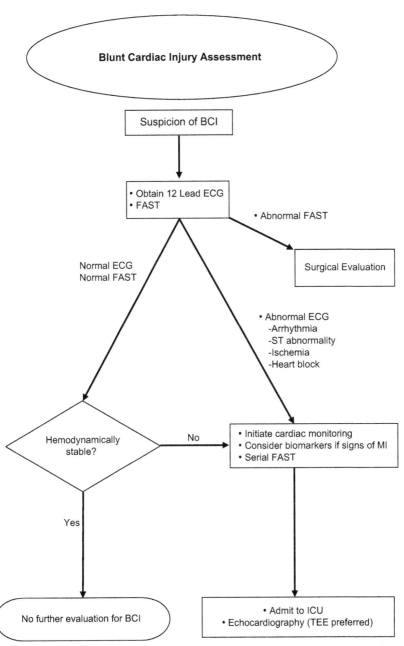

Fig. 1. Assessment of blunt cardiac injury (BCI). ECG, electrocardiography; FAST, focused assessment with sonography for trauma; ICU, intensive care unit; MI, myocardial infarction; TEE, transesophageal echocardiography.

evaluation in the ED (**Fig. 2**). After a thorough physical examination, patients require an immediate FAST examination of the heart, pericardium, and thorax to identify possible hemopericardium, tamponade, hemothoraces, and pneumothoraces.[132,133] The added benefit and need of a portable CXR in these patients must be weighed against

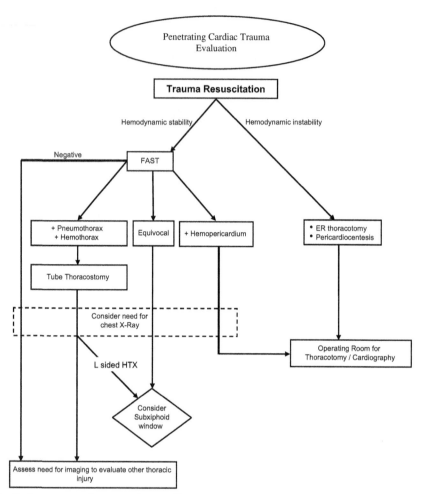

Fig. 2. Assessment of penetrating cardiac trauma. ER, emergency room; HTX, hemothorax.

the high sensitivity of bedside ultrasonography. The proficiency of the physician at performing the ultrasound procedure and the quality of the images generated must also be taken into account.

Patients with hemopericardium, even when stable, require urgent thoracotomy and cardiorrhaphy. Patients with left-sided hemothoraces could have a self-draining hemopericardium and are at risk of decompensating without warning. In such a case, a subxiphoid window can be performed to evaluate the pericardium. The same can be done if the result of the FAST is equivocal. If the patient becomes unstable at any time during the evaluation, an emergency thoracotomy can be performed in institutions that have the adequate surgical capacity to assume the care of these patients.

Aortic Injuries

Blunt aortic injuries usually occur when rapid deceleration produces sudden shearing forces on the aorta. The proximal descending aorta is the area most at risk because the ligamentum arteriosum is a transition point between the fixed descending aorta and the (relatively) mobile aortic arch. Although these injuries are not common, they are often lethal and are responsible for 15% of deaths in MVCs.[134]

Patients with blunt aortic injuries can be divided into 3 groups:

1. Complete transection of the aorta. These patients typically die at the scene or shortly after their arrival at the hospital.
2. Full-thickness injuries. These patients have ongoing bleeding and are hemodynamically unstable.
3. Partial-thickness injuries with contained hematomas. These patients can often present as hemodynamically stable.

In all cases, hemodynamic instability can also be present because of concomitant injuries and hemorrhage of other organs.

The challenge for the clinician is to identify the stable patients with incomplete injuries before the aortic lesion progresses to complete rupture. Unfortunately, there are no specific clinical signs that allow for the rapid identification of aortic injuries. For this reason they should be suspected in any patient with the proper mechanism, that is, rapid deceleration, high-speed MVC with frontal or side impact, and falls from a great height.[135,136]

Aortic injuries often result in some amount of mediastinal hemorrhage that can lead to disruption of mediastinal structures. Radiographic signs of such disruption include downward depression of the left main stem bronchus, deviation of the nasogastric tube to the right, apical pleural hematomas, disruption on the calcium ring in the aortic knob, and mediastinal hematoma. Ekeh and colleagues[137–139] found that CXR can miss 11% of aortic injuries and therefore is not an acceptable modality to rule out such injuries.

Angiography is the accepted gold standard for the diagnosis of aortic injuries. However, this modality is not available in all centers, and when it is present is rarely readily available. Furthermore, patients who require evaluation of the aorta typically need CT imaging of other organs and systems. Contrast CT has a reported sensitivity of greater than 97%, a specificity of greater than 85%, and a negative predictive value 100%.[137,140–142] For these reasons and because of the progress made in CT technology, CT with contrast is now the modality of choice for evaluation of aortic injuries. In the stable patient, angiography is still indicated when the CT result is equivocal. It can also be used for operative planning when the CT is positive. The need and timing of the angiography should usually be discussed with the consulting vascular surgeon.

The management of patients with aortic injuries includes: (1) prevention and control hypertension that can lead to progression of the injury; (2) control coagulopathy, including the prevention and treatment of hypothermia and acidosis; (3) correction of other life threatening injuries—it is important to prioritize which injuries need to be managed first because many aortic injuries do not require immediate treatment; and (4) definitive repair of the aortic injury.

Urgent repair is indicated for patients with hemodynamic instability attributed to the aortic injury, contrast extravasation on CT or with rapidly expanding hematoma, large hemorrhages from chest tubes, and penetrating aortic injuries.

Digestive Tract

Injuries to the esophagus are rare in blunt trauma because it is a well-protected structure due to its location in the posterior mediastinum. These injuries usually result from a rapid increase in esophageal luminal pressure. In penetrating trauma, esophageal injuries are also rare but must be suspected in all penetrating traumas that cross the mediastinum.[143]

The diagnosis of esophageal injuries is rarely evident at initial presentation. There are no specific clinical signs or specific radiographic findings that suggest the diagnosis. The risk of complications, namely sepsis from leakage of digestive track content, requires a high index of suspicion and early diagnosis. Basically any patient with air in the mediastinum of unclear origin should be evaluated for potential esophageal injury. Gastroscopy is avoided, as it increases mediastinal contamination if an injury exists. A water-soluble gastrografin swallow is the initial test of choice. A barium study can then be performed if the initial gastrografin test is negative, as barium has a greater sensitivity for small perforations.[144]

PUTTING IT ALL TOGETHER: INITIAL APPROACH AND RESUSCITATION OF THE UNSTABLE PATIENT
Data Gathering: Initial History and Physical Examination

The history should focus on determining the mechanism (blunt, penetrating, or a combination of both) and on estimating the severity of the forces to which the patient has been submitted. Blast mechanisms are for all purposes equivalent to blunt mechanisms, but with a much more rapid onset of symptoms.[63,145–147]

Immediate assessment of vital signs and physical examination structured along the usual ABCs (Airway, Breathing, Circulation) will allow the EP to rapidly identify respiratory and/or hemodynamic compromise, which mandate immediate action. In blunt trauma, tenderness to palpation will confirm thoracic involvement, but physical examination has shown poor sensitivity in ruling out specific injuries.[148] Clues to potential injuries should nonetheless be sought: asymmetry of chest rise (flail chest), crepitus on palpation (rib injury), decreased or absent air entry (splinting from rib fractures, hemothorax or pneumothorax), and subcutaneous emphysema (pneumothorax or tracheobronchial injury). It has been shown that physical examination is not reliable for the diagnosis of hemothorax or pneumothorax in blunt or penetrating trauma.[149–153]

In penetrating torso trauma, the initial goal of the EP should be to find the location of all wounds to better determine the pathway of potential injuries.[154] This step is critical, as important resuscitative decisions including ED thoracotomy may need to be taken within the first seconds of the patient's arrival in the ED. The protocol at the authors' institution is to rapidly expose (including bilateral log roll) the patient as soon (or simultaneously) as he or she is placed on the ED stretcher, which takes less than 20 seconds when done properly; waiting for the patient to be connected to monitors and intravenous catheters can delay this crucial step by several minutes. The authors have encountered cases whereby the discovery of unforeseen (posterior) thoracic wounds drastically altered initial management.

Management of the Unstable Patient

There is a paucity of scientific literature to support the exact sequence of actions to be performed in severe chest trauma, especially in blunt trauma cases. A previously planned algorithmic approach will help the physician who is confronted with a potentially dying patient.[155]

Airway compromise, a respiratory rate greater than 30, oxygen saturation below 90% to 92%, tachycardia above 120 beats per minute, and hypotension below 100 systolic are all ominous signs that mandate immediate resuscitative action. On identifying the unstable patient, physicians should attempt to differentiate between respiratory and circulatory issues, though this is not always possible. Hemorrhagic shock can present with important tachypnea and/or desaturation, mimicking respiratory compromise, so simultaneous interventions to restore oxygenation, ventilation, and circulation should be initiated. The use of E-FAST and CXR can be of tremendous value, but in true critical situations there may not be time to perform these procedures. It must be accepted that in critical patients the physician may need to perform therapeutic actions such as a thoracostomy, which in retrospect may not have been needed. Failure to perform these actions when indicated could result in much more significant consequences and patient's demise.

Blunt chest trauma
By answering a series of questions and taking the appropriate therapeutic actions, the physician will be able to successfully resuscitate the majority of severe, unstable chest trauma patients. Some of the steps may be done simultaneously. These questions include:

- Is the airway in jeopardy or is the patient nearing apnea? If so, immediate intubation is mandatory.
- Is the patient in respiratory distress of hypoxic? If so, the patient should receive high-flow oxygen by nonrebreather mask.
- Did the patient improve rapidly with high-flow oxygen? If yes, the clinician can pursue more calmly a more thorough diagnostic evaluation (with CXR and ultrasound evaluation of the chest).
- Is the patient also hypotensive? The combination of respiratory distress and hypotension in chest trauma highly suggests TPTX. Immediate chest decompression by thoracostomy is needed to salvage these patients[145,156] while simultaneous fluid resuscitation is undertaken.
  o Can the affected side be identified by the presence of deviated trachea, decreased air entry, obvious crepitus from rib fractures or subcutaneous emphysema, decreased chest expansion, or tenderness to palpation? If so, drain this side.
  o Is the patient still in distress after chest decompression or was the affected side not identifiable? Drain the contralateral side or perform bilateral thoracostomies from the start.[48]
- Examine the depth and pattern of breathing in combination with chest wall movement and integrity: is there compromise of respiratory mechanics from flail chest or multiple rib fractures? If yes, intubation and mechanical ventilation might benefit the patient.
- Is the patient still presenting gas exchange problems, as manifested by low oxygen saturation, or increased work of breathing? Obtaining bedside imaging can prove extremely useful as regards the diagnosis and appropriate treatment. Causes may include: lung collapse from hemothorax/pneumothorax; parenchymal damage from pulmonary contusions or lacerations; and alveolar filling with fluid, blood, or vomitus. Mechanical ventilation will benefit many of these injuries[145] except for pneumothoraces, which it may exacerbate. Major injuries to the chest such as pulmonary contusions and flail chest require time to improve, and the patient's status may often deteriorate in the subsequent hours, so aggressive management is warranted.[145] These patients should all be admitted to an ICU for proper monitoring.
- Is the patient hemodynamically unstable? TPTX as a cause should already have been dealt with. Fluid resuscitation, including blood products, should be well

under way through access by large-bore intravenous catheter. The sensitivity of the supine CXR for hemothorax is low, and as much as a liter of blood can be missed on such films.[24] E-FAST by well-trained operators can be used to assess the pleural spaces as well as the pericardial space; it is the most efficient way to rapidly assess the abdomen as well.

- Is there pleural fluid on E-FAST examination (or on CXR)? If so, insert a large-bore chest tube in the affected hemithorax and monitor blood output. The decision for urgent thoracotomy is based on the patient's physiologic status and response to volume resuscitation combined with the amount of immediate and ongoing blood drained from the chest.[24] Bilateral chest tube insertion may be indicated in a hypotensive patient to simultaneously diagnose and drain the chest cavities.[145,156] Taking this action would apply to the profoundly hypotensive patient or in pulseless electrical activity, to immediately relieve any tension physiology in the chest. It would also apply in cases where sonographic evaluation of the chest is impossible, the abdominal FAST is negative or equivocal, and the pelvis appears stable or has already been bound.
- Is there free abdominal fluid on the FAST examination? If so, involve immediately a general surgeon for possible laparotomy.

Penetrating trauma

Management of the unstable patient with penetrating chest trauma will be directly affected by the location of the wounds and types of injury (missile vs stab wound). It is therefore critical to identify all wounds very early on in the course of the resuscitation. Locations are referred to as transmediastinal, central (cardiac box), thoracoabdominal, or peripheral.[154] Decision branching points are also more straightforward.

Patients in respiratory distress or who are hypoxic are likely to have a large pneumothorax with or without associated hemothorax or tension physiology. These patients should be placed on high-flow oxygen and receive an immediate thoracostomy of the involved hemithorax. Intubation should be considered if the patient is too agitated to allow insertion of the chest tube. If insertion of the chest tube fails to improve the patient's condition, the physician should drain the contralateral hemithorax; this is especially important in gunshot wounds.

Managing hemodynamic instability in these cases revolves around rapidly obtaining large-bore intravenous access with immediate initiation of fluid resuscitation, with blood. The use of E-FAST is paramount to identify the presence of a pericardial effusion, which mandates operative exploration. If the patient is moribund or with worsening vital signs, an ED resuscitative thoracotomy should be done, as any delay decreases survival chances.[157] Otherwise it may be more appropriate to bring the patient immediately to the operating room for definitive surgical care.

Victims of gunshot wounds to the chest who are moribund but have a negative E-FAST for a pericardial effusion should be intubated and obtain bilateral thoracostomies, while simultaneously completing the rest of the FAST of the abdomen, because bullets can travel far from their point of entry. Urgent operative management is mandatory and should be directed according to the findings of the FAST and thoracostomies. Hypotensive but not moribund patients benefit from a similar approach, though a single chest tube can be inserted initially if the entry and exit wounds are on the same hemithorax. Transmediastinal gunshot wounds have a much higher likelihood of requiring a thoracotomy.[154]

In unstable stab wounds, the management is guided primarily by the location of the wound(s). Hypotensive patients with a central wound (in the cardiac box) who have a negative FAST of the pericardium should obtain a tube thoracostomy on the side of injury. The presence of a hemothorax should prompt immediate surgical exploration, as a ventricular laceration (with an associated pericardial laceration) could still be present and be draining blood directly into the chest cavity. In thoracoabdominal wounds a chest tube should be inserted in the wounded hemithorax, and a FAST should be done to identify the injured cavity and dictate the surgical approach.[154]

In all cases careful examination must be done to exclude other sources or areas of bleeding, as it is easy to be distracted by one obvious wound!

SUMMARY

Chest trauma is responsible for 25% of traumatic deaths. Rapid identification of injuries through an organized approach and stabilization based on patient physiology can prevent untimely death and morbidity. The incorporation of E-FAST will greatly facilitate the diagnostic approach. Therapeutic gestures such as tube thoracostomy and intubation play an important role in the initial stabilization of these patients. Further imaging with CT scanning allows for better definition of the majority of the injuries and has become the diagnostic modality of choice for aortic injuries. The majority of occult injuries (to CXR) can be easily observed. More than 80% of chest injuries may be managed nonoperatively, with supportive treatment. Prompt involvement of a thoracic surgeon is necessary in cases of ruptured airway, massive hemothorax, and penetrating cardiac trauma, as well as suspected esophageal injuries.

REFERENCES

1. Khandhar SJ, Johnson SB, Calhoon JH. Overview of thoracic trauma in the United States. Thorac Surg Clin 2007;17:1–9.
2. Centers for Disease Control and Prevention. Injury prevention and control: data and statistics (WISQARS). Available at: http://www.cdc.gov/injury/wisqars/index.html. Accessed January 8, 2010.
3. Boyd AD, Glassman LR. Trauma to the lung. Chest Surg Clin N Am 1997;7(2):263–84.
4. Swan KG, Reiner DS, Blackwood JM. Wound ballistics and principles of management. Mil Med 1987;152:29–34.
5. Jones JW, Kitchema A, Webb WR, et al. Emergency thoracotomy: a logical approach to chest trauma management. J Trauma 1981;21:280.
6. Kiser AC, O'Brien SM, Detterbeck FC. Blunt tracheobronchial injuries: treatment and outcomes. Ann Thorac Surg 2001;71:2059–65.
7. Gussack GS, Jurkovich GJ, Luterman A. Laryngotracheal trauma: a protocol approach to a rare injury. Laryngoscope 1986;96:660–5.
8. Graham JM, Mattox KL, Beall AC Jr. Penetrating trauma of the lung. J Trauma 1979;19:665–9.
9. Angood PB, Attia EL, Brown RA, et al. Extrinsic civilian trauma to the larynx and cervical trachea: important predictors of long-term morbidity. J Trauma 1986;26:869–73.
10. De La Rocha AG, Kayler D. Traumatic rupture of the tracheobronchial tree. Can J Surg 1985;28:68–71.
11. Kummer C, Netto FS, Rizoli S, et al. A review of traumatic airway injuries: potential implications for airway assessment and management. Injury 2007;38:27–33.
12. Barmada H, Gibbons JR. Tracheobronchial injury in blunt and penetrating chest trauma. Chest 1994;106:74–8.

13. Deslauriers J, Beaulieu M, Archambault G, et al. Diagnosis and long-term follow-up of major bronchial disruptions due to nonpenetrating trauma. Ann Thorac Surg 1982;33:32–9.
14. O'Connor JV, Adamski J. The diagnosis and treatment of non-cardiac thoracic trauma. J R Army Med Corps 2010;156(1):5–14.
15. Karmy-Jones R, Wood DE. Traumatic injury to the trachea and bronchus. Thorac Surg Clin 2007;17:35–46.
16. Richardson JD, Miller FB, Carrillo EH, et al. Complex thoracic injuries. Surg Clin North Am 1996;76(4):725–48.
17. Taskinen SO, Salo JA, Halttunen PE. Tracheobronchial rupture due to blunt chest trauma. Ann Thorac Surg 1989;48:846–9.
18. Round JA, Mellor AJ. Anaesthetic and critical care management of thoracic injuries. J R Army Med Corps 2010;156(3):145–9.
19. Hill SL, Edmisten T, Holtzman G, et al. The occult pneumothorax: an increasing diagnostic entity in trauma. Am Surg 1999;65:254–8.
20. Tam MM. Occult pneumothorax in trauma patients: should this be sought in the focused assessment with sonography for trauma examination? Emerg Med Australas 2005;17(5–6):488–93.
21. Ball CG, Ranson K, Dente CJ, et al. Clinical predictors of occult pneumothoraces in severely injured blunt polytrauma patients: a prospective observational study. Injury 2009;40(1):44–7.
22. Ouellet JF, Trottier V, Kmet L, et al. The OPTICC trial: a multi-institutional study of occult pneumothoraces in critical care. Am J Surg 2009;197:581–6.
23. Yadav K, Jalili M, Zehtabchi S. Management of traumatic occult pneumothorax. Resuscitation 2010;81(9):1063–8.
24. Mowery NT, Gunter OL, Collier BR, et al. Practice management guidelines for the management of hemothorax and occult pneumothorax. J Trauma 2011; 70(2):510–8.
25. Trupka A, Wadhas C, Hallfeldt K, et al. Value of thoracic computed tomography in the first assessment of severely injured patients with blunt chest trauma. J Trauma 1997;43:405–11.
26. Marx J, Hockberger R, Walls R. Rosen's emergency medicine. 7th edition. Philadelphia: Mosby; 2009.
27. Roberts JR, Hedges JR. Clinical procedures in emergency medicine. 5th edition. Philadelphia: Saunders; 2009.
28. Townsend CM Jr, Beauchamp RD, Evers MD, et al. Sabiston textbook of surgery. 18th edition. Philadelphia: Saunders; 2007.
29. American College of Surgeons. Advanced trauma life support, student course manual. 7th edition. Chicago: First Impression; 2004.
30. Leigh-Smith S, Harris T. Tension pneumothorax, time for a rethink? Emerg Med J 2005;22:8–16.
31. Rutherford RB, Hurt HH Jr, Brickman RD, et al. The pathophysiology of progressive, tension pneumothorax. J Trauma 1968;8:212–27.
32. Gustman P, Yerger L, Wanner A. Immediate cardiovascular effects of tension pneumothorax. Am Rev Respir Dis 1983;127:171–4.
33. Bennett RA, Orton EC, Tucker A, et al. Cardiopulmonary changes in conscious dogs with induced progressive pneumothorax. Am J Vet Res 1989;50:280–4.
34. Hurewitz AN, Sidhu U, Bergofsky EH, et al. Cardiovascular and respiratory consequences of tension pneumothorax. Bull Eur Physiopathol Respir 1986; 22:545–9.

35. Carvalho P, Hilderbrandt J, Charan NB. Changes in bronchial and pulmonary arterial blood flow with progressive tension pneumothorax. J Appl Physiol 1996;81:1664–9.

36. West J. The mechanics of breathing. Respiratory physiology—the essentials. 5th edition. Baltimore (MD): Williams and Wilkins; 1995. p. 31–50, 89–116.

37. Barton ED, Rhee P, Hutton KC, et al. The pathophysiology of tension pneumothorax in ventilated swine. J Emerg Med 1997;15:147–53.

38. Steier M, Ching N, Roberts EB, et al. Pneumothorax complicating continuous ventilatory support. J Thorac Cardiovasc Surg 1974;67:17–23.

39. Barton ED. Tension pneumothorax. Curr Opin Pulm Med 1999;5:269–74.

40. Beards SC, Lipman J. Decreased cardiac index as an indicator of tension pneumothorax in the ventilated patient. Anaesthesia 1994;49:137–41.

41. Coats TJ, Wilson AW, Xeropotamous N. Pre-hospital management of patients with severe thoracic injury. Injury 1995;2:581–5.

42. Eckstein M, Suyehara D. Needle thoracostomy in the prehospital setting. Prehosp Emerg Care 1998;2:132–5.

43. Barton ED, Epperson M, Hoyt DB, et al. Prehospital needle aspiration and tube thoracostomy in trauma victims: a six-year experience with aeromedical crews. J Emerg Med 1995;13:155–63.

44. Light RW. Tension pneumothorax. Intensive Care Med 1994;20:468–9.

45. ATLS. Advanced trauma life support. 6th edition. Chicago: American College of Surgeons; 1997.

46. McPherson JJ, Feigin DS, Bellamy RF. Prevalence of tension pneumothorax in fatally wounded combat casualties. J Trauma 2006;60(3):573–8.

47. Leigh-Smith S, Davies G. Pneumothorax: eyes may be more diagnostic than ears. Emerg Med J 2003;20:495–6.

48. Fitzgerald M, Mackenzie CF, Marasco S, et al. Pleural decompression and drainage during trauma reception and resuscitation. Injury 2008;39(1):9–20.

49. Clark S, Ragg M, Stella J. Is mediastinal shift on chest X-ray of pneumothorax always an emergency? Emerg Med (Fremantle) 2003;15(5–6):429–33.

50. Cullinane DC, Morris JA Jr, Bass JG, et al. Needle thoracostomy may not be indicated in the trauma patient. Injury 2001;32:749–52.

51. Available at: http://www.trauma.org/index.php/main/article/199/. Accessed April 6, 2011.

52. Britten S, Palmer SH. Chest wall thickness may limit adequate drainage of tension pneumothorax by needle thoracocentesis. J Accid Emerg Med 1996; 13:426–7.

53. Jenkins C, Sudheer PS. Needle thoracocentesis fails to diagnose a large pneumothorax. Anaesthesia 2000;55:925–6.

54. Jones R, Hollingsworth J. Tension pneumothoraces not responding to needle thoracocentesis. Emerg Med J 2002;19:176–7.

55. Mines D, Abbuhl S. Needle thoracostomy fails to detect a fatal tension pneumothorax. Ann Emerg Med 1993;22:863–6.

56. Butler KL, Best IM, Weaver W, et al. Pulmonary artery injury and cardiac tamponade after needle decompression of a suspected tension pneumothorax. J Trauma 2003;54(3):610–1.

57. Marinaro JL, Kenny CV, Rhett Smith S, et al. Needle thoracostomy in trauma patients: what catheter length is adequate? Acad Emerg Med 2003;10(5):495.

58. Lander OM, Sanchez LD, Pedrosa I. Anterior vs. lateral needle decompression of tension pneumothorax: comparison by computed tomography chest wall measurement. Acad Emerg Med 2005;12(5 Suppl 1):66.

59. Ferrie EP, Collum N, McGovern S. The right place in the right space? Awareness of site for needle thoracentesis. Emerg Med J 2005;22:788–9.

60. Rawlins R, Brown KM, Carr CS, et al. Life threatening haemorrhage after anterior needle aspiration of pneumothoraces. A role for lateral needle aspiration in emergency decompression of spontaneous pneumothorax. Emerg Med J 2003;20(4):383–4.

61. Cohn SM. Pulmonary contusion: review of the clinical entity. J Trauma 1997;42: 973–9.

62. O'Connor JV, Kufera JA, Kerns TJ, et al. Crash and occupant predictors of pulmonary contusion. J Trauma 2009;66:1091–5.

63. DePalma RG, Burris DG, Champion HR, et al. Blast injuries. N Engl J Med 2005; 352:1335–42.

64. Cohn SM, Dubose JJ. Pulmonary contusion: an update on recent advances in clinical management. World J Surg 2010;34(8):1959–70.

65. Oppenheimer L, Craven KD. Pathophysiology of pulmonary contusion in dogs. J Appl Physiol 1979;47:718–28.

66. Hellinger A, Konerding MA. Does lung contusion affect both the traumatized and the noninjured lung parenchyma? A morphological and morphometric study in the pig. J Trauma 1995;39:712–9.

67. Fulton RL, Peter ET. The progressive nature of pulmonary contusion. Surgery 1970;67:499–506.

68. Tyburski JG, Collinge JD, Wilson RF, et al. Pulmonary contusions: quantifying the lesions on chest X-ray films and the factors affecting prognosis. J Trauma 1999; 46(5):833–8.

69. Pape HC, Remmers D, Rice J, et al. Appraisal of early evaluation of blunt chest trauma: development of a standardized scoring system for initial clinical decision making. J Trauma 2000;49:496–504.

70. Schild HH, Strunk H, Wever W, et al. Pulmonary contusion: CT vs plain radiograms. J Comput Assist Tomogr 1989;13:417–20.

71. Wagner RB, Crawford WO Jr, Schimpf PP. Classification of parenchymal injuries of the lung. Radiology 1988;167:77–82.

72. Miller PR, Croce MA, Bee TK, et al. ARDS after pulmonary contusion: accurate measurement of contusion volume identifies high-risk patients. J Trauma 2001; 51:223–8.

73. Deunk J, Poels T, Brink M, et al. The clinical outcome of occult pulmonary contusion on multidetector-row computed tomography in blunt trauma patients. J Trauma 2010;68:387–94.

74. Gunduz M, Unlugenc H, Ozalevli M, et al. A comparative study of positive airway pressure (CPAP) and intermittent pressure ventilation (IPPV) in patients with flail chest. Emerg Med J 2005;22:325–9.

75. Antonelli M, Conti G, Moro ML, et al. Predictors of failure of noninvasive positive pressure ventilation in patients with acute hypoxemic respiratory failure: a multicenter study. Intensive Care Med 2001;27:1718–28.

76. Trinkle J, Richardson J, Franz J, et al. Management of flail chest without mechanical ventilation. Ann Thorac Surg 1975;19(4):355–63.

77. Richardson JD, Adams L, Flint LM. Selective management of flail chest and pulmonary contusion. Ann Surg 1982;196:481–7.

78. Ventilation with lower tidal volumes as compared with traditional tidal volumes for acute lung injury and the acute respiratory distress syndrome. The Acute Respiratory Distress Syndrome Network. N Engl J Med 2000; 342:1301–8.

79. Schreiter D, Reske A, Stichert B, et al. Alveolar recruitment in combination with sufficient positive end-expiratory pressure increases oxygenation and lung aeration in patients with severe chest trauma. Crit Care Med 2004;32: 968–75.
80. Sirmali M, Turut H, Topcu S, et al. A comprehensive analysis of traumatic rib fractures: morbidity, mortality and management. Eur J Cardiothorac Surg 2003;24:133–8.
81. Kroell CK, Schneider DC, Nahum AM. Impact tolerance and response to the human thorax II. Proceedings of the 18th Stapp Car Crash Conference. Pennsylvania: Society of Automotive Engineers; 1974. p. 383–457.
82. Cavanaugh JM. Bio mechanics of thoracic trauma. In: Nahum AM, Melvin JW, editors. Accidental injury: biomechanics and prevention. 2nd edition. New York: Springer Science; 2002.
83. Ziegler DW, Agarwal NN. The morbidity and mortality of rib fractures. J Trauma 1994;37:975–9.
84. Shweiki E, Klena J, Wood GC, et al. Assessing the true risk of abdominal solid organ injury in hospitalized rib fracture patients. J Trauma 2000;50:684–8.
85. Garcia VF, Gotschall CS, Eichelberger MR, et al. Rib fractures in children: a marker of severe trauma. J Trauma 1990;30:695–700.
86. Barnea Y, Kashtan H, Shornick Y, et al. Isolated rib fractures in elderly patients: mortality and morbidity. Can J Surg 2002;45(1):43–6.
87. Sharma OP, Oswanski MF, Jolly S, et al. Perils of rib fractures. Am Surg 2008; 74(4):310–4.
88. Bulger EM, Arneson MA, Mock CN, et al. Rib fractures in the elderly. J Trauma 2000;48:1040–7.
89. Flagel BT, Luchette FA, Reed RL, et al. Half-a-dozen ribs: the breakpoint for mortality. Surgery 2005;138(4):717–23 [discussion: 723–5].
90. Testerman GM. Adverse outcomes in younger rib fracture patients. South Med J 2006;99(4):335–9.
91. Holcomb JB, McMullin NR, Kozar RA, et al. Morbidity from rib fractures increases after age 45. J Am Coll Surg 2003;196(4):549–55.
92. Kshettry VR, Bolman RM. Chest trauma—assessment, diagnosis, and management. Clin Chest Med 1994;15:137–46.
93. Alexander JQ, Gutierrez CJ, Mariano MC, et al. Blunt chest trauma in the elderly patient: how cardiopulmonary disease affects outcome. Am Surg 2000;66(9): 855–7.
94. Velmahos GC, Chan LS, Murray JA, et al. Influence of flail chest on outcome among patients with severe thoracic cage trauma. Int Surg 2002;87:240–4.
95. Craven KD, Oppenheimer L, Wood LD. Effects of contusion and flail chest on pulmonary perfusion and oxygen exchange. J Appl Physiol 1979;47:729–37.
96. Freedland M, Wilson RF, Bender JS, et al. The management of flail chest injury: factors affecting outcome. J Trauma 1990;30(12):1460–8.
97. Bulger EM, Edwards T, Klotz P, et al. Epidural analgesia improves outcome after multiple rib fractures. Surgery 2004;136:426–30.
98. Kieninger AN, Bair HA, Bendick PJ, et al. Epidural versus intravenous pain control in elderly patients with rib fractures. Am J Surg 2005;189(3):327–30.
99. Simon BJ, Cushman J, Barraco R, et al. EAST Practice Management Guidelines Work Group. Pain management guidelines for blunt thoracic trauma. J Trauma 2005;59:1256–67.
100. Karmakar MK, Ho AM. Acute pain management of patients with multiple fractured ribs. J Trauma 2003;54:615–25.

101. Carrier FM, Turgeon AF, Nicole PC, et al. Effect of epidural analgesia in patients with traumatic rib fractures: a systematic review and meta-analysis of randomized controlled trials. Can J Anaesth 2009;56(3):230–42.

102. Sauaia A, Moore FA, Moore EE, et al. Epidemiology of trauma deaths: a reassessment. J Trauma 1995;38:185–93.

103. Miller LA. Chest wall, lung and pleural space trauma. Radiol Clin North Am 2006; 44:213.

104. Molnar TF. Surgical management of chest wall trauma. Thorac Surg Clin 2010; 20(4):475–85.

105. Hunt PA, Greaves I, Owens WA. Emergency thoracotomy in thoracic trauma: a review. Injury 2006;37:1–19.

106. Riskin DJ, Tsai TC, Riskin L, et al. Massive transfusion protocols: the role of aggressive resuscitation versus product ratio in mortality reduction. J Am Coll Surg 2009;209:198–205.

107. Parmley LF, Mattingly TW. Nonpenetrating traumatic injury of the heart. Circulation 1958;18:371–96.

108. Dubrow TJ, Mihalka J, Eisenhauer DM, et al. Myocardial contusion in the stable patient: what level of care is appropriate? Surgery 1989;106(2): 267–74.

109. DeMuth WE, Baue AE, Odom JA. Contusion of the heart. J Trauma 1967;7(3): 443–55.

110. Wisner DH, Reed WH, Riddick RS. Suspected myocardial contusion. Triage and indications for monitoring. Ann Surg 1987;206(2):200–5.

111. Shor RW, Crittenden M, Indeck M, et al. Blunt thoracic trauma. Analysis of 515 patients. Ann Surg 1990;212(1):82–6.

112. Mattox KL, Flint LM, Carrico CJ, et al. Blunt cardiac injury. J Trauma 1992;33(5): 649–50.

113. Sutherland GR, Driedger AA, Holliday RL, et al. Frequency of myocardial injury after blunt chest trauma as evaluated by radionuclide angiography. Am J Cardiol 1883;52(8):1099–103.

114. Paone RF, Peacock JB, Smith DL. Diagnosis of myocardial contusion. South Med J 1993;86(8):867–70.

115. Karalis DG, Victor MF, Davis GA, et al. The role of echocardiography in blunt chest trauma: a transthoracic and transesophageal echocardiographic study. J Trauma 1994;36(1):53–8.

116. Pasquale MD, Nagy K, Clarke J. Practice management guidelines for screening of blunt cardiac injury. The Eastern Association for the Surgery of Trauma. Available at: http://www.east.org/tpg/chap2.pdf. Accessed July 25, 2011.

117. Miller FB, Shumate CR, Richardson JD, et al. Myocardial contusion. When can the diagnosis be eliminated? Arch Surg 1989;124(7):805–8.

118. Foil MB, Mackersie RC, Furst, et al. The asymptomatic patient with suspected myocardial contusion. Am J Surg 1990;160(6):638–43.

119. Illig KA, Swierzewski MJ, Feliciano, et al. A rationale screening and treatment strategy based on the electrocardiogram alone for suspected cardiac contusion. Am J Surg 1991;161(6):537–43.

120. Biffl WL, Moore FA, Moore EE, et al. Cardiac enzymes are irrelevant in the patient with suspected myocardial contusion. Am J Surg 1994;168(6):523–8.

121. Bertichant JP, Polge A, Mohty D, et al. Evaluation of incidence, clinical significance, and prognostic value of circulating cardiac troponin I and T elevation in hemodynamically stable patients with suspected myocardial contusion after blunt chest trauma. J Trauma 2000;48(5):924–31.

122. Ferjani M, Droc G, Dreux S, et al. Circulating troponin T in myocardial contusion. Chest 1997;111(2):427–33.
123. Sybrandy KC, Kramer MJ, Burgersdijk C. Diagnosing cardiac contusion: old wisdom and new insights. Heart 2003;89(5):485–9.
124. Hossack KF, Moreno FA, Moore EE, et al. Frequency of cardiac contusion in non penetrating chest injury. Am J Cardiol 1988;61(4):391–4.
125. Chirillo F, Totis O, Cavarzerani A, et al. Usefulness of transthoracic and transesophageal echocardiography in recognition and management of cardiovascular injuries after blunt chest trauma. Heart 1996;75(3):301–6.
126. Demetriades D, Van Der Veen BW. Penetrating injuries of the heart: experience over two years in South Africa. J Trauma 1983;23:1034–41.
127. Rhee PM, Foy H, Kaufman C, et al. Penetrating cardiac injuries: a population-based study. J Trauma 1998;45(2):366–70.
128. Gunay C, Cingoz F, Kuralay E, et al. Surgical challenges for urgent approach in penetrating heart injuries. Heart Surg Forum 2007;10:E473.
129. Asensio JA, Berne JD, Demetriades D, et al. One hundred five penetrating cardiac injuries: a 2-year prospective evaluation. J Trauma 1998;44:1073.
130. Wall MJ, Mattox KL, Baldwin JC. Acute management of complex cardiac injuries. J Trauma 1997;42:905–12.
131. Altun G, Altun A, Yilmaz A. Hemopericardium-related fatalities: a 10-year medicolegal autopsy experience. Cardiology 2005;104(3):133–7.
132. Nagy KK, Lohman C, Kim DO, et al. Role of echocardiography in the diagnosis of occult penetrating cardiac injury. J Trauma 1995;38:859–62.
133. Rozycki GS, Feliciano DV, Ochsner MG, et al. The role of ultrasound in patient with possible penetrating cardiac wounds: a prospective multicenter study. J Trauma 1999;46(4):543–51.
134. Fabian TC, Richardson JD, Croce MA, et al. Prospective study of blunt aortic injury: multicenter trial of the American Association for the Surgery of Trauma. J Trauma 1997;43(3):374–80.
135. Katyal D, McLellan BA, Brenneman FD, et al. Lateral impact motor vehicle collisions: significant cause of blunt traumatic rupture of the aorta. J Trauma 1997; 42:769–72.
136. Brundage SI, Harrugg R, Jurkovich GJ, et al. The epidemiology of thoracic aortic injuries in pedestrians. J Trauma 1998;45:1010–4.
137. Demetriades D, Gomez H, Velmahos GC, et al. Routine helical tomography evaluation of the mediastinum in high-risk blunt trauma patients. Arch Surg 1998; 133(10):1084–8.
138. Ekeh AP, Peterson W, Woods RJ, et al. Is chest x-ray an adequate screening tool for the diagnosis of blunt thoracic aortic injury? J Trauma 2008;65(5):1088–92.
139. Benjamin ER, Tillou A, Hiatt JR, et al. Blunt thoracic aortic injury. Am Surg 2008; 74(10):1033–7.
140. Dyer DS, Moore EE, Ilke DN, et al. Thoracic injury: how to predictive is mechanism and is chest computed tomography a reliable screening tool? A prospective study of 1561 patients. J Trauma 2000;48(4):673–82.
141. Wintermark M, Vicky S, Schnyder P. Imaging of acute traumatic injuries of the thoracic aorta. Eur Radiol 2002;12(2):431–42.
142. Parjer MS, Matheson TL, Rao AV, et al. Making the transition: the role of the helical CT in the evaluation of the potentially acute thoracic aortic injury. Am J Roentgenol 2001;176(5):1267–72.
143. Cornwell EE 3rd, Kennedy F, Ayad IA, et al. Transmediastinal gunshot wounds. A reconsideration of the role of aortography. Arch Surg 1996;131(9):949–52.

144. James AE Jr, Montali RJ, Chaffee V, et al. Barium or gastrografin: which contrast media for diagnosis of esophageal tears? Gastroenterology 1975;68(5):1103–13.
145. Kiraly L, Schreiber M. Management of the crushed chest. Crit Care Med 2010; 38(Suppl 9):S469–77.
146. Guy RJ, Kirkman E, Watkins PE, et al. Physiologic responses to primary blast. J Trauma 1998;45:983–7.
147. American College of Surgeons Committee on Trauma. Advanced trauma life support for doctors, ATLS student course manual. Chicago: American College of Surgeons; 2008.
148. Dunlop MG, Beattie TF, Preston PG, et al. Clinical assessment and radiography following blunt chest trauma. Arch Emerg Med 1989;6:125–7.
149. Bokhari F, Brakenridge S, Nagy K, et al. Prospective evaluation of the sensitivity of physical examination in chest trauma. J Trauma 2002;53(6):1135–8.
150. Chen SC, Markman JF, Kauder DR, et al. Hemopneumothorax missed by auscultation in penetrating chest injury. J Trauma 1997;42:86–9.
151. Wormald PJ, Knottenbelt JD, Linegar AG. A triage system for stab wounds to the chest. S Afr Med J 1989;76:211–2.
152. Spiteri MA, Cook DG, Clark SW. Reliability of eliciting physical signs in examination of the chest. Lancet 1988;331:873–5.
153. Thompson SR, Huizinga WK, Hirshberg A. Prospective study of the yield of physical examination compared with chest radiography in penetrating thoracic trauma. Thorax 1990;45:616–9.
154. Mandal AK, Sanusi M. Penetrating chest wounds: 24 years experience. World J Surg 2001;25(9):1145–9.
155. Kirkpatrick AW, Ball CG, D'Amours SK, et al. Acute resuscitation of the unstable adult trauma patient: bedside diagnosis and therapy. Can J Surg 2008;51(1): 57–69.
156. Huber-Wagner S, Lefering R, Qvick M, et al. Outcome in 757 severely injured patients with traumatic cardiorespiratory arrest. Resuscitation 2007;75:276–85.
157. Moore EE, Knudson MM, Burlew CC, et al. Defining the limits of resuscitative emergency department thoracotomy: a contemporary western trauma association perspective. J Trauma 2011;70(2):334–9.

Emergency Airway Management: the Difficult Airway

Joe Nemeth, MD[a],*, Nisreen Maghraby, MD[a,b], Sara Kazim, MD[a,b]

KEYWORDS
- Airway • Emergency • Difficult • Review

Securing an airway is one of the many challenging procedures that a physician who deals with the critically ill needs to be competent to perform. However, this vital procedure is not a one-size-fits-all intervention but rather a carefully scripted and thought out maneuver that demands expertise and that is tailored to each patient.

Patients in the emergency department (ED) requiring airway management present a challenge because they are not usually optimized medically, are not fasting, and do not have the option of delaying/postponing the procedure because of imminent airway compromise.[1] The incidence of a difficult airway (DA) in the anesthesia literature ranges from 0.4% to 8.5%[2] of elective intubations. Furthermore, at the end of the anesthetist's DA algorithm there is either "cancel case" or "awaken patient," neither of which is a viable or realistic option in the ED.

The incidence of a DA in the ED is 3% to 5.3% for unanticipated difficult tracheal intubation and 0.5% to 1.2% for failed intubation.[3,4] However, in a recent United Kingdom audit of intubations, at least 1 in 4 major airway events was from the intensive care unit or the ED. The outcome of these events was more likely to lead to permanent harm or death than events in anesthesia. Analysis of the cases identified gaps in care that included poor identification of at-risk patients, poor or incomplete planning, inadequate provision of skilled staff and equipment to manage these events successfully, delayed recognition of events, and failed rescue because of lack or failure of interpretation of capnography.[5]

Therefore, emergency airway management in the ED requires not only a firm concept of techniques of securing the airway but also of dealing with the potential DA in which establishing a definite airway is not possible with the techniques routinely

Funding support: None.

The authors have nothing to disclose.

[a] Division of Emergency Medicine, Montreal General Hospital, McGill University Health Center, 1650 Cedar Avenue, Montreal, Quebec H3G 1A4, Canada

[b] Emergency Medicine Residency Training Program, McGill University, Montreal, Quebec, Canada

* Corresponding author.

E-mail address: joe.nemeth@mcgill.ca

Emerg Med Clin N Am 30 (2012) 401–420

doi:10.1016/j.emc.2011.12.005

0733-8627/12/$ – see front matter © 2012 Elsevier Inc. All rights reserved.

emed.theclinics.com

used. This article highlights the importance of recognition and management of the DA in emergent situations. Both awake and nonawake intubation are discussed. Indications and guidelines are given for the use of nonsurgical and surgical airway interventions.

THE DA

The term DA is succinct. It needs to be differentiated from a failed airway, because they are 2 distinct concepts. Furthermore, a DA needs to be evaluated in 2 distinct, but not necessarily exclusive, categories: (1) difficult bag-mask ventilation (BMV) and (2) difficult endotracheal intubation (ETI). A DA is understood to be an airway that is complicated to manage because of anatomic, physiologic, or injury-altering reasons. It is an airway for which a preintubation assessment has identified attributes that are likely to make laryngoscopy, ETI, BMV, the use of extraglottic devices, or surgical airway management more difficult than would be the case in an ordinary patient without those attributes.

A failed airway occurs when a provider has embarked on a certain course of airway management (eg, rapid-sequence intubation [RSI]) and has identified that intubation by that method is not going to succeed, requiring the immediate initiation of a rescue sequence. Definitions include but are not limited to:

- Failure to achieve ETI on 3 attempts by a skilled and experienced provider
- A cannot-intubate/can-oxygenate scenario (any failure at oral intubation with inability to maintain arterial oxygen saturation [Sao2] >90% using bag valve mask [BVM] resuscitator).

PREPARING FOR EMERGENCY AIRWAY MANAGEMENT
General Principles

Because management of a DA may necessitate certain interventions that are associated with potential significant harm to the patient, proper identification of indications for the intervention must be sought out. Indications for emergency airway management are in 3 main, but not necessarily exclusive, groups: (1) airway obstruction, (2) inability to maintain/protect an open intact airway, and (3) respiratory failure. Impending changes in the airway (eg, inhalation injury/anaphylaxis) must be expected and prepared for, in the ability to maintain the airway (eg, head trauma and potential deterioration in mental status) and in respiratory status (eg, severe asthma exacerbation). This expectant philosophy should further drive the physician to undertake emergency airway management earlier rather than later, even though the patient may not have any indications for emergency airway management at the time of initial assessment.

The patient should ideally have 2 established intravenous lines, be connected to a cardiac monitor, and be in a place where there is easy access to DA instruments if needed. Furthermore, if time permits, a time-out should be implemented. The time-out phrase was coined by the surgical/anesthesiology literature. It incorporates a process whereby potential error in patient identification, diagnosis, and treatment could be circumvented.[6] At this step in the preparatory phase, the team leader reconfirms with the other members of the resuscitation team the need, method, and backup plan for ETI.

Equipment, medications, and the presence of appropriate personnel needed for undertaking the ETI should also be confirmed. The mnemonic SOAPME is one way to remember the essentials needed for intubation: suction, oxygen, airway, pharmacology/personnel, monitoring, and equipment. For the airway, include the endotracheal tubes (ETTs), laryngoscopes, blades, stylets, and BVM. For pharmacology, select, draw up, and label the appropriate medications (sedative, neuromuscular blocker, ancillary drugs) based on the history, physical examination, and equipment available. Personnel adept at advanced airway management should be present. Monitoring should include pulse oximetry and cardiac monitoring at a minimum; also preferably with capnography. Other equipment should include advanced airway devices including surgical devices (discussed later).

PREPARING FOR EMERGENCY AIRWAY MANAGEMENT
History and Examination

In an acute setting it is rare to have the option of a preintubation interview. However, if possible, it should be undertaken to recognize potential challenges. Identification of previous difficult intubations and of any past/current illnesses that could compromise the integrity and anatomy of the upper airway, the jaw, and the neck is paramount (eg, maxillofacial trauma, surgery, or radiotherapy). Furthermore, hemorrhagic diasthesis should be identified, whether iatrogenic (medication) or disease related (eg, Von Willebrand disease), because any airway maneuver can entail mucosal bleeding.

An assessment of the patient's overall condition, focusing on the patient's mental status and adequacy of oxygenation and ventilation, should be performed because this may determine the urgency of airway intervention. If time allows, the examination should focus on predictors of a DA, as follows.

It is paramount to identify anatomy unfavorable for both ventilation (facial hair, obesity, edentulous, large tongue, advanced age) and directing laryngoscopy (distortion of the airway from the nasophayrnx/orophayrnx to the trachea [trauma, infection, neoplasm, edema, hemorrhage, foreign body], disproportion [tongue/pharynx, thyromental displacement space], dysmobility [atlantooccipital joint, neck mobility, temporomadibular joint], dentition [prominent incisors]).[7] If the physician has time, a checklist to identify potential anatomic challenges can be undertaken (**Box 1**). Besides inspection and palpation, listening/auscultation for dysphonia and/or stridor can alert the physician to potential periglottic/upper airway compromise.

PREPARING FOR EMERGENCY AIRWAY MANAGEMENT
Preparing the Patient

Is preoxygenation optimal? Is the patient's position optimal? Can the patient's condition be optimized any further before intubation? If the intubation is difficult, how will oxygenation be maintained (plans A, B, C, D)? Where is the relevant equipment, including alternative airway? Are any specific complications anticipated? These are the key questions the physician must ask before undertaking the emergency management of any airway, not necessarily a DA.

Box 1
Checklist to identify potential anatomic challenges

- BONES (beard, obese, no teeth, elderly, sleep apnea)

- SHORT (surgery, hematoma, obese, radiation, tumor)

- 4 Ds (distortion, disproportion, dysmobility, dentition) and 3-3-2 rule (3 fingers mouth open, 3 fingers mentum to hyoid cartilage, 2 fingers floor of mouth to thyroid cartilage)

- Mallamapti score (an objective assessment of oropharyngeal anatomy; a higher class is associated with more difficult intubation) **Fig. 1**.

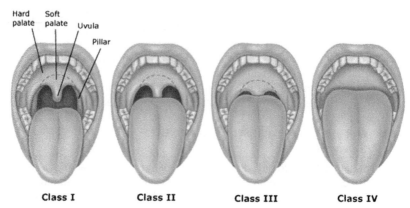

Fig. 1. The Mallampati classification for difficult laryngoscopy and intubation. Class I: full visibility of tonsils, uvula, and soft palate. Class II: visibility of hard and soft palate, upper portion of tonsils, and uvula. Class III: soft and hard palate and base of the uvula are visible. Class IV: only hard palate is visible. (*Reproduced with permission from* Walls RM, Murphy MF. The difficult airway in adults. In: UpToDate, Basow, DS (Ed), UpToDate, Waltham, MA 2011. Copyright © 2011 UpToDate, Inc.)

Preoxygenation and apneic oxygenation

Preoxygenation is an essential component in emergency airway management whether RSI is used or not. Its purpose is to replace the nitrogen in the patient's functional residual capacity with oxygen. Consequently, by increasing the oxygen reserve, the patient is more likely to be able to tolerate a longer apneic/bradypneic period.[8,9]

Recommendations for preoxygenation or denitrogenation in nonhypoxic patients are either breathing as close to 100% oxygen as possible (10–15 L/min O_2 by tight nonrebreather mask) for 3 to 5 minutes or 4 to 8 deep vital capacity breaths over 30 to 60 seconds.[8] It has been shown that more than 4 to 5 minutes of preoxygenation does not significantly increase the arterial oxygen tension in patients and may be harmful.[10] In healthy adult volunteers who have been preoxygenated for 3 to 5 minutes, the average time to desaturation (oxygen saturation <90%) is approximately 8 minutes. This time is significantly shorter in patients who are critically ill and have a higher metabolic demand for oxygen (**Fig. 2**).[11]

For patients in whom preoxygenation cannot be optimized by a nonrebreather face-mask, oxygenation may be improved further with the use of a ramped reverse Trendelenburg position (eg, in obesity)[12] (see later discussion) and/or with the use of noninvasive positive pressure ventilation (continuous positive airway pressure [CPAP]/biphasic positive airway pressure [BiPAP]) for short durations[13] just before undertaking intubation.

In patients already altered because of hypoxia and/or hypercapnia, precipitous attempts at intubation without adequate preoxygenation can lead to an existing DA becoming a failed airway. A novel term has been coined recently describing a method by which patients in whom preoxygenation has not been optimized: delayed-sequence intubation.

Delayed-sequence intubation consists of the administration of specific sedative agents that do not blunt spontaneous ventilations or airway reflexes, followed by a period of preoxygenation before the administration of a paralytic agent.[14] It is akin to procedural sedation, the procedure in this case being effective preoxygenation. After the completion of this procedure, the patient can be paralyzed and intubated.

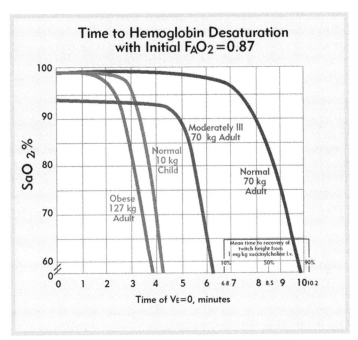

Time to Hemoglobin Desaturation with Initial $F_AO_2 = 0.87$

(Graph: y-axis "SaO$_2$ %" from 0 to 100; x-axis "Time of V$_E$=0, minutes" from 0 to 10. Curves labeled: Moderately Ill 70 kg Adult; Normal 10 kg Child; Normal 70 kg Adult; Obese 127 kg Adult. Inset: Mean time to recovery of twitch height from 1 mg/kg succinylcholine I.v. with 10%, 50%, 90% markers.)

Fig. 2. Time to desaturation. Preoxygenation prolongs the period between paralysis and oxygen desaturation in all patients, but to varying degrees depending on patient attributes. This diagram shows the time to desaturation for several different clinical conditions. F_AO_2, alveolar oxygen fraction; IV, intravenous; V_E, volume of expired gas; Sao$_2$, arterial oxygen saturation. (*From* Benumof JL, Dagg R, Benumof R. Critical hemoglobin desaturation will occur before return to an unparalyzed state following 1 mg/kg intravenous succinylcholine. Anesthesiology 1997;87:979, Lippincott Williams & Wilkins; with permission.)

The ideal agents to use are either ketamine, a dissociative agent, or dexmedetomidine, an α-2 agonist,[15] by slow intravenous push. Slow administration of both of these medications is unlikely to cause blunting of the patient's respiratory drive and airway reflexes, and both provide a dissociative/sedated state.[16,17] This allows proper preoxygenation of the patient with the application of a noninvasive mask connected to a ventilator with CPAP/BiPAP settings. After optimizing oxygenation (O$_2$ saturation >95%), a paralytic agent is administered and the patient can then be intubated.

Apneic oxygenation is also a key component in proper preoxygenation. It involves maintaining a patent upper airway passage (jaw thrust, placement of nasopharyngeal/oropharyngeal airway) for unobstructed oxygen flow from the pharynx through the glottis during the apneic period following induction. This step is crucial to maintaining oxygenation during the apneic period. Studies have shown that, during apnea, patients can maintain oxygen saturations of more than 98% for 18 to 55 minutes, which is thought to be caused by the capacity of oxygen to passively diffuse from the pharynx down its concentration gradient.[14,18]

Furthermore, high-flow oxygen (15 L/min) through a nasal cannula, in addition to 15 L/min by face mask, greatly improves the inspired forced inspiratory oxygen (Fio$_2$), eliminating the buildup of exhaled gas in the nasopharynx. Flushing the nasopharynx makes preoxygenation more effective. The nasal cannula is left on (and running) during mask ventilation (induction) and then during apnea while intubating through the mouth.

This maneuver decreases the likelihood of significant oxygen desaturation by the ability of the alveoli to entrain and absorb oxygen effectively from the upper airway, even during apnea following paralysis. There is also a theoretic potential to use this method to more rapidly reoxygenate a patient following desaturation during the intubation.[19]

Position During Intubation

If the patient does not have a potential cervical spine injury, the physician should try to achieve the ideal sniff position (which allows for optimal visualization of the glottic opening). This position is achieved by elevating the patient's head and extending the atlantooccipital joint. However, recent studies have questioned this maneuver, showing that simple head extension alone (without neck flexion) was as effective as the sniffing position in facilitating ETI.[20]

Placing the patient in a reverse Trendelenburg position (head elevated laryngoscopy position [HELP **Fig. 3**]) may also optimize the view of the airway by further aligning the airway (the sternal notch is aligned with the external auditory meatus) for a more direct view, especially in the morbidly obese (see **Fig. 3**).[21]

The so-called manual in-line cervical spine stabilization maneuver is the method proposed to achieve the goal of protecting the potentially injured cervical spine from further movement. Although, in theory, it has some merit in limiting movement and subsequent further injury, numerous studies have shown the opposite to be true. Evidence is mounting that manual in-line stabilization significantly impairs direct laryngoscopy without necessarily protecting against cervical movement.[22–24] For this reason, this practice must be vigorously scrutinized and abandoned if it negatively contributes to airway management.

Preparing for emergency airway management

Medications For simplicity, the medication armamentarium to be used for the DA can be divided into 2 basic groups of medications: the sedative/induction or nonparalyzing agents and the paralyzing agents. Depending on the strategy to be used for managing the DA, medications may be chosen from both groups (RSI) or from the former group only, as explained later. Although muscle paralysis is responsible for most of the improvement in ease of intubation with classic RSI,[25,26] it has been suggested that the use of a potent nonparalyzing agent can further improve the speed and success rate of paralyzing agent–facilitated ETI.[27,28]

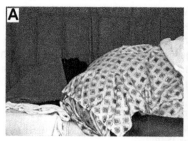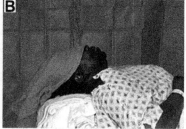

Fig. 3. Ramp position. (*A*) In the supine patient, access to the airway is obstructed. (*B*) With the patient propped on linens in the ramp position, access to the airway is improved. In this position, an imaginary horizontal line can be drawn from the external auditory meatus to the sternal notch. (*From* Wiser SH, Zane RD. The morbidly obese patient. In: Walls RM, Murphy MF, editors. Manual of emergency airway management. 3rd edition. Philadelphia: Lippincott Williams & Wilkins; 2008; with permission.)

Medications: pretreatment agents

A brief discussion is needed of the use of pharmaceutical agents labeled as pretreatment drugs. This group of medications was advocated in the past to blunt the physiologically untoward effects of direct laryngoscopy and paralysis[29] before RSI.

Lidocaine and opioids are traditionally administered to blunt the increase in intracranial pressure from the reflex sympathetic discharge and bronchospasm mitigated by direct laryngoscopy **Box 2**.[29–31]

There have been no studies of the effect of premedication with lidocaine on lowering intracranial pressure and improving outcome in patients with intracranial disorders undergoing RSI in the ED. Available studies in the operating room or the intensive care setting have shown a reduction in intracranial pressure with lidocaine pretreatment, but failed to show significant improvement in clinical outcome. A systematic review of the literature by Robinson and Clancy[31] failed to show any neuroprotective property for the use of lidocaine in patients with intracranial disorders undergoing ETI.

As a result, there is no conclusive evidence advocating the use of lidocaine to blunt the sympathetic surge in patients with intracranial disorders undergoing RSI. Lidocaine may result in an untoward lowering of mean arterial pressure, and consequently cerebral perfusion pressure, if not given slowly. Furthermore, although it does blunt cough reflexes, it may also cause bronchoconstriction. For these reasons, its use is not advocated.

Fentanyl in doses of 3 to 5 μg/kg has been found to have some beneficial effects in blunting sympathetic surge despite a lack of adequate studies proving that this has significant clinical benefit.[32] In addition, at high doses, fentanyl can precipitate the rigid chest syndrome, an acute onset of chest wall rigidity. The muscle wall rigidity is an idiosyncratic response to the opioid.

Atropine has been advocated for use in children less than 8 years of age to prevent vagal nerve–mitigated bradycardia provoked by direct laryngoscopy and the use of succinylcholine. Studies supporting its used are based on patients in the operating room who are also subjected to repeated dosing of succinylcholine, an event that is rare in the context of ED RSI. Studies showed that bradycardia related to intubation is a rare event, and the use of atropine does not confer protection against the development of bradycardia.[32]

Muscle fasciculation caused by succinylcholine[33,34] is thought to cause raised intracranial pressure and intraocular pressures. Pretreatment with a small dose of nondepolarizing neuromuscular blocking agents (NMBAs) is thought to reduce this

---

Box 2
Physiologic responses caused by laryngoscopy and intubation

- Increased mean arterial pressure
- Increased pulse
- Increase cerebral oxygen demand
- Increase myocardial oxygen demand
- Increase Intracranial pressure
- Increase intraocular pressure
- Laryngospasm
- Bronchospasm
- Dysrhythmia

incidence. Most of the evidence surrounding this practice originates from the operating theater[35] and is generally not transferable to the ED population. In addition, to achieve best results with the defasciculating agent, at least 3 minutes should elapse between the defasciculating agent administration and succinylcholine administration.[34] This time lapse is a luxury not often permitted when dealing with a DA. In addition, the use of a defasciculating dose of the nondepolarizing NMBA can cause pharyngeal muscle weakness in some patients while awake, leading to a distressing situation.[34] Furthermore, pretreatment with defasciculating agents can rarely cause premature apnea before the physician is ready to intubate. Overall, the use of defasciculating NMBA is not practical in the ED environment and has limited evidence of usefulness.

Medications: induction agents

The choice of which induction agent to use can be daunting. Although there are many options, an ideal agent does not exist and the choice needs to be individualized. The ideal induction agent for RSI should meet the following characteristics: it should have a fast onset of action; cause rapid loss of consciousness; have minimal hemodynamic effects, thereby stabilizing and even ameliorating the hemodynamic effects of intubation in patients with already compromised hemodynamic status; have a predictable onset of action; and have a duration of action that is sufficient to keep the patient sedated for the required period.[33,36,37]

Table 1 lists the most commonly used nonparalyzing agents in DA situations. The details of the pharmacodynamics and pharmacokinetics of each of these drugs is beyond the scope of this article. Instead, the clinical niche into which each drug ideally could fit is explored.

Hypotensive/normotensive patient scenario

Ketamine/etomidate/midazolam Whatever the cause of the hypotension, ketamine, etomidate, and midazolam exhibit, in descending order, the least untoward hemodynamic effects. Caution must be exercised in the use of each of these agents.

The use of ketamine has been regarded as a relative contraindication in the patient with potential head trauma. There is a theoretic increase in intracranial pressure from the increase in mean arterial pressure following ketamine infusion. However, the contrary has been shown.[36,38]

Ketamine should be used with caution in patients with coronary artery disease because of its effects on increasing myocardial oxygen demands.[39] Ketamine also has a negative inotropic effect in patients who are maximally adrenergically driven (eg, heart failure).[36,39,40] In patients with high blood pressure or tachycardia, the sympathomimetic effects of ketamine may be undesirable. Although these effects can be blunted with small doses of benzodiazepine and, perhaps, labetalol,[41] another agent should be considered for these hypertensive or tachycardic patients.

Concerns regarding etomidate-induced adrenocortical suppression has led to avoiding its use in the septic patient. Although current evidence suggests that etomidate suppresses adrenal function, it does so transiently, without having a significant effect on mortality. However, no studies to date have been powered to detect a difference in hospital, ventilator duration, ICU length of stay, or mortality.[42,43]

Midazolam is one of the most frequently used induction agents in the patient with a DA. However, the most common mistake observed is underdosing.[44] Physicians need to become familiar with the higher recommended doses for induction (at least in the range of 0.1–0.4 mg/kg) as well as its prolonged onset of action ($\sim$ 10 minutes), making it not suitable for RSI.[36]

Table 1
RSI induction agents

Dose (mg/kg)	Caution	Benefits	Class	Drug Name
0.3	None Known to suppress adrenal cortisol production	Excellent sedation with little hypotension	Imidazole derivative	Etomidate
1–2	Controversial regarding its use in pts with increased intracranial pressure and increased or high-normal blood pressure	Stimulates catecholamine release	Phencyclidine derivative, dissociative anesthetic	Ketamine
0.2–0.3	Dose-related myocardial depression can result in hypotension	Potent dose-related amnesic properties	Benzodiazepines	Midazolam
3	Dose-related hypotension	Bronchodilation	Alkylphenol derivative	Propofol
3–5	Potent venodilator and myocardial depressant; can cause hypotension Relatively contraindicated in reactive airway disease because of histamine release Acute intermittent and variegate porphyrias	Cerebroprotective and anticonvulsive properties	Ultra–short-acting barbiturate	Thiopental sodium

Data from Walls RM, Murphy MF. The difficult airway in adults. In: UpToDate, Basow, DS (Ed), UpToDate, Waltham, MA 2011.

Hypertensive patient scenario

Propofol/etomidate/midazolam/thiopental Propofol is an excellent induction agent in this patient population. It has fast onset (15–45 seconds), short duration of action (5–10 minutes), and provides the most favorable intubating conditions, compared with other induction agents,[39] by relaxing pharyngeal and laryngeal muscles. Its major side effect is its myocardial suppressive effect. It reduces stroke volume, cardiac output, and systemic vascular resistance.

Like propofol, thiopental can lower blood pressure through its vasodilatory effect.[33] It was the first induction agent used for RSI in the operating room; however, it became less favored because of its serious hemodynamic effects with repeated dosing, because it tends to redistribute and accumulate. When comparing propofol with thiopental, studies have shown that propofol produces more favorable intubating conditions compared with thiopental because of its muscle-relaxing effects.[33] Both agents are excellent in cases of suspected raised intracranial pressure, because they are known to suppress neuronal/oxygen-requiring metabolic activity in the brain.[33]

Awake intubation scenario

Midazolam/dexmedetomidine/ketamine The indications for awake intubation include the cannot-oxygenate/cannot-ventilate scenario. Awake intubation involves using local anesthetics in the upper airway with or without a small dose of a sedating agent, followed by intubation aided by fiberoptic visualization. By the nature of their pharmacocharacteristics, these drugs allow such an intervention.

Classic relative indications for awake intubation include, but are not limited to[45] (1) airway anomalies, acute severe upper airway disease; (2) cervical spine injury; (3) facial trauma; and (4) significant hemodynamic instability and fear of causing irreversible hemodynamic compromise with sedation/paralysis caused by loss of sympathetic tone.

In summary, the choice of induction agent for RSI/awake intubation depends on the patient's general condition, the indication for RSI/awake intubation, and the physicians comfort with differently available induction agents.

Medications: paralyzing agents

NMBA have long been used in anesthesia to optimize intubating conditions and reduce the risk of pharyngeal and vocal cord damage.[39] NMBA are fundamental in RSI to facilitate intubation and reduce the risk of gastric aspiration. They enhance rapid ETT placement following induction by the sedative agents and act synergistically with these agents.[33,46,47] The ideal NMBA should have a rapid onset of action (ideally within 60 seconds), possess a wide therapeutic range, have no significant hemodynamic effects, have a short duration of action ensuring rapid return to spontaneous breathing, and have no serious side effects.[48]

Table 2
The 2 most common NMBAs

Drug	Dose (mg/kg)	Onset of Action (min)	Duration of Action (min)	Benefits	Caution
Succinylcholine	0.3–2 IV push (average dose 1.5)	1	4–6	Depolarizing NMB; drug of choice for emergency pediatric intubation; rapid onset (<60 s) and brief duration of action; enhances nondepolarizing NMB effects	Increased serum potassium, muscle fasciculation; malignant hyperthermia; cardiac arrest in children with muscular dystrophy; dysrhythmia with multiple doses
Rocuronium	0.6–1 IV push	<1	30–60	Nondepolarizing NMBA; minimal effect on hemodynamics; low incidence of histamine release (0.8%)	Duration prolonged with hepatic impairment

Abbreviations: IV, intravenous; NMB, neuromuscular blocking.

The 2 most commonly used NMBA for ED RSI are the depolarizing NMBA succinylcholine and the nondepolarizing NMBA rocuronium (**Table 2**). Although other nondepolarizing NMBA exist, the favorable pharmacocharacteristics of rocuronium for acute airway intervention including reversibility with sugammadex[49] give it an advantage compared with the others (eg, pancuronium, vecuronium, rocuronium, rapacuronium).[48]

Succinylcholine (0.3–2 mg/kg intravenous push)

Aside from suspected contraindications, this is the paralyzing agent of choice for most DAs. The rapid onset of paralysis (1 minute) and the brief duration of action (4–6 minutes) make it the ideal paralytic agent. Furthermore, the ability to administer it intramuscularly is an added benefit if rapid intravascular access is not available. The physician should always err on the side of overdosing rather than underdosing. The insignificant increase in duration of paralysis is worth the risk to avoid incomplete muscle relaxation during intubation. If repeat dosing is needed, consider pretreatment with atropine to prevent significant bradycardia.

Rocuronium (0.6–1 mg/kg intravenous push)

The rapid onset of action (<1 minute) makes rocuronium the ideal substitute for succinylcholine in conditions when use of the latter is contraindicated.[39,48] However, its duration of action is longer than that of succinylcholine (30–60 minutes).

Preparing for emergency airway management: techniques/devices

The ultimate goal in managing the DA is to secure the airway with an ETT by any means possible. As in the case of selecting the proper pharmaceutical agent, a best technique does not exist. The physician must weigh the complexities of interplay between the patient's presentation, physiologic reserve, and the resources available to best individualize and optimize the most appropriate airway management strategy. Emphasis must be on identifying the DA and having a plan with a double setup ready for the cannot-intubate/cannot-ventilate scenario. The use of any supportive device does not increase one's ability; only one's options.

An outline of nonsurgical and surgical techniques is presented later along with the most appropriate clinical scenario in which to perform them. A detailed description of each technique/device is beyond the scope of this article.

Nonsurgical techniques/devices

Direct laryngoscopy Since Alfred Kirstein's attempt at the first direct laryngoscopy in 1895, this instrument has arguably been the most popular device for managing the DA. However, many novel devices have been developed recently, which has pushed this instrument's importance out of the mainstream. Furthermore, newer versions of the classic Macintosh laryngoscope have been recently shown to perform better in DA scenarios (**Fig. 4**).[50]

Tracheal intubation involves 3 distinct challenges: laryngeal sighting, delivering the tube to the glottic opening, and advancing the tube beyond the target and into the trachea.[51] With direct laryngoscopy, sighting of the larynx occurs through a direct line of sight by mechanically controlling the tongue and the epiglottis.

The Cormack-Lehane classification is broadly used to describe laryngeal view during direct laryngoscopy (**Fig. 5**).

The Sellick maneuver/cricoid pressure is a method by which regurgitation/aspiration is supposedly prevented during endotracheal intubation. It involves applying pressure on the cricoid cartilage to compress the esophagus between the cricoid cartilage anteriorly and the cervical spine posteriorly.[39] Controversy exists whether this maneuver is useful. There is evidence to suggest that cricoid pressure not only

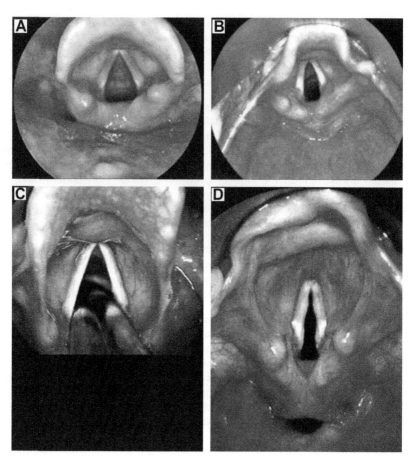

Fig. 4. Larynx appearance with videolaryngoscope. (*A*) Preintubation view of an adult airway. (*B*) Preintubation view of a pediatric airway. (*C*) ETT passing between the vocal cords. (*D*) The larynx and hypopharynx (note the horizontally oriented space below the laryngeal inlet, which is the esophagus). (*From* Nagdev A. Airway, breathing, circulation: normal airway. In: Greenberg MI, Hendrickson RG, Silverberg M, et al. editors. Greenberg's text-atlas of emergency medicine. Philadelphia: Lippincott Williams & Wilkins; 2005; with permission.)

increases the risk of gastric aspiration by reducing lower esophageal sphincter tone but it may also induce retching and vomiting if applied prematurely, and affects laryngeal visualization, thereby increasing the risk of failed intubation.[33,39]

However, external laryngeal manipulation has been shown to improve Cormack-Lehane grading. There are many different ways to accomplish this. The laryngeal lift has been used by anesthesiologists to enhance visualization of the cords.[52] This is done by applying a gentle displacement of the cricoid cartilage approximately 0.5 cm dorsally and 2.5 cm cephalad in a fluid lifting motion until mild resistance is met, similar to cricoid pressure. Another method involves the displacement of the larynx in 3 specific directions: (1) posteriorly against the cervical vertebrae, (2) as superiorly as possible, and (3) slightly laterally to the right (backward, upward to the right pressure [BURP]) *by the person intubating*. This method has been reported to improve the visualization of the larynx more easily than simple posterior pressure on the larynx.[53]

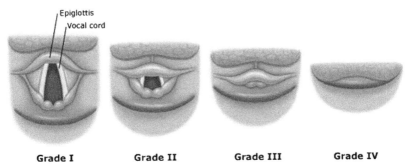

Epiglottis
Vocal cord

| Grade I | Grade II | Grade III | Grade IV |

Fig. 5. The Cormack-Lehane system for grading laryngoscopic view at intubation. Difficulty of direct laryngoscopy correlates with the best view of the glottis, as defined by the Cormack-Lehane scale. With this scale, a grade I view connotes a full view of the entire glottic aperture, grade II represents a partial glottic view, grade III represents visualization of the epiglottis only, and grade IV represents inability to visualize even the epiglottis. (*Reproduced with permission from* Walls RM, Murphy MF. The difficult airway in adults. In: UpToDate, Basow, DS (Ed), UpToDate, Waltham, MA 2011. Copyright © 2011 UpToDate, Inc.)

Bimanual laryngoscopy involves the manipulation of the larynx by the person intubating to directly view and improve the visualization of the cords while intubating. In a cadaveric study comparing bimanual laryngoscopy, the BURP technique, and cricoid pressure, bimanual laryngoscopy improved the percentage of glottic opening more than BURP or cricoid pressure.[54]

Although direct laryngoscopy is a good first choice for most cases of DA, it should be used with extreme caution in cases in which there is a potential for upper airway injury, specifically transection of the laryngotracheal region. Further injury to the airway by the blade of the laryngoscope, as well as during the passage of the ETT into a false lumen, could result in the DA rapidly progressing to an impossible airway by distortion of the already anatomically compromised airway.

Digital tactile intubation

Digital tactile intubation (DTI) is a tactile intubation technique in which intubators uses their fingers to direct an ETT into the larynx. The technique has gained limited usefulness in clinical practice. It is not easy to perform, especially if the intubator has small hands or short fingers. Because the procedure can be performed without movement of the head and neck, it was found particularly suitable in patients with trauma who might have suffered injury to the cervical spine. Added advantages are the ease of performance despite secretions or blood in the upper airway.[55]

Nasotracheal intubation

Nasotracheal intubation (NTI) has several serious drawbacks, and few advantages, compared with the other techniques that are now commonly used for emergency airway management. NTI has largely fallen out of favor in the ED because it takes longer, has a higher failure rate, has a higher complication rate, and requires smaller tube sizes than oral ETT. However, despite these inherent problems, NTI is still considered an important skill because it may be useful in certain DA situations (eg, limited mouth opening, indications for awake intubation).

Bougie-assisted endotracheal intubation

The bougie, otherwise known as an ETT introducer, remains one of the preferred devices for the management of the DA in which the vocal cords cannot be visualized.[56]

It is a 60-cm long, semirigid, narrow tube with a 35° angle 2.5 cm from the distal end, which facilitates blind insertion through the vocal cords. It is inserted blindly, the hook aimed anteriorly, with correct placement confirmed by feeling clicks as the device passes over the tracheal rings and a hold-up when entering the distal airways. The ETT is then threaded over the bougie into the trachea. The bougie may need to be rotated 90° for the ETT to pass. Extreme vigilance should be exercised with its use if there is suspicion of an injured/transected airway because the bougie may easily enter a false lumen, leading to catastrophic intubation of a false airway.[57]

Supraglottic airway devices

Supraglottic airway devices ventilate patients by delivering oxygen above the level of the vocal cords and are designed to aid in the management of the DA. The American Society of Anesthesiologists' Task Force on Management of the Difficult Airway suggests considering the use of supraglottic airway devices when intubation problems occur in patients with previously unrecognized DA, especially in a cannot-intubate/cannot-oxygenate situation.

There has been a significant evolution of these devices from the original laryngeal mask airway (LMA; **Fig. 6**), which was described as the missing link between the face-mask and the tracheal tube, to the more elaborate ones now available.

The Proseal laryngeal mask airway (PLMA) is a new LMA with a modified cuff designed to improve its seal and a drainage tube for gastric tube placement. These features are designed to improve safety of the LMA and broaden its scope, especially when used with positive pressure ventilation.[58]

Fastrach, a modification of the LMA (**Fig. 7**) is designed as a conduit for tracheal intubation in cases of poor visualization of the cords.[59] The esophageal-tracheal Combitube (ETC) **Fig. 8** is an easily inserted double-lumen/double-balloon supraglottic airway device that allows for ventilation independently of its position either in the esophagus or the trachea. The major indication of the ETC is a backup device for airway management. It is an excellent option for rescue ventilation in immediate life-threatening cannot-ventilate/cannot-intubate situations. The advantages of the Combitube include rapid airway control without the need for neck or head movement, minimized risk for aspiration, firm fixation of the device after inflation of the oropharyngeal balloon, and that it works equally well in either the tracheal or esophageal position.[60]

The unique quality of the Elisha device consists of its ability to combine 3 functions in a single device: ventilation, intubation (blind and/or fiberoptic-aided) without interruption of ventilation, and gastric tube insertion.[61]

Supraglottic devices

Lighted stylets Lighted stylets are mainly used in cases in which visualization of the vocal cords is difficult, and is a transillumination technique for blind orotracheal or

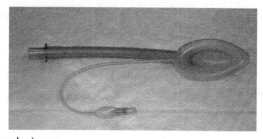

Fig. 6. Laryngeal mask airway.

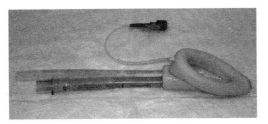

Fig. 7. Intubating laryngeal mask airway.

nasotracheal intubation.[62,63] The light at the tip of the stylet is positioned within 0.5 cm of the end of the ETT. The tube is guided by observing the anterior neck for transillumination through the soft tissue. A bright red glow in the midline at the level of the larynx indicates proper guidance of the tube. The tip of the tube is in the pyriform sinus if the bright red glow is off the midline. A dull diffuse glow represents passage of the tube into the esophagus. This technique is limited by overhead lighting and/or significant adiposity of the anterior neck, both of which create difficulty seeing the stylet light. In addition, because it is a blind technique, it is not recommended in patients with suspected anatomic abnormalities of the upper airway.

Fiberoptic-guided intubation/video-assisted devices

These devices aid in the visualization of the airway and thus are ideal for the DA with anatomic abnormalities. A video laryngoscope collects electronically processed images with a camera attached at its tip. Often, the success of these devices is unrelated to the traditional predictors of DA. Besides potentially less trauma to the airway and cervical spine, patients are also able to tolerate awake assessment of the airway, thereby increasing the safety margin in patients with limited respiratory reserve.

The flexibility of this device also makes it possible to perform tracheal intubation on patients in nonstandard positions if standing behind the head of the supine patient is not an option.[64]

An airway with potential blood/secretions/vomitus makes the use of these devices more difficult. Copious suctioning is recommended before undertaking this technique, with a low threshold for abandoning the attempt and using other nonfiberoptic aids.

Surgical techniques

This article discusses the most common surgical techniques. Formal tracheotomy (a technique that, arguably, is not favorable in the urgent management of the DA) is not discussed.

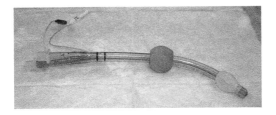

Fig. 8. ETC.

Translaryngeal-guided retrograde intubation

Although retrograde endotracheal intubation (REI) continues to be cited by the American Society of Anesthesiology as an alternative strategy for dealing with the DA,[65,66] there are no data available in the literature regarding indications for REI in the ED, or complications and outcomes of its use in the ED setting. The main drawback with this technique is the time it takes to accomplish the procedure.[67]

Percutaneous transtracheal jet ventilation

Percutaneous transtracheal jet ventilation is rarely, if ever, done in adults. It does not protect the airway and is grossly inferior to cricothyrotomy in terms of both airway protection and gas exchange. However, it is the surgical airway technique of choice for children less than 12 years of age. Indications are also the cannot-ventilate/cannot-intubate scenario.[68]

Cricothyroidotomy

"The hardest part of doing a 'cryc' is picking up the knife"— Peter Rosen.

Cricothyrotomy is the establishment of a surgical opening in the airway through the cricothyroid membrane and placement of a cuffed tracheostomy tube or ETT.

There may be little advantage to using a cricothyrotome rather than a formal, surgical cricothyrotomy set. Time of performance of the procedure, complication rates, degree of difficulty, and success rates are all comparable between the 2 methods.[69,70] Cricothyrotomy is nearly always performed as a last resort when orotracheal and nasotracheal intubation are impossible or contraindicated. Cricothyrotomy is easier and quicker to perform than tracheotomy, does not require manipulation of the cervical spine, and is associated with fewer complications. However, although cricothyrotomy may be lifesaving in extreme circumstances, this technique is only intended to be a temporizing measure until a definitive airway can be established.

Cricothyrotomy should never be started with the patient already hypoxic or in arrest; the outcome is usually unfavorable and time to ventilation is longer than with a rescue device, regardless of whether percutaneous methods are used. The only absolute contraindication is the age of the patient being younger than 10 years. There are a few relative contraindications with which the reader should be familiar: airway obstruction sufficiently distal to the cricoid membrane that a cricothyrotomy would not provide a secure airway with which to ventilate the patient; presence of a SHORT neck, which includes surgery (history or prior neck surgery), hematoma, obesity, radiation (evidence of radiation therapy), or trauma/burns, making it difficult to locate the patient's anatomic landmarks or producing an increased risk of further complications; tumor, infection, or abscess at the site of incision; and lack of operator expertise.[71,72]

SUMMARY

The management of the DA is fraught with permutations of preparatory techniques, medication armamentarium, and airway control instrumentation/techniques. The physician's choice of combination needs to be tailored to the clinical scenario encountered. The task is daunting, hence the onus on the acute care clinician to prepare theoretically and practically ahead of time.

REFERENCES

1. Christian S, Manji M. Indications for endotracheal intubation and ventilation. Trauma 2004;6(4):249–54.

2. Burkle CM, Walsh MT, Harrison BA, et al. Airway management after failure to intubate by direct laryngoscopy: outcomes in a large teaching hospital. Can J Anaesth 2005;52(6):634–40.

3. Wong E, Ng YY. The difficult airway in the emergency department. Int J Emerg Med 2008;1(2):107–11.

4. Sagarin MJ, Barton ED, Chng YM, et al. Airway management by US and Canadian emergency medicine residents: a multicenter analysis of more than 6,000 endotracheal intubation attempts. Ann Emerg Med 2005;46(4):328–36.

5. Cook TM, Woodall N, Frerk C. 4th National Audit Project of The Royal College of Anaesthetists and the difficult airway society. London: The Royal College of Anaesthetists; 2011. ISBN 978-1-900936-03-3.

6. McCafferty MH, Polk HC Jr. Patient safety and quality in surgery. Surg Clin North Am 2007;87(4):867–81, vii.

7. Janssens M, Hartstein G. Management of difficult intubation. Eur J Anaesthesiol 2001;18(1):3–12.

8. Mort TC. Preoxygenation in critically ill patients requiring emergency tracheal intubation. Crit Care Med 2005;33(11):2672–5.

9. Mort TC, Waberski BH, Clive J. Extending the preoxygenation period from 4 to 8 mins in critically ill patients undergoing emergency intubation. Crit Care Med 2009;37(1):68–71.

10. Reber A, Engberg G, Wegenius G, et al. Lung aeration. The effect of preoxygenation and hyperoxygenation during total intravenous anaesthesia. Anaesthesia 1996;51(8):733–7.

11. Reynolds SF, Heffner J. Airway management of the critically ill patient: rapid-sequence intubation. Chest 2005;127(4):1397–412.

12. Altermatt FR, Munoz HR, Delfino AE, et al. Pre-oxygenation in the obese patient: effects of position on tolerance to apnoea. Br J Anaesth 2005;95(5): 706–9.

13. El-Khatib MF, Kanazi G, Baraka AS. Noninvasive bilevel positive airway pressure for preoxygenation of the critically ill morbidly obese patient. Can J Anaesth 2007; 54(9):744–7.

14. Weingart SD. Preoxygenation, reoxygenation, and delayed sequence intubation in the emergency department. J Emerg Med 2011;40(6):661–7.

15. Riker RR, Shehabi Y, Bokesch PM, et al. Dexmedetomidine vs midazolam for sedation of critically ill patients: a randomized trial. JAMA 2009;301(5): 489–99.

16. Carollo DS, Nossaman BD, Ramadhyani U. Dexmedetomidine: a review of clinical applications. Curr Opin Anaesthesiol 2008;21(4):457–61.

17. Abdelmalak B, Makary L, Hoban J, et al. Dexmedetomidine as sole sedative for awake intubation in management of the critical airway. J Clin Anesth 2007;19(5): 370–3.

18. Baraka A, Salem MR, Joseph NJ. Critical hemoglobin desaturation can be delayed by apneic diffusion oxygenation. Anesthesiology 1999;90(1):332–3.

19. Ramachandran SK, Cosnowski A, Shanks A, et al. Apneic oxygenation during prolonged laryngoscopy in obese patients: a randomized, controlled trial of nasal oxygen administration. J Clin Anesth 2010;22(3):164–8.

20. Adnet F, Baillard C, Borron SW, et al. Randomized study comparing the "sniffing position" with simple head extension for laryngoscopic view in elective surgery patients. Anesthesiology 2001;95(4):836–41.

21. Zvara DA, Calicott RW, Whelan DM. Positioning for intubation in morbidly obese patients. Anesth Analg 2006;102(5):1592.

22. Santoni BG, Hindman BJ, Puttlitz CM, et al. Manual in-line stabilization increases pressures applied by the laryngoscope blade during direct laryngoscopy and orotracheal intubation. Anesthesiology 2009;110(1):24–31.

23. Thiboutot F, Nicole PC, Trepanier CA, et al. Effect of manual in-line stabilization of the cervical spine in adults on the rate of difficult orotracheal intubation by direct laryngoscopy: a randomized controlled trial. Can J Anaesth 2009;56(6): 412–8.

24. Turner CR, Block J, Shanks A, et al. Motion of a cadaver model of cervical injury during endotracheal intubation with a Bullard laryngoscope or a Macintosh blade with and without in-line stabilization. J Trauma 2009;67(1):61–6.

25. Dronen SC, Merigian KS, Hedges JR, et al. A comparison of blind nasotracheal and succinylcholine-assisted intubation in the poisoned patient. Ann Emerg Med 1987;16(6):650–2.

26. Adnet F, Minadeo JP, Finot MA, et al. A survey of sedation protocols used for emergency endotracheal intubation in poisoned patients in the French prehospital medical system. Eur J Emerg Med 1998;5(4):415–9.

27. Sparr HJ, Leo C, Ladner E, et al. Influence of anaesthesia and muscle relaxation on intubating conditions and sympathoadrenal response to tracheal intubation. Acta Anaesthesiol Scand 1997;41(10):1300–7.

28. McIndewar IC, Marshall RJ. Interactions between the neuromuscular blocking drug Org NC 45 and some anaesthetic, analgesic and antimicrobial agents. Br J Anaesth 1981;53(8):785–92.

29. Vaillancourt C, Kapur AK. Opposition to the use of lidocaine in rapid sequence intubation. Ann Emerg Med 2007;49(1):86–7.

30. Salhi B, Stettner E. In defense of the use of lidocaine in rapid sequence intubation. Ann Emerg Med 2007;49(1):84–6.

31. Robinson N, Clancy M. In patients with head injury undergoing rapid sequence intubation, does pretreatment with intravenous lignocaine/lidocaine lead to an improved neurological outcome? A review of the literature. Emerg Med J 2001; 18(6):453–7.

32. Schofer JM. Premedication during rapid sequence intubation: a necessity or waste of valuable time? Cal J Emerg Med 2006;7(4):75–9.

33. El-Orbany M, Connolly LA. Rapid sequence induction and intubation: current controversy. Anesth Analg 2010;110(5):1318–25.

34. Minton MD, Grosslight K, Stirt JA, et al. Increases in intracranial pressure from succinylcholine: prevention by prior nondepolarizing blockade. Anesthesiology 1986;65(2):165–9.

35. Stirt JA, Grosslight KR, Bedford RF, et al. "Defasciculation" with metocurine prevents succinylcholine-induced increases in intracranial pressure. Anesthesiology 1987;67(1):50–3.

36. Morris C, Perris A, Klein J, et al. Anaesthesia in haemodynamically compromised emergency patients: does ketamine represent the best choice of induction agent? Anaesthesia 2009;64(5):532–9.

37. Wilbur K, Zed PJ. Is propofol an optimal agent for procedural sedation and rapid sequence intubation in the emergency department? CJEM 2001;3(4): 302–10.

38. Albanese J, Arnaud S, Rey M, et al. Ketamine decreases intracranial pressure and electroencephalographic activity in traumatic brain injury patients during propofol sedation. Anesthesiology 1997;87(6):1328–34.

39. Gudzenko V, Bittner EA, Schmidt UH. Emergency airway management. Respir Care 2010;55(8):1026–35.

40. Pagel PS, Kampine JP, Schmeling WT, et al. Ketamine depresses myocardial contractility as evaluated by the preload recruitable stroke work relationship in chronically instrumented dogs with autonomic nervous system blockade. Anesthesiology 1992;76(4):564–72.

41. Aroni F, Iacovidou N, Dontas I, et al. Pharmacological aspects and potential new clinical applications of ketamine: reevaluation of an old drug. J Clin Pharmacol 2009;49(8):957–64.

42. Hohl CM, Kelly-Smith CH, Yeung TC, et al. The effect of a bolus dose of etomidate on cortisol levels, mortality, and health services utilization: a systematic review. Ann Emerg Med 2010;56(2):105–13.e105.

43. Kulstad EB, Kalimullah EA, Tekwani KL, et al. Etomidate as an induction agent in septic patients: red flags or false alarms? West J Emerg Med 2010;11(2): 161–72.

44. Sagarin MJ, Barton ED, Sakles JC, et al. Underdosing of midazolam in emergency endotracheal intubation. Acad Emerg Med 2003;10(4):329–38.

45. Benumof J. Airway management: principles and practice. St Louis (MO): Mosby; 1996.

46. Sivilotti ML, Filbin MR, Murray HE, et al. Does the sedative agent facilitate emergency rapid sequence intubation? Acad Emerg Med 2003;10(6):612–20.

47. Walls RM, Brown CA 3rd, Bair AE, et al. Emergency airway management: a multi-center report of 8937 emergency department intubations. J Emerg Med 2011; 41(4):347–54.

48. Mallon WK, Keim SM, Shoenberger JM, et al. Rocuronium vs. succinylcholine in the emergency department: a critical appraisal. J Emerg Med 2009;37(2): 183–8.

49. de Boer HD, Driessen JJ, Marcus MA, et al. Reversal of rocuronium-induced (1.2 mg/kg) profound neuromuscular block by sugammadex: a multicenter, dose-finding and safety study. Anesthesiology 2007;107(2):239–44.

50. Ong JR, Chong FC, Chen CC, et al. Comparing the performance of traditional direct laryngoscope with three indirect laryngoscopes: a prospective manikin study in normal and difficult airway scenarios. Emerg Med Australas 2011; 23(5):606–14.

51. Levitan RM, Heitz JW, Sweeney M, et al. The complexities of tracheal intubation with direct laryngoscopy and alternative intubation devices. Ann Emerg Med 2011;57(3):240–7.

52. Krantz MA, Poulos JG, Chaouki K, et al. The laryngeal lift: a method to facilitate endotracheal intubation. J Clin Anesth 1993;5(4):297–301.

53. Takahata O, Kubota M, Mamiya K, et al. The efficacy of the "BURP" maneuver during a difficult laryngoscopy. Anesth Analg 1997;84(2):419–21.

54. Levitan RM, Kinkle WC, Levin WJ, et al. Laryngeal view during laryngoscopy: a randomized trial comparing cricoid pressure, backward-upward-rightward pressure, and bimanual laryngoscopy. Ann Emerg Med 2006;47(6):548–55.

55. Stewart RD. Tactile orotracheal intubation. Ann Emerg Med 1984;13(3):175–8.

56. Marco CA, Marco AP. Airway adjuncts. Emerg Med Clin North Am 2008;26(4): 1015–27, x.

57. Lavery GG, McCloskey BV. The difficult airway in adult critical care. Crit Care Med 2008;36(7):2163–73.

58. Brimacombe J, Keller C, Brimacombe L. A comparison of the laryngeal mask airway ProSeal and the laryngeal tube airway in paralyzed anesthetized adult patients undergoing pressure-controlled ventilation. Anesth Analg 2002;95(3): 770–6.

59. Brimacombe J, Keller C. The ProSeal laryngeal mask airway: a randomized, crossover study with the standard laryngeal mask airway in paralyzed, anesthetized patients. Anesthesiology 2000;93(1):104–9.
60. Gaitini LA, Vaida SJ, Agro F. The esophageal-tracheal Combitube. Anesthesiol Clin North America 2002;20(4):893–906.
61. Vaida S. Airway management - supraglottic airway devices. 2004. Available at: http://www.atitimisoara.ro/_files/documents/files/2004/Airway%20management-supraglottic%20airway%20devices.pdf. Accessed December 9, 2011.
62. Manoach S, Paladino L. Manual in-line stabilization for acute airway management of suspected cervical spine injury: historical review and current questions. Ann Emerg Med 2007;50(3):236–45.
63. Birnbaumer DM, Pollack CV Jr. Troubleshooting and managing the difficult airway. Semin Respir Crit Care Med 2002;23(1):3–9.
64. Thong SY, Lim Y. Video and optic laryngoscopy assisted tracheal intubation–the new era. Anaesth Intensive Care 2009;37(2):219–33.
65. Practice guidelines for management of the difficult airway: an updated report by the American Society of Anesthesiologists Task Force on Management of the Difficult Airway. Anesthesiology 2003;98(5):1269–77.
66. Parmet JL, Metz S, Schwartz AJ. "Anesthesiology issues in general surgery: retrograde endotracheal intubation: an underutilized tool for management of the difficult airway". Contemp Surg 1996;49(5):300–6.
67. Gill M, Madden MJ, Green SM. Retrograde endotracheal intubation: an investigation of indications, complications, and patient outcomes. Am J Emerg Med 2005; 23(2):123–6.
68. Yealy DM, Stewart RD, Kaplan RM. Myths and pitfalls in emergency translaryngeal ventilation: correcting misimpressions. Ann Emerg Med 1988;17(7):690–2.
69. Spaite DW, Joseph M. Prehospital cricothyrotomy: an investigation of indications, technique, complications, and patient outcome. Ann Emerg Med 1990;19(3): 279–85.
70. Eisenburger P, Laczika K, List M, et al. Comparison of conventional surgical versus Seldinger technique emergency cricothyrotomy performed by inexperienced clinicians. Anesthesiology 2000;92(3):687–90.
71. American College of Surgeons. Advanced trauma life support for doctors. 7th edition. Chicago: American College of Surgeons; 2004.
72. Walls RM, Murphy MF, Luten RC, et al. Manual of emergency airway management, vol. 70. 2nd edition. Philadelphia: Lippincott Williams & Wilkins; 2004.

Invasive and Noninvasive Ventilation in the Emergency Department

Patrick M. Archambault, MD, MSc, FRCPC[a,b,c,d,*],
Maude St-Onge, MD, MSc, FRCPC[e,f]

KEYWORDS

- Invasive mechanical ventilation • Noninvasive ventilation
- Positive pressure ventilation
- Intermittent positive pressure ventilation
- Respiratory insufficiency • Closed-loop systems
- Dual-control modes

The Roman physician Galen (AD 129–217) may have been the first to describe mechanical ventilation using a bellows to inflate the lungs of a deceased animal.[1] However, it was not until the polio epidemic in the 1950s that mechanical ventilation was widely used. During this period, ventilation was performed by enclosing the thorax in an iron box, called the iron lung. It was designed to apply negative pressure that was transmitted to the intrapleural space, causing room air to enter through the mouth. However, increasing deaths from bulbar poliomyelitis led Engström[2] to

This work did not receive any funding support.
The authors have nothing to disclose.
[a] Department of Family Medicine and Emergency Medicine, Université Laval, 1050 Avenue de la Médecine, Quebec City, Quebec, G1V 0A6, Canada
[b] Division of Critical Care, Department of Anesthesiology, Université Laval, 1050 Avenue de la Médecine, Quebec City, Quebec, G1V 0A6, Canada
[c] Department of Emergency Medicine, Centre de santé et services sociaux Alphonse-Desjardins (CHAU de Lévis), 143 Rue Wolfe, Lévis, Quebec, G6V 3Z1, Canada
[d] Department of Anesthesiology, Centre de santé et services sociaux Alphonse-Desjardins (CHAU de Lévis), 143 Rue Wolfe, Lévis, Quebec, G6V 3Z1, Canada
[e] Department of Emergency Medicine, Centre hospitalier universitaire de Quebec, 2705, Boulevard Laurier, Quebec City, Quebec, G1V 4G2, Canada
[f] Adult Critical Care Medicine Residency Program, University of Toronto, Sunnybrook Health Sciences Center, 2075 Bayview Avenue, Room D134, Toronto, Ontario, M4N 3M5, Canada
* Corresponding author. CSSS Alphonse-Desjardins (CHAU de Lévis), 143 Rue Wolfe, Lévis, Quebec, G6V 3Z1, Canada.
E-mail address: patrick.m.archambault@gmail.com

Emerg Med Clin N Am 30 (2012) 421–449
doi:10.1016/j.emc.2011.10.008
0733-8627/12/$ – see front matter © 2012 Elsevier Inc. All rights reserved.

search for a better way to ventilate these patients. This need led to the invention of the modern positive pressure ventilator. These advances led to a reduction in mortality from bulbar polio from 90% to 20%, and the era of invasive positive pressure ventilation began.[3] Since this era, technological advances and computers have changed the way ventilators operate.[4] Currently, mechanical ventilation is used in many settings, including the Emergency Department (ED), where invasive and noninvasive ventilation (NIV) are essential tools for the treatment of critically ill patients. This article reviews the use of these modalities in the ED. Specifically, this review presents the goals of invasive and noninvasive positive pressure ventilation, the frequent ventilatory modes, and the physiologic principles underlying their use. Different case scenarios help apply these concepts in practice. This article will guide emergency physicians to resolve frequent problems and to prevent complications related to mechanical ventilation.

GOALS OF MECHANICAL VENTILATION AND GAS EXCHANGE PHYSIOLOGY
Goals of Mechanical Ventilation

The main goal of mechanical ventilation is to reduce the work of breathing (WOB) and reverse life-threatening hypoxemia and hypercarbia.[5] It can also support oxygenation and ventilation when patients fail to maintain or protect their airways (eg, coma, sedation, paralysis, poisoning).[6] Thus, it is useful to think of respiration as 2 separate processes: ventilation (alveolar ventilation is indirectly proportional to partial pressure of CO_2 in arterial blood [$PaCO_2$]) and oxygenation (assessed by partial pressure of O_2 in arterial blood [Pao_2] and by pulse oximeter [Spo_2]).

Gas Exchange Physiology

When trying to treat hypercarbia, an excess of CO_2 in the blood stream, it is useful to think of its determinants.[7] Hypercarbia is caused by increased CO_2 production (eg, sepsis, metabolic acidosis), hypoventilation (eg, narcotic overdose with low tidal volume [V_T] or low respiratory frequency) or high dead space (eg, pulmonary embolism). Dead space (V_D) is the volume of air that does not participate in CO_2 exchange.

Mechanical ventilation is helpful for treating hypoventilation by increasing respiratory frequency and V_T. However, mechanical ventilation can increase dead space with alveolar overdistention and excessive V_T or positive end-expiratory pressure (PEEP). Positive pressure ventilation can also increase dead space in the case of a pulmonary embolism or any low-output circulatory failure (eg, hemorrhagic shock). Caution is required when using positive pressure ventilation in these situations and appropriate treatment of the underlying cause is essential.

When trying to improve oxygenation, it is useful to think of the 6 different causes of hypoxemia to understand how mechanical ventilation can help: (1) low fractional inspired oxygen (Fio_2); (2) hypoventilation; (3) impaired diffusion; (4) ventilation-perfusion (V/Q) mismatching; (5) shunt; and (6) desaturation of pulmonary arterial (mixed venous) blood. Mechanical ventilation can help by solving hypoventilation and by increasing Fio_2 and PEEP. Increased Fio_2 can solve low Fio_2, impaired diffusion, V/Q mismatching, and desaturation of pulmonary arterial blood. Increasing PEEP can help reduce shunting by opening alveoli that are flooded with fluid or are atelectatic (PEEP is discussed further later). Increasing PEEP can also help reduce Fio_2 to nontoxic levels (<50%).[8]

POSITIVE PRESSURE VENTILATION

Positive pressure ventilation is divided into invasive mechanical ventilation and NIV.

Invasive Mechanical Ventilation

Ventilator variables

To understand the many different modes of ventilation, it is important to understand the 3 key ventilator phase variables[9] that determine (1) when a breath is delivered (trigger), (2) what limits gas delivery (limit), and (3) what ends gas delivery (cycle). **Table 1** describes each mode of ventilation with its respective trigger, limit, and cycle.

The trigger variable determines breath initiation and is set by the mode on the ventilator. The patient can initiate the breath (patient triggered) or the ventilator can deliver a breath after an elapsed amount of time (time triggered) (**Fig. 1**).

Assisted breaths in assist control (A/C) are patient triggered. Other patient-triggered modes include spontaneous breaths in synchronized intermittent mandatory ventilation (SIMV) and pressure-support ventilation (PSV). Examples of time-triggered breaths are controlled breaths in A/C or mandatory breaths in SIMV. With time triggering, the rate of breathing is controlled by the ventilator, which means the patient receives mandatory breaths at a prespecified frequency determined by the clinician. For most modes of ventilation, a preset trigger sensitivity has to be reached before a ventilator delivers flow. Pressure and flow are the most frequently used triggers. With pressure triggering, a set negative pressure must be attained for the ventilator to deliver a breath. This pressure is usually set at -2 cm H_2O. The higher (more negative) the trigger sensitivity, the harder the patient has to work to trigger a breath. With flow triggering, 2 variables must be set: the base flow rate (usually set between 5 and 20 L/min) and the flow sensitivity (usually set between a minimum of 1 L/min and one-half of the base flow). If the trigger sensitivity is set too low (too sensitive), the ventilator can autotrigger because of oscillating water in the ventilator tubing, or by hyperdynamic heartbeats, or when the patient moves.

To control the delivery of gas to the patient during the inspiratory phase, a limit variable is added. This limit variable is usually set as a volume limit (eg, A/C and mandatory breaths in SIMV), a pressure limit (eg, pressure A/C [PAC], PSV, or spontaneous breath in SIMV), a flow limit (eg, A/C or mandatory breaths in SIMV), or a time limit (eg, high-frequency oscillation ventilation [HFOV]). The limit variable does not terminate the breath. For example, a ventilator can be set for pressure ventilation with a limit of 25 cm H_2O and an inspiratory time set at 2 seconds. Such a breath is described as pressure limited and time cycled.

In the breath termination, a cycle variable is chosen (volume, flow, or time). Traditional ventilators were classified according to their cycling method. However, new ventilators have microprocessors that allow them to function in many different modes. Volume-cycled ventilation (eg, A/C, SIMV) has a predetermined V_T set for the patient that is delivered with each inspiration. The amount of pressure necessary to deliver this volume fluctuates based on the resistance and elastance of the patient and ventilator circuit. Flow-cycled ventilation (eg, PSV and spontaneous breaths in SIMV) allows the ventilator to begin the expiratory phase once the flow has decreased to a predetermined value during inspiration. The flow and volume remain unchanged, but the pressure fluctuates from breath to breath based on the resistance and elastance of the respiratory system. Time-cycled ventilation has a predetermined inspiration and expiration time set. The volume and pressure fluctuate. For example, it is used with airway pressure–release ventilation (APRV) and with HFOV (these modes are discussed later).

Inspiratory Flow Patterns

Most ventilators offer at least 3 different types of inspiratory flow patterns for volume-cycled breaths. These flow patterns include a square wave, a sinusoidal wave, and

Table 1
Advantages and disadvantages of different modes of mechanical ventilation

Ventilator Mode	Trigger	Limit	Cycle	Advantages	Disadvantages
VAC	Patient or time	Flow, volume	Time	Reduces WOB Guarantees delivery of set V_T (unless PIP limit exceeded)	Potential adverse hemodynamic effects (with auto-PEEP) May lead to inappropriate hyperventilation and excessive inspiratory pressures
PAC	Patient or time	Pressure	Time	Allows limitation of PIP	Same as VAC Potential hyperventilation or hypoventilation with changes in airway resistance or elastance
SIMV	Patient or time	Pressure (patient-triggered breaths) Flow/volume (VC breaths) Pressure (P-SIMV)	Flow (patient-triggered breaths) Volume or time for VC breaths	Less interference with normal cardiovascular function	Increased WOB compared with A/C Asynchrony Poor weaning mode
PRVC	Patient or time	Dual control: pressure-limited mode using a target V_T for feedback control	Time, flow (patient-triggered breaths)	Minimum MV at the lowest PIP possible; Maintains similar V_T with varying resistance and elastance Intelligent closed-loop ventilation that automatically transitions from controlled breathing to spontaneous when patient is ready	When patients attempt to breathe at a V_T greater than the clinician-set target V_T, the burden of inspiratory work is shifted onto the patient Absence of high-level evidence of its superiority on patient-oriented outcomes

			Trigger	Advantages	Disadvantages
ASV	Patient or time	Dual control: pressure-limited mode that uses a target MV for feedback control	Time, flow (patient-triggered breaths)	Same as PRVC. In addition, the microprocessor calculates the ideal V_T and RR to deliver minimizing WOB and targeting a lung protection strategy. Decreases workload	When patients attempt to breathe at an MV greater than the clinician-set target MV, the burden of inspiratory work is shifted onto the patient. Absence of high-level evidence of its superiority on patient-oriented outcomes
PSV	Patient	Pressure	Flow	Patient comfort. Improved patient-ventilator synchrony. Decreased WOB	Apnea alarm is only backup (newer microprocessor ventilators have a backup mode if patient apneic)

Abbreviations: A/C, assist control; ASV, adaptive support ventilation; MV, minute ventilation; PAC, pressure assist control; PC, pressure control; PIP, peak inspiratory pressure; PRVC, pressure-regulated volume control; P-SIMV, pressure SIMV (time-triggered breaths are pressure limited); PSV, pressure-support ventilation; RR, respiratory rate; SIMV, synchronized intermittent mandatory ventilation; VAC, volume assist control; VC, volume control; V_T, tidal volume.

Data from Parillo JE, Dellinger P, editors. Critical care medicine, principles of diagnosis and management in the adult. 3rd edition. Philadelphia: Mosby Elsevier; 2001.

Pressure-limited ventilation

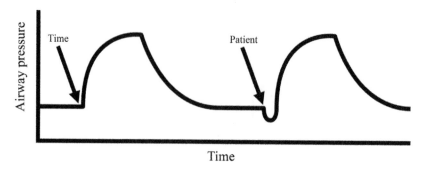

Volume-limited ventilation

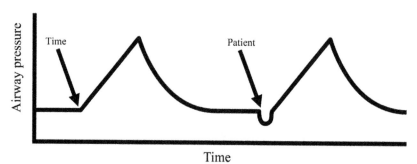

Fig. 1. Comparison of pressure-limited and volume-limited breaths and patient-triggered and time-triggered breaths. (*Adapted from* Pilbeam SP, Cairo JM. Mechanical ventilation: physiologic and clinical applications. 4th edition. St Louis (MO): Mosby Elsevier; 2006. p. 52; with permission.)

a descending ramp wave. In practice, the descending ramp wave is the most popular because it mimics the normal inspiratory pattern with flow increasing rapidly and then decreasing gradually until the end of inspiration.

Initial Ventilator Settings After Intubation

According to the clinical setting, ventilator variables are set depending on the mode chosen, the desired V_T, inspiratory pressure, inspiratory flow rate, and respiratory rate. Some ventilators also allow the operator to set the inspiratory/expiratory (I/E) ratio directly. For most adults, a normal I/E ratio of 1:2 or 1:3 is used. **Table 2** summarizes the basic initial settings for a multitude of clinical situations that are discussed later.

Conventional Modes

Basic modes used to ventilate patients are A/C ventilation, SIMV, and PSV. Refer to **Table 1** for the advantages and disadvantages of each mode.

A/C ventilation

With A/C, breath initiation can be patient or time triggered, depending on which occurs first. For patients who are paralyzed, comatose, or deeply sedated, this mode can be used for full ventilatory support. Breaths can be volume limited (volume A/C with

Table 2
Comparison of initial ventilator settings for different clinical situations

Clinical Example	Modes	Respiratory Rate (Breaths/min)	Tidal Volume (mL/kg IBW[a])	Flow Rate (L/min)	Fio$_2$	PEEP (cm H$_2$O)
Normal lung mechanics	Poisoning	VAC PAC SIMV PRVC ASV	10–15 (100%–110% MV)	8–10	60	<0.4	3–5
Severe airflow obstruction	Acute asthma	VAC PRVC ASV	8–10 (100%–110% MV)	4–8 (then adjust)	≥60	0.3–0.5	<80% of intrinsic PEEP
Acute/chronic respiratory failure	COPD exacerbation	VAC PRVC ASV	10–12 (100%–110% MV)	6–8	≥60	0.3–0.5	<80% of intrinsic PEEP
Acute hypoxemia	Cardiogenic pulmonary edema	VAC PAC PSV PRVC ASV	10–15 (spontaneous) (100%–110% MV)	8–10 (PS to maintain V$_T$ 8–10 mL/kg)	~60	1.0	10
Acute hypoxemia	Pneumonia and ARDS	VAC	20–35	6–8 and lower to 4–6 subsequently if Ppl >30	~60	1.0	5–24 (ARDS Network PEEP- Fio$_2$ chart)
Neuromuscular weakness and chest wall trauma	Myelopathy and chest wall trauma	PAC VAC PRVC ASV	15–25 (100%–110% MV)	8–10	60–80	≤0.5	5–8

Abbreviations: ARDS, acute respiratory disease syndrome; ASV, adaptive support ventilation; COPD, chronic obstructive pulmonary disease; IBW, ideal body weight; MV, minute ventilation (when using ASV, a percentage of MV is set instead of setting respiratory rate and V$_T$); PRVC, pressure-regulated volume control; PSV, pressure-support ventilation; SIMV, synchronized intermittent mandatory ventilation; VAC, volume assist control.

[a] Female IBW = 45.5+(0.91×[height in cm − 152.4]). Male IBW = 50+(0.91×[height in cm − 152.4]).

Data from Pilbeam SP, Cairo JM. Mechanical ventilation: physiologic and clinical applications. 4th edition. St Louis (MO): Mosby Elsevier; 2006.

a set V$_T$) or pressure limited (see **Fig. 1**). To prevent hypoventilation, a backup respiratory rate is set on the ventilator. This backup determines a minimum breathing rate, but the patient has the option of breathing at a faster rate. Thus, every breath is fully supported and has a set V$_T$. **Table 2** also presents the different clinical situations where A/C is often used.

SIMV

With SIMV, breath initiation can be patient or time triggered (similar to A/C) (**Fig. 2**). Furthermore, breath termination can be volume cycled (mandatory breaths) or flow cycled (spontaneous breaths).

The ventilator delivers a mandatory breath at a clinician-determined rate and V$_T$. After delivering a mandatory breath, the ventilator then allows the patient to breath spontaneously without receiving another mandatory breath until the next mandatory breath is due. Thus, the ventilator synchronizes its mandatory breaths with the patient's spontaneous breaths. When taking a spontaneous breath, patients breathe through the ventilator circuit at a V$_T$ and rate that is determined according to need. Pressure support can be added to spontaneous breaths to decrease the WOB. SIMV has been used in patients with severe respiratory alkalosis, to prevent auto-PEEP (auto-PEEP is discussed later), and to wean patients from the ventilator. This mode is commonly used in the ED after intubation[10] because it ensures that a patient

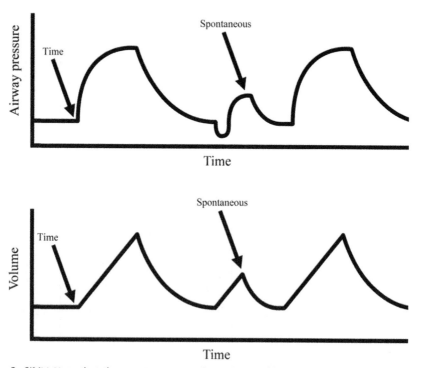

Fig. 2. SIMV. Note that the spontaneous patient-triggered breath is indicated by an arrow. This patient-triggered breath has a different inspiratory pressure determined by the pressure support set by the clinician. The volume generated by this breath is thus different than the other 2 mandatory time-triggered, volume-limited breaths. (*Adapted from* Pilbeam SP, Cairo JM. Mechanical ventilation: physiologic and clinical applications. 4th edition. St Louis (MO): Mosby Elsevier; 2006. p. 93; with permission.)

receives a minimal mandatory rate and V_T. When patients start recovering from neuro-muscular blockade and sedation, SIMV allows patients to breath spontaneously with pressure support, which is better tolerated in spontaneously breathing patients. However, studies[11,12] have shown that SIMV prolongs weaning and favors dyssyn-chrony. Dyssynchrony occurs when there is a mismatch between the patient's breaths and ventilator-assisted breaths, as well as the inability of the ventilator's flow delivery to match the patient's flow demand. This dyssynchrony increases agitation and respi-ratory distress. Clinicians must closely monitor the V_T of pressure-supported breaths because changing lung elastance and resistance can reduce air entry.

PSV

Pressure support is a ventilatory mode that supports a spontaneously breathing patient. The ventilator delivers a predetermined level of positive pressure (determined by the clinician) once the patient triggers a breath. The patient alone determines the respiratory rate, flow rate, inspiratory time, and V_T. A constant pressure is maintained until the patient's inspiratory flow decreases to a specific level (flow cycled) (**Fig. 3**).

Because patients must be spontaneously breathing, patients receiving PSV need close monitoring because neither their V_T nor their minute ventilation is assured. Clini-cians are able to adjust the slope of the pressure and flow curves during inspiration with PSV.[4] This feature has many different names: rise time, flow acceleration percent, inspiratory rise time, inspiratory rise time percent, and slope adjustment. These terms

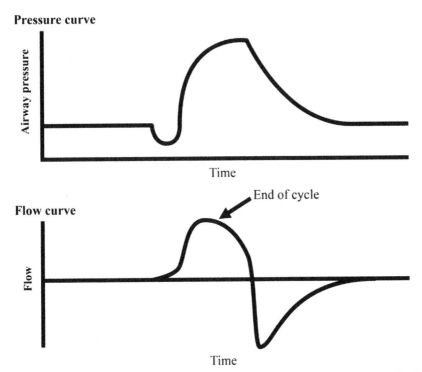

Fig. 3. Pressure-support ventilation. (*Adapted from* Pilbeam SP, Cairo JM. Mechanical ventilation: physiologic and clinical applications. 4th edition. St Louis (MO): Mosby Elsevier; 2006. p. 95; with permission.)

refer to the time required for the ventilator to rise to the set pressure at the beginning of inspiration. A rise time set too short (with a higher initial flow) can cause a pressure overshoot, and inspiratory flow may end prematurely. A rise time set too long (flow set too low), may not meet a patient's needs, and asynchrony develops.[4]

PEEP

PEEP is provided to the patient's airway throughout the respiratory cycle (**Fig. 4**).

Even though PEEP can be used by itself as an NIV mode for spontaneously breathing patients (in which case it is called continuous positive airway pressure [CPAP]) (**Fig. 5**), PEEP is often used in addition to other modes of ventilation to improve oxygenation.

PEEP shifts the pressure-volume curve toward normal, increases compliance, recruits alveoli, and increases functional residual capacity (FRC). PEEP is also helpful for left ventricular function because it decreases preload, afterload, and WOB. However, PEEP is detrimental for right ventricular function because it increases right ventricular afterload and might even cause cardiovascular collapse in patients with pulmonary embolism, severe pulmonary hypertension, and right ventricle infarction. Applying low levels of physiologic PEEP (5 cm H_2O) decreases the risk of atelectasis and pneumonia.[13] PEEP is indicated in cardiogenic pulmonary edema, acute lung injury (ALI), acute respiratory distress syndrome (ARDS), and to prevent atelectasis in obese patients. The contraindications to applying PEEP are bullous lung disease and preload-dependent shock.

The best level of PEEP to use is called best PEEP. Many different methods exist to try to identify the best level of PEEP to administer to a patient. There are both mechanical and gas exchange approaches. The most pragmatic approach in the ED is to use a gas exchange technique like the one used in the ARDS Network trial (**Table 3**),[14] which used a predetermined PEEP-Fio_2 algorithm designed to provide adequate values for Pao_2 while minimizing Fio_2. The choice between a high and a low PEEP-Fio_2 algorithm is still the subject of ongoing debate[15–17] even though a recent systematic review suggested that higher PEEP levels (open-lung ventilation strategy[18,19]) decreased mortality but increased barotrauma.[20] Moreover, no comparative studies have been conducted in the ED, where patients are often hypovolemic and unstable hemodynamically after intubation.[21] Because adding extrinsic PEEP can decrease preload, this urges clinicians to be prudent when choosing a high-PEEP strategy immediately after intubation for patients with possible ALI/ARDS. However, a high-PEEP strategy could be useful in hemodynamically stable patients with refractory hypoxemia.

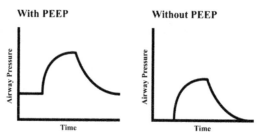

Fig. 4. PEEP. (*Adapted from* Pilbeam SP, Cairo JM. Mechanical ventilation: physiologic and clinical applications. 4th edition. St Louis (MO): Mosby Elsevier; 2006. p. 59; with permission.)

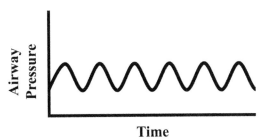

Time

Fig. 5. CPAP. (*Adapted from* Pilbeam SP, Cairo JM. Mechanical ventilation: physiologic and clinical applications. 4th edition. St Louis (MO): Mosby Elsevier; 2006. p. 58; with permission.)

Lung Protection Strategies

Since the publication of the ARDS Network trial in 2000,[14] a lung protection ventilation strategy is the norm for all patients with ALI and ARDS. Using such a strategy decreases mortality by 9% (number needed to treat = 11). It is essential that the emergency physician uses initial ventilator settings that protect the lung from further ventilator-induced injury. These settings include a low V_T (4–8 mL/kg of ideal body weight [IBW]), aiming for a plateau pressure (Ppl) less than 30 cm H_2O and the use of an appropriate PEEP-Fio_2 scale (proposed in the ARDS Network trial; see **Table 3**). Calculating every patient's IBW is essential to target the appropriate V_T, and is easily performed by measuring the height of every patient after intubation and applying the appropriate formula based on the patients' gender (see **Table 2**).

The open-lung ventilation strategy combines low V_T (4–8 mL/kg) with prevention of atelectrauma using recruitment maneuvers and higher PEEP levels than the ARDS Network trial (for more information on this topic, read the LOVS[19] and ExPress[18] trials). Modes like APRV and HFOV have been developed to offer alternative strategies to maintain higher average airway pressures to improve recruitment and oxygenation. Because the evidence for these modes is still considered weak and they are mostly used in the intensive care unit (ICU) when a basic lung-protective ventilation strategy is not working, this article only briefly reviews these modes.

APRV

APRV is a time-triggered, pressure-limited, time-cycled mode of ventilation that allows unrestricted spontaneous breathing throughout the ventilatory cycle. With APRV, the ventilator cycles between 2 different levels of pressure (**Fig. 6**).

Table 3
ARDS PEEP-Fio_2 charts. Note that 2 PEEP-Fio_2 charts (high and low PEEP) are presented. The decision to choose one chart rather than the other is still a matter of debate (see text). Note that both charts aim for a Pao_2 between 55 and 80 mm Hg or a Spo_2 between 88% and 95%

Lower PEEP/higher Fio_2							
Fio_2	0.3	0.4	0.5	0.6	0.7	0.8	0.9	1.0
PEEP (cm H_2O)	5	5–8	8–10	10	10–14	14	14–18	18–24
Higher PEEP/lower Fio_2							
Fio_2	0.3	0.4	0.5	0.6	0.7	0.8	0.9	1.0
PEEP (cm H_2O)	5–10	10–18	18–20	20	20	20–22	22	22–24

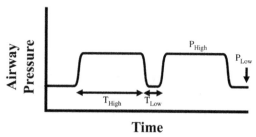

Fig. 6. Airway pressure–release ventilation. T_{High}, time spent at high pressure level; T_{Low}, release time; P_{High}, high pressure level; P_{Low}, low pressure level. (*Adapted from* Pilbeam SP, Cairo JM. Mechanical ventilation: physiologic and clinical applications. 4th edition. St Louis (MO): Mosby Elsevier; 2006. p. 99; with permission.)

The ventilator maintains a high pressure setting for most of the respiratory cycle (P_{High} 20–25 cm H_2O), which is followed by a periodic release to a low pressure (P_{Low} 5–10 cm H_2O).[22] The purpose of cycling between P_{High} and P_{Low} is to remove CO_2. The theoretic advantages of APRV are that it protects the lung (favors alveolar recruitment, decreases overinflation, and enhances gas exchange). However, there is little evidence about its safety and efficacy. To date, low-level evidence suggests that promoting spontaneous breathing with APRV may not be appropriate in patients with severe ALI/ARDS.[23] There is also a fear that APRV might not be protective because of high transpulmonary pressures generated when a patient breathes at P_{High}.[23,24] APRV should not be used with patients with chronic obstructive pulmonary disease (COPD), asthma, or diseases for which permissive hypercapnia is contraindicated.

HFOV
HFOV is an emerging ventilatory strategy for adults that has been used successfully in the neonatal and pediatric population. This mode uses high mean airway pressures (25–35 cm H_2O) to maintain an open lung, and low V_T (1–4 mL/kg[25]) at a high frequency (3–10 Hz).[26] This allows for adequate ventilation and prevents alveolar overdistension. The application of HFOV has mainly been reported as a rescue ventilatory mode in patients with ARDS in the ICU setting when conventional ventilation has failed. Thus, HFOV is not a ventilatory mode used in the ED. Ongoing studies are evaluating the use of HFOV earlier in the course of ARDS.[27]

Closed-loop ventilation
Because of technological advances in computing and in artificial intelligence, intelligent modes with complex closed loops have been developed.[28–30] Proportional assist ventilation (PAV)[31,32] and neurally adjusted ventilatory assist (NAVA[33]) are 2 modes that can deliver ventilation proportional to the instantaneous patient effort and seem to improve patient-ventilator interaction.[34] Dual-control modes (eg, pressure-regulated volume control [PRVC] and adaptive support ventilation [ASV[35]]) refer to ventilation modes that allow the clinician to set a volume target and the ventilator delivers pressure-controlled breaths.[28,36] The common characteristic of these new closed-loop modalities of ventilation is their adaptation to the patient, which explains the improvement in patient-ventilator interaction. Each of these modes changes the level of assistance in response to the patient's breathing pattern. These modes are promoted as helping the work of a respiratory therapist, who would typically have to remain at the bedside to offer the same level of adaptation to patients.[30]

Nevertheless, and despite their attractiveness, all these new methods of ventilation must show their clinical benefits before being recommended in routine practice.[28]

PAV

PAV delivers an inspiratory pressure proportional to the instantaneous effort of the patient and is amplified according to the patient respiratory mechanics (pulmonary compliance and airway resistance) and the chosen level of assistance (0%–100% assistance for the respiratory muscles).[28,37–39] Technical improvements made recently (under the name PAV+, available with the Puritan Bennett 840 ventilator, Puritan Bennett, Boulder, CO) allow intermittent and automated measurements of the patient's compliance and resistance[40,41] and make this mode easier to use.[42] Despite its potential, there is currently no evidence that PAV or PAV+ changes the clinical course of patients in comparison with pressure support.[28,43,44]

Neurally adjusted ventilatory assist (NAVA)

NAVA is a new mode of ventilation[30,33] that is available on Servo-i ventilators (MAQUET Critical Care, Solna, Sweden). As for PAV, the level of ventilatory assistance is proportional to the patient's effort. Its main feature is that the signal used by the ventilator to deliver assistance is not a pressure signal but the diaphragmatic electromyogram signal collected from electrodes placed on an esophageal catheter. Despite these potential benefits, several questions remain concerning the practical use of NAVA. In particular, the ease of placement of the esophageal catheter to record diaphragmatic electromyograms remains uncertain.[30] Thus, NAVA remains a promising mode of ventilation that needs more evidence of benefit for large-scale use.

Dual-control Breath-to-Breath, Pressure-limited, Time-cycled Ventilation

Volume-targeted, pressure-regulated modes of ventilation control V_T through variable levels of pressure and are referred to as dual-control modes. Pressure-regulated, volume control ventilation (PRVC) (AVEA, CareFusion, San Diego, CA, USA; Servo-i and Servo 300, MAQUET Critical Care, Solna, Sweden), AutoFlow (Evita 4, Dräger Medical, Lübeck, Germany), Volume Ventilation Plus (VV+) (Puritan Bennett 840, Puritan Bennett, Boulder, CO, USA), and variable pressure control (VPC) and variable pressure support (VPS) (Venturi Ventilator, Cardiopulmonary Corp., Milford, CT, USA) all possess similar proprietary modes. Breath initiation is patient or time triggered and breath termination is volume cycled, but each breath is pressure limited. All use a pressure-targeted algorithm in which the ventilator determines after each breath whether the pressure applied to the airway was sufficient to deliver the desired V_T. For example, if the V_T did not meet the set target, the ventilator will adjust the pressure applied to the airway on the next breath.

A similar but more complex dual-control mode, adaptive support ventilation (Hamilton G5, Hamilton C2, Galileo, Raphael, Hamilton Medical, Bonaduz, Switzerland) provides automatic ventilation in which minute volume (MV) is controlled through a V_T-respiratory rate (V_T-RR) combination based on respiratory mechanics. Clinicians must set a MV depending on the IBW (0.1 L/kg IBW per minute). The setting is expressed as a percentage of the target (% MV). The % MV can be adjusted later according to the target $Paco_2$ in passive patients and according to the clinical condition in active patients.[30] In patients unable to trigger a breath (passive or paralyzed patients), the ventilator generates a pressure-controlled breath, automatically adjusting inspiratory pressure and timing to achieve the target V_T and respiratory rate. Based on the Otis equation[45] and on the patient's own expiratory flow-volume curve,[46–48] the target V_T-RR combination minimizes WOB for a clinician-set MV.[45,46] ASV automatically determines the V_T and respiratory rate that minimizes auto-PEEP[30] and maintains the peak airway pressure at less than the target level.[45]

Even if these dual modes are promising, clinical studies have not shown a clear clinical benefit in comparison with other modes of ventilation.[48,49] Certain investigators have suggested that ASV could be appropriate for patients with ARDS, but others have found inappropriate tidal volumes for this population.[49] Other investigators have raised the possibility that patients' WOB increase when patients attempt to breathe at a V_T or MV greater than the clinician-set target V_T or MV with different dual-control modes.[50]

SmartCare

The SmartCare system (Evita XL; Dräger, Lübeck, Germany) uses pressure support as primary mode[30] and integrates an algorithm that (1) maintains the patient in a respiratory comfort zone by adapting the level of pressure support; (2) gradually decreases the level of the pressure support in case of stability; and (3) implements automated spontaneous breathing trials performed with minimal levels of pressure support. The first multicenter study comparing this system of automated weaning with usual weaning was published recently[51] showing shorter weaning periods, duration of mechanical ventilation, and duration of ICU stay.

NIV

Since the introduction of CPAP to treat obstructive sleep apnea in the 1980s[52,53] and the discovery that masks were a convenient conduit to assist ventilation, noninvasive positive pressure ventilation has become an important modality to treat acute respiratory failure and to prevent the need for invasive mechanical ventilation.[3] NIV is postulated to improve physiologic effects of various diseases by reducing the WOB and improving oxygenation and alveolar ventilation.[54] In the acute care setting, NIV has been proven to reduce the need for intubation[55,56] and its related complications, reduce mortality,[57] and shorten the hospital stay for certain patients requiring mechanical ventilation.[58,59] It also provides flexibility in initiating and removing mechanical ventilation, reduces sedation requirements, and preserves airway defenses, speech, and swallowing mechanisms. However, NIV can cause gastric distension, pressure sores, facial pain, nose dryness, eye irritation, discomfort, claustrophobia, and poor sleep.

In this article, NIV includes both noninvasive bilevel positive pressure ventilation (NPPV) and noninvasive CPAP. NIV can be delivered via a variety of portable NIV ventilators and adult acute care ventilators.[60]

Most portable NIV ventilators are microprocessor controlled and use a blower to regulate gas flow into the patient's circuit to maintain the preset pressure.[60] They have a single-circuit gas delivery system that uses an intentional leak port for patient exhalation instead of a true exhalation valve. This system allows the continuous flow of gas to help maintain pressure levels and flush exhaled gases from the circuit. NIV ventilators are often pressure-limited, flow-triggered and time-triggered, flow-cycled and time-cycled ventilators. They deliver an inspiratory positive airway pressure (IPAP) and an expiratory positive airway pressure (EPAP) (**Fig. 7**).

The IPAP level set on most NIV ventilators is equivalent to the total inspiratory pressure (pressure-support + PEEP) found in the PSV mode used on acute care ventilators. Most portable NIV ventilators can offer the following modes: CPAP, assist mode (similar to PSV), and an A/C mode (similar to pressure A/C). NIV ventilators have the ability to compensate for air leaks[61] that make breaths easier to trigger and terminate[60] compared with ICU ventilators. One of the limitations of portable NIV ventilators is

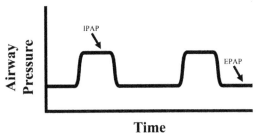

Time

Fig. 7. NPPV. IPAP and EPAP are presented as 2 different levels of airway pressure. (*Adapted from* Pilbeam SP, Cairo JM. Mechanical ventilation: physiologic and clinical applications. 4th edition. St Louis (MO): Mosby Elsevier; 2006. p. 60; with permission.)

that oxygen delivery can be difficult. Because most NIV ventilators do not have an integrated oxygen blender, supplemental oxygen must be blended into the system. In the past, Respironics BiPAP Vision (Philips, Amsterdam, Netherlands) was the only NIV ventilator with this feature.[60] However the newer high-performance NIV ventilators now include oxygen blenders.

Indications and contraindications
Recently, Keenan and colleagues[62] produced clinical practice guidelines about the use of NIV in acute care settings based on a comprehensive review of the literature. These investigators recommend that NPPV be used for patients with severe exacerbation of COPD (pH <7.35 and relative hypercarbia) (grade 1A recommendation)[55,56] and that either NPPV or CPAP be used for patients with respiratory failure caused by cardiogenic pulmonary edema in the absence of shock or acute coronary syndrome requiring urgent coronary revascularization (grade 1A recommendation).[57–59,63] They also suggest that NPPV be used for immunosuppressed patients who have acute respiratory failure (grade 2B recommendation).[64,65] No recommendation was made about the use of NPPV for acute asthma exacerbations, because of inconclusive studies. They recommend not to use CPAP for patients who have ALI (grade 1C recommendation), but no recommendation about the use of NPPV for ALI was made. The recommendation not to use CPAP for patients with ALI comes from an RCT comparing the use of CPAP plus usual therapy versus usual therapy alone.[66] In a subgroup of patients with ALI, the addition of CPAP did not affect endotracheal intubation or hospital mortality, but was associated with more adverse events (including 4 cardiac arrests). Other contraindications to NIV include cardiorespiratory arrest, severe encephalopathy, severe upper gastrointestinal bleeding, hemodynamic instability or unstable cardiac arrhythmia, facial or neurologic surgery, trauma or deformity, upper airway obstruction, inability to cooperate or protect the airway, inability to clear secretions, or high risk for aspiration.[67]

Interfaces (nasal, oronasal, full face, helmet)
To prevent skin pressure lesions, discomfort, and mask leaks, the choice of interface is important. Keenan and colleagues[62] suggest the use of an oronasal mask rather than a nasal mask for patients in acute respiratory failure (grade 2C recommendation). No other recommendation was made regarding other interfaces currently available (helmet interface or full face). Modifications to the interfaces are available to avoid pressure sores to the nasal bridge, such as forehead spacers, masks with ultrathin silicon seals, or heat-sensitive gels that minimize skin trauma.[53] A heated humidifier should be used to prevent drying of the airway during prolonged NIV. In addition, further research is

needed to determine the optimal period of rest to allow oral intake, speech, and pressure relief on skin surfaces.[54]

Initiation and monitoring of NIV

Several factors are vital to the success of NIV: careful patient selection; properly timed initiation; comfortable, well-fitting interface; coaching and encouragement; and careful monitoring.[53] Initial ventilator pressure settings should be started at low to maximize patient compliance and comfort and then can be increased to alleviate respiratory distress.[53] Typical starting pressures are an IPAP of 10 to 12 cm H_2O and an EPAP of 4 to 5 cm H_2O, maintaining a gradient of at least 5 cm H_2O. IPAP can be increased to 20 cm H_2O, and EPAP to 10 or 12 cm H_2O. However, these higher pressures are limited by air leaks and by the amount of pressure needed to keep a tight fit of the mask on the patient's face. Most importantly, monitoring the V_T is essential in determining whether adequate ventilation is generated by these settings.

Once NIV is initiated, patients should be closely monitored in the ED, a critical care unit, or a step-down unit. Improving signs of respiratory distress (abdominal paradox, accessory muscle use, and tachypnea) and improving pH within the first 2 hours of NIV are indications of success.[53] However, if these signs of distress persist, adjustments must be made. Leaks should be sought and corrected, patient-ventilator synchrony should be optimized, and pressures may have to be increased.[53] Improvement in mental status, gas exchange, respiratory rate, and heart rate is expected in the first 1 or 2 hours. If this does not occur, clinicians must consider immediate intubation because delays are associated with worse outcomes.[57,62]

Sedation during NPPV

Patient agitation has been considered a relative contraindication for the use of NPPV because of the fear of using sedation. A cross-sectional Web-based survey[68] performed on American and European physicians concluded that most physicians infrequently use sedation and analgesic therapy for patients receiving NPPV. If used, sedation was usually administered as an intermittent intravenous bolus, outside of a protocol. A benzodiazepine alone was the most preferred (33%), followed by an opioid alone (29%). Short-acting narcotics like remifentanil[69] and newer agents like dexmedetomidine[70] have been reported to help agitated patients cooperate with mask ventilation without inducing respiratory depression. Although sedation can help reduce anxiety and respiratory rate (notably helping reduce auto-PEEP with patients who have COPD), it must be administered with caution in a monitored setting. Sedation levels, breathing amplitude, respiratory rates, and blood gases must be monitored closely.

Boussignac CPAP system and other portable CPAP systems

The Boussignac CPAP system includes a valve capable of delivering a PEEP level ranging from 2.5 to 10 cm H_2O without using a generator. The valve is a small plastic tube attached to a face mask that creates continuous positive pressure. It has been proven to be equivalent to NPPV for the treatment of acute pulmonary edema in the ED[71] and is used to treat acute pulmonary edema in certain prehospital settings.[72] Other portable CPAP systems also exist, like the WhisperFlow Fixed CPAP Generator (Philips Respironics, Andover, MA, USA), and PORTO2VENT CPAP device (Emergent Respiratory, LLC, Anaheim, CA, USA), which are mainly used in prehospital settings because they offer a portable CPAP system offering a low consumption of oxygen.

High-flow nasal oxygen

High-flow nasal (HFN) oxygen delivery is also a potential alternative to CPAP because it delivers air and oxygen via a humidified circuit at greater flow rates than those traditionally used with a nasal interface (up to 40 L/min).[73] Similar to CPAP, this therapy may provide augmented airway pressures that can improve oxygenation. However, more research is needed to define the ideal population for this modality.

Case Scenarios

Normal lung mechanics: poisonings

Following ingestion of benzodiazepines and antidepressants, a 30-year-old woman without any past medical history is intubated for airway protection. This patient has normal lung mechanics and gas exchange, but remains apneic after intubation. The following modes could all be used to guarantee adequate minute ventilation: volume or pressure A/C, SIMV and dual-control modes (PRVC, ASV). An extrinsic PEEP set at 5 cm H_2O is often used to offset the gradual loss of functional residual volume (FRC) in the supine mechanically ventilated patient. Adequate minute ventilation must be ensured to maintain normocarbia. **Table 2** presents the initial ventilator settings (including V_T and respiratory rate) that are suggested for this patient.

Severe airflow obstruction: acute asthma

A 16-year-old boy known for severe asthma is brought to the ED with a progressively worsening asthma exacerbation. At arrival, the patient is unresponsive and presents obvious signs of respiratory failure with abdominal paradox. The patient is intubated using ketamine and a neuromuscular blocker. After intubation, the peak inspiratory pressure (PIP) is measured at 50 cm H_2O and the Ppl is measured at 25 cm H_2O. This situation is an example of an airway resistance problem with normal compliance. In asthma, bronchospasm, mucosal edema, and secretions contribute to an increase in airway resistance. Increased airway resistance causes an increase in the PIP. PIP is the sum of the pressure required to force gas through the resistance of the airways and the pressure of gas in the alveoli. The Ppl reflects the effect of the elastic recoil on the gas volume inside the alveoli. If the peak pressure during a mechanical breath is 50 cm H_2O and the Ppl is 25 cm H_2O, the pressure lost in the airway because of airway resistance is 25 cm H_2O (**Fig. 8**). Normally this should measure less than 10 cm H_2O with a proper-sized endotracheal tube.

Another problem with airflow obstruction is auto-PEEP. Gas can be trapped in the lungs during mechanical ventilation if not enough time is allowed for exhalation. When

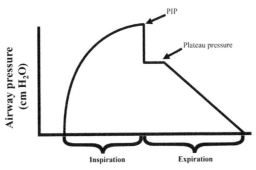

Fig. 8. Effect of an increase in airway resistance on the peak pressure. (*Adapted from* Pilbeam SP, Cairo JM. Mechanical ventilation: physiologic and clinical applications. 4th edition. St Louis (MO): Mosby Elsevier; 2006. p. 159; with permission.)

air trapping occurs, the increased alveolar pressure reduces venous return and cardiac output. Because the cause of auto-PEEP in the asthmatic is edema in the bronchi, applying extrinsic PEEP to these patients remains controversial.[62]

Intrinsic or auto-PEEP is related to hyperinflation caused by air trapping and is most often found in patients with acute asthma, COPD, or in patients with normal lungs when insufficient time is allowed to exhale. The simplest way of detecting auto-PEEP is to examine the expiratory flow rate waveform (**Fig. 9**), because flow never returns to zero at the moment of taking the next breath.

Auto-PEEP can also be measured by performing the end-expiratory airway occlusion method, which consists of occluding the inspiratory and expiratory valves at the end of expiration for 3 to 5 seconds. Pressure then equalizes and any positive pressure remaining in the circuit is auto-PEEP. This maneuver must be performed in patients without any spontaneous inspiratory effort because this interferes with the measurement.

This problem can be prevented by an optimal treatment of the underlying cause of obstruction, a lower respiratory frequency, and allowing the patient to exhale. Therefore, asthmatic patients require a shorter inspiratory time, higher inspiratory flow, and a longer time for expiration. In patients with normal airway resistance, the normal I/E ratio is 1:2 or 1:3. In patients with obstructive airway disease, the goal is to have an I/E ratio closer to 1:4 or 1:5. This ratio is achieved by decreasing the respiratory rate (8–10 breaths per minute), decreasing the VT (4–8 mL/kg) and increasing the flow rate (>60 mL/min). Typical settings for a patient with severe airflow obstruction are found in **Table 2**. Volume-limited or pressure-limited modes may be used, but

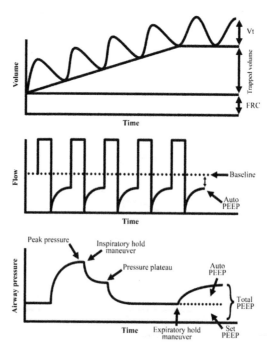

Fig. 9. Auto-PEEP. (*Adapted from* Pilbeam SP, Cairo JM. Mechanical ventilation: physiologic and clinical applications. 4th edition. St Louis (MO): Mosby Elsevier; 2006. p. 373; with permission.)

a volume-limited mode may be preferable to ensure a minimal V_T. It may be acceptable to allow permissive hypercapnia (pH>7.10–7.20) except if the patient has severe pulmonary hypertension, ventricular dysfunction, or increased intracranial pressure. Plateau pressure has to be maintained at less than 30 cm H_2O. A dual-control mode like PRVC or ASV may also be an option if the physician wants to limit the pressure delivered with each breath. Deep sedation and paralysis are often required to gain rapid control of the patient's breathing pattern and to allow a prolonged I/E ratio.

Acute/chronic respiratory failure: COPD exacerbation

The same principles as for asthmatic patients apply to patients with COPD except that the application of extrinsic PEEP is indicated for patients with COPD. For patients with COPD, the cause of air trapping is more related to dynamic expiratory airway collapse than the fixed severe distal airway edema that is found in asthmatic patients. NPPV is also the initial intervention strategy to favor in acute respiratory failure caused by COPD because this often responds well.

If intubation is necessary, a common mistake (as discussed for acute asthma) is to set a respiratory rate too high, causing auto-PEEP. If this mistake is not recognized, hypotension and cardiovascular collapse will occur. If this happens, an important step is to simply disconnect the patient from the ventilator and allow the patient to exhale. Then, resetting a lower respiratory rate, minimizing inspiratory time, and applying extrinsic PEEP help prevent the formation of auto-PEEP.

Extrinsic PEEP can also be used to prevent the formation of auto-PEEP in patients with COPD, which is especially important when treating patients with COPD who are having difficulty in triggering the ventilator. Auto-PEEP imposes extra work on patients because patients must generate enough inspiratory pressure to overcome auto-PEEP (see **Fig. 9**). Applying extrinsic PEEP (up to 80% of measured auto-PEEP) to the ventilator circuit can balance expiratory pressure throughout the ventilator circuitry to reduce the triggering load. A more pragmatic approach is simply to titrate extrinsic PEEP until every inspiratory effort made by a patient triggers the ventilator.

Acute hypoxemia: cardiogenic pulmonary edema

A 75-year-old man presents with rapidly progressive shortness of breath. He is known to have congestive heart failure. He is tachypneic with a saturation of 89% on a nonrebreather mask, and has a normal blood pressure, ECG, and mental status. NIV using CPAP in addition to other therapies (nitroglycerine and furosemide) is attempted first. However, increasing the CPAP level and changing the mode to bilevel positive pressure ventilation with an IPAP of 15 cm H_2O and EPAP of 5 cm H_2O could not decrease the signs of respiratory failure. After an hour of treatment, the patient's mental status is decreased. Considering that the patient is failing NIV therapy, the clinician decides to intubate. Initial settings for patients with acute pulmonary edema are found in **Table 2**. PSV (if the patient is breathing spontaneously), pressure and volume A/C, pressure and volume SIMV, and the dual-control modes can be used with higher PEEP levels to improve oxygenation and decrease preload and left ventricle afterload.

Acute hypoxemia: pneumonia and ARDS

A 60-year-old man with severe pneumonia is intubated on arrival to the ED because of hypoxemic respiratory failure. His postintubation chest radiograph shows diffuse bilateral infiltrates. The patient is not known for any cardiac problems and a bedside ultrasound reveals normal left ventricular contractility. He is diagnosed with ARDS with a Pao_2/Fio_2 less than or equal to 200.

Known to have decreased compliance, patients with ARDS benefit from a lung-protective ventilation strategy. This strategy is used to prevent pulmonary barotraumas and ventilator-induced lung injury (VILI) by minimizing airway pressures. The goals of ventilation in ALI/ARDS are found in **Table 2**. As previously stated, the low V_T (6–8 mL/kg IBW and 4–6 mL/kg IBW if Ppl>30) and low Ppl (<30 cm H_2O) are desired. PEEP is set according to Fio_2 requirement as per ARDS Network guidelines (see **Table 3**) aiming for arterial saturation to be more than 88%. Once the patient is stabilized, the Fio_2 can be titrated down to maintain a Pao_2 >60 mm Hg.

The management of refractory hypoxemia in patients with ARDS includes decreasing oxygen consumption (antipyretics, sedatives, analgesics, and paralytics[74–77]), improving oxygen delivery, and manipulating mechanical ventilatory support. These interventions include rescue therapies like recruitment maneuvers,[78] HFOV, prone ventilation,[79,80] and inhaled nitric oxide.[81,82]

Neuromuscular weakness and chest wall trauma

A 40-year-old woman is brought to the ED after falling off a horse. She has a saturation of 85% with 100% Fio_2 and is unable to move her arms or legs. She is intubated to correct her hypoxia. She is also found to have multiple rib fractures and lung contusions.

When initiating mechanical ventilation in patients with polytrauma, the physician must take into account the implications of potential hypovolemia, poor lung compliance, and, in the patient with traumatic brain injury (TBI), increased intracranial pressure. Determining a safe PEEP level in TBI is difficult without intracranial pressure monitoring. Even so, low levels of PEEP seem to be safe. PEEP can also exacerbate hypotension. In cases of TBI, hypercapnia and acidosis should be avoided. A Pco_2 between 35 and 40 mm Hg is recommended.[83] However, patients with significant thoracic trauma can have poor pulmonary compliance, increasing the risk of barotrauma.

The patient in the present case scenario has neuromuscular weakness (quadriplegia), restriction of her chest wall (rib fractures), and decreased lung compliance (pulmonary contusions). This patient remains a challenge to ventilate because she may require larger V_T and respiratory rates to minimize the air hunger and atelectasis that she may experience with her neuromuscular weakness. The same principles apply with neuromuscular diseases such as Guillain-Barré syndrome or myasthenia gravis. However, with the reduced compliance, Ppl must be monitored to avoid inducing VILI or barotrauma. Initial settings for patients with neuromuscular disorders are shown in **Table 2**.

Complications

Although mechanical ventilation is lifesaving, it is associated with several complications that can be related to the direct effects of the ventilator, the endotracheal tube, the toxicity of the oxygen, as well as systemic complications.[5]

VILI encompasses barotrauma, volutrauma, atelectrauma, biotrauma, and oxygen toxicity. Barotrauma (eg, pneumothorax, pneumomediastinum, pneumopericardium) occurs when the transalveolar pressure increases to a degree that disrupts the structural integrity of the alveolus. Volutrauma (eg, ALI) occurs when the lung parenchyma is damaged by overdistending the alveoli. To prevent these complications, the physician should try to keep Ppl at less than 30 cm H_2O and V_T between 4 and 8 mL/kg IBW. Atelectrauma and biotrauma are caused by cyclic opening and closing of lung units. Application of a PEEP to keep the lung open may attenuate these problems.

Oxygen toxicity is explained by production of free radicals causing a spectrum of lung injury, ranging from mild tracheobronchitis to diffuse alveolar damage. To prevent this, the physician may accept Pao_2 as low as 50 mm Hg.

Complications related to the endotracheal tube include vocal cord or airway edema, mucosal ulceration, airway granulomas, tracheal stenosis, tracheoesophageal fistula, and vocal cord paralysis. Ventilator-associated pneumonia (VAP) represents another major problem.

Troubleshooting

In urgent situations, when a patient develops severe respiratory distress or hemodynamic instability while receiving mechanical ventilation, the physician should immediately know what to do. **Fig. 10** presents an algorithm of the various steps to troubleshoot a patient who has decompensated.

The first step is to disconnect the patient from the ventilator and provide manual bagging ventilation with 100% Fio_2. This step removes a large number of potential ventilator-related problems and enables the clinician to concentrate on the patient.

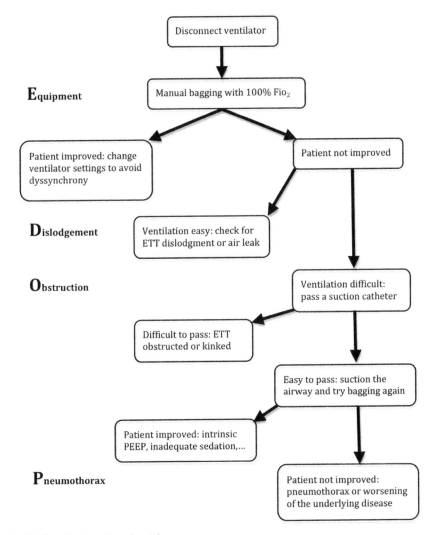

Fig. 10. Troubleshooting algorithm.

If the patient gets better with this simple maneuver, the physician should try to change the ventilator settings to match patients' effort to the required support.

If the patient continues to deteriorate, this may be a sign of tension pneumothorax, displaced or obstructed endotracheal tube, intrinsic PEEP, failure in oxygen supply, or dysrhythmia. A useful mnemonic for the causes of unexpected acute decompensation of mechanically ventilated patients is DOPE: dislodgement of the endotracheal tube, obstruction of the endotracheal tube, pneumothorax, and equipment failure.

Consulting any alarms that were triggered can also be helpful in determining the cause of distress. Alarms warn of possible danger related to the patient-ventilator system. Low-pressure alarms are used to detect ventilator disconnection and leaks in the system. High-pressure alarms ring when the patient coughs, when there is high resistance, or when there is a drop in compliance. Apnea alarms are used to monitor mandatory and/or spontaneous breaths. The low gas source alarms notify the operator that the available high-pressure gas source is no longer functional. It cannot be silenced if gas is critical to ventilator operation.

Important bedside respiratory mechanics

In addition to the DOPE mnemonic and assessing the alarms, it is also essential to understand basic respiratory system mechanics to decide what to do with patients who are difficult to ventilate.[84] An easy way to remember these basic concepts is to represent the respiratory system by a block attached to a wall with a spring, acted on by a unidirectional force (**Fig. 11**).[84,85]

The spring represents the elastance of the system (lungs and chest wall), the friction offered by moving the block represents the resistive element (mainly airway resistance), the distance the block is moved represents the volume of lung inflation, the velocity of moving the block represents the flow of air, and the unidirectional force represents the sum of the pressure generated by the mechanical ventilator and by the diaphragm's effort to inflate the lungs.

At the bedside, clinicians can easily measure these pressures to guide their assessment of any patient who is difficult to ventilate. PIP represents the pressure needed to overcome both the resistive and elastic elements. The difference between PIP and Ppl is the pressure required to overcome airway resistance. Ppl is the pressure generated by the elastance of the lung filled with a certain V_T. Patients must first be put in a volume-preset mode to control the volume administered. Patients must not generate any spontaneous breathing (ie, deeply sedated) that would falsify these measures.

Assuming inflation onset with a constant flow, an initial change in pressure is recorded, which precedes alveolar filling, and corresponds with the resistive pressure (PIP−Ppl) related to gas flow in the airways.[84] At the end of inspiration, a step-off in

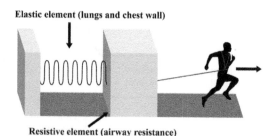

Elastic element (lungs and chest wall)

Resistive element (airway resistance)

Fig. 11. Respiratory system represented by a block attached to a spring. (*From* an unpublished presentation by Pierre Cardinal, Royal College of Physicians and Surgeons of Canada; with permission.)

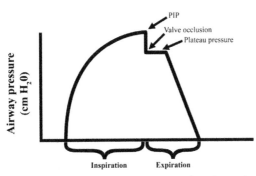

Fig. 12. Plateau pressure measured after a breath delivered to the patient before exhalation begins. (*Adapted from* Pilbeam SP, Cairo JM. Mechanical ventilation: physiologic and clinical applications. 4th edition. St Louis (MO): Mosby Elsevier; 2006. p. 159; with permission.)

resistive pressure occurs during an applied airway occlusion (**Fig. 12**). When the flow of gas falls to zero, the remaining pressure is called the Ppl and represents the static summation of elastic recoil forces corresponding with the applied V_T.

In the clinical setting, peak airway pressures that differ by more than 10 cm H_2O from the Ppl should prompt the clinician to look for a cause of increased resistance in the airways (kinked endotracheal tube, inspissated secretions, right mainstem intubation, bronchospasm, patient biting the endotracheal tube). If Ppl is increased (>30 cm H_2O), clinicians should look for causes of increased elastance (tension pneumothorax, ARDS, pulmonary edema, obesity, and abdominal compartment syndrome). Auto-PEEP can also be a cause of increased Ppl.

If signs of respiratory distress persist without any abnormal change in the PIP or Ppl, the clinician must then consider a pulmonary embolism. In situations of respiratory distress, clinicians should also ensure that the triggers are not too sensitive (triggering frequent breaths) or not sensitive enough (failing to trigger). Adequate sedation and analgesia are essential in managing a patient who is difficult to ventilate.

As previously stated, the main goal of mechanical ventilation is to reduce the WOB. In acute respiratory failure, the inability of the respiratory pump, mainly the diaphragm and extrinsic respiratory muscles, to meet metabolic demands is a result of either increased ventilatory load at more than the critical level or inability of these respiratory muscles to generate sufficient force to overcome the elastic and resistive forces previously presented. Measuring the WOB is still difficult at bedside, but careful clinical examination is paramount in determining whether sufficient ventilatory support is offered. This determination consists in assessing the breathing pattern, the use of extrinsic respiratory muscles, and the presence of paradoxic motion of the thorax and abdomen. If there are signs of persistent increased WOB, physicians must attempt to correct the underlying cause and adapt the ventilatory support to target the resistive or elastic components of respiratory failure.

SUMMARY

To reduce WOB and reverse life-threatening hypoxemia and hypercarbia, emergency physicians need to understand basic lung mechanics, the patient's underlying disease, and the different modes of invasive ventilation and NIV. Following the initiation of ventilatory support, the emergency physician must then evaluate the interaction between the patient and the ventilator to see whether hypoxemia and/or hypercarbia are resolving.

Basic modes used to ventilate patients are A/C, SIMV, and PSV. In cases of ALI/ARDS, it is recommended to ventilate patients in volume A/C, to set low V_T (4–8 mL/kg IBW), and to maintain low Ppl (<30 cm H_2O). For patients with acutely decompensated COPD (pH<7.35 and relative hypercarbia), NIV should be started early. Starting NIV early helps to avoid unnecessary intubation. If invasive mechanical ventilation is needed, it is essential to decrease the set respiratory rate because air trapping occurs (auto-PEEP) with high respiratory rates. Increasing inspiratory flow to decrease inspiratory time and prolong expiratory time also helps to avoid auto-PEEP formation. Extrinsic PEEP is also essential in patients with COPD to prevent distal airway collapse, thus preventing more air trapping. NIV should also be started early for patients with acute cardiogenic pulmonary edema, but only in the absence of shock or acute coronary syndrome. NIV is also recommended for immunosuppressed patients who have acute respiratory failure.

Although mechanical ventilation is lifesaving, it is associated with several complications. Therefore, avoiding mechanical ventilation when NIV is indicated and having a systematic approach to initiating ventilation, making adjustments, and troubleshooting is essential. Emergency physicians must also understand how airway resistance and elastance affect the ventilated patient. This understanding helps them perform basic bedside measurements (inspiratory occlusion pressure and expiratory occlusion pressure) to identify the cause of a patient difficult to ventilate.

ACKNOWLEDGMENTS

We would like to thank Jean-François Smith for his editorial support in preparing this article and for his help in creating the figures. We also thank Mélany Grondin for contributing her clinical expertise as a clinical educator in respiratory care therapy, Dr Christine Drouin, Dr Neill Adhikari, and Andrea Bilodeau (research professional) for reviewing the final version of this article. We must also thank Drs Todd Gorman and Pierre Cardinal (Royal College of Physicians and Surgeons of Canada) for allowing us to adapt some of their original figures. We also extend our gratitude to Dr Joel Turner for his leadership in the coordination of this edition of the *Emergency Medicine Clinics of North America*.

REFERENCES

1. Sternbach GL, Varon J, Fromm RE, et al. Galen and the origins of artificial ventilation, the arteries and the pulse. Resuscitation 2001;49(2):119–22.
2. Engström CG. Treatment of severe cases of respiratory paralysis by the Engström universal respirator. Br Med J 1954;2(4889):666–9.
3. Goldberg AI. Noninvasive mechanical ventilation at home: building upon the tradition. Chest 2002;121(2):321–4.
4. Pilbeam SP, Cairo JM. Mechanical ventilation: physiological and clinical applications. 4th edition. St Louis (MO): Mosby Elsevier; 2006.
5. Gebreab F, Saleh A. Introduction to mechanical ventilation. In: Raoof S, editor. Manual of critical care. New York: McGraw-Hill; 2009. p. 150–65.
6. Walls RM, Murphy MF. Manual of emergency airway management. 3rd edition. Philadelphia: Lippincott Williams & Wilkins; 2008.
7. Gross RL, Dellinger RP. Arterial blood gas interpretation. In: Fink MP, editor. Textbook of critical care. 5th edition. Philadelphia: Elsevier Saunders; 2005. p. 463–70.
8. Sevitt S. Diffuse and focal oxygen pneumonitis. A preliminary report on the threshold of pulmonary oxygen toxicity in man. J Clin Pathol 1974;27(1):21–30.

9. Marik PE. Handbook of evidence-based critical care. 2nd edition. New York: Springer; 2010.

10. Rose L, Gerdtz MF. Use of invasive mechanical ventilation in Australian emergency departments. Emerg Med Australas 2009;21(2):108–16.

11. Esteban A, Frutos F, Tobin MJ, et al. A comparison of four methods of weaning patients from mechanical ventilation. Spanish Lung Failure Collaborative Group. N Engl J Med 1995;332(6):345–50.

12. Brochard L, Rauss A, Benito S, et al. Comparison of three methods of gradual withdrawal from ventilatory support during weaning from mechanical ventilation. Am J Respir Crit Care Med 1994;150(4):896–903.

13. Manzano F, Fernandez-Mondejar E, Colmenero M, et al. Positive-end expiratory pressure reduces incidence of ventilator-associated pneumonia in nonhypoxemic patients. Crit Care Med 2008;36(8):2225–31.

14. Ventilation with lower tidal volumes as compared with traditional tidal volumes for acute lung injury and the acute respiratory distress syndrome. The Acute Respiratory Distress Syndrome Network. N Engl J Med 2000; 342(18):1301–8.

15. Rubenfeld GD. How much PEEP in acute lung injury. JAMA 2010;303(9):883–4.

16. Briel M, Meade M, Mercat A, et al. Higher vs lower positive end-expiratory pressure in patients with acute lung injury and acute respiratory distress syndrome: systematic review and meta-analysis. JAMA 2010;303(9):865–73.

17. Burns KE, Adhikari NK, Slutsky AS, et al. Pressure and volume limited ventilation for the ventilatory management of patients with acute lung injury: a systematic review and meta-analysis. PLoS One 2011;6(1):e14623.

18. Mercat A, Richard JC, Vielle B, et al. Positive end-expiratory pressure setting in adults with acute lung injury and acute respiratory distress syndrome: a randomized controlled trial. JAMA 2008;299(6):646–55.

19. Meade MO, Cook DJ, Guyatt GH, et al. Ventilation strategy using low tidal volumes, recruitment maneuvers, and high positive end-expiratory pressure for acute lung injury and acute respiratory distress syndrome: a randomized controlled trial. JAMA 2008;299(6):637–45.

20. Phoenix SI, Paravastu S, Columb M, et al. Does a higher positive end expiratory pressure decrease mortality in acute respiratory distress syndrome? A systematic review and meta-analysis. Anesthesiology 2009;110(5):1098–105.

21. Rady MY, Rivers EP, Nowak RM. Resuscitation of the critically ill in the ED: responses of blood pressure, heart rate, shock index, central venous oxygen saturation, and lactate. Am J Emerg Med 1996;14(2):218–25.

22. Rose L, Hawkins M. Airway pressure release ventilation and biphasic positive airway pressure: a systematic review of definitional criteria. Intensive Care Med 2008;34(10):1766–73.

23. Kallet RH. Patient-ventilator interaction during acute lung injury, and the role of spontaneous breathing: part 2: airway pressure release ventilation. Respir Care 2011;56(2):190–203 [discussion: 203–6].

24. Neumann P, Golisch W, Strohmeyer A, et al. Influence of different release times on spontaneous breathing pattern during airway pressure release ventilation. Intensive Care Med 2002;28(12):1742–9.

25. Sedeek KA, Takeuchi M, Suchodolski K, et al. Determinants of tidal volume during high-frequency oscillation. Crit Care Med 2003;31(1):227–31.

26. Ritacca FV, Stewart TE. Clinical review: high-frequency oscillatory ventilation in adults—a review of the literature and practical applications. Crit Care 2003;7(5): 385–90.

27. Sud S, Sud M, Friedrich JO, et al. High frequency oscillation in patients with acute lung injury and acute respiratory distress syndrome (ARDS): systematic review and meta-analysis. BMJ 2010;340:c2327.

28. Branson RD, Johannigman JA. What is the evidence base for the newer ventilation modes? Respir Care 2004;49(7):742–60.

29. Wysocki M, Brunner JX. Closed-loop ventilation: an emerging standard of care? Crit Care Clin 2007;23(2):223–40, ix.

30. Lellouche F, Brochard L. Advanced closed loops during mechanical ventilation (PAV, NAVA, ASV, SmartCare). Best Pract Res Clin Anaesthesiol 2009;23(1):81–93.

31. Younes M. Proportional assist ventilation. In: Tobin MJ, editor, Principles and practice of mechanical ventilation, vol. 15. New York: McGraw-Hill; 1994. p. 1300.

32. Younes M, Puddy A, Roberts D, et al. Proportional assist ventilation. Results of an initial clinical trial. Am Rev Respir Dis 1992;145(1):121–9.

33. Sinderby C, Navalesi P, Beck J, et al. Neural control of mechanical ventilation in respiratory failure. Nat Med 1999;5(12):1433–6.

34. Sinderby C, Beck J. Proportional assist ventilation and neurally adjusted ventilatory assist–better approaches to patient ventilator synchrony? Clin Chest Med 2008;29(2):329–42, vii.

35. Laubscher TP, Heinrichs W, Weiler N, et al. An adaptive lung ventilation controller. IEEE Trans Biomed Eng 1994;41(1):51–9.

36. Branson RD, Davis K Jr. Dual control modes: combining volume and pressure breaths. Respir Care Clin N Am 2001;7(3):397–408, viii.

37. Mols G, von Ungern-Sternberg B, Rohr E, et al. Respiratory comfort and breathing pattern during volume proportional assist ventilation and pressure support ventilation: a study on volunteers with artificially reduced compliance. Crit Care Med 2000;28(6):1940–6.

38. Wrigge H, Golisch W, Zinserling J, et al. Proportional assist versus pressure support ventilation: effects on breathing pattern and respiratory work of patients with chronic obstructive pulmonary disease. Intensive Care Med 1999;25(8):790–8.

39. Wysocki M, Meshaka P, Richard JC, et al. Proportional-assist ventilation compared with pressure-support ventilation during exercise in volunteers with external thoracic restriction. Crit Care Med 2004;32(2):409–14.

40. Younes M, Kun J, Masiowski B, et al. A method for noninvasive determination of inspiratory resistance during proportional assist ventilation. Am J Respir Crit Care Med 2001;163(4):829–39.

41. Younes M, Webster K, Kun J, et al. A method for measuring passive elastance during proportional assist ventilation. Am J Respir Crit Care Med 2001;164(1):50–60.

42. Kondili E, Prinianakis G, Alexopoulou C, et al. Respiratory load compensation during mechanical ventilation–proportional assist ventilation with load-adjustable gain factors versus pressure support. Intensive Care Med 2006;32(5):692–9.

43. Fernandez-Vivas M, Caturla-Such J, Gonzalez de la Rosa J, et al. Noninvasive pressure support versus proportional assist ventilation in acute respiratory failure. Intensive Care Med 2003;29(7):1126–33.

44. Gay PC, Hess DR, Hill NS. Noninvasive proportional assist ventilation for acute respiratory insufficiency. Comparison with pressure support ventilation. Am J Respir Crit Care Med 2001;164(9):1606–11.

45. Otis AB, Fenn WO, Rahn H. Mechanics of breathing in man. J Appl Physiol 1950;2(11):592–607.

46. Jaber S, Sebbane M, Verzilli D, et al. Adaptive support and pressure support ventilation behavior in response to increased ventilatory demand. Anesthesiology 2009;110(3):620–7.

47. Lourens MS, van den Berg B, Aerts JG, et al. Expiratory time constants in mechanically ventilated patients with and without COPD. Intensive Care Med 2000;26(11):1612–8.

48. Brunner JX, Laubscher TP, Banner MJ, et al. Simple method to measure total expiratory time constant based on the passive expiratory flow-volume curve. Crit Care Med 1995;23(6):1117–22.

49. Arnal JM, Wysocki M, Nafati C, et al. Automatic selection of breathing pattern using adaptive support ventilation. Intensive Care Med 2008;34(1): 75–81.

50. Mireles-Cabodevila E, Chatburn RL. Work of breathing in adaptive pressure control continuous mandatory ventilation. Respir Care 2009;54(11):1467–72.

51. Lellouche F, Mancebo J, Jolliet P, et al. A multicenter randomized trial of computer-driven protocolized weaning from mechanical ventilation. Am J Respir Crit Care Med 2006;174(8):894–900.

52. Sullivan CE, Issa FG, Berthon-Jones M, et al. Reversal of obstructive sleep apnoea by continuous positive airway pressure applied through the nares. Lancet 1981;1(8225):862–5.

53. Rajan T, Hill NS. Noninvasive positive-pressure ventilation. In: Fink MP, Abraham E, Vincent JL, et al, editors. Textbook of critical care. 5th edition. Philadelphia: Elsevier Saunders; 2005. p. 519–26.

54. Bersten AD. Best practices for noninvasive ventilation. CMAJ 2011;183(3):293–4.

55. Keenan SP, Sinuff T, Cook DJ, et al. Which patients with acute exacerbation of chronic obstructive pulmonary disease benefit from noninvasive positive-pressure ventilation? A systematic review of the literature. Ann Intern Med 2003;138(11):861–70.

56. Ram FS, Picot J, Lightowler J, et al. Non-invasive positive pressure ventilation for treatment of respiratory failure due to exacerbations of chronic obstructive pulmonary disease. Cochrane Database Syst Rev 2004;1:CD004104.

57. Vital FM, Saconato H, Ladeira MT, et al. Non-invasive positive pressure ventilation (CPAP or bilevel NPPV) for cardiogenic pulmonary edema. Cochrane Database Syst Rev 2008;3:CD005351.

58. Gray A, Goodacre S, Newby DE, et al. Noninvasive ventilation in acute cardiogenic pulmonary edema. N Engl J Med 2008;359(2):142–51.

59. Winck JC, Azevedo LF, Costa-Pereira A, et al. Efficacy and safety of non-invasive ventilation in the treatment of acute cardiogenic pulmonary edema–a systematic review and meta-analysis. Crit Care 2006;10(2):R69.

60. Gramlich T. Basic concepts of noninvasive positive pressure ventilation. In: Pilbeam SP, Cairo JM, editors. Mechanical ventilation. St Louis (MO): Mosby Elsevier; 2006. p. 417–41.

61. Criner GJ, Brennan K, Travaline JM, et al. Efficacy and compliance with noninvasive positive pressure ventilation in patients with chronic respiratory failure. Chest 1999;116(3):667–75.

62. Keenan SP, Sinuff T, Burns KE, et al. Clinical practice guidelines for the use of noninvasive positive-pressure ventilation and noninvasive continuous positive airway pressure in the acute care setting. CMAJ 2011;183(3):E195–214.

63. Peter JV, Moran JL, Phillips-Hughes J, et al. Effect of non-invasive positive pressure ventilation (NIPPV) on mortality in patients with acute cardiogenic pulmonary oedema: a meta-analysis. Lancet 2006;367(9517):1155–63.

64. Hilbert G, Gruson D, Vargas F, et al. Noninvasive ventilation in immunosuppressed patients with pulmonary infiltrates, fever, and acute respiratory failure. N Engl J Med 2001;344(7):481–7.

65. Antonelli M, Conti G, Bufi M, et al. Noninvasive ventilation for treatment of acute respiratory failure in patients undergoing solid organ transplantation: a randomized trial. JAMA 2000;283(2):235–41.

66. Delclaux C, L'Her E, Alberti C, et al. Treatment of acute hypoxemic nonhypercapnic respiratory insufficiency with continuous positive airway pressure delivered by a face mask: a randomized controlled trial. JAMA 2000;284(18):2352–60.

67. International Consensus Conferences in Intensive Care Medicine: noninvasive positive pressure ventilation in acute respiratory failure. Am J Respir Crit Care Med 2001;163(1):283–91.

68. Devlin JW, Nava S, Fong JJ, et al. Survey of sedation practices during noninvasive positive-pressure ventilation to treat acute respiratory failure. Crit Care Med 2007;35(10):2298–302.

69. Rocco M, Conti G, Alessandri E, et al. Rescue treatment for noninvasive ventilation failure due to interface intolerance with remifentanil analgosedation: a pilot study. Intensive Care Med 2010;36(12):2060–5.

70. Takasaki Y, Kido T, Semba K. Dexmedetomidine facilitates induction of noninvasive positive pressure ventilation for acute respiratory failure in patients with severe asthma. J Anesth 2009;23(1):147–50.

71. Moritz F, Brousse B, Gellee B, et al. Continuous positive airway pressure versus bilevel noninvasive ventilation in acute cardiogenic pulmonary edema: a randomized multicenter trial. Ann Emerg Med 2007;50(6):666–75, 675 e661.

72. Dieperink W, Weelink EE, van der Horst IC, et al. Treatment of presumed acute cardiogenic pulmonary oedema in an ambulance system by nurses using Boussignac continuous positive airway pressure. Emerg Med J 2009;26(2):141–4.

73. Kernick J, Magarey J. What is the evidence for the use of high flow nasal cannula oxygen in adult patients admitted to critical care units? A systematic review. Aust Crit Care 2010;23(2):53–70.

74. Devlin JW, Garpestad E, Hill NS. Neuromuscular blockers and ARDS. N Engl J Med 2010;363(26):2562 [Letter: author reply: 2563–64].

75. Gusmao D. Neuromuscular blockers and ARDS. N Engl J Med 2010;363(26):2562–3 [Letter: author reply: 2563–64].

76. Puthucheary Z, Hart N, Montgomery H. Neuromuscular blockers and ARDS [letter]. N Engl J Med 2010;363(26):2563.

77. Papazian L, Forel JM, Gacouin A, et al. Neuromuscular blockers in early acute respiratory distress syndrome. N Engl J Med 2010;363(12):1107–16.

78. Hodgson C, Keating JL, Holland AE, et al. Recruitment manoeuvres for adults with acute lung injury receiving mechanical ventilation. Cochrane Database Syst Rev 2009;2:CD006667.

79. Gattinoni L, Tognoni G, Pesenti A, et al. Effect of prone positioning on the survival of patients with acute respiratory failure. N Engl J Med 2001;345(8):568–73.

80. Sud S, Sud M, Friedrich JO, et al. Effect of mechanical ventilation in the prone position on clinical outcomes in patients with acute hypoxemic respiratory failure: a systematic review and meta-analysis. CMAJ 2008;178(9):1153–61.

81. Ferguson ND. Inhaled nitric oxide for acute respiratory distress syndrome. BMJ 2007;334(7597):757–8.

82. Ferguson ND, Granton JT. Inhaled nitric oxide for hypoxemic respiratory failure: passing bad gas? CMAJ 2000;162(1):85–6.

83. The Brain Trauma Foundation. The American Association of Neurological Surgeons. The Joint Section on Neurotrauma and Critical Care. Hyperventilation. J Neurotrauma 2000;17(6–7):513–20.

84. Caples SM, Hubmayr RD. Respiratory system mechanics and respiratory muscle function. In: Fink MP, editor. Textbook of critical care. 5th edition. Philadelphia: Elsevier Saunders; 2005. p. 471–82.

85. Rodarte JR, Rehder K. Dynamics of respiration. In: Macklem PT, Mead J, editors. Handbook of physiology. Baltimore (MD): Williams & Wilkins; 1986. p. 131–44.

Thoracic Ultrasound

Joel P. Turner, MD, MSc, FRCP[a,b,c,d,*], Jerrald Dankoff, MDCM, CSPQ[e]

KEYWORDS

- Ultrasound • Thoracic • Pneumothorax • Pleural effusion
- Pneumonia • Blue • B-lines • Pleural line

Patients with thoracic emergencies can present a diagnostic dilemma to the emergency physician. Furthermore, there are often situations of severe respiratory distress in which an urgent diagnosis is required within minutes to direct potentially life-saving therapy. Traditionally, the emergency physician has relied on historical and physical examination findings to help in the initial differential diagnosis of dyspnea. These have often been found to be unreliable.[1–3] A bedside chest radiograph (CXR) can provide useful information but it has been shown to be inaccurate in many situations. Circumstances often arise in which one experienced physician evaluates the same patient as another physician and comes to diametrically different diagnoses; wet versus dry, pneumonia versus heart failure, pleural effusion versus pneumonia versus chronic obstructive pulmonary disease (COPD), and so forth. CT scan could resolve many of these issues but involves transporting potentially unstable patients out of the department, larger radiation doses (typically 200 times that of a CXR), the use of contrast, and cannot routinely be used in pregnancy. Clearly, there is a need for more exact tools.

Lung ultrasound is a new method of emergency patient assessment. So new in fact, that the latest editions of some North American emergency ultrasound textbooks do not even mention the lung as an organ that can be evaluated using ultrasound, except for passing discussions concerning the detection of traumatic pneumothorax.[4,5] The 2008 edition of *Harrison's Principles of Internal Medicine*[6] continues to state that ultrasound imaging is not useful for pulmonary parenchyma imaging. However, thanks to pioneering work of French intensivist Daniel Lichtenstein, and others, we now can confidently use ultrasound to evaluate patients with respiratory complaints.

Disclosure: Dr Turner is coauthor and presenter of the EDE-2 Course©.
a McGill Emergency Medicine, McGill University, Montreal, Quebec, Canada
b Royal College Emergency Medicine Residency Training Program, McGill University, Montreal, Quebec, Canada
c Emergency Medicine Ultrasound Training Program, McGill University, Montreal, Quebec, Canada
d Emergency Department, Jewish General Hospital, Montreal, Quebec, Canada
e Emergency Department, Jewish General Hospital, McGill University, Montreal, Quebec, Canada
* Corresponding author. Department of Emergency Medicine, Jewish General Hospital, 3755 Côte-Sainte-Catherine Road, Room D-010, Montreal, Quebec, Canada H3T 1E2, Canada.
E-mail address: joel.turner@mcgill.ca

Emerg Med Clin N Am 30 (2012) 451–473
doi:10.1016/j.emc.2011.12.003
0733-8627/12/$ – see front matter © 2012 Elsevier Inc. All rights reserved.

emed.theclinics.com

This article reviews the basic technical and anatomic principles of thoracic ultrasound, describes the important evidenced-based sonographic features found in a variety of pathologic conditions, and provides a framework of how to use thoracic ultrasound to aid in assessing a patient with severe dyspnea.

PRINCIPLES OF THORACIC ULTRASOUND

The basis and utility of thoracic ultrasound is attributed to several important principles first proposed by Lichtenstein[7]:

1. The intimate relationship between air and water in the lung causes a variety of artifacts seen by ultrasound. Because air (and, by extension, the lung) cannot be visualized by sonography, thoracic ultrasound is based primarily on the analysis of these artifacts.
2. Air and water have opposing gravitational dynamics. Consequently, a variety of pathologic conditions (pleural effusions, consolidations) is predominantly "water-rich" and, thus, considered "dependent disorders." These pathologies are generally found in the posterior aspects of a supine patient. On the other hand, there are several "air-rich" conditions (pneumothorax) that are considered "nondependent" disorders and, as a result, are predominantly found in the anterior aspects of a supine patient (**Fig. 1**).
3. All sonographic lung patterns arise from the "pleural line." The pleural line is a bright echogenic line approximately 0.5 to 1.0 cm below the ribs, corresponding to the apposition of the parietal and visceral pleura. Most acute lung disorders abut the lung surface, which explains the wide-ranging utility of thoracic ultrasound. The pathologic condition not attached to the pleural line is necessarily visualized by lung ultrasound (eg, tumor, other hilar processes).

PROBE SELECTION

There are several probe options when performing thoracic ultrasound, each with its inherent advantages and disadvantages. The curved array probe has the advantage of allowing rapid assessment of the lateral thoracic cavity for signs of pleural fluid in

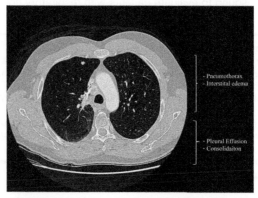

Fig. 1. Water-rich pathology such as pleural effusion and consolidation will tend to occur in the dependent (ie, posterior) regions of the supine patient. Pneumothorax and severe interstitial edema tend to occur in the anterior portions of the lung.

the supine patient. This is often the case in trauma (for example as part of the Extended Focused Assessment with Sonography for Trauma [EFAST] examination). However, due to its large footprint, only a small portion of the intercostal space (ICS) is accessible. Furthermore, the low frequency does not allow for detailed assessment of the main area of interest in thoracic ultrasound—the pleural line.

The high-frequency linear array probe allows for detailed examination of the pleura and provides rapid assessment of superficial lesions, such as pneumothorax. Its large footprint, however, hinders access to larger areas of lung tissue because of the interference of the ribs. Furthermore, the high-frequency sacrifices depth-of-penetration, preventing assessment of deeper structures such as atelectasis, consolidation, and large pleural effusions. Some investigators find the phased array cardiac probe convenient for simultaneous heart and lung examinations.[8] The relatively large dead-zone area in the near field may prevent clear assessment of superficial structures.

In the authors' opinion, the best probe to use for lung ultrasound is the 5 Mhz microconvex probe (**Fig. 2**). This probe design allows access to the ICS and facilitates examination of patients unable to cooperate by sitting. The probe can slide behind the patients back and aim up roughly perpendicular to the chest wall, even with the patient supine. Although sacrificing some resolution compared with the linear 10 Mhz probe, the microconvex has good depth of field, which is important for imaging deeper chest structures. All filters should be turned off to maximize real-time dynamic images. It is preferable not to smooth or suppress artifacts associated with lung movement or tissue impedance characteristics.

PATIENT POSITION AND LUNG FIELDS

Thoracic ultrasound can be performed either in the seated or, in sick patients unable to cooperate, in the supine position. The seated patient allows for the methodical assessment of all important lung fields: anterior, lateral, and posterior. It also allows the assessment of patients unable to lie supine (eg, severe COPD exacerbation, congestive heart failure [CHF]). When examining the supine patient who is unable to sit, each hemithorax should be divided into five zones; two anterior zones (separated by the third ICS), two lateral zones, and one posterior zone (**Fig. 3**).[9,10]

To begin the examination, the probe is placed between the ribs perpendicular to the chest wall, oriented in the longitudinal axis of the patient. The image generated will

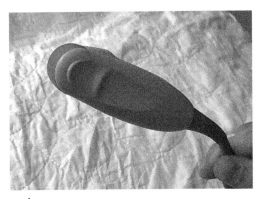

Fig. 2. Microconvex probe.

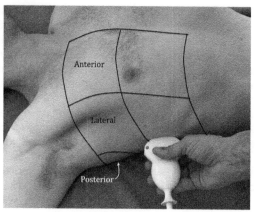

Fig. 3. In the supine patient, each hemithorax is divided into five zones; each should be interrogated by ultrasound depending on the indications.

show the upper rib on the left side of the screen and the lower rib at the right. The ribs cast a shadow framing the rest of the image. Approximately, 0.5 to 1.0 cm below and between the rib shadows will be the pleural line, a bright, slightly curved line. This is the key area of interest in almost all lung pathology of concern to the emergency physician and, as such, is the primary landmark to identify on the screen (**Fig. 4**).

In the normal lung, one will appreciate a shimmering or lung sliding representing the movement of the visceral on the parietal pleura during respiration. Note that, as one scans caudally down the chest wall, this should be more pronounced, whereas there is less lung movement or sliding near the apex of the lung.

Lung sliding is the first sonographic finding one should identify in the normal lung. Below the pleura, at regular intervals, are horizontal reverberation artifacts referred to as A lines (see **Fig. 4**).

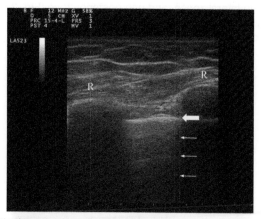

Fig. 4. Characteristic thoracic view showing adjacent ribs (R) with corresponding shadow artifact. Notice the white echogenic pleural line (*block arrow*), approximately 0.5 cm below the level of the ribs. A-line artifacts (*line arrows*) are seen at equidistant spaces below the pleural line.

Another artifact that may be seen both in normal and in diseased lung is the B-line (also known as a comet-tail artifact). Related to the sonographic interaction between small water-rich structures at the periphery of the lung surrounded by air, B lines have a very specific appearance that differentiates them from other, clinically unimportant artifacts. B lines are well-defined echogenic artifacts fanning out from the pleural line right down to the edge of the screen. They do not fade, they erase the A-lines, and they move in time with respiration (**Fig. 5**).

The number, location, and characterization of B-lines are important to differentiate normal lung from pathologic conditions. A solitary B-line is often a normal finding in any region of the lung and is found in the lower dependant areas of the lung in 28% of normal patients.[11] B-lines are not seen in all patients. The appearance of B-lines provides clinically important information with respect to pathologic diagnoses such as pneumothorax, pneumonia, and alveolar interstitial syndrome.

The physician should also be aware of the anatomic boundaries of the lung cavities and not mistake abdominal viscera or cardiac structures for pathologic condition. Anteriorly, the abdominal cavity usually starts at the fifth ICS and the pericardium and heart will be seen to the left of the sternum up to the midclavicular line. The liver and spleen are situated approximately at the sixth and fifth ICS, respectively, laterally and eighth ICS posteriorly. The diaphragm on both sides must always be identified to verify that intra-abdominal viscera are not being mistaken for an intrathoracic patho-logic condition.

PATHOLOGIC STATES
Pneumothorax

Bedside radiography has a notoriously inconsistent accuracy in detecting pneumo-thorax, regardless of the cause, with sensitivities ranging between 50% and 90%.[12–16] Through the recognition of specific dynamic sonographic artifacts at the pleural line, bedside ultrasound can detect pneumothorax with the sensitivity similar to a CT scan.

There have been several studies years comparing the accuracy of ultrasound to CXR and/or CT scan for the diagnosis of pneumothorax.[16–24] Alrajhi and colleagues[25] recently published a systematic review of eight high-quality studies. Overall, in 1047 patients, ultrasound had a sensitivity of 90.0% (95% CI; 86.5–93.9) and a specificity of 98.2% (95% CI; 97.0–99.0). This translates into a positive likelihood ratio (LR⁺)

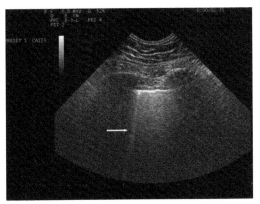

Fig. 5. B-line, or comet-tail artifact, extending from the pleural line to the edge of the screen, erasing the A-line. Solitary B-lines have no pathologic significance.

of 50 and a negative likelihood ratio (LR⁻) of 0.1. The comparative sensitivity and specificity of CXR in theses studies was 50.2% (95% CI; 43.5–57.0) and 99.4% (95% CI; 98.3–99.8), respectively. Among the 766 patients who had developed a traumatic pneumothorax, bedside ultrasound was 90.2% sensitive and 98.8% specific (LR⁺ = 75; LR⁻ = 0.1). The time to perform the examination ranged between 2 and 7 minutes.

Because an air-containing pneumothorax is a nondependent entity, sonographic assessment of the lungs is initiated on the most anterior portion of the supine patient, usually at the third-fourth intercostal space, at the parasternal-midclavicular line (**Figs. 6** and **7**). It is sometimes necessary to scan more than one intercostal space to ensure that the most nondependent region is assessed. The landmark to identify is the pleural line. The diagnosis, or exclusion of pneumothorax, relies on a stepwise approach to assess the existence of various dynamic signs.

The most important initial sign to look for is lung sliding, which is the back-and-forth movement of the bright echogenic parietal and visceral pleura occurring during respiration, often resembling marching ants along the pleural line. The confirmation of lung sliding has a 100% negative predictive value for the absence of pneumothorax.[26] In cases where lung sliding may not be clearly appreciated, power Doppler may help in confirming movement of the pleural line.[27]

The use of M-mode can also objectify the presence or absence of lung sliding. In the normal lung, the familiar "sandy beach" or "sea-shore sign" appearance will confirm the presence of lung sliding (**Fig. 8**). In the context of a pneumothorax, the characteristic "bar code" or stratosphere sign is seen (**Fig. 9**).[7]

It is important to recognize that, although the presence of lung sliding effectively rules out pneumothorax, its absence does not necessarily rule it in, with the specificity of the absence of lung sliding ranging from 60% to 90%. Several clinical entities may also present with the absence of lung sliding (**Box 1**).

Therefore, to safely rule in a pneumothorax, the following sonographic signs must be relied on. B-lines are caused by the reflections of the ultrasound beam between the alveolar air and the fluid of the interlobular septa. Therefore, the appearance of a single B-line confirms the apposition of both pleural and effectively rules out a pneumothorax.[4]

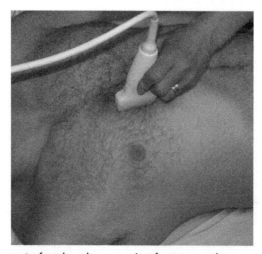

Fig. 6. Initial placement of probe when assessing for pneumothorax.

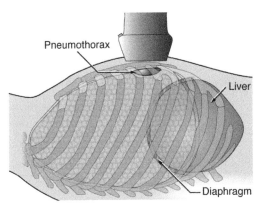

Fig. 7. Even small pneumothoraces can be identified anteriorly by lung ultrasound—a finding often missed in the supine CXR. (*Courtesy of* The EDE 2 Course, Sudbury, Ontario, Canada; with permission.)

The lung point refers to the point on the chest wall where the visceral pleura has separated from the parietal pleura and, therefore, defines where the pneumothorax begins. Visualization of the lung point is 100% specific for the diagnosis of pneumothorax.[28] Once the absence of lung sliding has been confirmed on the anterior chest wall, the physician should slide the probe laterally until the lung point comes into view with the reappearance of either lung sliding and/or B-lines (**Fig. 10**). This indicates the degree of extension of the pneumothorax.

Not only does the lung point confirm the presence of a pneumothorax, but its location may be able to predict its approximate size.[16,18,29] Although there has been not strict criteria comparing bedside ultrasound with CT scans regarding pneumothorax size, it is reasonable to suggest that the more lateral the lung point is found, the larger the extension of the pneumothorax. This information may be enough to drive treatment decision in most cases of pneumothorax.[30] A lateral lung point has been shown

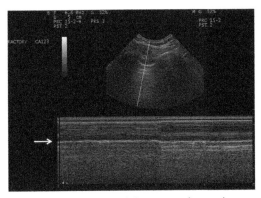

Fig. 8. M-mode appearance of normal lung sliding. Note that at the transition of the pleural line (*arrow*), the linear pattern (corresponding to the immobile muscle and subcutaneous tissue) is replaced by the grainy pattern (corresponding to the motion of lung tissue).

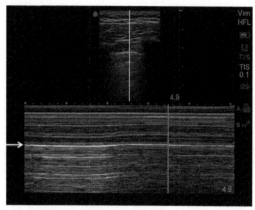

Fig. 9. M-mode appearance of absent lung sliding. The linear pattern remains distal to the pleural line (*arrow*), confirming lack of motion above and below the parietal pleura.

to correlate with a 90% need for chest tube drainage in the ICU, compared with 8% with an anterior lung point.[29] It should be noted that in the setting of a complete lung collapse there would be no lung point visualized. It should also be emphasized that in the setting of traumatic injury causing respiratory distress, impending cardiovascular collapse, or cardiac arrest the absence of both lung sliding and B-lines is enough to be necessitate immediate chest tube insertion. The extra time to identify the lung point is not advocated.

Occasionally, when lung sliding is absent, a vertical vibration at the pleural line is visualized and is noted to be in rhythm with the patient's heartbeat. This is known as the lung pulse and it can only occur if there is lung that extends to the pleural line allowing for the mechanical transmission of the heartbeat. Situations in which one might find absent lung sliding and the presence of the lung pulse include: apnea, pharmacologic paralysis, massive atelectasis, consolidation, and mainstem intubation.[30,31] Because air

---

Box 1
Differential diagnosis of absent lung sliding

Pneumothorax

Massive atelectasis or consolidation

Main stem intubation

Pulmonary contusion

Acute respiratory distress syndrome

Pleural adhesion or pleurodesis

Severe fibrosis

Phrenic nerve palsy

Apnea or cardiac arrest

Data from Volpicelli G. Sonographic diagnosis of pneumothorax. Intensive Care Med 2010;37(2):224–32; and Lichtenstein DA, Lascols N, Prin S, et al. The "lung pulse": an early ultrasound sign of complete atelectasis. Intensive Care Med 2003;29(12):2187–92.

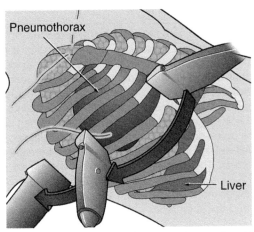

Fig. 10. The approximate size of the pneumothorax can be predicted by sliding the probe laterally until the lung point is visualized. (*Courtesy of* The EDE 2 Course, Sudbury, Ontario, Canada; with permission.)

(ie, of a pneumothorax) cannot transmit the movements of the heartbeat to the parietal pleura, visualization of the lung pulse rules out pneumothorax.

Putting together the various dynamic sonographic signs required to either rule out or rule in pneumothorax, a flow chart can provide the necessary steps to take to make an accurate diagnosis (**Fig. 11**).

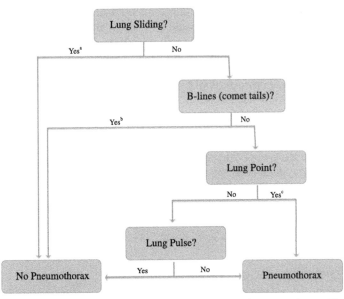

Fig. 11. Proposed flow chart for the sonographic assessment of pneumothorax. The presence of lung sliding ([a]) rules out pneumothorax with a PPV of 100%.[26] The presence of any comet tail ([b]) or B-line rules out pneumothorax with a sensitivity of 100%.[4] The presence of a lung point ([c]) confirms pneumothorax with 100% specificity.[28] (*Adapted from* Volpicelli G. Sonographic diagnosis of pneumothorax. Intensive Care Med 2010;37(2):224–32; with permission.)

Alveolar Interstitial Syndrome

First described in the mid 1990s, alveolar interstitial syndrome (AIS) constitutes a group of diseases that is caused by an increase in lung fluid and/or a reduction in its air content. The result of this engorgement or thickening of the interlobular septa causes a particular artifact that is seen arising from the pleural line. The major causes of AIS are summarized in **Box 2**. By far, the most common cause of acute AIS presenting to the emergency department (ED) is cardiogenic pulmonary edema. The sonographic appearance of AIS is a vertical artifact, called a B-line. When compared with CT scan images, B-lines correspond to edema of the interlobular septa.[11] As described above, B lines are well-defined vertical artifacts generated from the pleural line, reaching the edge of the screen. They do not fade, they erase the A-lines, and they will move synchronously with lung sliding. It is believed that B-lines are caused by multiple reflections of the ultrasound beam between the air-rich and water-rich structures, such as the alveoli and the edematous interlobular septa, generating the resonance phenomenon.[32]

The number, location, and characterization of B-lines are important to note. An isolated B-line (often defined as located >7 mm from an adjacent B-line) is a normal finding. In fact, B-lines are found in the lower dependant areas of the lung in up to 28% of normal patients.[11,33] Lichtenstein and colleagues[34] also suggest that B-lines extend up the back of bedridden patients so frequently that their absence suggests severe dehydration.

To be considered an abnormal finding, some investigators suggest that there must be at least three B-lines on a single scan using a microconvex probe or at least six B-lines using a linear probe.[33]

When diffuse B-lines are visualized, this gives the appearance of lung rockets (or B+ pattern), and suggests a diagnosis of AIS (**Fig. 12**).[10,11]

There is some controversy when diagnosing cardiogenic pulmonary edema using lung ultrasound. Lichtenstein and colleagues[11] and Lichtenstein and Meziére[35] originally categorized a positive scan when diffuse B-lines are found on both sides of the anterior chest (referred to as the B-Profile). In this scenario, bilateral diffuse B-lines had a specificity of 95% and a sensitivity of 97% for the diagnosis of pulmonary edema. It is suggested, however, that this may be true of only severe cases. Others have suggested that in milder cases multiple bilateral B-lines need only be visualized at several intercostal spaces along the anterolateral or lateral surfaces of the chest.[10,36] Using these criteria, diffuse B lines had a sensitivity of 85.7% and a specificity of 97.7% for AIS. This translates into an LR$^+$ of 37.3 and an LR$^-$ of 0.15.

In the bedside assessment of a patient with CHF, it has been shown that the number of B-lines is directly related to the severity of cardiogenic pulmonary edema when compared with CXR findings and pulmonary wedge pressure.[37–40] The number of

---

Box 2
Differential diagnosis of AIS

Acute

Pulmonary edema

Acute respiratory distress syndrome

Interstitial pneumonia

Chronic

Pulmonary Fibrosis

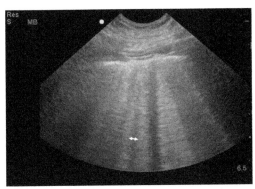

Fig. 12. Multiple B-lines, greater than three in a single scan, each less than 7 mm apart from adjacent one (*double arrow*), suggestive of AIS.

B-lines is also directly correlated with B-type natriuretic peptide levels, which may aid in the diagnosis of cardiogenic pulmonary edema.[41,42] In addition, the appearance of B-lines may precede any abnormalities on CXR, which may aid in the determining the aggressiveness of fluid resuscitation in critically ill.[43]

In addition to its utility in diagnosing pulmonary edema, lung ultrasound can also be used to monitor the effects of treatment. Several studies have demonstrated that B-lines clear rapidly after medical treatment as well as dialysis.[44–46] Because this effect has been shown to occur in real time, lung ultrasound has a significant advantage over CXR to evaluate the response to therapy.

Over the past 15 years, the use of lung ultrasound at the bedside to assess for the presence of B-lines has become has become universally accepted in both the critical care as well as ED setting. Recently, the ability to use this technique has been endorsed by various scientific bodies such as the American College of Chest Physicians and La Societe de Reanimation de Langue Française, in their joint Statement on competence in critical care ultrasonography, as well as the Heart Failure Association of the European Society of Cardiology.[47,48]

Pleural Effusion

The ability to diagnose pleural effusion by ultrasound has existed for almost 50 years. Despite this, its routine use at the ED bedside remains low. Ultrasound is, in fact, the diagnostic modality of choice in cases of suspected pleural effusion and hemothorax and is considered the standard of care in the safe localization, characterization, and aspiration of pleural fluid. Several studies have confirmed the relative ease in acquiring the skill to perform thoracic ultrasound for the detection of a pleural effusion.[49–51]

Ultrasound is exquisitely sensitive for the presence of pleural effusions even when the CXR is normal (may miss up to 500 cc).[52] Lung ultrasound can detect as little as 20 cc of pleural fluid,[53] whereas an upright posteroanterior CXR requires 100 to 200 mL of fluid before blunting of the costophrenic angle can be seen.[54] The supine CXR, in trauma situations or in the setting of a critically ill patient, is even less accurate.

There are two possible methods to ascertain the presence of a pleural effusion. When used as an extension of the FAST examination, simply sliding the probe from the right upper quadrant or left upper quadrant areas of the abdomen cephalad, past the identified diaphragm, allows access to the lungs. The presence of a pleural effusion is confirmed by the anechoic appearance in the postero-lateral recesses of the thoracic cavity (**Fig. 13**).

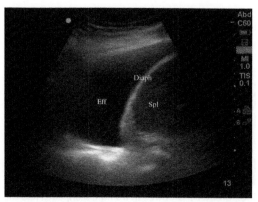

Fig. 13. Moderate left-sided pleural effusion. Diaph, diaphragm; Eff, pleural effusion; Spl, spleen.

A second method, as described by Lichtenstein,[55] is to simply place the probe directly along the posterolateral aspect of the thorax. Other than the obvious anechoic fluid appearance distal to the ribs, two additional signs that confirm the presence of a pleural effusion are described. The static sharp sign (or quad sign) refers to the four boundaries that delineate the appearance on the screen: the superior and inferior rib shadows on either side of the screen, the superficial parietal pleura, and the deep boundary, usually the lung. The dynamic sinusoid sign refers to the sinusoidal pattern of the effusion seen on M-Mode corresponding to the centrifugal movement of the visceral pleura during respiration (**Fig. 14**). This sinusoidal movement of fluid also confirms the low viscosity of the effusion (eg, transudate). The presence of these two signs has a specificity of 96% in identifying effusion and it should prevent the physician from misidentifying, for example, a large hiatus hernia or a breast implant as effusion.[56]

Trauma-related hemothorax is a condition that requires urgent bedside diagnosis. The accuracy of the supine CXR is quite low, leading to possible delayed or unnecessary chest tube insertions. Bedside trauma ultrasound has now expanded its role to include the lung (ie, EFAST). The sensitivity of ultrasound to diagnose a hemothorax ranges between 92% and 96% and has a specificity of over 99%.[57–59]

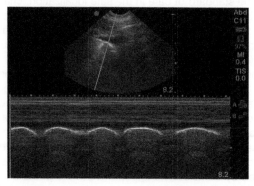

Fig. 14. Sinusoid sign.

Recently, Grimberg and colleagues[60] performed a systematic review comprising 924 patients who underwent lung ultrasound to diagnose pleural effusion. In the four studies included, CT scan and/or chest tube drainage was used as the gold standard.[3,57,59,61] They reveal that lung ultrasound has a sensitivity of 93% (95% CI; 89%–96%) and a specificity of 96% (95% CI; 95%–98%). This translates into an LR^+ of 23.25 and an LR^- of 0.07. These same four studies revealed that the sensitivity of the comparative CXR ranged between 24% and 100%.

Although not replacing the need for a diagnostic thoracentesis, the composition of the effusion can also be predicted with the use of ultrasound.[62] Transudates will be almost completely black in most cases, whereas an exudate will be more echogenic. A hemothorax and empyema have often been described as having a "snow flurry" appearance. An empyema can also reveal complex loculations and bright echogenic traces comparable to "Swiss cheese."[63] The presence of septations can also be assessed by ultrasound, sometimes with higher accuracy than CT scan.[64]

With the presence of a pleural effusion acting as an acoustic window, the lung will have an appearance of a bright line moving back and forth with respiration. If the pleural effusion is abundant enough to be compressive, the lung is seen consolidated and floating in the pleura effusion.

Examining the use of ultrasound in the ED to diagnose nontraumatic pleural effusion, it has been shown to be a rapid test to perform (<2 minutes) and that it changes management in 41% of symptomatic patients.[65] To determine whether bedside ultrasound to diagnose pleural effusion decreases the need for radiography and chest CT scans. Peris and colleagues[66] examined 376 mechanically ventilated patients admitted to the ICU. The use of daily bedside ultrasound led to a 26% reduction in CXRs and a 47% decrease in CT scans.

Pneumonia

Pneumonia causes significant morbidity and mortality, with an estimated 15% mortality rate in those admitted to hospital. Early diagnosis is essential for rapid initiation of therapy. The accuracy of CXR has shown to be extremely variable and is especially low in dehydrated, immunocompromised, and elderly patients. Campbell and colleagues[67] found that in 671 cases where an emergency physician diagnosed pneumonia on radiograph, the radiologist agreed in only 57% of cases. Furthermore, postero-anterior and lateral CXR's are often difficult to obtain in many patients, especially the critically ill and the elderly. Anteroposterior CXRs performed portably often fail to show an infiltrate. Over the past 15 to 20 years, lung ultrasound has developed as an important modality for the bedside diagnosis of pneumonia both in the ED and ICU setting.

The sonographic characteristic of an alveolar consolidation is one of a hypoechoic structure, whose appearance is "liver-like" (ie, hepatisation), with irregular deep boundaries. The superficial boundary corresponds to the level of the pleural line; the deep boundary is in direct connection with either the aerated lung giving an irregular, shredded boundary (the shred sign) (**Fig. 15**) or a corresponding pleural effusion.

In more than one-third of cases, pneumonia is accompanied by a pleural effusion.[68,69] The absence of the "sinusoid sign" helps distinguish alveolar consolidation from an associated pleural effusion. The presence of these signs has 90% sensitivity and 98% specificity for the diagnosis of alveolar consolidation.[9]

In most cases, the consolidation will also show corresponding hyperechoic punctiform images signifying air bronchograms arborizing within (**Fig. 16**). Centrifugal movement of these air bronchograms during respirations, referred to as "dynamic air bronchograms," confirms the presence of a consolidation and differentiates this

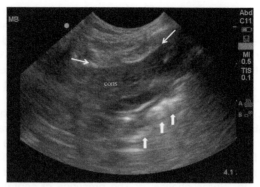

Fig. 15. Left lower lobe pneumonia showing hepatization of consolidation (cons), shred sign at the deep boundary of the consolidation (*block arrows*), and apposition of consolidation along the pleural line (*arrows*).

from atelectasis (static air bronchograms) with a specificity of over 94%.[70] The presences of B-lines can aid in the diagnosis of pneumonia. Often, the consolidation area is surrounded by multiple localized B lines, consistent with alveolar interstitial syndrome. Finally, it has been shown that diffuse B-lines found on a single lung is highly predictive of interstitial pneumonia with a specificity of 99%.[35] The sensitivity, however, remains quite low (14.5%) and should not be used to rule out pneumonia.

Because pulmonary consolidation consists mostly of fluid, with little air, these lesions are found mostly in the lateral and posterior aspects of the lung. When sonographic signs of pneumonia appear anteriorly, they often represent whole lung involvement.[9]

In several case control and retrospective studies, lung ultrasound was found to accurately detect the characteristic findings of a consolidation.[71,72] In a nonblinded study of 342 patients admitted with pneumonia, ultrasound was able to detect 92% of the consolidations.[69] In a prospective study of ICU patients, ultrasound was found to have a sensitivity of 90% and a specificity of 98% in diagnosing consolidation when compared with CT scan.[9]

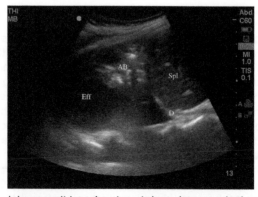

Fig. 16. Left, lower lobe consolidate showing air bronchograms (AB), and pleural effusion (Eff). D, diaphragm; Spl, Spleen.

Two ED-based prospective studies found that lung ultrasound has a high concordance rate with CXR to diagnose pneumonia and often demonstrated higher sensitivities than CXR when compared with CT scan findings. In 49 adult patients with suspected pneumonia, Parlamento and colleagues[73] revealed that lung ultrasound was diagnostic in 97% of cases. In eight cases where ultrasound and CXR were discordant, CT scan confirmed the sonographic findings. More recently, 120 patients with suspected pneumonia were evaluated in the ED.[74] Using the CT scan result and discharge diagnosis, ultrasound was found to have a sensitivity and specificity of 98% and 95%, respectively. The CXR in this study had a sensitivity of only 67%. When assessing the ultrasound's ability to diagnose pneumonia in ED patients presenting with dyspnea of unknown cause, ultrasound was found to be more reliable than CXR when using CT scan as the gold standard.[75]

Although these early ED and ICU-based studies provide strong evidence for the use of lung ultrasound to diagnose pneumonia, these studies were performed by a limited number of expert physician ultrasonographers. The generalizability of these results requires further confirmation.

Pulmonary Embolism

The use of lung ultrasound for the diagnosis of pulmonary embolism (PE) is a relatively new concept compared with the other indications. The most common positive sonographic finding in PE is a wedge-shaped hypoechoic lesion that extends to the pleural surface.[76] These have been referred to as C-lines by Lichtenstein.[77] Most lesions will be localized in the area of the pleuritic chest pain and adopt a triangular shape. A localized fluid collection may eventually develop adjacent to the affected lung. The pleural line may then become convex, bulge outward, and appear less echogenic and fragmented.[76,78] A localized subpleural effusion is seen in about 40% of patients with confirmed PE. Basal pleural effusions are seen in 50% to 60% of cases.

The literature examining the sensitivity of lung ultrasound to diagnose PE is sparse and limited by significant referral bias. Furthermore, the criteria used to diagnose PE are not standard. Mathis[78] used the following criteria: PE was *likely* when two or more characteristic triangular or rounded pleura-based lesions were demonstrated; PE was *probable* when one typical lesion with a corresponding low-grade pleural effusion; PE was *possible* if nonspecific subpleural lesions less than 5 mm in size or a single pleural effusion alone; and PE was *unlikely* if the lung ultrasound was normal. Using the first two criteria as diagnostic for PE, lung ultrasound showed a sensitivity of 74% and a specificity of 95%.

Lichtenstein simplified the sonographic criteria to diagnose PE. According to his Bedside Lung Ultrasound in Emergency (BLUE) protocol, in the severely dyspneic patient not in shock, a normal lung ultrasound (presence of A-lines throughout) plus signs of deep vein thrombosis (DVT) is 81% sensitive and 99% specific for PE.[35] This translates to a LR^+ of 81 and a LR^- of 0.19.

There are several limitations of lung ultrasound to diagnose PE. Only two-thirds of the lung area is accessible to ultrasound examination because the remainder is covered by bony structures. However, almost 80% of lesions are located in the lower lobes, which are accessible to examination.[79] Only thromboembolic lesions extending to the pleura can be detected. It has been demonstrated that central and peripheral lesions occur concurrently in 80% of cases.[76,78] As is the case with lung ultrasound for the diagnosis of pneumonia, studies on PE are limited to an exclusive group of expert sonographers and as such, its reproducibility and generalizability remains to be seen.

It should be added that in addition to performing lung ultrasound, the ability of the emergency physician to perform a bedside cardiac echocardiogram as well as compression ultrasound (looking for DVT) greatly improves the diagnostic power of ultrasound.

In a patient presenting with symptoms suggestive of PE, 50% have a documented DVT with no appreciable evidence on physical examination.[80] Lichtenstein and Meziére[35] reported that, in the BLUE protocol of patients with severe dyspnea, 85% of patients with a diagnoses of PE had a documented DVT.

In a patient with shock and severe shortness of breath, a normal lung ultrasound (or presence of C-lines) and signs of right ventricular overload on echocardiography rules in massive PE; therefore, intravenous thrombolytics or thrombectomy should be considered. A normal cardiac examination of the right heart rules out massive PE only in hemodynamically unstable patients.[81]

The most common differential diagnoses of such hypoechoic peripheral lesions include pneumonia, malignancy (primary or metastatic), and pleurisy. The description of these lesions is beyond the scope of the article.

PUTTING IT TOGETHER: THE DYSPNEIC PATIENT

The severely dyspneic patient often presents a challenge to the emergency physician as well as to associated consultants—often resulting in dichotomous impressions.

One of the most difficult challenges lies in differentiating patients with cardiogenic respiratory failure (ie, pulmonary edema) with those caused by primary lung disease (ie, COPD, asthma, PE). All too often, the CXR in the supine or poorly cooperative patient results in uninterruptable or nondiagnostic impressions that possibly lead to delays in treatment or in the wrong treatment being started.

Several studies have looked at the ability of bedside ultrasound to help differentiate the cause of respiratory symptoms when presenting to the ED or once admitted to an ICU. With the high sensitivity of lung ultrasound in recognizing alveolar interstitial syndrome described above, the diagnoses of CHF and COPD can be easily differentiated. For example, when originally describing the existence of B-lines, Lichtenstein and Mezière[82] concluded that the appearance of diffuse, bilateral B-line artifacts was 100% sensitive and 92% specific in diagnosing pulmonary edema versus COPD. As part of a landmark BLUE protocol study, lung ultrasound was found to distinguish patients with COPD and CHF with similarly high precision.[35]

Two recent ED-based studies were published evaluating the use of lung ultrasound in assessing the cause of patients presenting with dyspnea. Volpicelli and colleagues[10] performed lung ultrasound on 300 consecutive patients within 48 hours of arrival to the ED. They reported a sensitivity and specificity of 85.7% and 97.7%, respectively, of diffuse B-lines to diagnose AIS. More recently, Cibinel and colleagues[83] performed bedside lung ultrasound on 56 patients presenting to the ED with dyspnea. Ultrasound was performed by the emergency physician during the patient's initial assessment. The presence of diffuse B-lines was highly predictive for cardiogenic pulmonary edema, with a sensitivity and specificity of 93.6 and 84%, respectively (LR^+ of 5.6, LR^- of 0.08).

In 2008, Lichtenstein and Mezière[35] published the BLUE protocol, with the goal of determining the cause of a patient's respiratory failure. Just as the Rapid Ultrasound in SHock (RUSH) protocol revolutionized the assessment of the undifferentiated shock patient,[84] the BLUE protocol aimed to improve the speed and accuracy of the bedside diagnosis of patients with severe breathlessness. The study, which was performed on patients on admission to ICU, is pertinent to the emergency assessment of patients with respiratory failure. For a detailed description of the protocol, the reader is encouraged to refer to Ref.[35]

The results of the BLUE protocol are summarized in **Table 1**. The examination of the lower extremities for evidence of DVT is a crucial aspect of the protocol for the diagnosis of PE. Furthermore, PE cannot be ruled out using the BLUE protocol and should be treated on speculation, if the pretest probability is not extremely low, until a definitive test can be performed. However, if another diagnosis such as CHF or pneumothorax can be established with confidence, this lowers the pretest probability of PE below the test threshold because none of the patients with diffuse bilateral B-lines or with absent lung sliding had a PE. A complete pneumothorax (no lung point) needs to be confirmed on CXR.

It should be noted that neither the emergency nor the ICU physicians had access to the information in the study and that 26% of the diagnoses made in the ED were incorrect compared with the discharge diagnosis. The incorrect diagnoses chiefly included under-calling pneumonia, missing PE, and over-calling and under-calling CHF. The overall accuracy of the BLUE protocol was 90.5% for reaching the correct diagnosis.

This study was performed by the world's experts in lung ultrasound on the sickest patients presenting to the ED with respiratory failure. It is not yet known how the BLUE protocol will perform in other settings, in different spectrums of illness, and by other physicians. There have not been any validation studies at the time of this writing.

PEDIATRIC LUNG ULTRASOUND

The use of bedside ultrasound in the pediatric population is slowly increasing in the ED and intensive care environments. Studies have been focused mainly on the use of ultrasound in obtaining vascular access in children.[85–88] There remain several obstacles to its widespread use because there are no well-founded indications specifically for children. Much of its current use in pediatrics has simply been extended from well-established indications in the adult population (eg, assessment of free fluid following

Table 1
Results of the BLUE protocol

	Sensitivity (%)	Specificity (%)	Positive LR	Negative LR
Cardiogenic pulmonary edema[a]	97	95	19.4	0.03
COPD or asthma[b]	89	97	29.6	0.11
Pulmonary embolism[c]	81	99	81[g]	0.19
Pneumothorax[d]	88	100	∞	0.12
Pneumonia[e]	14	100	∞	0.86
Pneumonia[f]	21	99	21.0	0.80

[a] Diffuse bilateral anterior B-lines.
[b] Predominant anterior A-lines, lung sliding, and no posterior or lateral abnormalities; or with absent lung sliding without lung point.
[c] Predominant anterior A-lines with signs of DVT.
[d] No anterior lung sliding, no anterior B-lines and present lung point.
[e] Predominant anterior B-lines on one side, predominant anterior A-lines on the other.
[f] Anterior alveolar consolidation (C profile).
[g] A specificity of 100% indicates a theoretical positive likelihood ratio (LR) of infinity.
Data from Lichtenstein DA, Meziére GA. Relevance of lung ultrasound in the diagnosis of acute respiratory failure: the BLUE protocol. Chest 2008;134(1):117–25.

trauma, first trimester pregnancy, and limited echocardiography) but without the same number of dedicated studies in children.[89] The use of abdominal ultrasound in pediatric abdominal trauma remains controversial because studies have revealed varied results. In the literature, promising research has emerged on the role of inferior vena cava diameter and collapsibility to predict dehydration in children,[90,91] several orthopedic pathologies such as the diagnosis of clavicle fractures,[92] and the presence of hip joint effusions.[93–95]

The literature on lung ultrasound in the pediatric population is also sparse. Similar to other indications, the sensitivity of ultrasound for the diagnosis of conditions such as pneumothorax, pleural effusion, interstitial edema, and pneumonia is extrapolated mostly from findings in adults. The belief is that the same lung artifacts observed in the adult lung are seen equally in the pediatric lung. In fact, Lichtenstein[96] reported from a 3-year experience in the neonatal ICU that all basic signs (eg, A-lines, B-lines, lung sliding, sinusoid sign, shred sign) were present and found to be identical in critically ill newborns. Neonatal studies do suggest that lung ultrasound is a valuable tool for the diagnosis of transient tachypnea of the newborn[97] as well as respiratory distress syndrome.[98]

Examining the role of lung ultrasound to diagnose pediatric lung infections, Copetti and colleagues[99] examined 79 children between 6 months and 16 years of age presenting with clinical signs suggesting pneumonia. Among the 79 patients, 60 had lung ultrasound findings consistent with pneumonia, 10 of which also had a pleural effusion. Interestingly, while CXR "confirmed" the diagnosis of pneumonia in 53 of the 60 cases, there were four patients with a negative CXR and positive ultrasound who underwent CT scan imaging. In all four cases, CT scans confirmed the sonographic pneumonia diagnosis. These results reinforce the low sensitivity of CXR to diagnose pneumonia reported in the adult literature. Iuri and colleagues[100] also examined the role of lung ultrasound in 28 children presenting with a clinical suspicion of pneumonia. All 22 patients with subpleural consolidation found on CXR were also confirmed by ultrasound. Seven cases of perihilar consolidation were not detected by ultrasound. Lung ultrasound did seem to detect more pleural effusions (15) than CXR (8).

In a recent study comparing CXR and lung ultrasound in bronchiolitis, Caiulo and colleagues[101] performed a case control study of 52 children between 1 and 16 months of age. In their control group, lung ultrasound revealed 0 out of 52 consolidations, all had normal pleural lines, and 5 out of 52 revealed isolated B-lines (a normal finding). In contrast, 44 out of 52 infants with bronchiolitis had subpleural lung consolidation (only 16 out of 52 were found on CXR), 34 out of 52 had the presence of diffuse B-lines, and one infant had a small pneumothorax (not found on CXR). These initial findings suggest that bedside ultrasound is able to identify lung abnormalities not seen on CXR. The area of pediatric lung ultrasound shows much promise but requires much more vigorous studies.

SUMMARY

Bedside lung ultrasound has revolutionized the way emergency physicians and intensivists assess and reassess patients with a variety of respiratory conditions. It has been said that lung ultrasound has become the "stethoscope" of the twenty-first century.

This article is intended to provide an up-to-date review of the critical role of lung ultrasound for diagnosing pneumothorax, pleural effusion, PE, cardiogenic pulmonary edema, COPD, and pneumonia, all with accuracies far beyond what the physical examination and CXR can provide. Lung ultrasound is a rapid, safe tool that aids in diagnosis as well as monitors the effect of therapy.

REFERENCES

1. Wang CS, FitzGerald JM, Schulzer M, et al. Does this dyspneic patient in the emergency department have congestive heart failure? JAMA 2005;294(15):1944–56.
2. Reilly BM. Physical examination in the care of medical inpatients: an observational study. Lancet 2003;362(9390):1100–5.
3. Lichtenstein D, Goldstein I, Mourgeon E, et al. Comparative diagnostic performances of auscultation, chest radiography, and lung ultrasonography in acute respiratory distress syndrome. Anesthesiology 2004;100(1):9–15.
4. Lichtenstein D, Meziére G, Biderman P, et al. The comet-tail artifact: an ultrasound sign ruling out pneumothorax. Intensive Care Med 1999;25(4):383–8.
5. Cosby K, Kendall J. Practical guide to emergency ultrasound. Philadelphia (PA): Lippincott Williams & Wilkins; 2005. p. 367.
6. Fauci AS, Eugene B, Stephen L, et al. Harrison's principles of internal medicine. Ann Arbor (MI): McGraw-Hill Professional Publishing; 2008. p. 2754.
7. Lichtenstein DA. Ultrasound in the management of thoracic disease. Crit Care Med 2007;35(Suppl):S250–61.
8. Koenig SJ, Narasimhan M, Mayo PH. Thoracic ultrasonography for the pulmonary specialist. Chest 2011;140(5):1332–41.
9. Lichtenstein DA, Lascols N, Meziére G, et al. Ultrasound diagnosis of alveolar consolidation in the critically ill. Intensive Care Med 2004;30(2):276–81.
10. Volpicelli G, Mussa A, Garofalo G, et al. Bedside lung ultrasound in the assessment of alveolar-interstitial syndrome. Am J Emerg Med 2006;24(6):689–96.
11. Lichtenstein D, Meziére G, Biderman P, et al. The comet-tail artifact. An ultrasound sign of alveolar-interstitial syndrome. Am J Respir Crit Care Med 1997; 156(5):1640–6.
12. Ball CG, Kirkpatrick AW, Laupland KB, et al. Factors related to the failure of radiographic recognition of occult posttraumatic pneumothoraces. Am J Surg 2005;189(5):541–6 [discussion: 546].
13. Chiles C, Ravin CE. Radiographic recognition of pneumothorax in the intensive care unit. Crit Care Med 1986;14(8):677–80.
14. Ball CG, Kirkpatrick AW, Feliciano DV. The occult pneumothorax: what have we learned? Can J Surg 2009;52(5):E173–9.
15. Hill SL, Edmisten T, Holtzman G, et al. The occult pneumothorax: an increasing diagnostic entity in trauma. Am Surg 1999;65(3):254–8.
16. Soldati G, Testa A, Sher S, et al. Occult traumatic pneumothorax: diagnostic accuracy of lung ultrasonography in the emergency department. Chest 2008; 133(1):204–11.
17. Rowan KR, Kirkpatrick AW, Liu D, et al. Traumatic pneumothorax detection with thoracic US: correlation with chest radiography and CT—initial experience. Radiology 2002;225(1):210–4.
18. Blaivas M. A prospective comparison of supine chest radiography and bedside ultrasound for the diagnosis of traumatic pneumothorax. Acad Emerg Med 2005;12(9):844–9.
19. Zhang M, Liu ZH, Yang JX, et al. Rapid detection of pneumothorax by ultrasonography in patients with multiple trauma. Crit Care 2006;10(4):R112.
20. Soldati G, Testa A, Pignataro G, et al. The ultrasonographic deep sulcus sign in traumatic pneumothorax. Ultrasound Med Biol 2006;32(8):1157–63.
21. Dente CJ, Ustin J, Feliciano DV, et al. The accuracy of thoracic ultrasound for detection of pneumothorax is not sustained over time: a preliminary study. J Trauma 2007;62(6):1384–9.

22. Chung MJ, Goo JM, Im JG, et al. Value of high-resolution ultrasound in detecting a pneumothorax. Eur Radiol 2005;15(5):930–5.
23. Garofalo G, Busso M, Perotto F, et al. Ultrasound diagnosis of pneumothorax. Radiol Med 2006;111(4):516–25.
24. Kirkpatrick AW, Sirois M, Laupland KB, et al. Hand-held thoracic sonography for detecting post-traumatic pneumothoraces: the Extended Focused Assessment with Sonography for Trauma (EFAST). J Trauma 2004;57(2):288–95.
25. Alrajhi K, Woo MY, Vaillancourt C. Test characteristics of ultrasonography for the detection of pneumothorax: a systematic review and meta-analysis. Chest 2011. [Epub ahead of print].
26. Lichtenstein DA, Menu Y. A bedside ultrasound sign ruling out pneumothorax in the critically ill. Lung sliding. Chest 1995;108(5):1345–8.
27. Cunningham J, Kirkpatrick AW, Nicolaou S, et al. Enhanced recognition of "lung sliding" with power color Doppler imaging in the diagnosis of pneumothorax. J Trauma 2002;52(4):769–71.
28. Lichtenstein D, Meziére G, Biderman P, et al. The "lung point": an ultrasound sign specific to pneumothorax. Intensive Care Med 2000;26(10):1434–40.
29. Lichtenstein DA, Mezi re G, Lascols N, et al. Ultrasound diagnosis of occult pneumothorax. Crit Care Med 2005;33(6):1231–8.
30. Volpicelli G. Sonographic diagnosis of pneumothorax. Intensive Care Med 2010; 37(2):224–32.
31. Lichtenstein DA, Lascols N, Prin S, et al. The "lung pulse": an early ultrasound sign of complete atelectasis. Intensive Care Med 2003;29(12):2187–92.
32. Cardinale L, Volpicelli G, Binello F, et al. Clinical application of lung ultrasound in patients with acute dyspnoea: differential diagnosis between cardiogenic and pulmonary causes. Radiol Med 2009;114(7):1053–64.
33. Reissig A, Kroegel C. Transthoracic sonography of diffuse parenchymal lung disease: the role of comet tail artifacts. J Ultrasound Med 2003;22(2): 173–80.
34. Lichtenstein DA, Pinsky MR, Jardin F. General ultrasound in the critically ill. Heidelberg (Germany): Springer Verlag; 2007. p. 199.
35. Lichtenstein DA, Meziére GA. Relevance of lung ultrasound in the diagnosis of acute respiratory failure: the BLUE protocol. Chest 2008;134(1):117–25.
36. Volpicelli G, Caramello V, Cardinale L, et al. Detection of sonographic B-lines in patients with normal lung or radiographic alveolar consolidation. Med Sci Monit 2008;14(3):CR122–8.
37. Jambrik Z. Usefulness of ultrasound lung comets as a nonradiologic sign of extravascular lung water. Am J Cardiol 2004;93(10):1265–70.
38. Picano E, Frassi F, Agricola E, et al. Ultrasound lung comets: a clinically useful sign of extravascular lung water. J Am Soc Echocardiogr 2006;19:356–63.
39. Frassi F, Gargani L, Gligorova S, et al. Clinical and echocardiographic determinants of ultrasound lung comets. Eur J Echocardiogr 2007;8(6):474–9.
40. Agricola E, Bove T, Oppizzi M, et al. "Ultrasound comet-tail images": a marker of pulmonary edema: a comparative study with wedge pressure and extravascular lung water. Chest 2005;127(5):1690–5.
41. Gargani L, Frassi F, Soldati G, et al. Ultrasound lung comets for the differential diagnosis of acute cardiogenic dyspnoea: a comparison with natriuretic peptides. Eur J Heart Fail 2008;10(1):70–7.
42. Manson WC, Bonz JW, Carmody K, et al. Identification of sonographic B-lines with linear transducer predicts elevated B-type natriuretic peptide level. West J Emerg Med 2011;12(1):102–6.

43. Lichtenstein DA, Meziere GA, Lagoueyte JF, et al. A-lines and B-lines: lung ultrasound as a bedside tool for predicting pulmonary artery occlusion pressure in the critically ill. Chest 2009;136(4):1014–20.
44. Volpicelli G, Caramello V, Cardinale L, et al. Bedside ultrasound of the lung for the monitoring of acute decompensated heart failure. Am J Emerg Med 2008; 26(5):585–91.
45. Noble VE, Murray AF, Capp R, et al. Ultrasound assessment for extravascular lung water in patients undergoing hemodialysis. Time course for resolution. Chest 2009;135(6):1433–9.
46. Mallamaci F, Benedetto FA, Tripepi R, et al. Detection of pulmonary congestion by chest ultrasound in dialysis patients. JACC Cardiovasc Imaging 2010;3(6):586–94.
47. Mayo PH, Beaulieu Y, Doelken P, et al. American College of Chest Physicians/ La Société de Réanimation de Langue Française statement on competence in critical care ultrasonography. Chest 2009;135:1050–60.
48. Gheorghiade M, Follath F, Ponikowski P, et al. Assessing and grading congestion in acute heart failure: a scientific statement from the acute heart failure committee of the heart failure association of the European Society of Cardiology and endorsed by the European Society of Intensive Care Medicine. Eur J Heart Fail 2010;12(5):423–33.
49. Joyner CR, Herman RJ, Reid JM. Reflected ultrasound in the detection and localization of pleural effusion. JAMA 1967;200(5):399–402.
50. Eibenberger KL, Dock WI, Ammann ME, et al. Quantification of pleural effusions: sonography versus radiography. Radiology 1994;191(3):681–4.
51. Chalumeau-Lemoine L, Baudel JL, Das V, et al. Results of short-term training of naïve physicians in focused general ultrasonography in an intensive-care unit. Intensive Care Med 2009;35(10):1767–71.
52. Colins JD, Burwell D, Furmanski S, et al. Minimal detectable pleural effusions. A roentgen pathology model. Radiology 1972;105(1):51–3.
53. Röthlin MA, Näf R, Amgwerd M, et al. Ultrasound in blunt abdominal and thoracic trauma. J Trauma 1993;34(4):488–95.
54. Juhl JH, Crummy AB. Paul and Juhl's essentials of radiologic imaging. Philadelphia (PA): J.P. Lippincott; 1993. p. 1245.
55. Lichtenstein D. Lung ultrasound in the critically ill. Yearbook of Intensive care and Emergency Medicine. Heidelberg: Springer; 2004. p. 624–44.
56. Lichtenstein D, Hulot JS, Rabiller A, et al. Feasibility and safety of ultrasound-aided thoracentesis in mechanically ventilated patients. Intensive Care Med 1999;25(9):955–8.
57. Ma OJ, Mateer JR. Trauma ultrasound examination versus chest radiography in the detection of hemothorax. Ann Emerg Med 1997;29(3):312–6.
58. Brooks A, Davies B, Smethhurst M, et al. Emergency ultrasound in the acute assessment of haemothorax. Emerg Med J 2004;21(1):44–6.
59. Rocco M, Carbone I, Morelli A, et al. Diagnostic accuracy of bedside ultrasonography in the ICU: feasibility of detecting pulmonary effusion and lung contusion in patients on respiratory support after severe blunt thoracic trauma. Acta Anaesthesiol Scand 2008;52(6):776–84.
60. Grimberg A, Shigueoka DC, Atallah AN, et al. Diagnostic accuracy of sonography for pleural effusion: systematic review. Sao Paulo Med J 2010;128(2): 90–5.
61. Kataoka H, Takada S. The role of thoracic ultrasonography for evaluation of patients with decompensated chronic heart failure. J Am Coll Cardiol 2000; 35(6):1638–46.

62. Yang PC, Luh KT, Chang DB, et al. Value of sonography in determining the nature of pleural effusion: analysis of 320 cases. AJR Am J Roentgenol 1992; 159(1):29–33.

63. Reissig A, Copetti R, Kroegel C. Current role of emergency ultrasound of the chest. Crit Care Med 2011;39(4):839–45.

64. Kearney SE, Davies CW, Davies RJ, et al. Computed tomography and ultrasound in parapneumonic effusions and empyema. Clin Radiol 2000;55(7):542–7.

65. Tayal V, Nicks B, Norton H. Emergency ultrasound evaluation of symptomatic nontraumatic pleural effusions. Am J Emerg Med 2006;24(7):782–6.

66. Peris A, Tutino L, Zagli G, et al. The use of point-of-care bedside lung ultrasound significantly reduces the number of radiographs and computed tomography scans in critically ill patients. Anesth Analg 2010;111(3):687–92.

67. Campbell S, Murray D, Hawass A, et al. Agreement between emergency physician diagnosis and radiologist reports in patients discharged from an emergency department with community-acquired pneumonia. Emerg Radiol 2005;11:242–6.

68. Reissig A, Kroegel C. Sonographic diagnosis and follow-up of pneumonia: a prospective study. Respiration 2007;74(5):537–47.

69. Sperandeo M, Carnevale V, Muscarella S, et al. Clinical application of transthoracic ultrasonography in inpatients with pneumonia. Eur J Clin Invest 2010; 41(1):1–7.

70. Weinberg B, Diakoumakis EE, Kass EG, et al. The air bronchogram: sonographic demonstration. AJR Am J Roentgenol 1986;147(3):593–5.

71. Targhetta R, Chavagneux R, Bourgeois JM, et al. Sonographic approach to diagnosing pulmonary consolidation. J Ultrasound Med 1992;11(12): 667–72.

72. Yang PC, Luh KT, Chang DB, et al. Ultrasonographic evaluation of pulmonary consolidation. Am Rev Respir Dis 1992;146(3):757–62.

73. Parlamento S, Copetti R, Di Bartolomeo S. Evaluation of lung ultrasound for the diagnosis of pneumonia in the ED. Am J Emerg Med 2009;27(4):379–84.

74. Cortellaro F, Colombo S, Coen D, et al. Lung ultrasound is an accurate diagnostic tool for the diagnosis of pneumonia in the emergency department. Emerg Med J 2010. [Epub ahead of print].

75. Zanobetti M, Poggioni C, Pini R. Can chest ultrasonography replace standard chest radiography for evaluation of acute dyspnea in the ED? Chest 2011; 139(5):1140–7.

76. Reissig A. Sonography of lung and pleura in pulmonary embolism: sonomorphologic characterization and comparison with spiral CT scanning. Chest 2001; 120(6):1977–83.

77. Lichtenstein DA. Lung sonography in pulmonary embolism. Chest 2003;123(6): 2154–5.

78. Mathis G. Thoracic ultrasound for diagnosing pulmonary embolism: a prospective multicenter study of 352 patients. Chest 2005;128(3):1531–8.

79. Reissig A, Heyne JP, Kroegel C. Ancillary lung parenchymal findings at spiral CT scanning in pulmonary embolism. Relationship to chest sonography. Eur J Radiol 2004;49(3):250–7.

80. Hunt JM, Bull TM. Clinical review of pulmonary embolism: diagnosis, prognosis, and treatment. Med Clin North Am 2011;95(6):1203–22.

81. Torbicki A, Perrier A, Konstantinides S, et al. Guidelines on the diagnosis and management of acute pulmonary embolism: the Task Force for the Diagnosis and Management of Acute Pulmonary Embolism of the European Society of Cardiology (ESC). Eur Heart J 2008;29(18):2276–315.

82. Lichtenstein D, Meziére G. A lung ultrasound sign allowing bedside distinction between pulmonary edema and COPD: the comet-tail artifact. Intensive Care Med 1998;24(12):1331–4.

83. Cibinel GA, Casoli G, Elia F, et al. Diagnostic accuracy and reproducibility of pleural and lung ultrasound in discriminating cardiogenic causes of acute dyspnea in the Emergency Department. Intern Emerg Med 2011. [Epub ahead of print].

84. Perera P, Mailhot T, Riley D, et al. The RUSH exam: Rapid Ultrasound in SHock in the evaluation of the critically ill. Emerg Med Clin North Am 2010;28(1):29–56, vii.

85. Pirotte T, Veyckemans F. Ultrasound-guided subclavian vein cannulation in infants and children: a novel approach. Br J Anaesth 2007;98(4):509–14.

86. Froehlich CD, Rigby MR, Rosenberg ES, et al. Ultrasound-guided central venous catheter placement decreases complications and decreases placement attempts compared with the landmark technique in patients in a pediatric intensive care unit. Crit Care Med 2009;37(3):1090–6.

87. Grebenik CR, Boyce A, Sinclair ME, et al. NICE guidelines for central venous catheterization in children. Is the evidence base sufficient? Br J Anaesth 2004;92(6):827–30.

88. Chuan WX, Wei W, Yu L. A randomized-controlled study of ultrasound prelocation vs anatomical landmark-guided cannulation of the internal jugular vein in infants and children. Paediatr Anaesth 2005;15(9):733–8.

89. Chen L, Baker MD. Novel applications of ultrasound in pediatric emergency medicine. Pediatr Emerg Care 2007;23(2):115–23. [quiz: 124–6].

90. Ayvazyan S, Dickman E, Likourezos A, et al. Ultrasound of the inferior vena cava can assess volume status in pediatric patients. J Emerg Med 2009;37(2):219.

91. Chen L, Kim Y, Santucci KA. Use of ultrasound measurement of the inferior vena cava diameter as an objective tool in the assessment of children with clinical dehydration. Acad Emerg Med 2007;14(10):841–5.

92. Chien M, Bulloch B, Garcia-Filion P, et al. Bedside ultrasound in the diagnosis of pediatric clavicle fractures. Pediatr Emerg Care 2011;27(11):1038–41.

93. Vieira RL, Levy JA. Bedside ultrasonography to identify hip effusions in pediatric patients. Ann Emerg Med 2010;55(3):284–9.

94. Tsung JW, Blaivas M. Emergency department diagnosis of pediatric hip effusion and guided arthrocentesis using point-of-care ultrasound. J Emerg Med 2008;35(4):393–9.

95. Shavit I, Eidelman M, Galbraith R. Sonography of the hip-joint by the emergency physician: its role in the evaluation of children presenting with acute limp. Pediatr Emerg Care 2006;22(8):570–3.

96. Lichtenstein DA. Ultrasound examination of the lungs in the intensive care unit. Pediatr Crit Care Med 2009;10(6):693–8.

97. Copetti R, Cattarossi L. The "double lung point": an ultrasound sign diagnostic of transient tachypnea of the newborn. Neonatology 2007;91(3):203–9.

98. Copetti R, Cattarossi L, Macagno F, et al. Lung ultrasound in respiratory distress syndrome: a useful tool for early diagnosis. Neonatology 2008;94(1):52–9.

99. Copetti R, Copetti R, Cattarossi L, et al. Ultrasound diagnosis of pneumonia in children. Radiol Med 2008;113(2):190–8.

100. Iuri D, De Candia A, Bazzocchi M. Evaluation of the lung in children with suspected pneumonia: usefulness of ultrasonography. Radiol Med 2009;114(2):321–30.

101. Caiulo VA, Gargani L, Caiulo S, et al. Lung ultrasound in bronchiolitis: comparison with chest X-ray. Eur J Pediatr 2011;170(11):1427–33.

Pleural Disease in the Emergency Department

Erin Weldon, MD, FRCPC (EM)[a],*, Jen Williams, BScPT, MDCM, FRCPC (EM)[b]

KEYWORDS

- Pleura • Pleural effusion • Spontaneous pneumothorax
- Primary pneumothorax • Secondary pneumothorax

PLEURAL DISEASES

Introduction

The pleural cavity is traditionally considered a potential space. When disease processes cause this potential space to become a true space (filled with fluid, air, or tumor) the vital role of the pleura in lung mechanics becomes evident. Complaints related to pleural disease are common in the emergency department, with severity ranging from mild to life threatening.

Pleural Anatomy

The normal pleural anatomy consists of 2 thin layers of mesothelium that envelop a space containing a small amount of fluid on the order of 7 to 16 mL.[1,2] The pleura have 2 membranous components: the visceral and parietal pleura. The visceral pleura envelops the lung surface and invaginates between the lobes, creating the interlobar fissures. The parietal pleura lines the chest wall, diaphragm, and mediastinum and spares the hila. The superior aspect of the pleura extends 2 to 3 cm above the first rib, and the inferior aspect of the pleura ends at the sixth or seventh rib anteriorly but may extend beyond the twelfth rib posteriorly. The fact that the pleural space exists beyond the ribcage has important implications for injury during emergency procedures.[2–4] The main function of the pleural fluid and space is to allow movement of the lungs in relation to the chest wall. The pleural fluid provides a means of mechanical coupling, ensuring effective respiratory mechanics. For effective coupling to occur the volume of pleural liquid must be minimal.[5–7]

The blood supply of the parietal pleura originates from the systemic arteries that anatomically cover it. The visceral pleura is supplied by the pulmonary and bronchial

[a] Department of Emergency Medicine, University of Manitoba, T258E Old Basic Science Building, 770 Bannatyne Avenue, Winnipeg, Manitoba R3E 0W3, Canada
[b] Kingsway Emergency Agency, #541 CSC, Royal Alexandra Hospital, 10240 Kingsway Avenue, Edmonton, Alberta T5H 3V9, Canada
* Corresponding author.
E-mail address: weldy@mac.com

Emerg Med Clin N Am 30 (2012) 475–499
doi:10.1016/j.emc.2011.10.012
0733-8627/12/$ – see front matter © 2012 Elsevier Inc. All rights reserved.

emed.theclinics.com

arterial systems.[3] Sensory innervation of the parietal pleura is provided mostly by somatic intercostal nerves, with the exception of the central diaphragm, which is innervated, by the phrenic nerve. The visceral pleura has no specific nociceptors, therefore the presence of pleuritic chest pain indicates parietal pleural involvement. Pleural inflammation in the region of the central diaphragm is often referred to the ipsilateral shoulder.[8]

The lymphatic anatomy of the pleura consists of parietal pores that transfer fluid and particulate matter directly to the lymphatic system.[4,9] These lymphatic channels are a major route of drainage from the pleural space because the visceral pleura lymphatics do not connect directly to the pleural space.[3]

Pleural Effusion

Physiology and pathophysiology

Pleural fluid originates from systemic pleural vessels as well as the interstitium; homeostasis within the pleural space follows Starling's law. Intrapleural pressure is lower than the interstitial pressure of pleural tissues, favoring flow of pleural fluid into the pleural space.[7] Because pleural fluid is effectively a filtrate, the protein and cellular concentration in the fluid is typically low.[4] Normally, the influx of fluid into the pleural space is balanced by its removal via the lymphatic system. Any pathologic process that results in a loss of this homeostasis ultimately causes fluid accumulation (**Box 1**). In disease states the normal composition of pleural fluid is altered, which allows for diagnosis via pleural fluid analysis.

Cause of pleural effusion

The most common disease processes resulting in pleural effusion include congestive heart failure, malignancy, and infection.[10] The differential diagnosis of pleural effusion is extensive (**Box 2**).

Clinical features

The clinical presentation along with radiographic assessment guides diagnostic workup as well as treatment. Symptoms related to pleural effusion are dependent on the underlying disease process and the overall health of the patient's respiratory system, as well as the volume, type, and rate of accumulation of liquid occupying the pleural space. When excess volume enters the pleural space, the lungs respond by recoiling inward and the chest wall recoils outward. If the compensatory response is minimal and the lung and chest wall are of normal compliance, symptoms may be minimal. Larger effusions result in restrictive respiratory impairment with low total lung capacity, functional residual capacity, and forced vital capacity (FVC). As a result hypoxemia and ventilation-perfusion mismatch may occur.[11] Dyspnea typically occurs in the presence of large amounts of excess volume in the pleural space or if the respiratory system has abnormal underlying mechanics. Chest pain is resultant

---

Box 1
Mechanisms of fluid accumulation in the pleura

1. Increase in hydrostatic pressure

2. Decrease in oncotic pressure

3. Decrease in pleural space pressure

4. Increased permeability of vascular microcirculation

5. Blocked lymphatic drainage

6. Fluid movement from peritoneum

Box 2
Differential diagnosis of pleural effusion

Transudate

Congestive heart failure

  Nephrotic syndrome

  Liver cirrhosis

  Peritoneal dialysis

  Atelectasis

  Hypoalbuminemia

  Urinothorax

Exudate

Infectious

  Parapneumonic

  Tuberculous pleurisy

  Hepatic abscess

  Hepatitis

  Splenic abscess

  Esophageal rupture

Pulmonary embolism

Malignancy

  Mesothelioma

  Lymphoma

  Leukemia

  Metastatic

Drug-induced

  Amiodarone

  Nitrofurantoin

  Dantrolene

  Churg-Strauss syndrome

  Wegener granulomatosis

Connective tissue disease

  Lupus pleuritis

  Rheumatoid arthritis

Thoracic duct disruption

Abdominal disease

  Pancreatitis

  Esophageal perforation

Other

  Postcoronary surgery

  Ovarian hyperstimulation syndrome

  Meigs syndrome

  Dressler syndrome

  Central venous catheter migration

from inflammation of the parietal pleura[8] and cough is caused typically by lung distortion and inflammation. Classic signs of effusion include decreased breath sounds, decreased vocal fremitus, and dullness to percussion,[12] which is used to landmark for invasive procedures. Patients may also present with general signs and symptoms related to the overarching disease process underlying the pleural abnormalities. Fever is often present when effusion is secondary to an infectious process, whereas weight loss is more commonly seen in malignant and tuberculous effusions. Hemoptysis may result from neoplastic processes, tuberculosis, and pulmonary embolism. Past or recent history of trauma, pneumonia, renal failure, heart failure, liver disease, or cancer is helpful in determining a probable diagnosis.

Diagnosis

Chest radiography The initial diagnostic test is chest radiography because it is quick, readily available, and inexpensive. The effusion appearance is related to patient positioning and the cause of the fluid, as well as the stage of evolution of the collection.[2,13] A standard posteroanterior (PA) radiograph may be diagnostic of pleural effusion depending on the location and amount of pleural fluid (**Fig. 1**). Typically 175 to 200 mL of fluid are necessary to result in blunting of the costophrenic angle on PA radiography.[1,9] However, large subpulmonic collections may be present without any evidence of abnormality on radiograph.

Lateral radiography requires only 50 mL of fluid to result in posterior costodiaphragmatic angle blunting[1]; however, the lateral decubitus position is even more sensitive for fluid detection because it identifies as little as 5 to 10 mL of fluid.[2] An evolved inflammatory effusion may become loculated over time. Loculations between the lung and chest wall appear D-shaped, and loculations within fissures appear biconvex.[9] A particular challenge in the emergency department is that often patients are relatively immobile (especially in the setting of trauma or the critically ill patient), limiting imaging options to the supine view. The supine view is only moderately sensitive (67%) for the detection of pleural effusion, with an overall accuracy of 67%.[14] An indistinct hemidiaphragm, typical costophrenic angle blunting, veillike opacification

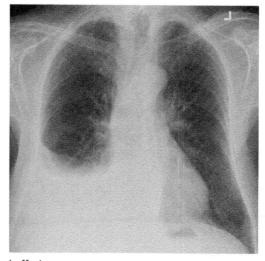

Fig. 1. Right pleural effusion.

not obscuring pulmonary arteries, thickening of fissures, and apical capping help identify effusions on a supine radiograph.[2]

Important features to note on radiography is whether the effusion is unilateral or bilateral, the general size of the effusion, and the presence or absence of other findings suggestive of diagnosis. Bilateral effusions are more consistent with the diagnosis of a transudate, typically caused by cardiac, hepatic, and renal failure. In the case of a bilateral effusion further diagnostic workup is often not needed unless there is clinical uncertainty such as with unequal bilateral effusions, nonresponse to appropriate therapy, and presence of fever or pleuritic chest pain. Large and massive pleural effusions occupying more than two-thirds of the hemithorax carry a higher incidence (55%) of malignancy.[15]

Note should also be made of radiographic findings suggestive of an underlying diagnosis such as pneumonia, cardiomegaly, mediastinal or peritoneal free air, parenchymal abnormalities, infarcts, or masses. A unilateral effusion carries a wide differential diagnosis (see **Box 2**), and thoracocentesis is typically indicated in a first presentation.[10]

Computed tomography scanning Multidetector computed tomography (CT) allows contiguous 1-mm to 3-mm sections through the chest, permitting imaging of the entire pleural space. CT is more sensitive than chest radiography and ultrasonography for differentiating pleural fluid from pleural thickening[1,2,13] and for the identification of focal pleural masses.[1] For differentiating parenchymal disease from a pleural collection and for determining the extent of pleural infection CT is unparalleled.[9,13] Disadvantages to CT include radiation exposure, the lack of availability in some emergency departments, the requirement for the patient to be able to lie supine, and, most importantly, the need to transport a potentially unstable patient out of the emergency department.[16] These limitations often preclude patients who are critically ill or in severe respiratory distress from being optimal candidates for CT scanning of the pleura.

Ultrasonography Bedside ultrasonography has become an important tool for pleural effusion detection, with advantages over conventional radiography, including real-time definitive results and no ionizing radiation exposure.[16] Ultrasonography shows higher sensitivity than radiography in the detection of free pleural effusions and may detect very small effusions with as little as 5 mL of pleural fluid.[1,16] In addition, ultrasonography can aid in differentiating transudates from exudates based on variability in echogenicity[2,13] and can be used for landmarking before thoracocentesis. In diseases of the pleura, as well as other pulmonary diseases, the diagnostic accuracy of portable ultrasonography is greater than 90% and concordance between ultrasonography and radiography is high.[16] The usefulness of portable ultrasonography is incomparable with any other diagnostic modality in the detection of pleural fluid in traumatized or critically ill supine patients and may become the routine imaging method for suspected pleural disease in the emergency department.

Magnetic resonance imaging Magnetic resonance imaging (MRI) has a limited role to play in the workup of pleural disease because of poor spatial resolution and motion artifacts.[1] MRI may be useful in select cases in which radiation is to be avoided or in patients with contrast allergies.[2]

Pleural fluid analysis The acquisition of pleural fluid for analysis is an essential step in diagnosing pleural effusions of unknown cause; however, given the many possible causes of pleural effusion, it is important for the emergency physician to develop a pre-thoracocentesis differential diagnosis based on history, physical, and diagnostic imaging because pleural fluid analysis in isolation results in a low diagnosis rate.[17] A 30-mL to 50-mL pleural fluid sample should be obtained by thoracocentesis to allow analysis of protein, lactate dehydrogenase (LDH), white blood cell count and differential, and either glucose or pH.[5] Other tests should be ordered based on clinical impression.

Thoracentesis guided by chest percussion and auscultation is safe so long as a standard chest radiograph shows a large effusion or one that layers to more than 1 cm depth on decubitus views.[13] No absolute contraindications exist for thoracentesis and the procedure is indicated for a pleural effusion when diagnosis is uncertain. Unguided thoracentesis has a pneumothorax rate of 10% to 39% and a dry tap rate of 12% to 15%.[13] For these reasons, ultrasound-guided thoracentesis is gaining momentum as the standard of care, and should be considered as an essential tool.[13]

The appearance and odor of the pleural fluid may aid in the formulation of a differential diagnosis. Empyema is the sole diagnosis that can be made at the bedside, heralded by the aspiration of pus.[5] A putrid odor is diagnostic of anaerobic infected fluid. Bloody pleural fluid suggests malignancy, pulmonary embolism, or trauma. If the pleural fluid is turbid or cloudy the diagnoses to consider are chylothorax and empyema. Transudates classically are clear straw-yellow fluid; green fluid may be suggestive of a rheumatoid effusion.[1,18] The smell of ammonia or urine indicates a pleural effusion secondary to obstructive uropathy called a urinothorax.[5] Although the appearance and odor of the fluid are often suggestive of the diagnosis, the definitive next step in confirmation is biochemical, microbiological, and cytologic pleural fluid analysis.

Light's criteria for distinguishing transudative from exudative pleural effusion The criteria used most often to distinguish a transudate from an exudate are the Light criteria and the diagnostic accuracy of these criteria is unsurpassed by any other methods.[1,18] Light's criteria consist of measurements of the LDH and protein concentration in pleural fluid and serum. Fluid is considered exudative if one of the following criteria is present.

Pleural fluid protein/serum protein ratio	>0.5
Pleural fluid LDH concentration/serum LDH concentration ratio	>0.6
Pleural fluid LDH concentration	>two-thirds the upper limit of normal serum LDH concentration

These criteria are nearly 100% sensitive for diagnosing exudates; however, the Light criteria may occasionally identify an exudate when the fluid is transudative. If clinical correlation suggests the fluid is likely transudative, either a serum-effusion gradient or a pleural fluid cholesterol measurement can be performed. A serum-effusion albumin gradient greater than 12 g/L suggests a transudate. A pleural fluid cholesterol value greater than 60 mg/dL (1.55 mmol/L) suggests an exudate.[1,10,18]

Although the Light criteria are historically the method of choice for discrimination of exudates and transudates, a meta-analysis by Heffner and colleagues[19] showed good sensitivity and specificity of alternate diagnostic test strategies. The 2-test and 3-test rules require a single criterion to be met to diagnose an exudate. With the 2-test rule either a pleural fluid cholesterol of greater than 45 mg/dL or pleural fluid LDH greater than 0.45 times the upper limit of the laboratory's normal serum LDH indicates the presence of an exudate (sensitivity 97.5%; specificity 70.4%). With the 3-test rule one of the following must be met to indicate the presence of an exudate: pleural fluid protein greater than 2.9 g/dL (29 g/L), pleural fluid cholesterol greater than cholesterol 45 mg/dL (1.165 mmol/L), pleural fluid LDH greater than 0.45 times the upper limit of the normal serum LDH level of the laboratory test (sensitivity 98.4%: specificity 70.4%).[20] The benefits of these alternate strategies include time and cost-effectiveness given that the criteria are based solely on pleural fluid tests without the requirement of serum values. Regardless of which criteria are chosen, further analysis is required if the fluid is determined to be an exudate.

Exudative pleural fluid analysis

Pleural fluid protein Pleural fluid protein is increased to a variable degree in all exudative processes and, except in the setting of tuberculosis, is not helpful in further defining the origin of an exudate. In tuberculous effusions the protein level is invariably more than 4.0 g/dL (40 g/L).[5]

Pleural fluid LDH LDH is not a sensitive or specific diagnostic marker in elucidating the cause of an effusion. LDH does generally reflect the degree of inflammation in the pleural space and therefore may be useful if serial thoracocentesis occurs. Although LDH is of limited value in the emergency department, baseline LDH and subsequent measurements can aid assessment of treatment effectiveness over time.

Pleural fluid glucose A reduced pleural fluid glucose defined as less than 60 mg/dL (3.33 mmol/L) or pleural fluid/serum of less than 0.5 is found in a limited number of disease states. These states include empyema/complicated parapneumonic effusion, malignant effusion, rheumatoid effusion, esophageal rupture, tuberculous effusion, and lupus pleuritis.[5]

Pleural fluid pH Pleural fluid pH has the greatest usefulness in parapneumonic effusions as an indicator of the need for invasive intervention. Chest tube drainage is indicated in a parapneumonic effusion with a pleural pH of less than 7.2.[21] Pleural fluid pH must be processed in the same fashion as arterial blood gases: in an anaerobic heparinized syringe, which is placed on ice and measured with a blood gas machine. Inaccuracies result when the sample is left open to air or is measured with a pH meter or indicator.

Pleural fluid amylase Pleural fluid amylase in the emergency department is most clinically useful in the setting of suspected esophageal perforation or pancreatic effusion. Pleural fluid amylase is considered increased if the pleural fluid to serum amylase ratio is greater than 1. An increased pleural fluid amylase in combination with a low pH ($\leq$6) is diagnostic of esophageal rupture, whereas pancreatic pleural effusions have pH values typically greater than 7.3.[5]

Pleural fluid hematocrit Traditionally, the hematocrit of the pleural fluid needed to be greater than 50% of blood to be considered a hemothorax.[5] Once the hematocrit of the fluid is greater than 5%, it is visually indistinguishable from blood. Within a few days of a true hemothorax, dilution of the fluid may occur, thereby reducing its hematocrit less than 50%. Thus the definition of hemothorax has been expanded to include fluid with hematocrits between 25% and 50%.[22]

Pleural fluid cell count and differential The total pleural fluid nucleated cell count is neither specific nor sensitive in the diagnosis of pleural effusion. In general counts greater than 50,000/μL indicate empyema or complicated parapneumonic effusions.[5] Total nucleated counts of greater than 10,000/μL are found in parapneumonic effusion, empyema, collagen vascular disease, and pulmonary embolism. Pleural fluid eosinophilia (defined as $\geq$10% eosinophils) may be seen in hemothorax, pneumothorax, drug-induced effusion (nitrofurantoin and dantrolene), benign asbestos effusion, parasitic and fungal infection, and malignancy. If lymphocytes predominate with greater than 80% of the total cell count, the differential may include lymphoma, chylothorax, acute lung rejection, sarcoidosis, rheumatoid pleurisy, or tuberculosis. A lymphocyte-predominant exudate indicates the need for referral for pleural biopsy.[17] The presence of mesothelial cells is uncommon in tuberculous effusions, and their presence should indicate an alternate diagnosis.[5]

Pleural fluid triglycerides, cholesterol, and chylomicrons Cholesterol and triglyceride levels are important in diagnosing lipid effusions. A chylothorax is highly likely when the pleural fluid triglyceride level is greater than 110 mg/dL (1.25 mmol/L) and unlikely if the level is less than 50 mg/dL (0.565 mmol/L). If an intermediate value is obtained, a test for chylomicrons is warranted. Identification of chylomicrons in pleural fluid indicates the presence of a chylothorax caused by the disruption of the thoracic duct. The presence of chylomicrons or triglyceride levels that are greater than 110 mg/dL (1.25 mmol/L) establishes the diagnosis.[23,24] Chylothorax is most often a result of trauma and malignancy.[25] Pseudochylothorax is usually associated with chronic diseases (such as tuberculosis), and although the fluid is also milky white, it contains cholesterol crystals instead of chylomicrons.

A cholesterol level greater than 250 mg/dL (3.075 mmol/L) identifies a cholesterol effusion, which is an effusion secondary to chronic lung entrapment in tuberculosis or rheumatoid pleuritis.[17]

Culture and gram stain Bacterial, fungal, and mycobacterial culture should be obtained for all undiagnosed exudative effusions or whenever infection is suspected. A Gram stain should be routinely performed in combination with cultures. In addition to collecting standard pleural fluid cultures it is important to inoculate blood culture bottles at the bedside because this increases the number of culture positive cases by 20.8%.[26]

Pleural fluid cytology Cytopathology is often positive in effusions caused by pleural malignancy and therefore should be performed in all patients with an undiagnosed exudate. Diagnostic yield is variable but increases with multiple separate specimens submitted.[17] Although often outside the purview of emergency department follow-up, cytologic studies should be performed if malignancy is suspected, in consultation with the appropriate specialty.

Management
Decisions regarding the management and disposition of patients with pleural effusions in the emergency department are multifactorial and dependent on the suspected disease process, the type of effusion, and the clinical acuity of the patient (**Fig. 2**). Treatment in general can be thought of in terms of (1) treatment of the underlying disease, and (2) conservative versus invasive treatment of the effusion itself. Transudates are typically managed by treating the underlying disease process, and invasive procedures are not normally indicated unless the patient requires therapeutic relief of symptoms. A symptomatic exudative effusion in which diagnostic thoracocentesis is indicated should be drained therapeutically during the same procedure unless it is determined at the bedside to be an obvious traumatic hemothorax or empyema, in which case tube thoracostomy is the definitive treatment. Once pleural fluid analysis has occurred invasive treatment with chest tube may be indicated based on the biochemical profile of the fluid, indicating the presence of hemothorax, chylothorax, or empyema. If the effusion is asymptomatic and has no indication for immediate drainage, observation and conservative management can be considered, particularly in malignant effusions.

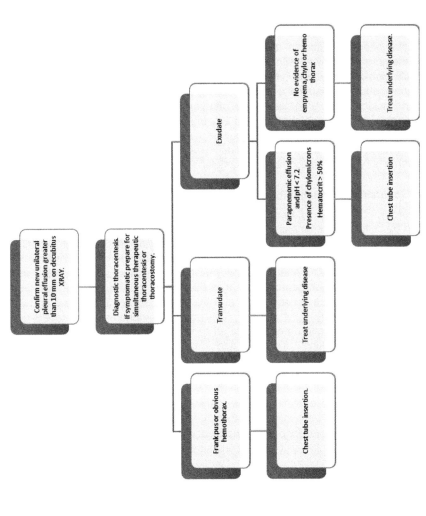

Fig. 2. Approach to new unilateral effusion in the emergency department.

The decision regarding the invasive treatment of parapneumonic effusions is of particular importance in the emergency department. Most cases of empyema are complications of ipsilateral lung infection; other causes include infection after thoracic surgery, and intra-abdominal infection.[4] Forty percent of all bacterial pneumonias are associated with pleural effusion.[27] Timeliness of definitive chest tube insertion is paramount, because a delay in intervention may lead to evolution of the collection, with loculation formation within 12 to 24 hours, thereby increasing morbidity and mortality.[21] If pleural fluid analysis suggests a complicated parapneumonic effusion/empyema a chest tube should be inserted without delay. Indications for chest tube drainage include frank pus, positive Gram stain, pleural fluid pH less than 7.2, multi-loculated effusion, and large parapneumonic effusion.[28] Traditionally, large-bore chest tubes have been indicated in the drainage of empyemas. The current literature suggests empyemas may be successfully treated with 8-F to 12-F pigtail catheters, with positioning of the catheter in the dependent part of the effusion.[21] A loculated parapneumonic effusion requires a specialized approach best addressed by CT or ultrasound-guided chest tube placement, often in combination with thrombolysis or thoracoscopy.[18] Antimicrobial therapy in the treatment of empyema should cover the most common organisms, which include anaerobes, gram-negative aerobes, and *Staphylococcus aureus*.[5] A comprehensive review of treatment and management of empyema is beyond the scope of this article.

Primary Spontaneous Pneumothorax

Epidemiology, etiology, and pathophysiology of primary spontaneous pneumothorax

Although by definition primary spontaneous pneumothorax (PSP) is a pneumothorax occurring in an individual without any apparent underlying lung disease, studies suggest there are both anatomic and histologic abnormalities that may contribute to the development of PSP.[29] Anatomic abnormalities such as subpleural blebs and bullae, referred to as emphysemalike changes (ELC), may rupture, resulting in pneumothorax. These ELCs have been found at the lung apices on CT scanning and on thoracoscopy in up to 90% of cases.[30] The major contributing factor to PSP is smoking, and bleb formation may be related to the degradation of elastic fibers in the lung induced by smoking.[31] There are additional risk factors predisposing patients to PSP that may heighten the emergency physician's suspicion for this disease process (**Box 3**). Histologic changes, termed pleural porosities, have been reported in studies[29]; however, there remains some controversy as to whether ELC or pleural porosities are the cause of PSP, given that they are not found in every individual with PSP.

The final common pathway for pneumothorax occurs once there is a break in the parietal pleura, resulting in air traveling down a pressure gradient into the intrapleural space until pressure equilibrium occurs with either partial or total lung collapse. Bleb rupture causes an air leak and releases irritant material into the pleural cavity, eosinophilic infiltration, and stimulates inflammation of the parietal pleura, resulting in chest pain.[34] Accumulation of air in the pleural space decreases vital capacity (VC) and increases the alveolar-arterial oxygen (O_2) gradient. This situation results in hypoxemia from increased shunting and a lower ventilation/perfusion ratio.[4,31,36] The amount of shunting increases with the size of pneumothorax.

Clinical features

The symptoms of PSP, which may include chest pain, dry cough, fatigue, hyperpnea, and dyspnea, are often subtle or even absent, requiring the emergency physician to maintain a high index of suspicion. Signs of PSP are also typically subtle, and may

Box 3 Risk factors for PSP	
Risk Factor	**Comments**
Male gender	• Male gender 6:1 relative risk compared with female gender[32]

Smoking	• 12% lifetime risk[3,30,31]
	• Relative risk of PSP:
	  ○ 7 times higher in light smokers (1–12 cigarettes/d)
	  ○ 21 times higher in moderate smokers (13–22 cigarettes/d)
	  ○ 80 times higher in heavy smokers (>22 cigarettes/d)[33]

Tall stature	• Taller individuals have more distending pressure at the lung apices, potentially predisposing them to apical blebs
Low body mass index (BMI, calculated as weight in kilograms divided by the square of height in meters)	• Patients with BMI <18.5 kg/m^2 have a higher risk of developing blebs[29]
Environmental factors	• Statistically significant increase in PSP 48 h after a 10-mbar drop in atmospheric pressure over 24 h[29] • Exposure to rapid environmental pressure changes such as flying and scuba diving[34]
Genetic predisposition	• Clusters of familial cases • Birt-Hogg-Dubé syndrome: autosomal-dominant condition involving skin tumors, renal carcinoma, and PSP[33]
Inhalant use	• Case reports of PSP after inhalation of nitrous oxide, marijuana, and hydrocarbons
Music	• Case series of 5 patients with PSP after exposure to loud music[35]

include reduced lung expansion, ipsilateral hyperresonance, and decreased breath sounds. Added sounds, such as clicking, may also be appreciated at the cardiac apex (**Box 4**). The size of pneumothorax cannot be judged based on the magnitude of presenting symptoms. Given the minimal symptoms, patients often delay seeking medical care, potentially increasing the risk of developing reexpansion pulmonary edema (REPE) after therapeutic lung reexpansion. Tension pneumothorax must be suspected in any patient whose signs and symptoms of respiratory distress are severe. These symptoms include cyanosis, diaphoresis, severe tachypnea, tachycardia, hypotension, distended neck veins, and reversible Horner syndrome.

Diagnosis of PSP
Imaging
Standard erect chest radiograph Standard erect chest radiograph is recommended for the initial diagnosis of pneumothorax rather than expiratory films.[37] The

Box 4
Clinical features of PSP

Symptoms:
- Chest pain
- Cough
- Hyperpnea
- Dyspnea/shortness of breath (SOB)
- Fatigue
- May be minimal/absent
- Size cannot be judged based on symptoms

Signs:
- Tachycardia (most common)
- Reduced lung expansion
- Hyperresonance
- Ipsilateral decreased breath sounds
- May have added sounds such as clicking audible at cardiac apex
- Often subtle
  - In the presence of severe respiratory distress, tachycardia, hypotension, tracheal deviation, or cyanosis tension pneumothorax must be considered

identification of displacement of the pleural line on radiography confirms the diagnosis of pneumothorax (**Fig. 3**). Up to 50% of cases may show an air-fluid level in the costophrenic angle; occasionally this is the only abnormality. Limitations of radiography include difficulty in accurately quantifying pneumothorax size and misdiagnosis of bullae as a pneumothorax. Pneumothorax size tends to be underestimated on chest radiography because it is a two-dimensional image of a three-dimensional structure.[37] The overall sensitivity of chest radiograph for pneumothorax is up to 80%.[38]

Several methods of pneumothorax measurement exist (**Tables 1** and **2**). These methods may either overestimate or underestimate the size of pneumothorax. Displacement of the pleural line by 2 cm on chest radiograph approximates a large pneumothorax occupying 50% of the hemithorax volume (**Figs. 4** and **5**). This general rule does not account for the possibility of a localized, as opposed to uniform, pneumothorax. Emergency physicians on average tend to overestimate pneumothorax size based on chest radiograph findings.[40] Lateral, expiratory, supine, and decubitus films are not routinely indicated for diagnosis.

Ultrasonography Ultrasonography provides a rapid, sensitive, and specific tool for the diagnosis of pneumothorax in the hands of an experienced operator. Patients may be scanned in the supine or sitting position. The anterior, lateral, and posterior zones must all be scanned from the apex to base using a convex probe.[41] The presence of lung sliding effectively rules out the presence of pneumothorax, with a negative predictive value of 100%.[42] The absence of lung sliding alone has 100% sensitivity but only 78% specificity for diagnosing an occult pneumothorax. When an A line is seen with the absence of lung sliding, there is 95% sensitivity and 94% specificity. The presence of comet-tail artifacts also effectively rules out a pneumothorax. The

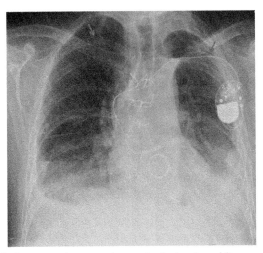

Fig. 3. Bilateral apical pneumothoraces. Arrows indicate pleural line.

presence of a lung point confers 100% specificity for occult pneumothorax.[43] Ultrasonography can also provide an accurate estimation of the size of the pneumothorax.

CT scanning Although considered the gold standard for diagnosis and size estimation of pneumothoraces, there is currently no evidence to support the use of CT scan in a first episode of PSP.[33] CT should be reserved for uncertain or complex cases of PSP, particularly in differentiating pneumothorax from bullous lung disease as well as identifying aberrant chest tube placement.[37]

Management

The goals of treatment in PSP are to remove air from the pleural space, achieve pleural-pleural apposition, and to prevent recurrences.[36] The clinical presentation is the most important determinant for management, as opposed to the pneumothorax size calculated from the chest radiography. Patients who show clinical SOB require active intervention and supportive treatments, including oxygen. All patients require referral to a respirologist for follow-up until there is full resolution, and patients must be strongly encouraged to quit smoking.[37]

Conservative management Observation is considered the treatment of choice for small PSP without any significant dyspnea.[37,44–47] Stable patients are observed in the emergency department for 3 to 6 hours while receiving supplemental oxygen. Supplemental high flow O_2 decreases the partial pressure contribution of nitrogen, thereby generating a partial pressure gradient between the pleural cavity and end capillary blood flow. O_2 alone increases the rate of pneumothorax reabsorption up to 4 times compared with room air.[30,33] Discharge from the emergency department is indicated if a repeat chest radiograph, after 3 to 6 hours of observation, fails to show any increase in size, assuming the patient or caregiver is reliable, and lives within a reasonable distance to definitive medical care. Follow-up with respiratory medicine within 12 to 48 hours must be ensured, and explicit written instructions about when to return to the emergency department (increased dyspnea) should be given.[37,44] If follow-up cannot be ensured or the patient does not live within a reasonable distance of an appropriate treatment facility, patients should be admitted to hospital or the

Table 1
Radiograph calculation methods for pneumothorax

Method	Calculation	Comments
Rhea (ACCP Guidelines [a])	Size = [interpleural distance (cm) at apex + midpoint of upper half of lung + midpoint of lower half of lung]/3 A normogram is used to convert the pneumothorax size to a volume[33,34]	The advantages of this method include standardized measurement points. The measurement is based on an absolute value, and has not been validated with digital radiography. However, this measurement may overestimate the size in a localized pneumothorax[30] and may underestimate the size of a larger pneumothorax compared with the Collins method.[33] This method requires both a PA and lateral chest radiograph for calculation
Light Index (BTS guidelines [b])	Volume of pneumothorax (%) = 100 − [(average diameter of lung)^3/(average diameter of hemothorax)^3 × 100]	The Light index is a simple measure based on proportions, making it suitable for digital radiography and the method requires only a PA chest radiograph. There is no standard level of the lung used for measurement. It may underestimate the size of small pneumothorax by up to 10% compared with the Collins method. It is more accurate in moderate and large pneumothorax
Collins	Size (%) = 4.2 + 4.7 [sum of interpleural distances at apex, midpoint upper half of collapsed lung, and midpoint lower half of collapsed lung]	This method was developed using data from helical CT scanning. It requires only a PA chest radiograph. It has not yet been validated for digital radiography and may overestimate the size of larger pneumothoraces[39]

Table 2
Large pneumothorax definitions

Guideline	Definition Large Pneumothorax	Comments
BTS	≥2 cm margin between the lateral lung edge and the chest wall	Does not allow for large apical collections
ACCP	≥3 cm intrapleural distance from the apex to cupola of the lung	Does not account for more uniform collections
Belgian	Complete dehiscence of the lung edge from the chest wall	

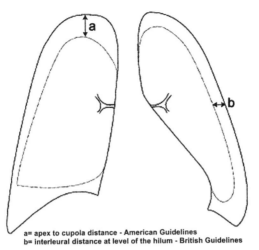

a= apex to cupola distance - American Guidelines
b= interleural distance at level of the hilum - British Guidelines

Fig. 4. Depth of pneumothorax. (*From* MacDuff A, Arnold A, Harvey J. Management of spontaneous pneumothorax: British Thoracic Society Pleural Disease Guideline 2010. Thorax 2010;65(Suppl 2):ii20. doi:10.1136/thx.2010.136986; with permission.)

emergency department observation unit.[44,48] Air travel must be avoided until complete resolution.[37]

Invasive management The British Thoracic Surgery guidelines (2010) recommend simple needle aspiration as first-line treatment of PSP.[37] The American College of Chest Physicians (ACCP) guidelines (2001) recommend either aspiration or small chest tube placement as acceptable choices.[6] A recent systemic review and meta-analysis by Aguinagalde and colleagues[49] suggested that mini-tube thoracostomy is superior to simple aspiration initially; however, there were no differences between

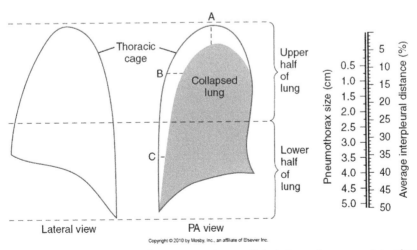

Fig. 5. Determining the size of a pneumothorax. Calculation of average interpleural distance to predict pneumothorax size. (*From* Koswsky J. Pleural disease. In: Marx J, editor. Rosen's emergency medicine, vol. 1. 7th edition. Philadelphia: Mosby Elsevier; 2010. p. 941; with permission.)

outcomes at 1 week, and minichest tubes result in greater rates of admission, with a similar recurrence rate found in both groups. A Cochrane review in 2011 looked at simple aspiration versus intercostal chest tube drainage for PSP in adults. A total of 1239 articles were identified, but only 6 met inclusion criteria, with another 5 studies excluded. The 1 study of 60 patients included, by Noppen and colleagues,[50] reported no difference in the immediate success rate or early failure of simple aspiration compared with intercostal tube drainage. However, simple aspiration did reduce the proportion of patients hospitalized (relative risk [RR] = 0.52, 95% confidence interval [CI] 0.36–0.75). There was also no significant difference in the groups with regards to duration of admission, the number of patients undergoing any lung pleurodesis procedure within 1 year of PSP, or 1-year success rate. These investigators concluded that simple aspiration is associated with a decrease in hospitalization rates compared with to chest tube thoracostomy.[51]

The initial use of suction is not recommended in PSP because of the risk of REPE. Suction is currently recommended only if an air leak persists or if lung reexpansion has not occurred at 48 to 72 hours. However, failure to reexpand or a persistent air leak may be an indication for early surgical consultation and intervention rather than initiation of suction.[37]

Large-bore chest tubes are not recommended in the initial management of PSP.[37] Certain populations and presentations of spontaneous pneumothorax may benefit from further subspecialized invasive intervention (**Box 5**). These interventions include video-assisted thoracoscopic surgery, limited axillary thoracotomy surgery, open thoracotomy, and chemical pleurodesis.

Complications

REPE REPE is a rare complication of rapid reexpansion of the lung after a more prolonged period of collapse (>3 days) occurring in less than 1% of patients. Typically

---

Box 5
Factors in the management of pneumothorax

Factors that should be taken into account when determining the management of pneumothorax include:

- Age
- Primary versus secondary
- Presence of significant SOB
- Pneumothorax size
- Operator experience
- Patient choice

Indications for surgical intervention[33]:

- Second ipsilateral pneumothorax
- First contralateral pneumothorax
- Bilateral pneumothorax
- Persistent air leak
- Spontaneous hemothorax
- Professions at risk
  - Includes pilots and scuba divers

REPE occurs in younger patients, aged 20 to 39 years;, however, the mortality is upwards of 20%. Clinical features include coughing, hypoxia, and hypotension usually within 1 hour of lung reinflation. Negative suction pressures of more than 20 cm H_2O have been implicated and thus should be avoided. Treatment is primarily supportive, including O_2, mechanical ventilation, and diuretics.[52]

Secondary Spontaneous Pneumothorax

Epidemiology, etiology, and pathophysiology of secondary spontaneous pneumothorax

By definition, secondary spontaneous pneumothorax (SSP) requires underlying lung disease as a precipitant of pneumothorax. These patients have chronic respiratory symptoms, impaired pulmonary function, and abnormalities seen on chest radiography or other imaging studies.[36] The most common underlying condition is chronic obstructive pulmonary disease (COPD), accounting for 70% of cases.[53] The incidence of SSP is similar to that of PSP amongst the general population.[36] Patients tend to be older than 50 years, and the occurrence of a pneumothorax in these patients suggests potentially more severe disease. Patients with a forced expiratory volume in 1 second (FEV$_1$) less than 1 L or an FEV$_1$/FVC ratio of less than 40% are at greater risk of SSP.[11,36,53] The most common underlying cause in COPD is the rupture of blebs or bullae. The morbidity and mortality of SSP in patients with COPD is significant, with 1 case series reporting a mortality of 16%.[36]

Another important cause of SSP is human immunodeficiency disease (HIV) disease. SSP is a frequent complication in untreated HIV infection as a complication of opportunistic infections and tumors.[34] Pneumothorax occurs in 2% to 5% of patients with AIDS in association with subpleural necrosis from *Pneumocystis* infection.[31,54]

An important cause of SSP in women is catamenial pneumothorax, also known as thoracic endometriosis syndrome. Endometrial implants on the diaphragm or thoracic cavity may occur[31] and are underdiagnosed in women with pneumothorax.[30] Other underlying conditions that have been implicated in SSP are found in **Box 6**.

Clinical features

The signs and symptoms of SSP are similar to, but often more severe than, those of PSP. SSP can be a life-threatening complication of the patient's underlying lung disease. Dyspnea of rapid and progressive onset is typical and is usually associated with pleuritic chest pain. The dyspnea is often out of proportion to the size of pneumothorax because of the poor underlying cardiorespiratory reserve. Patients may become cyanotic and hypotensive; sudden death has been reported before chest tube insertion.[36] Physical signs are often more subtle compared with PSP because hyperinflation is already present, and breath sounds are usually distant across all lung fields. Thus hyperresonance and decreased tactile fremitus are more difficult to appreciate. Subcutaneous emphysema, seen in patients with severe COPD, may also obscure pneumothorax physical findings.

Diagnosis of SSP
Imaging
Chest radiography Chest radiograph is less reliable in diagnosing pneumothorax in patients with underlying lung disease. The radiographic appearance of pneumothorax is altered by the loss of elastic recoil and the presence of air trapping in the diseased lung.[36] Bullous emphysematic changes can be mistaken for pneumothorax and vice versa. A distinguishing feature is the presence of a visceral pleural line in pneumothorax. The visceral pleural line is also difficult to distinguish because the lungs are already hyperlucent, and there is minimal difference in radiographic density between the

---

Box 6
Etiology of SSP[54]

- Airway disease
  - COPD
  - Status asthmaticus
  - Cystic fibrosis
  - Neonates with hyaline membrane disease
- Interstitial lung disease
  - Sarcoidosis
  - Idiopathic pulmonary fibrosis
  - Lyphangiomyomatosis
  - Tuberous sclerosis
  - Pneumoconiosis
- Infectious (leading cause in developing countries)
  - Tuberculosis
  - Necrotizing bacterial pneumonia/lung abscess
  - HIV/AIDS
    - *Pneumocystis jirovecii*
- Neoplasm
  - Primary lung cancers
  - Pulmonary and pleural malignancies
- Vascular
  - Pulmonary infarct
- Drug use
- Connective tissue disease
- Catamenial pneumothorax /thoracic endometriosis

From Koswsky J. Pleural disease. In: Marx J, editor. Rosen's emergency medicine, vol. 1. 7th edition. Philadelphia: Mosby Elsevier; 2010. p. 941; with permission.

---

emphysematous lung and the pneumothorax. The absence of air bronchograms should be noted, because these suggest the presence of an obstructing lesion.

Ultrasonography Ultrasonography is the easiest, fastest, and most accurate manner to diagnose pneumothorax from any cause. Theoretically, comet tailing on ultrasonography may help distinguish bullae from pneumothorax because it confirms the presence of pleural sliding and the absence of pneumothorax; however, accuracy is affected by the number of places on the chest wall that are scanned.[52] The presence of lung sliding in multiple fields confirms the absence of pneumothorax.

CT scanning Because of the difficulties both clinically and radiographically in determining bullous disease from SSP, CT of the chest is the diagnostic modality of choice if the presence of pneumothorax is in question. In addition to diagnosis, CT of the chest aids with management because it can guide the best location to insert a chest tube as well as identifying the presence of obstructing lesions, such as mucous plugging or mass, which should be managed with bronchoscopy rather than chest tube drainage.[36]

Management Management options of SSP are the same as PSP. However, because pneumothorax is a potentially life-threatening complication of the underlying lung disease, management is more aggressive in SSP. There is greater consensus amongst the available guidelines, indicating the need for admission and chest tube thoracostomy. Recent studies have suggested that a small chest tube is as effective as a large-bore chest tube for drainage in SSP.[37] In general all patients with SSP should be admitted to hospital for at least 24 hours and receive supplemental O_2, with most patients requiring insertion of a small chest tube.[30] Aspiration is less likely to be successful, but can be considered in symptomatic patients with a small pneumothorax in the effort to avoid placing a chest tube.[30] Approximately 20% of patients with COPD and SSP fail to reexpand the lung or have a persistent air leak at 15 days after chest tube insertion, and the use of suction has not been shown to improve this.[36] Despite this situation, ACCP guidelines recommend the use of suction if the pneumothorax fails to resolve with water-seal alone.[6] In addition, the risk of recurrence is higher in SSP than PSP. As a result, consideration of additional invasive treatments including video-assisted thoracoscopic surgery, open thoracotomy, or pleurodesis is suggested. The British Thoracic Society algorithm for the management of primary and secondary spontaneous pneumothoraces is seen in **Fig. 6**.

Pediatric Considerations in Spontaneous and Secondary Pneumothorax

Epidemiology and cause
Most information on pediatric spontaneous pneumothorax has been extrapolated from adult studies.[33] The exact incidence in the pediatric population of PSP is unknown. PSP can occur in all age groups, including in neonates, with a mean age of 14 to 15.9 years at presentation. There is a male predominance (range 65%–81%)[33]; however, there may be no gender difference in patients less than 9 years.[33] As with adults, there is preponderance for left-side PSP. Recurrence of PSP seems to be higher in children, occurring in 50% to 61% of cases; however, only 1 study separated SSP cases from PSP.

Pathophysiology
Blebs and bullae have a lower incidence in pediatric cases of PSP: 28% compared with the 56% to 88% incidence reported in the adult literature.[33] However, in bilateral PSP, there seems to be a larger association of emphysemalike changes in children (78%) compared with adults (15%–66%).

Clinical features
PSP occurs most commonly at rest, or may be precipitated by any maneuver increasing intrathoracic pressure. Signs and symptoms are similar to those found in adults. However, in children symptoms often resolve within 24 hours even with persistent pneumothorax.[33]

Diagnosis
Erect chest radiography helps confirm the clinical presentation of PSP. Expiratory, lateral, and lateral decubitus views may be of some benefit for small PSP, but they are not routinely indicated.[33] It is unknown if the calculations given for adult pneumothorax size on chest radiograph may be applied to a pediatric chest radiograph.

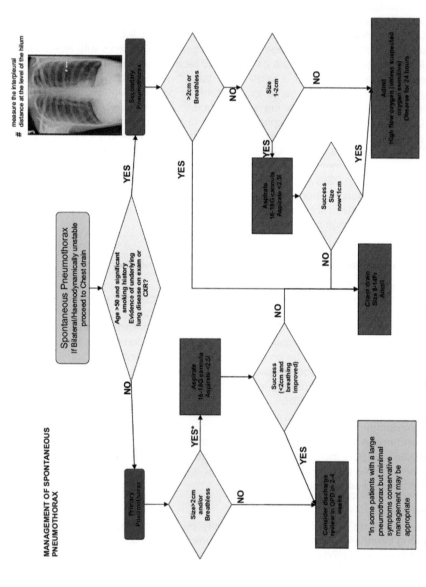

Fig. 6. Management of spontaneous pneumothorax. (*From* MacDuff A, Arnold A, Harvey J. Management of spontaneous pneumothorax: British Thoracic Society Pleural Disease Guideline 2010. Thorax 2010;65(Suppl 2):ii21. doi:10.1136/thx.2010.136986; with permission.)

Management and disposition

There are no pediatric specific management guidelines for PSP. The speed of resolution has not been documented in the pediatric population. Options are the same as described in the section on adult management.

SSP

Similar to adults, there is a lower threshold for hospital admission and need for chest tube thoracostomy in children with SSP because there is a higher failure rate of simple aspiration. The mortality may be especially high in SSP related to underlying cystic fibrosis.[33]

Spontaneous Hemothorax and Spontaneous Hemopneumothorax

Epidemiology and cause

Most hemothoraces results from trauma: blunt, penetrating, or iatrogenic. Spontaneous hemothorax is relatively rare, with approximately 300 cases in the literature in the form of case reports or case series.[22]

Spontaneous hemothorax associated with PSP occurs in 2% to 7% of cases. It is typically characterized by a large amount of blood in the pleural cavity, sometimes in excess of 400 mL.[31] It generally occurs in younger patients, with a mean age of 22 to 34 years.[22,55] Other causes include drug-induced spontaneous hemothorax secondary to warfarin or heparin, vascular causes such as aortic dissection or arteriovenous malformation, and thoracic endometriosis. Any bilateral spontaneous hemothorax should be considered a manifestation of tumor, especially angiosarcoma, until proved otherwise.[22] Aortic dissection is the most predominant vascular cause for spontaneous hemothorax. Thoracic endometriosis is shown by recurrent signs, symptoms, and radiographic changes associated with menstruation, including chest pain, dyspnea, pneumothorax, hemothorax, hemoptysis, or pulmonary nodules.[22]

Clinical features

The signs and symptoms of spontaneous hemothorax include sudden-onset pleuritic chest pain or dyspnea, diaphoresis (cold sweat), and potentially hemodynamic instability or shock depending on the extent of blood loss or accompanying tension.

Diagnosis

The diagnosis is made using the same modalities as described in spontaneous pneumothorax. Spontaneous hemopneumothorax shows a pneumothorax associated with an air-fluid line.[55] Pleural fluid should be tapped and sent for hematocrit to confirm hemothorax.

Management

Spontaneous hemopneumothorax General treatment of spontaneous hemopneumothorax requires either immediate chest tube drainage or surgical management by thoracic surgery. Specific management is determined by the most likely underlying cause. A large chest tube should always be used (36–42F) to aid with complete drainage and avoid clot formation or retention. Empiric antibiotics are recommended after chest tube insertion as prophylaxis against empyema formation and pneumonia.[56] Generally, if bleeding persists less than 24 hours, chest tube drainage is considered adequate treatment.[57]

If the patient is hemodynamically unstable, drains greater than 500 mL/h in the first hour, or drains greater than 200 to 300 mL/h, early surgical intervention is required in addition to ongoing resuscitation. In addition, patients who rebleed after lung expansion or fail conservative management after 24 hours also require surgical intervention.

Generally spontaneous hemopneumothorax is considered a potential surgical emergency because the bleeding can continue without physiologic control.

Spontaneous tension pneumothorax Traditionally the diagnosis of tension pneumothorax was considered only in the context of trauma or iatrogenic causes such as a misplaced chest tube or in a patient undergoing positive pressure ventilation. However, the diagnosis of spontaneous tension pneumothorax should be considered even in a patient who is clinically well. Young patients with good physiologic reserve often seem clinically stable, but have the potential for rapid deterioration and cardiac arrest.[58]

Tension pneumothorax is not necessarily easily defined. The definition of positive intrapleural pressure present throughout the respiratory cycle[59] cannot be applied to awake patients because the intrapleural pressure must be less than atmospheric pressure for at least part of the respiratory cycle for the pneumothorax to continue to develop (ie, air must continue to enter the pleural cavity).[58] Varying definitions of tension pneumothorax in the literature include severe clinical manifestations, hearing a hiss of air on thoracic needle decompression, mediastinal shift or diaphragmatic depression on chest radiography, hemodynamic compromise that improves with air release on tube thoracostomy, or expanding pneumothorax.[58]

A better term than tension pneumothorax may be expanding pneumothorax: Any pleural defect communicating with the atmosphere and functioning as a 1-way valve allows air to enter the pleural cavity on inspiration. This air cannot exit with expiration, resulting in further lung collapse, ipsilateral chest wall expansion, diaphragmatic depression, and eventual contralateral lung compression (depending on mediastinal distensability).

Clinically, a pneumothorax should be considered to be under tension when it results in significant and progressive respiratory or hemodynamic compromise that reverses on decompression alone (ie, without thoracostomy tube placement).

Signs and symptoms of tension pneumothorax in an awake patient universally include chest pain and respiratory distress. Other reliable early findings include air hunger, tachypnea, tachycardia, agitation, and decreased oxygen saturations. Ipsilateral decreased air entry occurs commonly (50%–75% of cases). Inconsistent findings (<25%) include decreased oxygen saturations, tracheal deviation, and hypotension. Rare findings (<10%) include cyanosis, hyperresonance, distended neck veins, decreasing level of consciousness, ipsilateral chest hyperexpansion and hypomobility, acute epigastric pain, cardiac apical displacement, and sternal resonance.[58]

In patients who are hemodynamically unstable, immediate needle thoracostomy should be attempted while preparing for tube thoracostomy, the definitive treatment, before imaging studies. If patients are stable, imaging (as discussed in previous sections) may occur before the diagnosis. Chest tube thoracostomy and admission are required in all patients with spontaneous tension pneumothorax.

SUMMARY

The crucial role of the pleura in respiratory function often becomes evident only when disease processes cause pain or an imbalance in intrapleural pressure and fluid homeostasis. The emergency physician has an important role to play in the acute assessment, diagnosis, and treatment of pleural disease, which often involves invasive maneuvers such as thoracocentesis and thoracostomy. Timeliness of interventions and treatment can improve morbidity and mortality, especially in critically ill patients, and it is incumbent on the emergency physician to have a systematic approach to pleural disease that allows for rapid recognition, diagnosis, and definitive management.

REFERENCES

1. Froudarakis M. Diagnostic work-up of pleural effusions. Respiration 2008;75(1): 4–13.
2. Ayres J, Gleeson F. Imaging of the pleura. Semin Respir Crit Care Med 2010;31(6): 674–88.
3. Finley DJ, Rusch VW. Anatomy of the pleura. Thorac Surg Clin 2011;21(2): 157–63.
4. English JC, Leslie KO. Pathology of the pleura. Clin Chest Med 2006;27(2): 157–80.
5. Sahn SA. State of the art. The pleura. Am Rev Respir Dis 1988;138(1):184–234.
6. Baumann MH, Strange C, Heffner JE, et al. Management of spontaneous pneumothorax: an American College of Chest Physicians Delphi consensus statement. Chest 2001;119(2):590–602.
7. Zocchi L. Physiology and pathophysiology of pleural fluid turnover. Eur Respir J 2002;20(6):1545–58.
8. Brims FJ, Davies HE, Lee YC. Respiratory chest pain: diagnosis and treatment. Med Clin North Am 2010;94(2):217–32.
9. Quigley RL. Thoracentesis and chest tube drainage. Crit Care Clin 1995;11(1): 111–26.
10. McGrath EE, Anderson PB. Diagnosis of pleural effusion: a systematic approach. Am J Crit Care 2011;20(2):119–27 [quiz: 128].
11. Ferrer J, Roldán J. Clinical management of the patient with pleural effusion. Eur J Radiol 2000;34(2):76–86.
12. Lombardi G, Zustovich F, Nicoletto M, et al. Diagnosis and treatment of malignant pleural effusion. Am J Clin Oncol 2010;33(4):420–3.
13. Heffner J, Klein J, Hampson C. Diagnostic utility and clinical application of imaging for pleural space infections. Chest 2010;137(2):467–79.
14. Ruskin J, Gurney J. Detection of pleural effusions on supine chest radiographs. AJR Am J Roentgenol 1987;148(4):681–3.
15. Porcel JM. Etiology and pleural fluid characteristics of large and massive effusions. Chest 2003;124(3):978–83.
16. Zanobetti M, Poggioni C, Pini R. Can chest ultrasonography replace standard chest radiography for evaluation of acute dyspnea in the ED? Chest 2011; 139(5):1140–7.
17. Sahn S. The value of pleural fluid analysis. Am J Med Sci 2008;335(1):7–15.
18. Light RW. Management of pleural effusions. J Formos Med Assoc 2000;99(7): 523–31.
19. Heffner J. Discriminating between transudates and exudates. Clin Chest Med 2006;27(2):241–52.
20. Heffner JE, Brown LK, Barbieri CA, et al. Diagnostic value of tests that discriminate between exudative and transudative pleural effusions. Chest 1997;111(4): 970–80.
21. Light RW. Parapneumonic effusions and empyema. Proc Am Thorac Soc 2006; 3(1):75–80.
22. Ali HA, Lippmann M, Mundathaje U, et al. Spontaneous hemothorax: a comprehensive review. Chest 2008;134(5):1056–65.
23. Skouras V, Kalomenidis I. Chylothorax: diagnostic approach. Curr Opin Pulm Med 2010;16(4):387–93.
24. Light R. Pneumothorax. In: Light R, editor. Pleural diseases. Baltimore (MD): Williams & Wilkins; 1991. p. 242–77.

25. Huggins JT. Chylothorax and cholesterol pleural effusion. Semin Respir Crit Care Med 2011;31(06):743–50.
26. Menzies SM, Rahman NM, Wrightson JM, et al. Blood culture bottle culture of pleural fluid in pleural infection. Thorax 2011;66(8):658–62.
27. Light RW, Rodriguez RM. Management of parapneumonic effusions. Clin Chest Med 1998;19(2):373–82.
28. Lim TK. Management of parapneumonic pleural effusion. Curr Opin Pulm Med 2001;7(4):193–7.
29. Porcel JM, Lee YC. Pleural disease. 2011. Available at: http://www.wiley.com/bw/vi.asp?ref=1323-7799#706. Accessed July 7, 2011.
30. MacDuff A, Arnold A, Harvey J. Management of spontaneous pneumothorax: British Thoracic Society Pleural Disease Guideline 2010. Thorax 2010;65(Suppl 2): ii18–31.
31. Humphries Roger L , Young JW. Spontaneous and iatrogenic pneumothorax. In: Tintinalli JE, Stapczynski JS, Cline DM, et al, editors. Tintinalli's emergency medicine: a comprehensive study guide. 7th edition. New York (NY): McGraw-Hill Medical; 2010. p. 471–4.
32. Hassani B, Foote J, Borgundvaag B. Outpatient management of primary spontaneous pneumothorax in the emergency department of a community hospital using a small-bore catheter and a Heimlich valve. Acad Emerg Med 2009; 16(6):513–8.
33. Robinson PD, Cooper P, Ranganathan SC. Evidence-based management of paediatric primary spontaneous pneumothorax. Paediatr Respir Rev 2009; 10(3):110–7 [quiz: 117].
34. Yazkan R, Han S. Pathophysiology, clinical evaluation and treatment options of spontaneous pneumothorax. Tuberk Toraks 2010;58(3):334–43.
35. Haynes D, Baumann MH. Pleural controversy: etiology of pneumothorax. Respirology 2011;16(4):604–10.
36. Shen KR, Cerfolio RJ. Decision making in the management of secondary spontaneous pneumothorax in patients with severe emphysema. Thorac Surg Clin 2009; 19(2):233–8.
37. Maskell N. British Thoracic Society pleural disease guidelines–2010 update. Thorax 2010;65(8):667–9.
38. Harrigan R, DeAngelis M. Evaluation and management of patients with chest syndromes. In: Mattu A, Goyal D, editors. Emergency medicine: avoiding the pitfalls and improving the outcomes. 1st edition. Maldon (MA): Blackwell Publishing; 2007. p. 1–16.
39. Druda D, Kelly AM. What is the difference in size of spontaneous pneumothorax between inspiratory and expiratory x-rays? Emerg Med J 2009;26(12):861–3.
40. Paoloni R. Management and outcome of spontaneous pneumothoraces at three urban EDs. Emerg Med Australas 2007;19(5):449–57.
41. Barillari A, Kiuru S. Detection of spontaneous pneumothorax with chest ultrasound in the emergency department. Intern Emerg Med 2010;5(3):253–5.
42. Lichtenstein DA. Ultrasound in the management of thoracic disease. Crit Care Med 2007;35(Suppl):S250–61.
43. Lichtenstein DA, Mezi re G, Lascols N, et al. Ultrasound diagnosis of occult pneumothorax. Crit Care Med 2005;33(6):1231–8.
44. Baumann MH. Pneumothorax. Semin Respir Crit Care Med 2001;22(6):647–56.
45. Kelly AM. Review of management of primary spontaneous pneumothorax: is the best evidence clearer 15 years on? Emerg Med Australas 2007;19(4): 303–8.

46. Marquette CH, Marx A, Leroy S, et al. Simplified stepwise management of primary spontaneous pneumothorax: a pilot study. Eur Respir J 2006;27(3):470–6.
47. Kelly AM, Kerr D, Clooney M. Outcomes of emergency department patients treated for primary spontaneous pneumothorax. Chest 2008;134(5):1033–6.
48. Kuan WS, Lather KS, Mahadevan M. Primary spontaneous pneumothorax–the role of the emergency observation unit. Am J Emerg Med 2011;29(3):293–8.
49. Aguinagalde B, Zabaleta J, Fuentes M, et al. Percutaneous aspiration versus tube drainage for spontaneous pneumothorax: systematic review and meta-analysis. Eur J Cardiothorac Surg 2010;37(5):1129–35.
50. Noppen M, Alexander P, Driesen P, et al. Manual aspiration versus chest tube drainage in first episodes of primary spontaneous pneumothorax: a multicenter, prospective, randomized pilot study. Am J Respir Crit Care Med 2002;165(9):1240–4.
51. Wakai AP. Spontaneous pneumothorax. Clin Evid (Online) Jan. 2010. Available at: http://clinicalevidence.bmj.com.proxy1.lib.umanitoba.ca/ceweb/conditions/rda/1505/1505.jsp. Accessed July 7, 2011.
52. Wills CP, Young M, White DW. Pitfalls in the evaluation of shortness of breath. Emerg Med Clin North Am 2010;28(1):163–81, ix.
53. Nakajima J. Surgery for secondary spontaneous pneumothorax. Curr Opin Pulm Med 2010;16(4):376–80.
54. Koswsky J. Pleural disease. In: Marx J, editor. Rosen's emergency medicine, vol. 1. 7th edition. Philadelphia: Mosby Elsevier; 2010. p. 939–46.
55. Hsu NY, Shih CS, Hsu CP, et al. Spontaneous hemopneumothorax revisited: clinical approach and systemic review of the literature. Ann Thorac Surg 2005;80(5):1859–63.
56. Reddy NS, Hornick P. Haemothorax. Br J Hosp Med (Lond) 2007;68(4):M71–3.
57. Patterson BO, Itam S, Probst F. Spontaneous tension haemopneumothorax. Scand J Trauma Resusc Emerg Med 2008;16:12.
58. Holloway VJ, Harris JK. Spontaneous pneumothorax: is it under tension? J Accid Emerg Med 2000;17(3):222–3.
59. Brims FJ. Primary spontaneous tension pneumothorax in a submariner at sea. Emerg Med J 2004;21(3):394–5.

Diagnosis and Management of Environmental Thoracic Emergencies

Paul D. Tourigny, MD, FRCPC[a,b,]*, Chris Hall, MD, FRCPC[a]

KEYWORDS

- Diving • Drowning • Altitude • Pulmonary • Environmental
- Toxins

Environmental thoracic illness encompasses a diverse set of conditions. Physiologic sequelae from increasing ambient pressure in underwater activities, decreasing ambient pressure while at altitude, or the consequences of drowning present a unique set of challenges to emergency physicians. In addition, several environmental toxins cause significant respiratory morbidity; whether they be pulmonary irritants, simple asphyxiants, or systemic toxins. It is important for emergency physicians to understand the pathophysiology of these illnesses, as well as to apply this knowledge to the clinical arena either in the prehospital setting or in the emergency department.

This review examines the pathophysiology underlying each of these processes and marries this pathophysiology to their clinical presentations. Current treatment paradigms and controversies within these regimens are discussed.

DIVING-RELATED THORACIC EMERGENCIES

Dive-related illness will become increasingly common in North America as more people access this recreational opportunity and as technology allows commercial divers to attain ever greater depths. More than 7 million people are known to participate in submersion-based activities worldwide, and more than 500,000 new divers are trained each year.[1]

The thoracic presentations of diving-related emergencies related to breath-hold diving and scuba diving are reviewed to provide emergency physicians with a working

The authors have nothing to disclose.
a Division of Emergency Medicine, Foothills Medical Centre, University of Calgary, 1403-29 Street Northwest, Calgary, Alberta, Canada T2N2T9
b Shock Trauma Air Rescue Society, Calgary, Alberta, Canada
* Corresponding author. Division of Emergency Medicine, Foothills Medical Centre, University of Calgary, 1403-29 Street Northwest, Calgary, Alberta, Canada T2N2T9.
E-mail address: pauldtourigny@mac.com

Emerg Med Clin N Am 30 (2012) 501–528
doi:10.1016/j.emc.2011.10.006
0733-8627/12/$ – see front matter © 2012 Elsevier Inc. All rights reserved.

emed.theclinics.com

understanding of the consequences of these activities. Diagnostic and treatment paradigms for immersion pulmonary edema, arterial gas embolism (AGE)/decompression sickness, and pulmonary barotrauma comprising respiratory tract hemorrhage, pneumothorax, pneumomediastinum, pneumopericardium, and subcutaneous emphysema are discussed.

Pathophysiology

Unlike altitude, small changes in underwater depth result in profound changes in ambient pressure. At the 8850-m (29,035-ft) summit of Mount Everest, atmospheric pressure is one-third that of sea level. Conversely, 1 additional atmosphere of pressure is added with each 10 m (33 ft) increase in depth once submerged.

Most thoracic injury that occurs during submersion is a consequence of gas laws that describe the physical behavior of liquids and gases. Dalton's law states that the total pressure exerted by a mixture of gases is equal to the partial pressures of each individual gas within the mixture and that each gas acts as if it alone occupied the entire volume.[2] Henry's law states that the amount of a given gas that dissolves in a given type and volume of liquid is directly proportional to the partial pressure of that gas in equilibrium with that liquid.[2] Boyle's law states that the pressure of a gas and the volume of a gas are inversely related. Pascal's law reminds us that a pressure applied to any part of a liquid is applied throughout that liquid equally. The human body at depth acts predominantly as a liquid.[2] The physical manifestations of these laws allow us to interpret the phenomena that occur during descent, at depth, during ascent, and during the postdive period. **Table 1** outlines the clinical implications of these laws.

Increased Work of Breathing

Although technically not an injury, physicians should understand the pathophysiology underlying the increased work required to breathe while using an underwater

Table 1
Clinical implications of submersion-related gas laws

Gas Law	Clinical Significance
Boyle's law: the pressure and volume of a gas are inversely related at a constant temperature. As pressure decreases, the volume of the inspired gas increases	AGE Pulmonary barotrauma: pneumothorax, pneumomediastinum, pneumopericardium, respiratory tract hemorrhage
Dalton's law: the pressure exerted by a gas mixture is the sum of the partial pressures of each different gas making up the mixture but each gas acts as if it alone occupies the entire volume. At depth, more molecules of gas are inspired	Decompression sickness
Henry's law: the partial pressure of a gas is directly proportional to the amount of that gas that dissolves in a liquid at a given temperature. At increasing depths, more nitrogen is taken into serum and tissues	Decompression sickness
Pascal's law: pressure applied to any part of a liquid is applied throughout that liquid equally. At depth, the human body acts as a liquid	Respiratory hemorrhage from compression of the entire respiratory tract during breath-hold diving

breathing apparatus. Thoracic venous return is increased immediately on immersion, causing a decrease in pulmonary compliance.[3] Increased density of breathing gas at depth (Boyle's law) as well as the resistance inherent to the breathing apparatus cause increased airway resistance and ventilation/perfusion mismatch.[1] This combination of factors results in an increased work of breathing.[1] Simple fatigue remains in the differential diagnosis for postdive dyspnea presentations but must remain a diagnosis of exclusion.

IMMERSION PULMONARY EDEMA
Pathophysiology and Incidence

Believed to be similar to swimming-induced pulmonary edema, immersion pulmonary edema can be lethal.[4–6] The mechanism behind this form of pulmonary edema is unclear. Capillary stress failure from the increased pulmonary blood volume seen in immersion and release of cardiac peptides causing diuretic, natriuretic, and vasodilatory responses resulting in increased capillary permeability have been proposed as possible causes.[4,6] The increased work of breathing secondary to higher inspiratory resistance may help breach the alveolar-capillary barrier and contribute to this phenomenon.[7,8]

The pulmonary edema seen in breath-hold diving may have a different pathogenesis. Within breath-hold diving, most injury is caused by mechanical compression as a result of increased ambient pressure. As pressure increases, atelectasis, compression of alveoli, and further distortion to pulmonary architecture occur. This situation results in fluid filtration into extraluminal spaces and disruption of the alveolar-capillary junction.[3] The 2 latter mechanisms, along with increased thoracic blood flow from immersion, are believed to be responsible for cases of pulmonary edema in breath-hold divers.[5,9–12]

Immersion pulmonary edema remains a rare phenomenon; in 2007, 9 dive injuries reported to the Divers Alert Network were believed to be immersion pulmonary edema.[13]

Clinical Features

Cold water, exertion, predive fluid loading, inspiratory resistance, and low vital capacity are all believed to predispose to this condition.[4,14–17] The incidence of diving-related pulmonary immersion is unknown but has been described for 30 years.[18] Immersion pulmonary edema invariably begins submersed, allowing for the distinction of this entity from decompression illness (DCI) (see **Table 1**).[19] Hemoptysis may be of the initial presenting features of immersion pulmonary edema, but hypoxia, dyspnea, tachycardia, and chest pain should lead the clinician to consider this diagnosis.[20]

DCI AND PULMONARY BAROTRAUMA

As depth increases, greater absolute amounts of the gases that comprise the dive-gas mixture (nitrogen, oxygen, and sometimes helium) are inspired and increased quantities of those gases are dissolved in body tissues and fluids. As a diver ascends toward the surface, these gases begin to come out of solution. If the rate of ambient pressure reduction is greater than the rate of washout of gas from tissues and fluid, supersaturation occurs and bubbles can form in the intravascular and extravascular spaces.[21] As ascent occurs and pressure decreases, the size of these bubbles increases in accordance with Boyle's law. Decompression sickness I and II (DCS I and II), AGE, and pulmonary barotraumas (hemoptysis, pneumothorax, pneumopericardium, and pneumomediastinum) can all result from this supersaturation.

DCI

Pathophysiology and incidence

Historically, decompression sickness was divided in to 2 groups. Cutaneous symptoms, pain, and constitutional symptoms comprised DCS I, whereas all more serious manifestations were considered DCS II. This distinction offered little predictive value as to who required recompression therapy or who would evolve to have a worse outcome. Along with AGE, DCS I and DCS II are now grouped under the common term DCI because the treatment of all 3 is essentially the same.

AGE as well as DCS I and II are caused by the appearance of bubbles (predominantly nitrogen) within tissues or vascular spaces. Aside from mechanical compression of tissue, bubbles can cause emboliclike obstruction of vascular structures and can activate an inflammatory cascade.[22,23] Endothelial damage results in capillary leak, extravasation of plasma, and hemoconcentration, platelet activation, and deposition as well as leukocyte-endothelial adhesion.[21,22] The complement, kinin, fibrinolytic, and coagulation cascades are activated, resulting in a complex inflammatory response.[1] Although grouped together with DCS I and II because of the significant overlap in pathophysiology and clinical presentation, the most extreme clinical presentation of AGE acts more like pulmonary barotrauma and is considered in a separate section of this review.

In a sample of 135,000 dives by 9000 recreational divers, the Divers Alert Network found a rate of DCI of 0.03%.[13,21] This rate reflects the safety parameters built in to modern recreational dive tables. US Navy (USN) divers have shown rates of DCI of 0.03% for operational dives to 4.4% when designing new protocols for decompression.[24,25] More than 100 reports exist in case-report literature with symptoms consistent with decompression sickness after repeated breath-hold dives; these are predominantly noted amongst commercial breath-hold divers.[26] Theoretic calculations using the USN Dive Tables show that it is possible for breath-hold divers to violate no-decompression limits using repeated dives with limited surface intervals.[27]

Risk factors

Many factors can influence the likelihood of DCS I and II. The appearance of decompression sickness is directly affected by the length and depth of a dive because its occurrence is the physiologic consequence of Henry's law. Nearly 80% of all reported cases of DCI involved the proper adherence to dive tables through the use of dive charts or dive computers.[13] The act of immersion (as opposed to dry hyperbaric environments) seems to increase the risk for DCI. The increased thoracic venous return and cardiac output are believed to be responsible for this risk.[21] Temperature can have an effect in 2 separate ways: warm dive environments promote vasodilation, leading to an increased risk of inert gas uptake on ascent; cool environments after dive can promote vasoconstriction and venous pooling, leading to an increased postdive risk of decompression sickness.[21,28] Body mass index (calculated as weight in kilograms divided by the square of height in meters) and age may slightly increase the risk of decompression sickness.[21,29,30]

Clinical features

DCI is a clinical diagnosis. Any new symptom that manifests itself after decompression or ascent from depth should be viewed as a potential variant of DCI.[21] The emergency physician needs to be aware of several unusual clinical variants of DCI: pulmonary DCI, spinal DCI, and AGE.

Pulmonary DCI, historically referred to as the chokes or as cardiorespiratory decompression sickness, is a rare phenomenon. The lungs act as a filter for venous bubbles.[1] In the chokes, the pulmonary vasculature is overloaded by a massive bubble burden, leading to acute respiratory distress manifested by hypoxia, cough, and dyspnea.[21] Some investigators believe that this form of DCI results in increased pulmonary artery pressure and right ventricular pressures.[31]

The existence of thoracic pain or back pain after dive should prompt an emergency physician to consider spinal cord DCI, which can lead to a variety of presentations ranging from trivial paresthesias to paraplegia.[14] Preferentially affecting the lower cervical or lower thoracic regions of the cord, spinal DCI is believed to be caused by obstruction of venous outflow from the epidural plexus followed by bubble formation within the spinal cord tissue itself.[31–33] Patients may initially complain of a vague, girdlelike pain before the onset of more specific syndromes such as ascending paresthesias and paralysis as well as bowel and bladder dysfunction. Contrary to the immediate loss of function seen with a spinal artery syndrome, spinal DCS slowly progresses over several minutes.[31]

The cascade of secondary effects caused by bubbles can result in DCI presenting 24 to 48 hours after diving.[1,21] DCI must be considered several days after flying if the patient has subsequently flown or ascended to altitude.[19,21] The lengthy decompression involved in saturation diving means that symptoms can appear during or after the decompression process; decompression sickness must be considered in the differential diagnosis of any patient presenting after having undergone a saturation dive cycle.

AGE

Pathophysiology and incidence

As a diver ascends, the intrapulmonary gas expands in volume. If a diver's glottis is closed, or if there is bronchospasm or excessive mucous plugging, excessive transpulmonary pressures could result within the now-closed pulmonary air spaces. Alveoli and small airways can rupture, allowing gas to be displaced into the pulmonary venules and subsequently into the systemic circulation.[1] Alternatively, the presence of a patent foramen ovale permits the passage of bubbles into the systemic circulation.[21] Although most symptoms are neurologic in nature because of the buoyancy of bubbles and blood flow, 5% of patients with AGE suffer complete cardiovascular collapse.[1,34] The mechanism resulting in cardiac arrest is unknown. Neither accidental coronary artery air embolization in humans nor experimental injection of air into the left ventricle of a dog has resulted in sudden cardiac death.[28]

Of all cases of DCIs reported to the Divers Alert Network, only 3.9% were attributed to AGE.[13,21]

Risk factors

Almost all cases of AGE are caused by a rapid or uncontrolled ascent from depth. Obstructive lung disease, emphysema, mucous plugging, and a patent foramen ovale are all believed to contribute to the risk of developing AGE.[2]

Clinical features

Although AGE and DCS are grouped together as DCI for purposes of treatment, it is important to remember a few distinguishing features. Almost all cases of AGE present within 5 minutes of surfacing.[34] Although AGE results in catastrophic cardiovascular collapse in only 5% of cases, dyspnea, hemoptysis, and pleuritic chest pain may be seen in half of all cases of AGE.[34,35]

Because the largest change in lung volume occurs in the shallowest of dives, the clinician should not use depth of dive to rule out AGE in the hemodynamically unstable patient after dive. Length of time at depth does affect the likelihood of AGE because its occurrence is the physiologic consequence of Boyle's law.

Pulmonary Barotrauma

Pathophysiology and incidence

Like AGE, pulmonary barotrauma in breathing-apparatus diving is the consequence of the inverse relationship between pressure and volume. Gas escaping from ventilatory units ruptured during the ascent from depth can result in pneumomediastinum, pneumothorax, pneumopericardium, or subcutaneous emphysema.[21] Pulmonary barotrauma has been documented with ascents from as shallow as 1.2 m (4 ft) in divers maintaining maximum lung volume against a closed glottis.[36]

A respiratory technique known as glossopharyngeal insufflation or lung packing is used to add air to the lungs after full inspiration in breath-hold diving. The glossopharyngeal muscles are used to pump as much as an additional 50% of vital capacity into the lungs.[4] The increased transpulmonary pressures caused by lung packing may be responsible for the clinical appearance of pneumomediastinum and AGE within the breath-hold diving population.[37–39]

Believed to be caused by similar mechanisms as seen in the pulmonary edema of breath-hold diving, hemoptysis from alveolar hemorrhage has been described in both scuba divers and breath-hold diving athletes.[3,14,19] Hemoptysis may arise from other structures within the respiratory tract; during descent the entire tracheobronchial tree collapses, with resultant mechanical trauma.[3] In addition, the mucosal vessels of the sinuses may bleed as they become engorged from increased venous return from increased ambient pressure.

The incidence of pulmonary barotrauma is more common than other immersion-related thoracic injuries. Of 411 injuries reported to the Divers Alert Network in 2008, 51 (14.1%) were attributed to pulmonary barotrauma. Five of these cases were confirmed via radiography to show either subcutaneous emphysema or pneumothorax; a further 6 cases had subcutaneous emphysema documented by telephone history.[13]

Risk factors

Pulmonary barotrauma, like AGE, is the physiologic consequence of Boyle's law. Uncontrolled or rapid ascent allows for the passage of bubbles into a variety of potential or actual spaces within the human body.

Clinical features

These clinical entities are readily distinguished from most others on history. Symptoms begin during ascent from depth or shortly after surfacing. Like decompression sickness, IPE and AGE, dyspnea, cough, and chest pain are common symptoms. Physical examination findings are identical to other causes of hemoptysis, pneumothorax, pneumomediastinum or pneumopericardium. Pneumomediastinum may present with fullness in the neck or a change in voice timbre secondary to submucosal emphysema or recurrent laryngeal nerve injury.[40] One caveat to remember is that subcutaneous emphysema related to diving does not necessarily imply pneumothorax but may be a diagnosis in and of itself.

DIVE HISTORY AND DIFFERENTIAL DIAGNOSIS

The most important element in treating patients with diving-related illness is a proper, focused dive history. Although it is unreasonable to expect all emergency physicians to be able to perform a detailed dive history, a short history based on dive profile and appearance of symptoms helps determine if the physician is dealing with a diving-related emergency. **Box 1** details the most important elements of this history; if assistance is required, the Divers Alert Network Emergency Hotline provides 24-hour-a-day support to emergency physicians for DCI, AGE, pulmonary barotraumas, or other serious diving-related emergencies.[13]

The dive history is essential in sorting out the differential diagnosis. Most of the thoracic dive-related emergencies have potentially overlapping clinical presentations. **Box 1** and **Table 2** should allow for the differentiation of most of these conditions from each other. Included in the differential diagnosis is water aspiration (see section on drowning), cardiac dysrhythmia, cardiac ischemia/infarction, pulmonary embolus, pulmonary infection, intoxication, oxygen toxicity, and nitrogen narcosis.

TREATMENT

In general, treatment of most diving-related illness is supportive. Advanced cardiac life support (ACLS), hemodynamic monitoring, intravenous fluids, and, most importantly, 100% oxygen should be used in the treatment of most dive-related injuries. Oxygen administered during first aid resulted in fewer recompression treatments in 1

Box 1
Focused dive history for thoracic emergencies

1. What type of diving was being practiced (breath-hold, scuba, saturation)?
2. At what point in the dive cycle did symptoms appear (on descent, at depth, on ascent, after surfacing)?
3. If the symptoms appeared on ascent or after surfacing, have they been progressive?
4. If the symptoms appeared after surfacing, how long after surfacing did they appear?
5. What was the nature of the dive (commercial, recreational, military/research)?
6. How was the dive time established (dive charts, dive computer)?
7. How deep was the dive?
8. Was the patient intoxicated during the dive?
9. Was the patient dehydrated?
10. What was the water temperature?
11. How strenuous was the dive?
12. Was the decompression limit approached or exceeded?
13. Were decompression stops used?
14. If decompression stops were used, were they of appropriate length?
15. Was in-water decompression attempted?
16. Was there in-water loss of consciousness?
17. How many dives were performed in the 72 hours leading up to the appearance of symptoms? What were those dive profiles (depth achieved, bottom time, total dive time, surface intervals)?
18. What is the patient's past medical history (obstructive airway disease/restrictive airway disease, history of pneumothorax, coronary artery disease, dysrhythmia, patent foramen ovale, neurologic illness including seizure disorder, pregnancy)?
19. What treatment was performed at the dive site/en route to the emergency department?

Table 2
Historical features and treatment modalities in various dive-related illnesses

Clinical Condition	Appearance in Dive Cycle	Timeline After Dive	Affected by Depth of Dive?	Affected by Length of Dive?	Therapies
Pulmonary edema	At depth	Not applicable	No	No	Oxygen Continuous positive airway pressure Diuretics[a] β-agonists
DCI	Ascent At surface	48 h[b]	Yes	Yes	Oxygen Recompression
AGE	Ascent At surface	Minutes[b]	No	No	Oxygen Recompression
Hemoptysis	Any point	Minutes to hours	No	No	Conservative
Pneumothorax	Ascent	Minutes[b]	No	No	Conservative Needle/tube thoracostomy
Pneumopericardium Pneumomediastinum	Ascent	Minutes[b]	No	No	Conservative

[a] Controversial; please see body of text.
[b] Longer if the patient is a saturation diver or has taken a flight.

observational study.[41] **Table 1** summarizes treatment modalities and historical features to help distinguish important causes of thoracic dive illness.

Immersion Pulmonary Edema

Most cases of pulmonary edema caused by breath-hold diving or from immersion can be observed and treated conservatively. The use of β-agonists, diuretics, as well as continuous positive airway pressure has been described in case reports.[6,19,42] However, diuretic use is controversial: not only does it seem to increase the risks of DCI, but most divers are volume deplete at the end of a dive.[4,6] If the diagnosis of pulmonary edema is equivocal, computed tomography (CT) scanning of the chest can be of use. In a case series of 19 divers, 4 had normal chest radiographs but all showed evidence of edema on chest CT.[6]

DCI Including AGE

Recompression therapy is the universally accepted standard of care for DCI. Since 1944, 100% oxygen breathing has been used to increase the concentration gradient allowing for washout of inert gases solubilized in body tissues and fluids. The most commonly used treatment paradigm was developed by the USN; USN Treatment Table 6 recompresses patients to 2.8 ATA maximum pressure using a 100% oxygen breathing schedule over 4.75 hours.[43]

There are no completed randomized controlled trials as of September 2011 examining different recompression therapy paradigms; the only trial published in abstract form seems to have been abandoned before completion.[44] Given the inherent ethical implications of a sham recompression strategy, there are unlikely to be any trials approved comparing recompression strategies with placebo.[45]

With respect to adjunct therapies, 1 randomized controlled trial has been published regarding the role of nonsteroidal antiinflammatory medications in the treatment of

DCI. Tenoxicam (Mobiflex) may reduce the number of recompressions needed but does not improve the odds of recovery.[45,46] Expert opinion recommends maintaining the patient in a horizontal position to prevent increased bubble load from entering the cerebral circulation, but this has not been borne out clinically.[21] Massive fluid resuscitation is not recommended in isolated AGE before recompression therapy.[47]

Transportation of patients suffering DCI is a concern for emergency physicians. Air transportation is often necessary to minimize time between symptom onset and recompression therapy, but air travel can exacerbate symptoms of DCI.[48] Commercial airplanes are typically pressured to ~2400 m (~8000 ft), and most aeromedical transport helicopters cannot be pressurized. No clinical trials examining air transport of patients with DCI exist, but a consensus statement outlining flight-path criteria for these patients has been published.[49] A cabin altitude of 152 m (500 ft) above pick-up location is recommended, with increases to less than 355 m (1000 ft) above pick-up location considered acceptable depending on flying conditions or terrain. This discussion should involve the transport physician, the hyperbaric specialist, and the pilots of the transport aircraft.

After recompression, patients should not fly for at least 72 hours. If residual symptoms persist at this time, consultation with a hyperbaric specialist is recommended.[21,43] With complete recovery, recreational divers may resume diving 4 weeks after treatment.[21] Commercial and military divers may return to diving after a few days for milder symptoms (ie, joint pain) but require a similar prolonged hiatus and detailed examinations for AGE or neurologic decompression sickness before a return to diving is allowed.[21,43]

Pulmonary Barotrauma

Pneumothorax is treated as per a spontaneous pneumothorax. Subcutaneous emphysema, pneumomediastinum, and pneumopericardium can typically be observed without intervention. Similarly, pulmonary hemorrhage should be managed as in nonsubmersion-related cases.

DROWNING

Although the clinical phenomenon of drowning is one that seems intuitively easy to understand, the medical community has historically struggled to establish a clear definition of this term. Because of the heterogeneity of clinical findings and outcomes associated with accidental submersion in water, the literature is crowded with a variety of confusing or misleading terms intended to address this issue of taxonomy. For these reasons, the World Congress on Drowning met in 2002 to provide a universal definition of drowning; specifically, it is "a process resulting in primary respiratory impairment from submersion/immersion in a liquid medium."[50] This definition is conspicuously devoid of any reference to the eventual outcome of the event; drowning, therefore, may be either a fatal or nonfatal event. Terms such as near-drowning, dry/wet drowning, secondary drowning, and active/passive drowning are now avoided.[50]

Although deaths because of drowning have decreased steadily since 1970, they remain the fifth most common cause of accidental deaths in the United States, with more than 3500 fatalities recorded in 2009.[51] Worldwide estimates of incidence vary, with the most recent data available from the World Health Organization estimating approximately 305,000 deaths in 2008, although this is likely an underestimate.[52] Young children are at particularly high risk of drowning, and males in general face a significantly greater risk than females.[53] Other risk factors for drowning vary among jurisdictions, but alcohol abuse and a history of seizure disorders are common themes.[54,55] Children drown more frequently in pools and bathtubs, whereas adults tend to drown more often in open water.[53,55,56] Patients surviving the initial resuscitation phase may face significant disability because of prolonged central nervous system hypoxia, thus further contributing to the morbidity burden of this illness.

Pathophysiology

When submerged in water, the initial response of the conscious victim is to attempt voluntary breath-holding. During this time, arterial pco_2 levels increase, whereas po_2 levels decrease.[57] The ensuing hypercarbia eventually reaches levels that compel the individual to take an involuntary breath, a moment known as the breath-hold breaking point.[58] Predrowning hyperventilation (resulting in hypocarbia) typically prolongs the delay until the break point is reached, potentially allowing hypoxic loss of consciousness to occur before the onset of involuntary respiration caused by hypercarbia.[57] Voluntary apnea combined with cold-water immersion may provoke a diving reflex of bradycardia and peripheral vasoconstriction, reducing oxygen consumption, and potentially delaying the onset of critical hypoxia and fatal drowning.[59] In contrast, physical exertion tends to increase CO_2 production, thus hastening the onset of involuntary respiration in struggling submersion victims.[57] In extreme circumstances, contact with cold water may induce ventricular dysrhythmias, prompting rapid loss of consciousness and preventing any attempts at self-rescue, a phenomenon known as the immersion syndrome.[60] Cold-water immersion may also provoke a gasp reflex, preempting any voluntary attempts at breath-holding.[61] As liquid involuntarily enters the pharynx, laryngospasm temporarily prevents pulmonary aspiration, resulting in the swallowing of large amounts of water.[58] Eventually, as hypoxia progresses laryngospasm ceases, resulting in fluid aspiration of varying degrees.[62] Drowning without aspiration, if it occurs at all, is now considered to be a rare phenomenon, with a recent case series documenting that less than 2% of drowning fatalities had not aspirated any liquid into their lungs.[60,62–64] As liquid enters the alveoli, gas exchange is further impaired, accelerating the decline in arterial po_2. Even in cases in which the aspirated volume of fluid is small, significant hypoxia can result, showing that simple mechanical consolidation of the airspaces is not the sole cause of respiratory insufficiency.[65,66] In the case of freshwater aspiration, the surfactant film within the alveoli is disrupted, leading to alveolar collapse, capillary hyperpermeability, and pulmonary edema.[58] Saltwater aspiration causes pulmonary edema largely because of osmotic fluid shifts into the alveolar space.[58] Irrespective of the immersion medium, secondary lung dysfunction and injury contribute significantly to respiratory dysfunction, potentially explaining why some patients develop delayed respiratory failure. Ultimately, if the process of drowning is not interrupted, hypoxia progresses to the point of complete circulatory collapse and cardiac arrest.

Clinical Presentation

Drowning victims may come into contact with health care personnel at any point along the pathologic continuum described earlier. If the drowning process has been interrupted quickly, patients may seem asymptomatic, whereas more advanced cases may present with severe hypoxia, altered mental status, coma, or cardiac arrest.[56,67,68] Pulmonary edema is a common finding, manifesting as low oxygen saturation, dyspnea, respiratory distress, and crackles on chest auscultation. Respiratory distress from pulmonary edema may occur in a delayed fashion, sometimes up to several hours after the drowning occurred.[69,70] Chest radiography may show variable degrees of pulmonary infiltrates, but these are not necessarily correlated with the clinical severity of the illness.[69,70] Hypothermia is often present, potentially resulting in faulty transcutaneous pulse oximetry because of peripheral vasoconstriction.[71–73] Serum electrolyte shifts may occur with massive amounts of aspirated fluid; however, this is uncommon and typically requires no specific therapy.[58,74] Pulmonary infections may occur in a delayed fashion from aspirated material, some of which may result from rare or atypical pathogens such as fungi.[68,75,76] Patients in cardiac arrest are more likely to display a nonshockable cardiac rhythm (ie, asystole or pulseless electrical activity).[56,77] Those who survive the initial resuscitation phase are at significant risk for developing serious delayed sequelae, such as acute respiratory distress syndrome (ARDS), pancreatitis, disseminated intravascular coagulation, or rhabdomyolysis during their subsequent hospital stay.[56,68]

Management

The initial, and perhaps most critical, phase of treatment of submersion victims occurs in the prehospital environment. Retrieval of the victim combined with rapid restoration of oxygenation is of paramount importance. Early arrival of emergency medical personnel to the scene and rapid initiation of assisted respiration are associated with improved rates of survival in pulseless drowning victims.[56,78] First responders should focus on the importance of activating emergency medical services and providing adequate artificial respiration to unresponsive drowning victims. Properly trained rescuers should initiate rescue breathing even as the victim is being retrieved from the water.[74,79] Although recent recommendations for basic life support protocols have shifted to emphasizing chest compressions as the initial step of cardiopulmonary resuscitation, the hypoxic nature of cardiac arrest secondary to drowning warrants adherence to the traditional airway-breathing-circulation (A-B-C) protocol.[74,79] In patients found unresponsive by a lone rescuer after an apparent drowning episode, initiating a single 2-minute cycle of rescue breaths and chest compressions before leaving to notify emergency medical services is reasonable because many patients may begin to breathe spontaneously with rescue breaths alone.[79] Other than these modifications, ACLS algorithms should be followed as usual in resuscitating pulseless drowning victims. Cervical spine immobilization during rescue efforts and initial resuscitation is recommended only in cases in which spinal trauma is suggested by the mechanism of injury or physical evidence of trauma.[74,79] Routine cervical immobilization in all drowning victims is not recommended because of the relative rarity of these injuries, and the potential for interference of the hard collar with effective ventilation.[80,81] Caution is still warranted in patients whose mechanism of injury is unknown. Prehospital personnel are discouraged from pronouncing death in the field in the absence of clear indications (eg, unsurvivable trauma, putrefaction, or rigor mortis), because of reports of neurologically intact survival even in moribund patients exposed to prolonged submersion.[74,79,82–84] In all patients, hypoxia and respiratory distress should be addressed with supplemental oxygen, and an advanced airway should be secured via endotracheal tube or supraglottic device if indicated, recognizing that obtunded patients are at significant risk of regurgitating and aspirating swallowed water.[85]

On arrival to hospital, care of the drowning victim remains largely supportive. Awake patients may have their ventilation supported with the use of noninvasive positive pressure ventilation techniques, thus avoiding intubation in some cases.[58,68] Intubation may be required if oxygenation does not improve with these measures. Intubated patients likely require a positive end-expiratory pressure setting of at least 5 to 10 cm H_2O (and perhaps as high as 20 cm H_2O) to overcome the ventilation-perfusion mismatch associated with acute lung injury (ALI) and ARDS.[86] Lung protective ventilation strategies using smaller tidal volumes (ie, 6 mL/kg) have shown improved outcomes in patients suffering from all-cause ARDS, and should therefore be considered in drowned patients with this complication.[74,87] Patients failing to improve with advanced ventilation strategies may be candidates for extracorporeal membrane oxygenation, which has been used with some success in pediatric case series.[82,88] Steroids have not been shown to have any benefit in the treatment of ARDS in drowned patients, and are not typically recommended.[59] Prophylactic antibiotics to prevent postdrowning pneumonia are not recommended unless there is evidence of active infection or the patient was submerged in grossly contaminated liquid.[58,74] Increases in intracranial pressure (ICP) often occur in patients resuscitated from cardiac arrest, likely secondary to hypoxic/ischemic cerebral injury.[89] Whereas some investigators believe invasive ICP monitoring coupled with active treatment of increased pressures is not unreasonable, others note that aggressive ICP treatment regimens have met with little success in the past, calling their usefulness into question.[58,77,89–91] In drowning patients resuscitated from cardiac arrest and who remain comatose, therapeutic hypothermia has been recommended to maintain a core temperature of 32 to 34°C.[74] For many drowning victims, this target temperature range may require careful rewarming, with continuous core temperature monitoring.

Prognosticating patient outcomes has proved difficult in cases of drowning, leading to various recommendations regarding disposition. In general, patients presenting with a normal level of consciousness and not showing any signs of respiratory distress or hypoxia at 6 to 8 hours after a drowning incident do not require admission to hospital.[69,70] Patients presenting in a comatose state have typically been shown to have poorer outcomes; however, normal neurologic recovery is still possible in these circumstances.[90,92] Prolonged submersion is also associated with poorer outcomes, but in pediatric cold-water drownings neurologically intact survival has been reported even in cases of submersion for longer than 1 hour.[83,84,92,93] Retrospective analysis of the pediatric risk of mortality score has shown some usefulness in pediatric drowning patients, with all patients having a score of 24 or less on presentation to the emergency department recovering with good neurologic function.[94] The score subsequently performed less precisely in patients admitted to the pediatric intensive care unit, suggesting it should not be used in isolation to predict outcomes.[95] The outcome may remain in doubt for an extended period and often is ascertainable during the emergency department stay. In cases of cardiac arrest after drowning, all efforts should be made to rewarm the patient to a core temperature as close to normothermia as possible before terminating resuscitation efforts.

Summary

Drowning remains a significant concern from a public safety perspective, and promises to challenge the skills of emergency physicians for the foreseeable future. Because our ability to resuscitate postdrowning anoxic brain injury has reached a plateau, a continued emphasis on public education and the implementation of appropriate safety standards for boaters, swimmers, and pool owners is likely to be the most effective way of reducing drowning-related injury and death in the future.[58] Numerous interventions have been associated with a reduced risk of drowning, including protective fencing around pools, banning alcohol use in recreational swimming areas, personal flotation device use among boaters, and swimming lessons for young children.[96–99] Future prevention strategies should continue to focus on these proven methods and other interventions targeted at specific demographic groups.[100,101]

HIGH-ALTITUDE PULMONARY EDEMA

As with diving, the popularity of outdoor pursuits involving the exposure of unacclimatized individuals to high altitudes is increasing. These activities carry with them the risk of developing a specific subset of altitude-related illnesses. The root cause of these conditions is hypoxia, which develops as a result of the declining po_2 found in the ambient air at progressively higher altitudes.[102] Ascending a mountain is analogous to decreasing one's atmospheric depth; therefore it follows that at higher altitudes less atmospheric gas is present above the climber to compress the surrounding air, resulting in diminished ambient air pressure. Given that the relative ratios of the constituent gases found in atmospheric air do not change at different altitudes, Dalton's law (detailed earlier) predicts that as atmospheric air pressure declines, the po_2 declines as well. This ambient hypoxia prompts an increase in the respiratory rate, a phenomenon known as the hypoxic ventilatory response (HVR), which results in improved alveolar and arterial po_2 levels. Hyperventilation also produces a respiratory alkalosis that blunts the HVR via medullary chemoreceptors. This process is offset by a gradual increase in renal bicarbonate diuresis over the course of several days, allowing the climber to acclimatize to progressively higher altitudes.[103,104] The effectiveness of these homeostatic compensatory mechanisms is highly variable amongst individuals, allowing some to acclimatize well to altitudes that others would not tolerate. Regardless of one's tolerance to altitude-related hypoxia, climbing too high or too quickly eventually results in a variety of pathophysiologic processes manifesting as illnesses of the cerebral and pulmonary systems. This review examines the latter of these.

High-altitude pulmonary edema (HAPE) consists of alveolar fluid accumulation in unacclimatized individuals who have recently ascended to altitudes greater than 2500 to 3000 m. First described in the literature by Hultgren and Spickard[105] and Houston,[106] HAPE is a condition that can develop in parallel with the cerebral forms of altitude illness, acute mountain sickness (AMS) and high-altitude cerebral edema (HACE). Approximately 50% of patients with HAPE also show symptoms of AMS/HACE, but these 2 forms of altitude illness can exist independently of each other.[107] The incidence of HAPE is highly dependent on the ascent profile adopted on any given climb; the rate of ascent and the ultimate altitude achieved affect the appearance of this illness. Recent estimates in the literature vary from an incidence of 1.6% at 3600 m to 2.5% at 4400 m, whereas historical figures have ranged as high as 15% at altitudes more than 5500 m.[108–110] HAPE may also be observed in high-altitude dwellers who return to their homes after a prolonged sojourn at low altitude, a phenomenon known as reentry HAPE.[110,111] If left untreated, HAPE is a potentially life-threatening illness, and given that many cases occur far from advanced medical care, careful clinical evaluation is the key to its early identification and treatment.

Pathophysiology

HAPE is believed to be a form of noncardiogenic pulmonary edema caused by exposure to the low po_2 found at high altitudes.[103,110] Hypoxia leads to uneven areas of vasoconstriction within the pulmonary vascular bed, resulting in a pattern of patchy overperfusion.[112] These foci of high vascular pressure lead to localized violation of the capillary endothelium, causing fluid extravasation.[113,114] The degree of hypoxic pulmonary vasoconstriction seems to be highly individual and is more pronounced among HAPE-prone individuals.[115] Decreased nitric oxide secretion in HAPE-prone individuals likely worsens this clinical picture.[116,117] The sympathetic discharge associated with hypoxia and exertion, as well as the hypoxia-induced impairment of the sodium-potassium adenosine triphosphatase (Na-K ATPase) responsible for alveolar fluid clearance, likely play a role in the development of HAPE.[118,119] Evaluation of the alveolar fluid in climbers with HAPE has shown that inflammation does not play a causative role in uncomplicated HAPE.[120] However, concomitant respiratory illness can increase the risk of HAPE, leading to speculation that the inflammatory component of such infections may have an instigating role.[121]

Risk Factors

The most modifiable risk factor for the development of HAPE is the rate of ascent to high altitude. Although it is universally accepted that slower rates of ascent pose a lower risk of developing altitude illness, no one regimen has been proved to be completely safe.[102,112,122] The 2010 Wilderness Medical Society Consensus Guidelines for the Prevention and Treatment of Altitude Illness recommend that climbers avoid increasing their sleeping altitude by more than 500 m per day after ascending beyond an altitude of 3000 m, and that every 3 to 4 days (or approximately every 600–1200 m) climbers should observe a rest day during which the sleeping altitude is not increased.[122] Additional risk factors for developing HAPE include a previous history of the disease, vigorous exercise, exposure to cold ambient temperatures, and lower respiratory tract infections.[119,121,123,124] Preexisting conditions affecting the pulmonary vasculature, such as congenital absence of 1 pulmonary artery and primary pulmonary hypertension, can also increase the risk of acquiring HAPE.[112,125]

Clinical Presentation

Patients suffering from HAPE initially show dyspnea at rest, along with exercise intolerance and a dry cough. These symptoms are often mild initially and can provide the astute clinician with an early warning of impending illness. Symptoms typically become apparent 2 to 4 days after ascending past the altitude that triggered the disease process. This delay sometimes causes patients to ascribe the cause of their illness to something other than high altitude, especially if they have not been actively gaining altitude during this time. As the illness progresses, dyspnea evolves into frank respiratory distress and cyanosis, the cough may eventually produce pink frothy sputum, and the patient may have a low-grade fever. The Lake Louise criteria have been derived to assist in the clinical diagnosis of HAPE: the presence of any 2 symptoms in combination with any 2 physical findings among those listed in **Box 2** satisfy a presumptive diagnosis in unacclimatized individuals who have recently ascended to high altitudes.[126] When available, chest radiography (**Fig. 1**) initially shows patchy, heterogeneous peripheral alveolar infiltrates progressing eventually to widespread, confluent airspace involvement.[127,128] Portable lung ultrasonography provides a more feasible imaging option in remote locations and shows progressively larger numbers of extravascular fluid comet tails in patients ascending to altitude and suffering from HAPE.[129,130]

DIFFERENTIAL DIAGNOSIS

A broad differential diagnosis needs to be entertained in patients with potential HAPE, including pulmonary embolism, asthma, respiratory tract infections, and cardiogenic pulmonary edema. Narrowing the differential becomes increasingly difficult considering the limited scope of resources available to physicians in the field. Distinguishing HAPE from the lower respiratory tract infections ubiquitous among trekkers, travelers, and climbers can be especially challenging, and clinicians should be cautious when attributing acute respiratory symptoms at high altitude to an infectious cause. Given

---

Box 2
Lake Louise criteria for HAPE

Symptoms (at least 2)

- Dyspnea at rest
- Chest tightness/congestion
- Marked decrease in exercise tolerance
- Cough

Signs (at least 2)

- Central cyanosis
- Tachypnea (>20 respirations/minute)
- Tachycardia (>100 beats per minute)
- Crackles/wheezing on chest auscultation

---

the potentially dire consequences of allowing a patient with early HAPE to continue their ascent, clinicians should adhere to the maxim that all illness at altitude is altitude illness until proved otherwise. All acute respiratory symptoms at high altitude should be considered to be potentially related to HAPE.

Management

The most important therapy in the treatment of suspected HAPE is descent to a lower altitude. No trials exist that establish the minimum altitude reduction required to effect a resolution of symptoms. The most commonly recommended regimen is to descend at least 1000 m from the patient's current altitude, or until the symptoms resolve.[112,122] Because of the delayed onset of symptoms typical of HAPE, the patient may have ascended beyond the altitude that initiated their symptoms, and this should be taken into account when estimating the magnitude of descent required. Environmental factors such as ambient temperature, active local weather, available hours of daylight, the availability of mechanized transport, and the ruggedness of the terrain to be

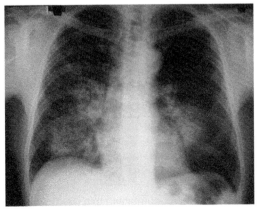

Fig. 1. Chest radiography showing asymmetric distribution of alveolar infiltrates in HAPE, focused in right middle lobe. (*Courtesy of* Buddha Basnyat, MD, Kathmandu, Nepal.)

traversed must also be factored into the timing of evacuation. Given that some cases of HAPE can be managed at altitude with supplemental oxygen and careful monitoring, the clinician must balance the patient's anticipated clinical course against the expected difficulties of transport.[131] In general, patients in developed areas whose symptoms respond well to supplemental oxygen alone can be monitored closely at altitude without the need for descent unless their condition deteriorates.[122] Patients experiencing severe symptoms in isolated locations and at extreme altitudes warrant consideration for immediate descent even in the face of difficult terrain or inclement weather. In cases requiring evacuation, the patient should be kept as warm as possible, and every effort should be made to avoid physical exertion on their part because this could further exacerbate the symptoms of HAPE.

In addition to descent, several adjunctive therapies exist that can be used to temporize patients for whom immediate descent is not a reasonable option. Supplemental oxygen, supplied via portable oxygen tanks or electrically powered ambient air oxygen concentrators, should be applied to all patients, and in select conditions may be adequate to obviate descent. Nifedipine has long been the pharmacologic adjunct of choice in HAPE, because of its ability to reverse pulmonary vasoconstriction. Evidence in favor of this therapy is limited to a small nonblinded trial, but extensive positive clinical experience continues to support its use.[132] Although their use has been reported in the literature, phosphodiesterase inhibitors such as tadalafil have been studied more closely in a prophylactic role, and no trials exist examining their use as an acute therapy for HAPE.[133,134] These drugs should be considered as substitute pulmonary vasodilators only if nifedipine is unavailable.[122] Inhaled β_2-agonists have also been proposed as a potential therapy for HAPE, because of their salutary effects on alveolar fluid clearance by way of increased Na-K ATPase function. However, although salmeterol has been shown to have prophylactic benefits, no trial has been performed to evaluate the role of these agents in acute treatment, making their role uncertain at this time.[135] Dexamethasone has also unexpectedly been shown to have prophylactic effects against HAPE, but no evidence exists to support its use acutely except as an adjunctive therapy for concomitant AMS/HACE.[134] Use of a portable hyperbaric chamber, known as a Gamow bag, can provide an opportunity to temporarily reverse some of the symptoms of HAPE.[136] This device may prove especially useful in remote locations, where access to supplemental oxygen may not be available. All of these adjuncts should be considered as secondary options only, and delaying descent in favor of their use should generally be avoided. **Table 3** summarizes the adjunctive treatments available for HAPE.

Once a patient with HAPE has been treated (with or without descent) to complete resolution of symptoms, careful resumption of ascent may be considered. In such cases, the ascent profile must remain conservative, and pharmacologic prophylaxis with nifedipine should be entertained.[122]

Prophylaxis

The most effective prophylaxis against the development of HAPE is to adhere to a conservative ascent profile, as detailed earlier. Although evidence exists to support the use of salmeterol, tadalafil, and dexamethasone in the prevention of HAPE, nifedipine remains the preferred first-line agent based on the preponderance of clinical experience as well as a single clinical trial.[123,134,135] If salmeterol is used for prophylaxis, current guidelines recommend combining this agent with additional oral agents and avoiding monotherapy.[122] Although most experts advocate prophylaxis only in those patients who have a history of HAPE, preventative therapies may also be

Table 3
Summary of HAPE treatment/prophylaxis

Agent	Role in Treatment	Role in Prophylaxis
Oxygen	First-line therapy	Effective; impractical in most cases
Nifedipine	First-line adjunct to oxygen Dose: 10 mg by mouth loading dose × 1; then 20 mg slow release by mouth every 8 h or 30 mg slow release by mouth every 12 h	Preferred agent. Significant clinical experience; single randomized controlled trial Dose: 20–30 mg slow release by mouth every 12 h
Tadalafil	No proven role; may be considered based on case reports	Effective; single small randomized controlled trial Dose: 10 mg by mouth on demand
Salmeterol	No proven role; may be considered based on case reports	Effective; single small randomized controlled trial; not recommended as monotherapy Dose: 125 µg inhaled twice a day
Dexamethasone	No proven role	Has shown benefit in single randomized controlled trial; not used routinely in HAPE prevention

extended to patients with a history of pulmonary hypertension, as well as rescue or military personnel for whom a gradual ascent profile may not be possible.[102,122,136,137]

Summary

HAPE is a potentially life-threatening illness that is completely preventable. Although the early clinical manifestations can be misinterpreted, the careful clinician possesses an opportunity to intervene at an early stage, thereby avoiding potential catastrophe. As the popularity of trekking and climbing grows among the general populace, physicians will be increasingly relied on as a source of education, prophylaxis, and treatment, making a working familiarity with altitude-induced illnesses such as HAPE an indispensable tool for emergency physicians.

INHALED TOXINS

Environmental toxins affecting the pulmonary system can be divided into 2 primary categories: pulmonary irritants and simple asphyxiants. The following is a discussion of these agents, their pathophysiologic effects, and the clinical management of the toxicities they create.

Pulmonary Irritants

A broad variety of inhaled toxins exist that can exert their effects via direct toxicity to the endothelial membrane of the respiratory tract (**Table 4**). These substances are nearly ubiquitous, resulting in exposures within the home, the workplace, and even in sporting venues.[138–141] Accidental large-scale industrial releases of inhaled irritants have caused widespread morbidity and mortality.[142] The total percentage of chronic obstructive pulmonary disease resulting from prolonged workplace exposures to inhaled irritants has been difficult to determine but has been estimated in the range of 15% to 20%, and likely contributes to the steady flow of chronic obstructive pulmonary disease presentations to emergency departments each year.[143]

Table 4
Common pulmonary irritants based on solubility

Pulmonary Irritant	Common Sources	Comments
Highly Water Soluble		
Ammonia	Household cleansers	
Hydrogen chloride	Tanning, electroplating	Consider nebulized $NaHCO_3$ therapy
Hydrogen fluoride	Industrial applications	May cause severe hypocalcemia
Chloramine	Inappropriate mixing of cleaning products (bleach + ammonia)	
Intermediate Solubility		
Chlorine	Industry, swimming pool disinfectants	Consider nebulized $NaHCO_3$ therapy
Hydrogen sulfide	Sewage, petroleum industry	Cellular asphyxiant
Poorly Water Soluble		
Phosgene	Chemical warfare, industrial applications	
Nitrogen oxides (NO_x)	Hydrocarbon combustion	

Pathophysiology
The toxicity of pulmonary irritants is caused by their dissolution within the aqueous secretions of the mucous membranes lining the respiratory tract, resulting in the creation of by-products that are directly toxic to pulmonary tissues. These by-products elicit a host inflammatory response that leads to tissue exudates and edema, further complicating the direct effects of the irritant itself.[144] The resultant inflammatory cascade can lead to upper airway obstruction, bronchospasm, and alveolar edema and may progress to respiratory insufficiency, hypoxia, and death.

Clinical presentation
The clinical manifestations observed after exposure to a specific pulmonary irritant are determined primarily by the water solubility of the gas. Highly water-soluble agents dissolve more quickly on inhalation and affect the more proximal portions of the respiratory tract. This process leads to pharyngeal irritation, cough, and stridor that may progress to complete airway obstruction. Poorly water-soluble gases are capable of bypassing the upper airways and penetrating deep into the alveoli. By interacting primarily with the alveolar membranes, these agents cause capillary leakage in the distal airways, resulting in a noncardiogenic form of pulmonary edema known as ALI. Patients may report experiencing cough, dyspnea, or chest pain, and the physical examination may reveal respiratory distress and wheezing or crackles on auscultation of the chest. The clinical manifestations of ALI may be delayed in onset by 6 to 8 hours after the initial exposure.[144,145]

Pulmonary irritants with intermediate solubility can produce a mixed clinical picture; whether upper or lower tract symptoms predominate depends on the duration and intensity of the exposure. Chlorine gas is a prototypical example of an intermediate-solubility irritant, and can produce a broad spectrum of clinical syndromes depending on the circumstances surrounding a given exposure.[144] Brief, high-intensity exposures typically result in more prominent upper airway involvement, whereas low-level or prolonged contact with the gas allows more distal airway involvement.[145,146] However, although these parameters can provide a general guide to the clinician, the possibility of lower airway involvement developing several hours after an apparent upper airway response should always be entertained after any exposure to an intermediate-solubility gas.

Several pulmonary irritants may also manifest systemic toxicities. Hydrogen sulfide acts as a cellular asphyxiant, arresting oxidative phosphorylation, whereas hydrogen fluoride is known to cause severe hypocalcemia.[145,147]

Management

The management of pulmonary irritant exposures begins with routine supportive measures. Supplemental oxygen or positive pressure ventilation should be applied as needed to maintain adequate oxygenation. Upper airway obstruction related to soft tissue edema may require invasive airway interventions, such as endotracheal intubation or surgical airway access.[138] Bronchodilators may be used to address bronchospasm and wheezing.[148] Corticosteroids are often used to counteract bronchospasm as well as the inflammatory processes underlying inhalational ALI, but most of the evidence regarding their use derives from animal studies or small, uncontrolled human studies and case reports. Although there is evidence to suggest that they may improve certain physiologic parameters in ARDS, they do not seem to improve clinical outcomes.[149] In addition to supportive care, neutralization therapy with dilute (2%) nebulized sodium bicarbonate solution has shown benefit in the treatment of chlorine gas inhalation, primarily with respect to symptom control.[150–152] Various antioxidant therapies (such as cysteine, glutathione, and N-acetylcysteine) have been examined as therapies for irritant-induced ALI, but their use remains largely anecdotal or research-based, with no definite clinical role.[153] Nebulized calcium gluconate may prove useful in reducing hypocalcemia after inhaled hydrogen fluoride exposures; however, current experience is isolated to case reports.[154,155] Systemic calcium administration is also often needed depending on serum calcium measurements.[146]

Disposition

Patients exposed to highly soluble gases whose symptoms are minimal or have resolved may be discharged home. Asymptomatic patients exposed to intermediate or poorly soluble gases should be observed and receive chest radiography at 6 to 8 hours after exposure to rule out the development of ALI. Patients already showing significant lower airway symptoms require admission for treatment.

Simple Asphyxiants

This class of toxins exerts its effects through the displacement of oxygen from the ambient air, resulting in a lower inhaled pO_2 and subsequent hypoxia in the exposed individual. By definition, a simple asphyxiant possesses no localized or systemic toxic effects but practically speaking many gases with pharmacologic effects can also produce simple asphyxia if they are present in quantities large enough to displace a significant percentage of oxygen from the air.[156] Common simple asphyxiants include nitrogen, carbon dioxide, simple hydrocarbons (eg, methane, propane), and the noble gases (eg, argon).[157] Fatalities caused by simple asphyxia often occur in an industrial or occupational setting, usually in confined spaces.[158] Common mechanisms include failure of respirator devices because of mechanical or operator error as well as coworkers or rescue personnel succumbing attempting to retrieve the victim from the low-oxygen environment. Many cases of simple asphyxia have also been reported in the outdoors, typically involving accidental exposures to volcanic exhaust, which is rich in carbon dioxide.[159–161]

Clinical presentation

The clinical presentation of simple asphyxia is predictably similar to that of acute hypoxia. As the po_2 decreases, symptoms progress from mild euphoria and headache to seizures, coma, and eventually death. Dyspnea, which is more strongly linked to hypercapnia than to hypoxia, is often a later symptom in simple asphyxia. In cases of simple asphyxia involving near-total displacement of oxygen from the surrounding air, the onset of symptoms may be rapid, progressing to a loss of consciousness within seconds.[162] Alternatively, if the reduction in the ambient pO_2 is not severe, patients may experience a more insidious progression.

Management and disposition

Immediate evacuation of the patient is the only specific therapy required in cases of simple asphyxia; often, symptoms resolve by the time the patient is evaluated in the emergency department.[156] Patients with minor exposures and rapidly resolving symptoms can be discharged home after brief observation; no specific investigations are necessary. Otherwise, management and disposition are directed toward the specific hypoxic complications experienced by the victim (eg, cardiac arrest, myocardial infarction, dysrhythmias, seizures, coma).

SUMMARY

Thoracic environmental emergencies represent a diverse group of illnesses, each requiring significant emphasis on a well-performed history and physical examination. Recognition of the importance of when symptoms appear during activities at depth or at altitude are of particular importance to the emergency physician. Understanding the need for recompression therapies or descent from altitude is essential to the treatment of these illnesses, and using various adjunct therapies helps the emergency physician competently manage these illnesses. Key to the management of the thoracic consequences from inhaled toxins is understanding the pathophysiology associated with various toxins. Similarly, an awareness of the delayed appearance of the thoracic sequelae of drowning or exposure to environmental toxins and pulmonary irritants is important to the management of these illnesses. With proper attention to history and physical examination and a recognition of the importance of pathophysiology to these illnesses, the practicing emergency physician should be able to adequately manage these illnesses.

REFERENCES

1. Levett DZ, Millar IL. Bubble trouble: a review of diving physiology and disease. Postgrad Med J 2008;84:571–8.
2. Byyny RL, Shockley LW. Scuba diving and dysbarism. In: Marx JA, Hockberger RS, Walls RM, et al, editors. Rosen's emergency medicine. 7th edition. Philadelphia: Mosby Elsevier; 2010. Chapter 141.
3. Muth CM, Ehrmann U, Radermacher P. Physiological and clinical aspects of apnea diving. Clin Chest Med 2005;26:381–94.
4. Moon RE, Cherry AD, Stolp BW, et al. Pulmonary gas exchange in diving. J Appl Physiol 2008;106:668–77.
5. Slade JB Jr, Hattori T, Ray CS, et al. Pulmonary edema associated with scuba diving: case reports and review. Chest 2001;120:1686–94.
6. Henckes A, Lion F, Cochard G, et al. L'oedème pulmonaire en plongée sous-marine autonome: fréquence et gravité à propos d'une série de 19 cas. Ann Fr Anesth Reanim 2008;27:694–9.

7. West JB, Mathieu-Costello O. Stress failure of pulmonary capillaries: role in lung and heart disease. Lancet 1992;340:762–7.

8. Janssens JP, Pache JC, Nicod LP. Physiological changes in respiratory function associated with ageing. Eur Respir J 1999;13:197–205.

9. Lindholm P, Lundgren CE. The physiology and pathophysiology of human breath-hold diving. J Appl Physiol 2009;106:284–92.

10. Cialoni D, Maggiorelli F, Sponsiello N, et al. Epidemiological investigation on hemoptysis in breath hold divers. In: Bedini R, Belardinelli A, Rale L, editors. Blue 2005 human behaviour and limits in underwater environment. Special conference on breath-hold diving. Pisa (Italy): University of Chiety; 2005. p. 103–4.

11. Fitz-Clarke JR. Adverse events in competitive breath-hold diving. Undersea Hyperb Med 2006;33:55–62.

12. Liner MH, Andersson JP. Pulmonary edema after competitive breath-hold diving. J Appl Physiol 2008;104:986–90.

13. Pollock NW. Annual diving report: 2008 edition. Durham (NC): Divers Alert Network; 2008.

14. Kiyan E, Aktas S, Toklu AS. Hemoptysis provoked by voluntary diaphragmatic contractions in breath-hold divers. Chest 2001;120:2098–100.

15. Shupak A, Weiler-Ravell D, Adir Y, et al. Pulmonary oedema induced by strenuous swimming: a field study. Respir Physiol 2000;121:25–31.

16. Thorsen E, Skogstad M, Reed JW. Subacute effects of inspiratory resistive loading and head-out water immersion on pulmonary function. Undersea Hyperb Med 1999;26:137–41.

17. Weile-Ravell D, Sjupak A, Goldenberg I, et al. Pulmonary oedema and haemoptysis induced by strenuous swimming. BMJ 1995;311:361–2.

18. Wilmshurst PT, Nuri M, Crowther A, et al. Cold-induced pulmonary oedema in scuba divers and swimmers and subsequent development of hypertension. Lancet 1989;1:62–6.

19. Boussages A, Pinet C, Thoms P, et al. Haemoptysis after breath-hold diving. Eur Respir J 1999;13:697–9.

20. Freiberger JJ, Denoble PJ, Pieper CF, et al. The relative risk of decompression sickness during and after air travel following diving. Aviat Space Environ Med 2002;73:980–4.

21. Vann RD, Bytler FK, Mitchel SJ, et al. Decompression illness. Lancet 2010;377:153–64.

22. Boussuges A, Blanc P, Molenat F, et al. Haemoconcentration in neurological decompression illness. Int J Sports Med 1996;17:351–5.

23. Bosco G, Yang ZJ, Savini F, et al. Environmental stress on diving-induced platelet activation. Undersea Hyperb Med 2001;28:207–11.

24. Temple DJ, Ball R, Weathersby PK, et al. The dive profiles and manifestations of decompression sickness cases after air and nitrogen-oxygen dives. Volume I: data set summaries, manifestation descriptions, and key files. Washington, DC: Naval Medical Research Center; 1999. NMRC 99–02.

25. Ladd G, Stepan V, Stevens L. The Abacus Project: establishing the risk of recreational scuba death and decompression illness. SPUMS J 2002;32:124–8.

26. Lemaitre F, Fahlman A, Gardette B, et al. Decompression sickness in breath-hold divers: a review. J Sports Sci 2009;27:1519–34.

27. Thorsen HC, Zubieta-Calleja G, Paulev PE. Decompression sickness following seawater hunting using underwater scooters. Res Sports Med 2007;15:225–39.

28. Gerth WA, Ruterbusch VL, Long ET. The influence of thermal exposure on diver susceptibility to decompression sickness. Panama City (FL): Navy Experimental Diving Unit; 2007. NEDU TR: 06–07.

29. Dunford RG, Vann RD, Gerth WA, et al. The incidence of venous gas emboli in recreational diving. Undersea Hyperb Med 2002;29:247–59.

30. Vann RD. Mechanisms and risks of decompression. In: Bove AA, editor. Bove and Davis' diving medicine. 4th edition. Philadelphia: Saunders; 2004. p. 127–64.

31. Neuman TS. Arterial gas embolism and decompression sickness. News Physiol Sci 2002;17:77–81.

32. Francis TJ, Griffin JL, Homer LD, et al. Bubble-induced dysfunction in acute spinal cord decompression sickness. J Appl Physiol 1990;68:1368–75.

33. Hallenbeck JM. Cinephotomicography of dog spinal vessels during cord-damaging decompression sickness. Neurology 1976;26:190–9.

34. Lynch JH, Bove AA. Diving medicine: a review of current evidence. J Am Board Fam Pract 2009;22:399–407.

35. Ball R. Effect of severity, time to recompression with oxygen, and re-treatment on outcome in forty-nine cases of spinal cord decompression sickness. Undersea Hyperb Med 1993;20:133–45.

36. Bove AA. Medical aspects of sport diving. Med Sci Sports Exerc 1996;28: 591–5.

37. Liner MH, Andersson JP. Suspected arterial gas embolism after glossopharyngeal insufflation in a breath-hold diver. Aviat Space Environ Med 2010;81:74–6.

38. Jacobson FL, Loring SH, Ferrigno M. Pneumomediastinum after lung packing. Undersea Hyperb Med 2006;33:313–6.

39. Loring SH, O'Donnell CR, Butler JP, et al. Transpulmonary pressures and lung mechanics with glossopharyngeal insufflation and exsufflation beyond normal lung volumes in competitive breath-hold divers. J Appl Physiol 2007;102:841–6.

40. Edmonds C, Lowry C, Pennefather J. Diving and subaquatic medicine. 3rd edition. Oxford (United Kingdom): Butterworth-Heinemann; 1992. p. 95–114.

41. Gorman DF, Browning DM, Parsons DW. Redistribution of cerebral arterial gas emboli: a comparison of treatment regimens. In: Bove AA, Bachrach AJ, Greenbaum LJ Jr, editors. Underwater and hyperbaric physiology IX proceedings of the ninth international symposium on underwater and hyperbaric physiology. Bethesda (MD): Undersea and Hyperbaric Medical Society; 1987. p. 1031–54.

42. Halpern P, Gefen A, Sorkine P, et al. Pulmonary oedema in scuba-divers: pathophysiology and computed risk analysis. Eur J Emerg Med 2003;10:35–41.

43. Navy Department. US Navy diving manual. Revision 6. NAVSEA 0910-LP-106–0957. Diving medicine and recompression chamber operations, vol. 5. Washington, DC: Naval Sea Systems Command; 2008.

44. Drewry A, Gorman DF. A progress report on the prospective randomized double blind controlled study of oxygen and oxygen-helium in the treatment of air-diving decompression illness. Undersea Hyperb Med 1994;21(Suppl):98.

45. Bennett MH, Lehm JP, Mitchell SJ, et al. Recompression and adjunctive therapy for decompression illness [review]. Cochrane Database Syst Rev 2007;2: CD005277.

46. Bennett M, Mitchell S, Dominguez A. Adjunctive treatment of decompression illness with a non-steroidal anti-inflammatory drug (tenoxicam) reduces compression requirement. Undersea Hyperb Med 2003;30:195–205.

47. Moon RE. Adjunctive therapy for decompression illness. Kensington (MD): Undersea and Hyperbaric Medical Society; 2003.

48. Vann RD, Denoble P, Emmerman MN, et al. Flying after diving and decompression sickness. Aviat Space Environ Med 1993;64:801–7.
49. MacDonald RD, O'Donnell C, Allan MG, et al. Interfacility transport of patients with decompression illness: literature review and consensus statement. Prehosp Emerg Care 2006;10:482–7.
50. Idris AH, Berg RA, Bierens J, et al. Recommended guidelines for uniform reporting of data from drowning: the "Utstein Style". Circulation 2003;108: 2565–74.
51. Kochanek K, Xu J, Murphy S, et al. Deaths: preliminary data for 2009. Natl Vital Stat Rep 2011;59:1–68.
52. World Health Organization. Causes of Death 2008 Summary Tables. Available at: http://www.who.int/evidence/bod. Accessed June 14, 2011.
53. Gilchrist J, Gotsch K, Ryan G. Nonfatal and fatal drownings in recreational water settings. MMWR Morb Mortal Wkly Rep 2004;53:447–52.
54. Driscoll TR, Harrison JA, Steenkamp M. Review of the role of alcohol in drowning associated with recreational aquatic activity. Inj Prev 2004;10:107–13.
55. Quan L, Cummings P. Characteristics of drowning by different age groups. Inj Prev 2003;9:163–8.
56. Youn CS, Choi SP, Yim HW, et al. Out-of-hospital cardiac arrest due to drowning: An Utstein Style report of 10 years of experience from St. Mary's Hospital. Resuscitation 2009;80:778–83.
57. Craig AB Jr. Causes of loss of consciousness during underwater swimming. J Appl Physiol 1961;16:583–6.
58. Layon AJ, Modell JH. Drowning: update 2009. Anesthesiology 2009;110: 1390–401.
59. Alboni P, Alboni M, Gianfranchi L. Diving bradycardia: a mechanism of defence against hypoxic damage. J Cardiovasc Med (Hagerstown) 2011;12: 422–7.
60. Orlowski J, Szpilman D. Drowning: rescue, resuscitation, and reanimation. Pediatr Clin North Am 2001;48:627–46.
61. Tipton MJ. The initial response to cold-water immersion in man. Clin Sci (Lond) 1989;77:581–8.
62. Lunetta P, Modell JH, Sajantila A. What is the incidence and significance of "dry-lungs" in bodies found in water? Am J Forensic Med Pathol 2004;25:291–301.
63. Salomez F, Vincent JL. Drowning: a review of epidemiology, pathophysiology, treatment and prevention. Resuscitation 2004;63:261–8.
64. Modell JH, Bellefleur M, Davis JH. Drowning without aspiration: is this an appropriate diagnosis? J Forensic Sci 1999;44:1119–23.
65. Modell JH, Moya F. Effects of volume of aspirated fluid during chlorinated fresh-water drowning. Anesthesiology 1966;27:662–72.
66. Modell JH, Moya F, Newby EJ, et al. The effects of fluid volume in seawater drowning. Ann Intern Med 1967;67:68–80.
67. Modell JH, Graves SA, Ketover A. Clinical course of 91 consecutive near-drowning victims. Chest 1976;70:231–8.
68. Gregorakos L, Markou N, Psalida V, et al. Near-drowning: clinical course of lung injury in adults. Lung 2009;187:93–7.
69. Causey A, Tilelli J, Swanson M. Predicting discharge in uncomplicated near-drowning. Am J Emerg Med 2000;18:9–11.
70. Noonan L, Howrey R, Ginsburg CM. Freshwater submersion injuries in children: a retrospective review of seventy-five hospitalized patients. Pediatrics 1996;98: 368–71.

71. Barbieri S, Feltracco P, Delantone M, et al. Helicopter rescues and prehospital care for drowning children: two summer season case studies. Minerva Anestesiol 2008;74:703–7.

72. Bruning C, Siekmeyer W, Siekmeyer M, et al. Retrospective analysis of 44 childhood drowning accidents. Wien Klin Wochenschr 2010;122:405–12.

73. Montenij LJ, de Vries W, Schwarte L, et al. Feasibility of pulse oximetry in the initial prehospital management of victims of drowning: a preliminary study. Resuscitation 2011;82(9):1235–8.

74. Soar J, Perkins G, Abbas G, et al. European Resuscitation Council guidelines for resuscitation 2010 Section 8. Cardiac arrest in special circumstances: electrolyte abnormalities, poisoning, drowning, accidental hypothermia, hyperthermia, asthma, anaphylaxis, cardiac surgery, trauma, pregnancy, electrocution. Resuscitation 2010;81:1400–33.

75. Katragkou A, Dotis J, Kotsiou M, et al. *Scedosporium apiospermum* infection after near-drowning. Mycoses 2007;50:412–21.

76. Chaney S, Gopalan R, Berggren RE. Pulmonary *Pseudallescheria boydii* infection with cutaneous zygomycosis after near drowning. South Med J 2004;7: 683–7.

77. Claesson A, Svensson L, Silfverstolpe J, et al. Characteristics and outcome among patients suffering out-of-hospital cardiac arrest due to drowning. Resuscitation 2008;76:381–7.

78. Venema AM, Groothoff JW, Bierens JJ. The role of bystanders during rescue and resuscitation of drowning victims. Resuscitation 2010;81:434–9.

79. Vanden Hoek T, Morrison L, Shuster M, et al. Part 12: cardiac arrest in special situations: 2010 American Heart Association Guidelines for cardiopulmonary resuscitation and emergency cardiovascular care. Circulation 2010;122(Suppl 3): S829–61.

80. Watson RS, Cummings P, Quan L, et al. Cervical spine injuries among submersion victims. J Trauma 2001;51:658–62.

81. Dodd FM, Simon E, McKeown D, et al. The effect of a cervical collar on the tidal volume of anaesthetized adult patients. Anaesthesia 1995;50:961–3.

82. Eich C, Brauer A, Timmermann A, et al. Outcome of 12 drowned children with attempted resuscitation on cardiopulmonary bypass: an analysis of variables based on the "Utstein Style for Drowning". Resuscitation 2007;75:42–52.

83. Schmidt U, Fritz KW, Kasperczyk W, et al. Successful resuscitation of a child with severe hypothermia after cardiac arrest of 88 minutes. Prehospital Disaster Med 1995;10:60–2.

84. Bolte RG, Black PG, Boweres RS, et al. The use of extracorporeal rewarming in a child submerged for 66 minutes. JAMA 1988;260:377–9.

85. Manolios N, Mackie I. Drowning and near-drowning on Australian beaches patrolled by life-savers: a 10-year study, 1973-1983. Med J Aust 1988;148: 165–7, 170–1.

86. Moran I, Zavala E, Fernandez R, et al. Recruitment manoeuvres in acute lung injury/acute respiratory distress syndrome. Eur Respir J Suppl 2003;42:37s–42s.

87. The Acute Respiratory Distress Syndrome Network. Ventilation with lower tidal volumes as compared with traditional tidal volumes for acute lung injury and the acute respiratory distress syndrome. N Engl J Med 2000;342:1301–8.

88. Guenther U, Varelmann D, Putensen C, et al. Extended therapeutic hypothermia for several days during extracorporeal membrane-oxygenation after drowning and cardiac arrest: two cases of survival with no neurological sequelae. Resuscitation 2009;80:379–81.

89. Frewen T, Sumabat W, Han V, et al. Cerebral resuscitation therapy in pediatric near-drowning. J Pediatr 1985;106:615–7.

90. Warner D, Knape J. Brain resuscitation in the drowning victim; consensus and recommendations. In: Bierens J, editor. Handbook on drowning. Heidelberg (Germany): Springer-Verlag; 2006. p. 436–9.

91. Szpilman D. Near-drowning and drowning classification: a proposal to stratify mortality based on the analysis of 1,831 cases. Chest 1997;112:660–5.

92. Orlowski JP. Prognostic factors in pediatric cases of drowning and near-drowning. JACEP 1979;8:176–9.

93. Suominen PK, Korpela RE, Silfvast TG, et al. Does water temperature affect outcome of nearly drowned children. Resuscitation 1997;35:111–5.

94. Zuckerman G, Gregory P, Santos-Damiani S. Predictors of death and neurologic impairment in pediatric submersion injuries: The Pediatric Risk of Mortality Score. Arch Pediatr Adolesc Med 1998;152:134–40.

95. Gonzalez-Luis G, Pons M, Cambra F, et al. Use of the Pediatric Risk of Mortality Score as predictor of death and serious neurologic damage in children after submersion. Pediatr Emerg Care 2001;17:405–9.

96. Thompson DC, Rivara FP. Pool fencing for preventing drowning in children. Cochrane Database Syst Rev 2000;2:CD001047.

97. Fenner P. Drowning awareness. Prevention and treatment. Aust Fam Physician 2000;29:1045–9.

98. Cummings P, Mueller BA, Quan L. Association between wearing a personal flotation device and death by drowning among recreational boaters: a matched cohort analysis of United States Coast Guard data. Inj Prev 2011;17:156–9.

99. Brenner RA, Taneja GS, Haynie DL, et al. Association between swimming lessons and drowning in childhood: a case-control study. Arch Pediatr Adolesc Med 2009;163:203–10.

100. Franklin RC, Scarr JP, Pearn JH. Reducing drowning deaths: the continued challenge of immersion fatalities in Australia. Aust Fam Physician 2010;192:123–6.

101. Weiss J, Committee on Injury, Violence, and Poison Prevention. Prevention of drowning. Pediatrics 2010;126:e253–62.

102. Hackett PH, Roach RC. High-altitude illness. N Engl J Med 2001;345:107–14.

103. Schoene RB. Illnesses at high altitude. Chest 2008;134:402–16.

104. Gallagher SA, Hackett PH. High-altitude illness. Emerg Med Clin North Am 2004;22:329–55.

105. Hultgren HN, Spickard W. Medical experiences in Peru. Stanford Med Bull 1960; 18:76–95.

106. Houston CS. Acute pulmonary edema of high altitude. N Engl J Med 1960;263: 478–80.

107. Hultgren HN, Honigman B, Theis K, et al. High altitude pulmonary edema at a ski resort. West J Med 1996;164:222–7.

108. Ren Y, Fu Z, Shen W, et al. Incidence of high altitude illnesses among unacclimatized persons who acutely ascended to Tibet. High Alt Med Biol 2010;11(1): 39–42.

109. Hackett PH, Rennie D. The incidence, importance, and prophylaxis of acute mountain sickness. Lancet 1976;7996:1149–55.

110. Bartsch P, Mairbaurl H, Maggiorini M, et al. Physiological aspects of high-altitude pulmonary edema. J Appl Phys 2005;98:1101–10.

111. Scoggin CH, Hyers TM, Reeves JT, et al. High-altitude pulmonary edema in the children and young adults of Leadville, Colorado. N Engl J Med 1977;297: 1269–72.

112. Hultgren HN. High-altitude pulmonary edema: current concepts. Annu Rev Med 1996;47:267–84.
113. Schoene RB, Swenson ER, Pizzo CJ, et al. The lung at high altitude: bronchoalveolar lavage in acute mountain sickness and pulmonary edema. J Appl Physiol 1988;64:2605–13.
114. West J, Mathieu-Costello O. High altitude pulmonary edema is caused by stress failure of pulmonary capillaries. Int J Sports Med 1992;13(Suppl 1): S54–8.
115. Kawashima A, Kubo K, Kobayashi T, et al. Hemodynamic responses to acute hypoxia, hypobaria, and exercise in subjects susceptible to high-altitude pulmonary edema. J Appl Physiol 1989;67:1982–9.
116. Busch T, Bartsch P, Pappert D, et al. Hypoxia decreases exhaled nitric oxide in mountaineers susceptible to high-altitude pulmonary edema. Am J Respir Crit Care Med 2001;163:368–73.
117. Duplain H, Sartori C, Lepori M, et al. Exhaled nitric oxide in high-altitude pulmonary edema: role in the regulation of pulmonary vascular tone and evidence for a role against inflammation. Am J Respir Crit Care Med 2000;162:221–4.
118. Duplain H, Vollenweider L, Delabays A, et al. Augmented sympathetic activation during short-term hypoxia and high-altitude exposure in subjects susceptible to high-altitude pulmonary edema. Circulation 1999;99:1713–8.
119. Stream JO, Grissom CK. Update on high-altitude pulmonary edema: pathogenesis, prevention, and treatment. Wilderness Environ Med 2008;19:293–303.
120. Swenson ER, Maggiorini M, Mongovin S, et al. Pathogenesis of high-altitude pulmonary edema: inflammation is not an etiologic factor. JAMA 2002;287: 2228–35.
121. Durmowicz AG, Noordweir E, Nicholas R, et al. Inflammatory processes may predispose children to high-altitude pulmonary edema. J Pediatr 1997;130: 838–40.
122. Luks AM, McIntosh SE, Grissom CK, et al. Wilderness Medical Society consensus guidelines for the prevention and treatment of acute altitude illness. Wilderness Environ Med 2010;21:146–55.
123. Bartsch P, Maggiorini M, Ritter M, et al. Prevention of high-altitude pulmonary edema by nifedipine. N Engl J Med 1991;325:1284–9.
124. Reeves J, Wagner J, Zafren K, et al. Seasonal variation in barometric pressure and temperature in Summit County: effect on altitude illness. In: Sutton J, Houston C, Coates G, editors. Hypoxia and molecular medicine. Burlington (VT): Charles S Houston; 1993. p. 275–81.
125. Schoene RB. Fatal high altitude pulmonary edema associated with absence of the left pulmonary artery. High Alt Med Biol 2001;2:405–6.
126. Roach RC, Bartch P, Hackett PH, et al. The Lake Louise consensus on the definition and quantification of altitude illness. In: Sutton JR, Coates G, Houston CS, editors. Hypoxia and mountain medicine. Burlington (VT): Queen City Printers; 1992.
127. Vock P, Fretz C, Franciolli M, et al. High-altitude pulmonary edema: findings at high-altitude chest radiography and physical examination. Radiology 1989; 170(3 Pt 1):661–6.
128. Vock P, Brutsche MH, Nanzer A, et al. Variable radiomorphologic data of high altitude pulmonary edema: features from 60 patients. Chest 1991;100:1306–11.
129. Fagenholz PJ, Gutman JA, Murray AF, et al. Chest ultrasonography for the diagnosis and monitoring of high-altitude pulmonary edema. Chest 2007;131: 1013–8.

130. Pratali L, Cavana M, Sicari R, et al. Frequent subclinical high-altitude pulmonary edema detected by chest sonography as ultrasound lung comets in recreational climbers. Crit Care Med 2010;38:1818–23.
131. Zafren K, Reeves JT, Schoene R. Treatment of high-altitude pulmonary edema by bed rest and supplemental oxygen. Wilderness Environ Med 1996;7:127–32.
132. Oelz O, Maggiorini M, Ritter M, et al. Nifedipine for high altitude pulmonary oedema. Lancet 1989;2:1241–4.
133. Fagenholz PJ, Gutman JA, Murray AF, et al. Treatment of high altitude pulmonary edema at 4240 m in Nepal. High Alt Med Biol 2007;8:139–46.
134. Maggiorini M, Brunner-La Rocca HP, Peth S, et al. Both tadalafil and dexamethasone may reduce the incidence of high-altitude pulmonary edema. Ann Intern Med 2006;145:497–506.
135. Sartori C, Allemann Y, Duplain H, et al. Salmeterol for the prevention of high-altitude pulmonary edema. N Engl J Med 2002;346:1631–6.
136. Freeman K, Shalit M, Stroh G. Use of the Gamow Bag by EMT-basic park rangers for treatment of high-altitude pulmonary edema and high-altitude cerebral edema. Wilderness Environ Med 2004;15:198–201.
137. Luks AM. Can patients with pulmonary hypertension travel to high altitude? High Alt Med Biol 2009;10:215–9.
138. Tanen DA, Graema KA, Raschke R. Severe lung injury after exposure to chloramine gas from household cleaners. N Engl J Med 1999;341:848–9.
139. Jajosky R, Harrison R, Reinisch F, et al. Surveillance of work-related asthma in selected U.S. states using surveillance guidelines for state health departments–California, Massachusetts, Michigan, and New Jersey, 1993-1995. MMWR CDC Surveill Summ 1999;48(SS03):1–20.
140. Kahan ES, Martin UJ, Spungen S, et al. Chronic cough and dyspnea in ice hockey players after an acute exposure to combustion products of a faulty ice resurfacer. Lung 2007;185:47–54.
141. Fisk MZ, Steigerwald MD, Smoliga JM, et al. Asthma in swimmers: a review of the current literature. Phys Sportsmed 2010;38:28–34.
142. Varma DR, Guest I. The Bhopal accident and methyl isocyanate toxicity. J Toxicol Environ Health 1993;40:513–29.
143. Balmes JR. Occupational contribution to the burden of chronic obstructive pulmonary disease. J Occup Environ Med 2005;47:154–60.
144. Nelson LS, Hoffman RS. Inhaled toxins. In: Marx JA, Hockberger RS, Walls RM, editors. Rosen's emergency medicine: concepts and clinical practice. 6th edition. Philadelphia: Mosby Elsevier; 2006.
145. White CW, Martin JG. Chlorine gas inhalation: human clinical evidence of toxicity and experience in animal models. Proc Am Thorac Soc 2010;7:257–63.
146. Centers for Disease Control and Prevention. Ocular and respiratory illness associated with an indoor swimming pool–Nebraska, 2006. MMWR CDC Surveill Summ 2007;56:929–32.
147. Tsonis L, Hantsch-Bardsley C, Gamelli RL. Hydrofluoric acid inhalation injury. J Burn Care Res 2008;29:852–5.
148. Russell D, Blaine PG, Rice P. Clinical management of casualties exposed to lung damaging agents: a critical review. Emerg Med J 2006;23:421–4.
149. De Lange DW, Meulenbelt J. Do corticosteroids have a role in preventing or reducing acute toxic lung injury caused by inhalation of chemical agents? Clin Toxicol 2011;49:61–71.
150. Aslan S, Kandis H, Akgrun M, et al. The effect of nebulized NaHCO3 treatment on "RADS" due to chlorine gas inhalation. Inhal Toxicol 2006;18:895–900.

151. Bosse GM. Nebulized sodium bicarbonate therapy in the treatment of chlorine gas inhalation. J Toxicol Clin Toxicol 1994;32:233–41.

152. Vinsel PJ. Treatment of acute chlorine gas inhalation with nebulized sodium bicarbonate. J Emerg Med 1990;8:327–9.

153. Pauluhn J, Hai CX. Attempts to counteract phosgene-induced acute lung injury by instant high-dose aerosol exposure to hexamethylenetetramine, cysteine, or glutathione. Inhal Toxicol 2011;23:58–64.

154. Kono K, Watanabe T, Dote T, et al. Successful treatments of lung injury and skin burn due to hydrofluoric acid exposure. Int Arch Occup Environ Health 2000;73: 93–7.

155. Lee DC, Wiley JF Jr, Snyder JW Jr. Treatment of inhalational exposure to hydrofluoric acid with nebulized calcium gluconate. J Occup Med 1993;35:470.

156. Nelson LS. Simple asphyxiants and pulmonary irritants. In: Flomenbaum NE, Goldfrank LR, Hoffman RS, et al, editors. Goldfrank's toxicologic emergencies. 8th edition. New York: McGraw-Hill; 2006.

157. Suruda A, Agnew J. Deaths from asphyxiation and poisoning at work in the United States 1984-6. Br J Ind Med 1989;46:541–6.

158. Dorevitch S, Forst L, Conroy L, et al. Toxic inhalation fatalities of US construction workers, 1990 to 1999. J Occup Environ Med 2002;44:657–62.

159. Hill M. Possible asphyxiation from carbon dioxide of a cross-country skier in eastern California: a deadly volcanic hazard. Wilderness Environ Med 2000; 11:192–5.

160. Cantrell L, Young M. Fatal fall into a volcanic fumarole. Wilderness Environ Med 2009;20:77–9.

161. Baxter PJ, Kapila M, Mfonfu D. Lake Nyos disaster, Cameroon, 1986: the medical effects of large scale emission of carbon dioxide? BMJ 1989;298: 1437–41.

162. Miller TM, Mazur PO. Oxygen deficiency hazards associated with liquefied gas systems: derivations of a program of controls. Am Ind Hyg Assoc J 1984;45: 293–8.

Common Pediatric Respiratory Emergencies

Joseph Choi, MD[a],*, Gary L. Lee, MD, CCFP-EM, FRCPC[b]

KEYWORDS

• Pediatric • Asthma • Bronchiolitis • Croup • Pneumonia

Acute respiratory distress is one of the most common reasons why parents bring their children to the emergency department (ED). Severity can range from mild, self-limiting illness to life-threatening disease. This article reviews the 4 most common of these conditions, namely asthma, croup, bronchiolitis, and pneumonia, to update the reader on the current state of evidence in the assessment and treatment of these conditions.

ASTHMA IN CHILDREN

Asthma is a chronic inflammatory condition of the airways leading to episodic wheezing, coughing, chest tightness, and shortness of breath. It is a common condition, with the highest prevalence occurring between the ages of 5 and 17 years.[1] Asthma afflicted 7.0 million children in this age group in the United States in 2008.[1] It led to 1.7 million ED visits in 2006, and children younger than 15 years accounted for 33% of those with a discharge diagnosis of asthma while this age group only represents 20% of the general population.[1]

Asthma is the most activity-limiting condition in children and accounts for 14.4 million lost school days. It is an expensive disease, with an annual burden of $15.6 billion in direct health care costs and $5.1 billion in indirect health care costs and lost productivity, for a total annual sum of $20.7 billion.[1]

Pathophysiology

Asthma is a chronic disease of the lower airways punctuated with episodic acute exacerbations. The clinical manifestations are caused by airway hyperresponsiveness to stimuli that are generally innocuous, leading to constriction of bronchial smooth

The authors have nothing to disclose.
[a] McGill University FRCP Emergency Medicine Residency Program, Royal Victoria Hospital, 687 Pine Avenue West, Room A4.62, Montreal, Quebec, Canada H3A 1A1
[b] Department of Emergency Medicine, Montreal Children's Hospital, Montreal General Hospital, McGill University, 1650 Cedar Avenue, Montreal, Quebec, Canada H3G 1A4
* Corresponding author.
E-mail address: joseph.choi@mail.mcgill.ca

Emerg Med Clin N Am 30 (2012) 529–563
doi:10.1016/j.emc.2011.10.009
0733-8627/12/$ – see front matter © 2012 Elsevier Inc. All rights reserved.

muscle (bronchospasm), the major cause of wheezing during an asthma exacerbation. Airway inflammation and edema in response to these stimuli further narrows the airway and restricts ventilation.[2,3]

These physiologic changes on the cellular level can occur through IgE-mediated pathways (allergen-triggered asthma)[4] and non–IgE-mediated pathways (asthma in response to nonsteroidal anti-inflammatory drugs,[5] certain other drugs, exercise, and cold temperatures).[3] Both pathways lead to a release of various cytokines and chemokines from inflammatory cells, which promote further migration and activation of inflammatory cells in the lower airways, thus perpetuating the cycle.[3]

Diagnosis

The diagnosis of asthma is particularly challenging in the pediatric population. Young children usually cannot be cooperative enough to undergo formal pulmonary function testing, which is the gold standard in the diagnosis of asthma. Thus they often must be diagnosed clinically.

Many first-time wheezers also present to the ED. Most instances of wheezing in young children presenting to the ED are solely related to upper respiratory infections (URI) causing inflammation of the lower airways rather than true asthma.[6] The majority of early wheezers do not go on to develop asthma in later childhood or adulthood.[6,7] This distinction is an important one, as it can affect the efficacy of certain therapeutic options.[8] Clues that increase the likelihood that the wheezing is due to asthma include the frequency of episodes (more than once a month), triggers (exercise, allergens, tobacco smoke), prolonged respiratory symptoms in the setting of URI (symptoms lasting more than 10 days suggest a viral trigger of asthma), personal or family history of atopy or asthma, and a history of a good and rapid response to bronchodilator therapy.[3,6,9]

Other historical features of the patient that may aid in predicting the severity of the asthma exacerbation include the frequency and compliance in using asthma medications at home, previous hospital visits for asthma exacerbations (requiring admission to the ward or intensive care unit [ICU]), and severity of asthma exacerbations (requiring intubation). Social attributes of the patient and caregivers, such as the ability to purchase medications and comply to their use, a household environment free of known or suspected asthma triggers, and ability to obtain follow-up and access medical services in the event of another exacerbation, have important discharge planning implications and should be elicited early.[2,3,7,9]

The physical examination may reveal any combination of the classic constellation of symptoms in the acute asthma exacerbation, which includes wheezing, cough, chest tightness, tachypnea, respiratory distress, intercostal indrawing, and accessory muscle use.[3,7,9] Of interest, the use of the scalene muscles and suprasternal retractions have the highest interrater reliability and correlation with asthma severity.[10] Clinical asthma assessment tools, such as the Pediatric Respiratory Assessment Measure (PRAM; **Table 1**)[10,11] and the Pediatric Asthma Severity Score (PASS),[12] have been independently shown to be predictive in discriminating a patient's length of stay in the hospital and admission.[10,12] The strength of these two scales is that they include preschool-aged children, in comparison with older severity scales such as the Pulmonary Index and the Pulmonary Score, which are only validated in older, school-aged children.[10–12] A recent head-to-head comparison of the two scores showed very similar performance in their ability to predict a prolonged stay (>6 hours) and/or admission when taken at triage.[13] However, a repeat score taken 90 minutes after treatment showed that the PRAM score was more responsive and predictive

Table 1
The Pediatric Respiratory Assessment Measure (PRAM) score

Signs	0	1	2	3
Suprasternal indrawing	Absent		Present	
Scalene use	Absent		Present	
Wheezing	Absent	Expiratory only	Inspiratory and expiratory	Audible without stethoscope or minimal air entry/silent chest
Air entry	Normal	Decreased at bases	Widespread decrease	Minimal air entry/silent chest
Pulse oximetry on room air	>95%	92%–94%	<91%	

Data from Ducharme F, Chalut D, Plotnick L, et al. The Pediatric Respiratory Assessment Measure: a valid clinical score for assessing acute asthma severity from toddlers to teenagers. J Pediatr 2008;152(4):476–80, 480.e471.

(area under the receiver-operator characteristic curve 0.82 vs 0.72).[13] These tools can be particularly useful when integrated into protocolized treatment regimens.[2,9,14]

Investigations should include measurement of oxygen saturation, with more severe exacerbations deserving continuous monitoring. A blood gas sample may be useful in severe exacerbations in addition to clinical signs to determine respiratory function and responsiveness to therapy. In particular, normocarbia or hypercarbia in a patient after a round of standard treatment is a worrisome sign.[3,9]

Peak expiratory flow (PEF) is an objective method of assessing the degree of airway obstruction. However, it is often exceedingly difficult (if not impossible) to obtain these measurements in children younger than 6 years, and even with a cooperative child the measurements may not be reliable in an acute exacerbation.[15,16] If PEF values are obtained, suggested categories include mild (PEF >80% predicted), moderate (PEF 60%–80% predicted), or severe (PEF <60%),[2] though different governing bodies have varying values.[3,9]

Additional blood work and imaging only aid in excluding complications or other diagnoses based on clinical suspicion,[3,9] and are not routinely recommended.

First-Line Treatment

Children with acute exacerbations should be rapidly assessed and triaged to a location in the ED where observation and frequent reassessment can be performed by medical and nursing staff. Reassessment of patients after each round of treatment is by far the most important aspect in the management of acute asthma exacerbations. Children, and especially infants, are particularly at risk for respiratory failure. Hypoxemia develops more rapidly in children than in adults; therefore monitoring of oxygen saturation is necessary.[3,9] Oxygen should be administered only to maintain a saturation of greater than 92%–94%,[3,9] as indiscriminate high-flow oxygen despite good saturations can lead to poorer outcomes.[17]

Short-acting β-agonist (SABA) treatment is the most effective method of relieving bronchospasm, and should be given to all patients with asthma exacerbations.[3,9] SABA can be administered as either intermittent therapy spaced 15 to 20 minutes apart via wet nebulizer or metered-dose inhaler (MDI) with a holding chamber, or as continuous therapy via a nebulizer.[18,19] In mild to moderate asthma, an MDI has been shown to be at least equivalent if not better in efficacy than a nebulizer in infants, children, and adults,[20–23] and is more cost effective.[24] Factors that influence the choice of MDI versus nebulizer include patient cooperation, response to treatment via MDI, and severity of the exacerbation. Salbutamol (albuterol, Ventolin) 2 to 4 puffs, can be given every 15 minutes via MDI with chamber, waiting 5 tidal volume breaths between puffs.[3,9] More puffs can be administered (up to 10) in more resistant exacerbations. Salbutamol can also be given at 0.15 to 0.3 mg/kg via nebulizer, with a minimum of 2.5 mg and maximum of 5 mg per nebulized mask. This volume is then diluted with normal saline for a total of 5 mL of fluid per nebulized mask. The most severe exacerbations may benefit from continuous therapy[19] with a nebulizer driven by oxygen if hypoxia is also present.[3,9,17] With continuous nebulization, salbutamol is recommended to be given at 0.5 mg/kg/h with the hourly dose not exceeding 10 to 15 mg/h.[3]

Levosalbutamol ((R)-salbutamol, also known as levalbuterol) is the pure (R)-enantiomer of the salbutamol molecule. In a typical salbutamol preparation, there is a 50:50 mixture of the (S)- and (R)-enantiomers, and it is the (R)-enantiomer that provides the vast majority of the bronchodilating effects, due to its 100-fold higher affinity for the β2-adrenergic receptor. The selectivity of levosalbutamol theoretically maximizes the bronchodilating effects while minimizing systemic side effects such as tachycardia[25] and hypokalemia.[26] Small trials have shown mixed results, with some trials showing benefit in pulmonary function,[27,28] reduction in hospital admission rates,[29] and reduced side effects[26,30]; whereas other studies have shown no difference.[30,31] Levosalbutamol is considerably more expensive than the conventional racemic mixture, and current guidelines do not recommend using one over the other. The dose of levosalbutamol is half that of salbutamol.

Ipratropium bromide (Atrovent) has been shown to be an effective adjunct in moderate to severe asthma in addition to inhaled β-agonists.[32,33] It is a muscarinic acetylcholine receptor blocker, which produces bronchodilation via smooth muscle relaxation. Ipratropium bromide can be given via MDI (4–8 puffs every 15–20 minutes) or nebulizer (0.25–0.5 mg, combined in the same nebulizer as the β-agonist).[3,9] Treatment can be tapered as the patient improves clinically.

Systemic corticosteroids (SCS) have been shown to decrease the need for hospital admission from the ED when given early[34,35] and to decrease the length of stay.[36] SCS should be considered in all but the mildest exacerbations.[3,9,34] However, there is evidence that shows administration of steroids to children with wheezing triggered by a URI and with no other history suggesting asthma provides no benefit in time to discharge, admission rate, morbidity, or mortality.[8] The efficacy of oral versus intravenous (IV) SCS has been shown to be equivalent in pediatric asthma exacerbations.[37,38] Parenteral SCS should be reserved for those who cannot tolerate oral steroids or have intestinal issues that would affect its absorption.[3,9] Oral prednisone or prednisolone, 1 to 2 mg/kg, should be given once daily, with a maximum dose of 60 mg/d for 3 to 5 days.[2,3] Studies suggest that a 2-day course of oral dexamethasone (dosed at 0.6 mg/kg daily, maximum of 16 mg) is as effective (measured by symptoms scores, admission rates, and 10-day relapse rate) and well tolerated (rates of nausea and vomiting) as a 5-day course of oral prednisone in adults[39] and children.[40,41] Another study even suggests that a single dose is non-inferior to a 5-day course of prednisone.[42] Intramuscular (IM) injection of depot steroids, such as dexamethasone acetate, has also been shown in small studies to be as effective as a 5-day course of prednisone.[43,44] IV steroids can be given as methylprednisolone, 2 mg/kg/d in two divided doses.[3] Inhaled corticosteroids (ICS) are not currently recommended as a replacement for SCS for the treatment of acute asthma exacerbations presenting to the ED,[3,9] because of the lack of efficacy when used alone.[34,35,45–48] Recent evidence suggests that the addition of inhaled budesonide to standard therapy including SCS does not improve outcomes.[49]

Second-Line Treatments

In children with severe or life-threatening asthma, the aforementioned therapies may not be sufficient. It is crucial to recognize refractory asthma and to treat it aggressively.

Magnesium sulfate is a safe drug with few side effects, which has been shown to have bronchodilating effects.[50–52] Its use has not been shown to be beneficial in mild to moderate asthma, but has demonstrated a reduction in admission rates for severe asthma, with minimal side effects.[53,54] A single IV dose of 25 to 75 mg/kg (not exceeding 2 g) can be given over 2 hours.[3,9] Inhaled magnesium sulfate has been shown in small studies to improve expiratory flow measures when used in addition to inhaled β-agonists in severe asthma exacerbations,[55,56] but confers no benefit in mild to moderate episodes.[57] A Cochrane review showed that nebulized magnesium sulfate provided significant improvement in pulmonary function tests and a nonsignificant trend to decreased hospital admission rates in severe asthma exacerbations, but no statistically significant difference when included in all severities of asthma attacks.[58] Inhaled magnesium sulfate is given as the diluent in place of normal saline (usually 2.5 mL of a 250 mmol/L solution) combined with salbutamol and ipratropium bromide in the same nebulized mask.

Oral leukotriene receptor antagonists (LTRA) such as montelukast (Singulair) have been shown to decrease symptoms of mild to moderate asthma exacerbations,[59,60] but their role in severe asthma is unknown because of their slow onset of action.[61] In moderate to severe asthma there is some evidence in the adult literature that IV administration may be effective,[62] but there are no corresponding studies done in children. The oral dosage of montelukast in children is 4 to 10 mg orally once per day.

Heliox is a blend of helium and oxygen, the use of which is based on the principle of increased ventilation into the lower airspaces in asthma, due to its low viscosity.[63] Some studies have shown modest benefit[63–65] whereas others show no benefit.[66] It has a level D recommendation as the driver of nebulized salbutamol in severe asthma,[3] mainly because of its lack of side effects.

Routine antibiotics are not recommended unless there is a suspicion of pneumonia (fever, purulent sputum) or bacterial sinusitis.[2,3,9] Mucolytics and sedation are not recommended.[2,3,9]

Status Asthmaticus and Imminent Respiratory Failure

One of the most terrifying prospects for an emergency physician is the sight of a child with asthma not responding to treatment and heading toward respiratory failure. Signs include increasing somnolence, tiring of breathing muscles, cyanosis, and a silent chest. Heralds of impending cardiac arrest are bradycardia, severe hypoxia, and hypercapnia.

If not already performed, IV access should be obtained and any hypovolemia should be corrected. This action is also taken to prevent hypotension that the induction drugs may cause during rapid sequence intubation and positive ventilation.

IV β-agonists have not been shown to be beneficial in severe exacerbations, and carry significant side effects.[3,67] Likewise, aminophylline has not been recommended, due to its considerable toxicity and lack of clear benefit,[68] though a study has shown some effect in children with life-threatening asthma already receiving maximum doses of conventional therapy.[69] However, in the setting of a status asthmaticus in extremis with no response to other therapies, guidelines still endorse consideration of their use as a last resort.[2,3,9]

Temporizing measures can include a trial of noninvasive positive-pressure ventilation (NPPV). There are small studies analyzing the ability of NPPV to avoid intubation and improve outcomes in children with status asthmaticus,[70–75] and a Cochrane review showed a trend toward benefit.[76] If the patient is unable to tolerate NPPV and continues to deteriorate, endotracheal intubation with mechanical ventilation is necessary.[3,9] Once the decision has been made, the most experienced physician should make the attempt, as asthmatic patients are often difficult to intubate and desaturate quickly. Traditionally the induction agent of choice is ketamine (1–2 mg/kg IV) because of its mild bronchodilating properties,[77] though the clinical significance of this bronchodilation is questionable,[77,78] and several trials using ketamine infusion as an adjunct in status asthmaticus have shown no benefit.[78,79] Ketamine can also increase oral and airway secretions[80] and trigger laryngospasm, and should be used in conjunction with a paralytic agent to counteract this possibility.[81] Other choices for induction include etomidate (0.3 mg/kg IV) and propofol (1.5–3 mg/kg IV). The paralytic agent of choice depends on patient characteristics, the presence of contraindications to particular agents, and physician preference and experience.

A ventilator strategy that has shown benefit is one of permissive hypercapnea.[3,82–86] With this strategy, Pco_2 is allowed to reach up to 70 mm Hg, providing high Fio_2 concentrations to maintain saturations greater than 92%, and manipulating ventilator settings (such as the prolonging the expiratory time to allow for complete exhalation) to minimize pressures and avoid barotrauma and other complications. Bicarbonate can be given to correct severe acidosis.[87]

Disposition

The decision to hospitalize children with severe asthma depends on the severity of the exacerbation and its response to ED therapy. Those who present with PEF less than 25%, or have a PEF less than 40% or significant symptoms after therapy, should be admitted for continued treatment and observation.[2,3] Unstable home situations or predicted poor compliance and follow-up are also indications for admission.[2,3,9]

Children receiving treatment in the ED should be monitored for at least 1 hour after their last round of treatment to ensure resolution of symptoms.[2,3,9] In those able to provide PEF measures, a general value of greater than 70% to 80% of expected value is acceptable for discharge. Those with a PEF of 40% to 69% with minimal symptoms can also be discharged if they have good follow-up and demonstrate good compliance, and if medical attention is readily accessible.[2,3]

Follow-up with a primary care provider or asthma specialist should be arranged within a month of discharge from the ED to reassess medications and treatment plans,[2,3] as this has been shown to improve outcomes and decrease ED visits.[88,89] The appointment should be scheduled before discharge from the ED, as this has been shown to increase compliance.[90,91]

Medications to be continued after discharge include inhaled salbutamol and oral steroids as already described, with no need for a tapering dose.[2,3,9] Current guidelines state that the initiation of ICS should be considered in those with moderate to severe exacerbations who were not previously on ICS.[2,3,9] Patients should be given a 1- to 2-month supply, as this has been shown to reduce the number of exacerbations and ED visits.[46,92,93] ICS should be continued if previously prescribed. Ipratropium bromide has not been shown to be of benefit after discharge from the ED.

Discharge home with a peak flow meter is also recommended for children older than 5 years,[3] especially in those who do not perceive mild symptoms well or have recurrent severe exacerbations.[94]

Children to be discharged should be provided a written action plan (WAP) that delineates clearly discharge medications, instructions in proper inhaler and peak flow meter technique, follow-up appointments, and warning signs that indicate a need to return to the ED.[2,3]

CROUP

Croup is a common cause of stridor in the young child. Croup is characterized by a harsh inspiratory stridor and a hoarse cough that is often described as barky or resembling a seal, secondary to upper airway inflammation and edema. Although usually benign and self-limiting, it can cause significant respiratory distress requiring intubation.

Croup is the most common cause of stridor in young children older than 6 months. It peaks between 6 and 36 months of life. At 2 years of age, 5% of all children will have had croup.[95] In a 14-year observational study in Ontario, Canada, its incidence seems to have a biennial mid-autumn peak and an annual summer trough, with boys being affected 1.5 times as often as girls.[96]

Pathophysiology

There has been much confusion in the use of the term croup. It has been used to describe different disease entities in which stridor and hoarse cough are the predominant symptoms,[95] such as spasmodic croup, laryngotracheobronchitis (LTB), laryngotracheobronchopneumonia (LTBP), bacterial tracheitis, and diphtheria. In this review croup specifically refers to laryngotracheitis, as the other entities have different presentations, treatment options, and prognoses.

Croup is commonly caused by parainfluenza virus (PIV)-1.[97] PIV-2 and PIV-3 are also implicated in croup, with type 2 causing a milder form and type 3 causing a more severe form. Other viruses that can lead to croup include influenza, respiratory syncytial virus (RSV), rhinoviruses, enteroviruses, and measles, among others.[95]

Viral infection often starts via inoculation of the nares and pharynx, which leads to typical URI symptoms of low-grade fever, coryza, and rhinorrhea. The infection then spreads down to the larynx and subglottic area, causing cough and inflammation and edema of the upper airway and leading to varying degrees of obstruction. According to Poiseuille's equation, resistance to flow is inversely proportional to radius to the fourth power. Therefore even slight decreases in diameter can cause significant resistance, especially in the already tiny airways of the young child. The lower airways are usually not affected in PIV-associated croup, though RSV and influenza can cause lower respiratory symptoms.

Diagnosis

The constellation of a barky cough, hoarseness, and stridor is common in many diseases, and differentiation between them is of utmost importance, as treatment and potential complications vary widely.

The onset and progression of symptoms leading to the ED visit should be explored. The history of a preceding URI in the last day or two is often elicited. In addition to cough and stridor, the child is often febrile. Combined with other features of the history, a suddenly stridorous child without fever or URI should raise a suspicion of foreign body aspiration or angioneurotic edema. An immunization and travel history should be elicited, since an unimmunized child is at higher risk of developing laryngeal diphtheria from *Corynebacterium diphtheriae* infection. Pharyngitis and dysphagia are features that are uncommon with croup, and may suggest retropharyngeal abscess, peritonsillar abscess, epiglottitis, or diphtheria. Finally, caution is required when diagnosing croup in a stridorous child younger than 6 months, due to the important differential diagnosis in this age group. The differential includes laryngomalacia (the most common cause, and a self-limited condition that 90% grow out of by 12–18 months),[98] vocal cord paralysis,[99] papillomatosis,[100] congenital causes (such as hemangiomas,[101] laryngeal webs,[100] and neurofibromas[102]), and iatrogenic causes (such as subglottic stenosis following intubation for prematurity,[103] or vocal cord paralysis caused by laryngeal nerve damage from thoracic or cardiac procedures[104]).

The child should otherwise appear well; a toxic-looking child should be investigated for alternative diagnoses such as bacterial tracheitis (which can be a complication of croup), LTB, LTBP, or epiglottitis. There should be no signs of lower airway involvement such as wheezing or crackles, which may suggest an alternative diagnosis. If hemangiomas are noted on the child, especially above the clavicles, a subglottic hemangioma should be considered along with historical features such as a lack of URI symptoms. A throat examination should identify pharyngeal causes of stridor easily, though caution should be exercised if the presentation is suspicious for epiglottitis. The epiglottis, if visualized, should be normal.

The diagnosis of croup remains a clinical one, with additional testing being useful in ruling out other differential diagnoses. Complete blood cell counts (CBC) may show a mildly elevated white cell count in croup, whereas it is usually markedly elevated or depressed in bacterial infections of the upper airway with increased neutrophils and band forms. Posterior-anterior neck radiographs in croup may show subglottic narrowing (steeple sign) with a smooth tracheal contour. Irregularity of this contour suggests bacterial tracheitis and other diagnoses.[95] Lower respiratory symptoms should be investigated with a chest radiograph (CXR) to assess for a possible pneumonia. A lateral neck radiograph showing a thickened mass at the level of the epiglottis (thumbprint sign) suggests epiglottitis.[105] Foreign bodies may appear on plain films, depending on the object.

Classification

Different classification scales based on physical examination findings have been devised. The Westley Croup Score[106] is the most widely known and used, although it is used more commonly in research protocols and less frequently in clinical practice.[107] Key criteria used in this score include level of consciousness, stridor, air entry, cyanosis, and chest wall retractions.[95,106,107]

A simplified classification, based from the original Westley Croup Score, has been suggested by several investigators.[95,107] Mild croup is defined by an absence of stridor at rest, minimal respiratory distress, and occasional cough. Moderate croup has stridor at rest and increased amount of respiratory distress, but behavior and mental status are normal. Severe croup has significant respiratory distress and mental status changes, with increasing somnolence and decreasing air entry signifying impending respiratory failure.

Treatment

As with all patients, the ABCs (Airway, Breathing, Circulation) must be prioritized. Patients with signs of impending respiratory failure should be intubated with an endotracheal tube 0.5 to 1 mm smaller than the expected size. Oxygen should be delivered to maintain oxygen saturation greater than 92% to 94%. Where possible, the child should be kept calm to decrease respiratory distress and improve airway dynamics.

The mainstays of pharmacotherapy in the ED management of croup are corticosteroids and nebulized epinephrine. Dexamethasone remains the corticosteroid of choice over prednisolone through its ability to decrease return visits and admissions.[108] In a recent Cochrane review, dexamethasone was shown to reduce symptoms in the ED, decrease length of stay, and result in fewer return visits.[109] Dexamethasone is given as a single dose of 0.6 mg/kg by mouth/IM/IV (oral is preferred, though parenteral routes have been shown to be equally effective[110]) to a maximum of 10 mg. There are several studies that show lower doses of dexamethasone (0.15–0.3 mg/kg) may be equally effective.[111–113] Inhaled budesonide can be used if available (2 mg via nebulizer) and has been shown to be similar in efficacy to dexamethasone,[109,114,115] though availability, cost, and convenience makes dexamethasone a more attractive option. There does not appear to be any additional benefit from combining oral and inhaled steroids in the setting of croup.[116] Corticosteroids should be considered in all severities of croup.

Nebulized epinephrine is used in moderate to severe croup, and has been shown to be highly efficacious in reducing symptom scores at 30 minutes after treatment and time spent in the ED.[117] However, the natural history of the disease is unchanged, and thus it is important to monitor children after epinephrine treatment for rebound reactions.[106,118] Despite the theoretical benefits of L-epinephrine over racemic epinephrine, studies did not show a benefit of choosing one over the other.[117] L-Epinephrine is given as 5 mL of a 1:1000 solution (racemic epinephrine is given as 0.5 mL of a 2.25% solution in 2.5 mL of normal saline) delivered via nebulizer every 15 minutes to effect. Although serious cardiac complications from epinephrine treatment are exceedingly rare, it is prudent to put children requiring multiple treatments on continuous cardiac monitoring.

Although cold, humid air anecdotally has been thought to improve croup symptoms, recent trials did not show this benefit in the ED setting.[119–121] A study evaluating the use of Heliox showed that it may be as effective as nebulized racemic epinephrine in moderate to severe croup.[122] Heliox also demonstrated a nonstatistically significant trend toward improvement in croup scores when combined with epinephrine and steroids.[123] However, a Cochrane review showed no significant difference in croup scores when Heliox was added to conventional therapy, and therefore did not routinely recommend its use at this time.[124] Antibiotics should be saved for suspected bacterial complications such as bacterial tracheitis or LTBP. Sedatives and antitussives are not indicated.[95,107]

Disposition

Most cases of croup are mild to moderate and respond well to steroid with or without nebulized epinephrine therapy, and the vast majority of patients are discharged home. Children with mild symptoms (ie, no stridor at rest) can be safely sent home. Patients receiving epinephrine should be observed for 4 hours to watch for any rebound phenomenon. Children who require multiple epinephrine doses should be admitted for observation. ICU admission may be required in cases of severe croup that fail to respond to treatment. On discharge, it is prudent to inform the parents that symptoms of croup usually peak between days 2 to 3.

BRONCHIOLITIS

Bronchiolitis is the most common lower respiratory tract condition in children younger than 2 years, and is the leading cause of hospitalization of infants. Its most common cause, RSV, is ubiquitous worldwide, affecting nearly all children by the age of 2, often causing dyspnea in its tiniest of victims with the potential to cause respiratory failure and death. Significant literature and practice guidelines have been published to guide practitioners. Active research in the field is ongoing, and even small improvements in therapy or resource use can make a major impact given the burden of disease.

Definition and Epidemiology

Bronchiolitis is typically caused by viral infection, characterized by bronchiolar inflammation in children usually younger than 2 years. Children from age 2 to 5 years with similar symptoms rarely have bronchiolitis, as asthma, recurrent viral wheeze, or pneumonia are more likely diagnoses. Wheezing is the hallmark of the American definition of bronchiolitis, where British and Australian definitions include inspiratory crackles as part of the diagnosis.[125,126] Most studies and guidelines define bronchiolitis as the first episode of wheezing or crackles. As the presentations of bronchiolitis, viral-associated wheeze, and asthma may appear similar, attention to the features of patients becomes very important given differing pathophysiology and responses to treatment.[125]

RSV continues to be the most common cause, responsible for approximately 50% to 80% of cases. The epidemiology of bronchiolitis follows closely that of RSV. A strongly seasonal virus, RSV causes outbreaks most commonly between November and March in the northern hemisphere and between May and September in the southern hemisphere. Up to half of infected children younger than 2 years will have lower respiratory tract symptoms, whereas older children and adults are more likely to have upper tract disease only. Peak age for bronchiolitis is 2 to 6 months old, with most cases occurring before age 9 months. Reinfection with RSV is common, given poor postinfection immunity.

Recent studies demonstrate an increasing role and frequency of other viruses causing bronchiolitis, including human metapneumovirus (10%–20%), human bocavirus, rhinovirus, parainfluenza, adenovirus, influenza, and coronavirus.[127–129] Although rhinovirus and human metapneumovirus infection has been shown to be generally less severe than RSV (Group A strains causing more severe disease than Group B strains), etiologic diagnosis is often not known in the ED and does not currently affect ED management.[127,130]

Bronchiolitis-associated hospitalizations have more than doubled over recent decades, likely attributable to several factors including increased spread of viral illnesses from daycare exposures, greater awareness of hospitalization criteria, routine oximetry use, and marginally larger numbers of higher-risk children afflicted because of higher survival rates of at-risk populations.[131] Associated mortalities for the condition fortunately have fallen from an alarming 4500 annually in the United States in 1985 to 390 in 1999.[132] Although a significant portion of the decrease in mortality is likely attributable to proper recognition and admission of high-risk infants and improvements in supportive care, a continuing challenge for emergency room providers remains predicting those children in true need of hospitalization as opposed to those requiring appropriate supportive outpatient care.

Clinical Presentation and Course

Nasopharyngeal viral invasion usually causes rhinorrhea and coryza. As infection spreads via inhalation and direct spread of the virus toward the lower respiratory tract, a dry wheezy cough develops. Low-grade fever (<39°C) may often occur. A high (>40°C) or prolonged fever is unusual, and should prompt consideration for coexistent infection. Lower respiratory symptoms typically start on the second to third day of symptoms and peak within the third to fifth day. Viral invasion proceeds distally, leading to the classic changes of bronchiolar inflammation, edema, increased mucus production, bronchospasm, and necrosis and sloughing of epithelial cells.[125,126] This process leads to bronchiolar airway obstruction, atelectasis, and hyperinflation. Tachypnea, increased respiratory effort, and wheezing become common reasons for ED presentation. Patients may or may not have audible crackles on examination.

The peak in symptom severity may be an important consideration with respect to ED disposition decisions and parental education. Although symptoms may improve substantially after 7 days, it is not uncommon for postbronchiolitic symptoms such as dry cough and wheeze to continue on to the second and third week for almost half of children, with up to 9% extending beyond 4 weeks.[133,134] This aspect is important to address with respect to parental anticipatory guidance and management of parental expectations. Education on duration may potentially affect the frequency of otherwise unwarranted return ED visits.[133,134]

The differential diagnosis of wheeze in the infant and young child must be considered, which includes asthma, episodic viral wheeze, bronchitis, pneumonia, congestive heart failure, gastroesophageal reflux, and foreign body aspiration. Patients not matching the traditional features of acute viral bronchiolitis may require diagnostic testing and management appropriate for the presumptive diagnosis.

For most patients, bronchiolitis will be a mild self-limited disease and will resolve without notable sequelae. Significant complications may occur in up to 10% to 20% of patients and may include dehydration, hypoxemia, coinfection, apneic periods, and respiratory failure. Rates of admission for bronchiolitis cases assessed in the ED range between 19% and 45% in some studies.[127] The duration of hospitalization is usually between 2 and 4 days for the average patient. Children more severely afflicted manifest with markedly increased respiratory effort, and rarely with altered mental status, sepsis syndrome, and cyanosis. Feeding difficulties and sleeping disturbances may occur secondary to the respiratory symptoms or occult hypoxemia, and are thus important additional markers of severity that should be inquired about in the ED.[130] It is crucial to recognize significant feeding difficulties, which may be harbingers of early respiratory failure. Approximately 3% of hospital admissions will require ICU admission[135] and as many as 1.5% may require assisted ventilation.[136] Although the mortality rate has recently remained stable, the potential lethality of the illness will always remain a key concern.

A common question of both parents and clinicians concerns future risk of asthma in children and infants presenting with bronchiolitis. Literature and expert opinion suggest that viral lower respiratory tract infections do not cause asthma, but that children affected remain at higher risk of future episodes of non-atopic wheezing as well as asthma exacerbations.[137–139]

Assessment and Management

The diagnosis of bronchiolitis can be made clinically in most children with classic signs and symptoms. Given that a very significant proportion of bronchiolitis cases are mild, they resolve with supportive care alone. Routine diagnostic tests such as CXR, viral cultures, and blood tests have rarely been shown to have an impact on the clinical course, and often add unnecessary and unjustified expense.

Multiple studies and guidelines have illustrated the low yield of CXR in the setting of bronchiolitis, particularly in the mildly ill child without risk factors. Moreover, routine CXR has been shown to increase the rate of unnecessary antibiotic prescription without improving outcomes.[140] Schuh and colleagues[141] reported on 265 cases of children with a clinical diagnosis of likely bronchiolitis who underwent CXR. Of these, 92.8% showed airway disease and another 6.9% showed airway and airspace disease, both patterns consistent with viral bronchiolitis. In only 0.75% of cases did CXR reveal lobar consolidation warranting antibiotics. This study concluded that the risk of airspace disease was particularly low in patients with O_2 saturation greater than 92% and only mild to moderate respiratory distress, and that CXR was unwarranted in this patient subgroup. Another study of 270 children found that the subset of patients with focal findings on CXR were more likely to present with fever, have temperature higher than 38.4°C in the ED, and were 4 times more likely to present with focal crackles on examination.[142] Settings whereby CXR has been shown to be more likely of value include prolonged or unusually high fevers, significant hypoxemia (<90%), previous cardiopulmonary disease, need for ICU admission or mechanical ventilation, and atypical cases.

Although rapid RSV identification is available in many centers and offers sensitivities up to of 90%, the added value over clinical diagnosis for patients well enough for discharge remains questionable, and therefore should not be routinely ordered. For those patients requiring admission, nasopharyngeal fluid testing may be of value. In some situations, testing of febrile young infants for RSV may decrease the extent of septic workup that would otherwise be undertaken. Rapid influenza testing may be warranted if treatment of a positive result would be indicated.

A CBC is not routinely recommended in the setting of bronchiolitis. Although often taken in patients being admitted, the use of an elevated white blood cell count (WBC) to predict bacterial superinfection in this setting has been shown to be unreliable. A study of 1920 patients with confirmed RSV infection showed that the WBC was unable to distinguish between those with and without serious bacterial infection.[143] WBC can also be significantly elevated in the setting of adenovirus infections.[144]

Coinfection should be considered in cases with unexpectedly high or prolonged fevers. Otitis media has been reported to be the most common coinfection with RSV, in the range of 53% to 62%.[130] Although the possibility of RSV etiology is possible in individual cases, bacterial isolation has been shown to be extremely common in this scenario and should be treated as such. The literature has also addressed the issue of the extent of workup necessary in infants 1 to 90 days old with a clinical diagnosis of bronchiolitis. It has been shown that the incidence of serious bacterial illness (SBI) is lower compared with controls without the diagnosis of bronchiolitis,[145] though a full septic workup is still recommended for patients younger than 1 month. In two case series of 42 and 187 children having blood, urine, and cerebrospinal fluid cultures sent despite the diagnosis of bronchiolitis, no cases of septicemia or meningitis were found and the incidence of urinary tract infection (UTI) in the latter study was 2%. One study of 282 infants younger than 60 days with bronchiolitis showed a 1.5% incidence of SBI including 3 UTI, 1 pneumococcal bacteremia, and 1 meningitis; however, the clinical presentations included shock, apnea/cyanosis, hypothermia, and resolving pneumonia.[146] These studies together suggest that the yield of a full septic workup in this scenario is very low, including the yield of urine culture, and that antibiotics should be used sparingly and with clear indications.[147] One notable caveat to this is that several studies have documented significantly higher rates of bacterial coinfection (mainly bacterial pneumonia) in bronchiolitic patients ill enough to require admission to the ICU,[148,149] so further testing in this population is likely warranted.

Treatment

Despite several studies and Cochrane reviews on the possible interventions to treat bronchiolitis, there has been little impact on the overall course and outcome in patients presenting to the ED.[150–156] Supportive care measures such as suctioning, supplemental oxygen, hydration, and respiratory monitoring remain the current cornerstones of treatment. Nasal suctioning is an easy, useful adjunctive treatment that may improve respiratory status, given the significant secretions in many younger infants who are obligate nose breathers; it is recommended before feeds.[157] No evidence currently exists to support deeper airway suctioning. Oxygen should be administered for saturation less than 90% according to American Academy of Pediatrics Guidelines,[130] and is an option in those with saturations of 90% to 94% and moderate signs of respiratory distress.[157,158] Non-invasive positive-pressure ventilation or intubation is indicated for those rare cases presenting with respiratory failure. IV hydration is necessary for those with dehydration and feeding difficulty. Attention to the risk of syndrome of inappropriate antidiuretic hormone secretion (SIADH) is necessary. Chest physiotherapy has been well studied in the inpatient setting and has not been shown to improve short-term clinical scores or hospital course, and is therefore discouraged.[130,157–159]

The benefit of bronchodilators such as epinephrine and salbutamol is controversial. A recent Cochrane review of more than 1912 infants showed no significant effect of bronchodilators on O_2 saturation, hospital admission rate, length of stay, and disease duration.[160] There was a small improvement in clinical scores in the outpatient studies; however, the clinical significance of this is questionable. Another systematic review included 48 trials using bronchodilators (and/or steroids).[151] Only epinephrine use was found to decrease hospital admissions on day 1 by 33% compared with placebo (relative risk [RR] of 0.67 with 95% confidence interval [CI] of 0.50–0.89). This figure translates into a number needed to treat of 15 for epinephrine to avoid 1 hospitalization (95% CI 10–45). However, a 2004 Cochrane review found the benefit of nebulized epinephrine in inpatients to be unproven.[150] Future studies will likely clarify the role of nebulized epinephrine ED treatments.

One cost estimate of bronchodilator use in 2003 in the United States for admitted patients was $37.5 million,[160] suggesting overutilization of these often temporizing treatments. Side effects such as tachycardia, agitation, hyperactivity, flushing, prolonged cough and tremor, and decreased oxygen saturation[160] are reported, although significant morbidity from their use is rare. As a result, routine use of bronchodilators in the setting of clear bronchiolitis is discouraged in all guidelines.[130,157–159]

However, because of the challenges in distinguishing bronchiolitis from asthma and episodic viral wheeze, an initial trial of bronchodilators remains an option.[130,158,159] Up to 25% of patients may respond to bronchodilators,[130] although the positive placebo response has been estimated at up to 43%.[161] Clinical scores such as the Respiratory Distress Assessment Index or Respiratory Assessment Change Score[130,162] before and after bronchodilator treatment is recommended.

Anticholinergics such as ipratropium bromide have been studied, often in conjunction with β-agonists, and have been shown not to add any benefit in the setting of bronchiolitis.[153]

In examining the role of steroids in the management of bronchiolitis, a 2010 Cochrane systematic review[154] of 17 controlled studies concluded no effect of systemic or inhaled glucocorticoids on the rate of admissions or length of hospitalization. Furthermore, a large, multicenter, randomized controlled trial of 600 patients in the United States showed no benefit from steroid treatment, including subgroup analysis of those with a personal or family history of atopy or asthma.[163] This finding refutes the theory proposed by some that a small asthmatic subgroup may benefit.

In a much debated study, the Pediatric Emergency Research Canada (PERC) group published a multicenter ED study of a series of 800 patients who were treated with nebulized epinephrine, dexamethasone, neither, or both, and outcome measures such as risk of hospitalization at 1 week were documented.[164] Unexpectedly, the combined treatment of inhaled epinephrine and dexamethasone demonstrated a significantly reduced admission rate versus placebo at day 7 (RR 0.65, 95% CI 0.44–0.95). Improvements in breathing and feeding were noted on subsequent days, without harmful outcomes. However, given the high doses of dexamethasone used (1 mg/kg day 1, 0.6 mg/kg days 2–6) and its potential side effects, lack of efficacy of dexamethasone alone, and the lack of other supporting studies, this treatment option needs further validation. Evidence for treatment synergy as well as rationale for potential efficacy via targeting various aspects of the pathophysiology of the disease exists.[126]

Nebulized hypertonic (3%) saline has emerged over the last decade as a potentially promising inpatient therapy for bronchiolitis. Given its proposed actions on improving clearance of mucus and cellular debris, initial studies in the setting of cystic fibrosis showed some benefit.[165] Multiple studies and a 2010 Cochrane review[155] have revealed that nebulized hypertonic saline consistently improves post-inhalation clinical scores and decreases length of stay in hospital by approximately 25% or 0.94 days.[166] In contrast to the inpatient data whereby nebulized hypertonic saline is given at intervals of every 8 hours or less over several days, ED studies using 1 to 3 consecutive doses with a bronchodilator have not to date shown statistically significant improvement in short-term clinical scores, nor decreased hospitalization rates (although trends to these outcomes are suggested and decreased severity is found at 24–72 hours).[135,151,155,162,166,167] Nebulized hypertonic saline may need to be given at adequate intervals, dose, and duration for a significant treatment benefit to be seen. It may also be possible that ED initiation followed by continuation of treatment may lead to later benefits in hospital. Further research is currently under way to better establish and clarify the roles of nebulized hypertonic saline in both the outpatient and inpatient settings.

Small studies looking at the effect of Heliox have demonstrated some benefits in improving short-term respiratory distress scores, but without clear reductions in the need for intubation or length of ICU stay.[156,168] The use of ventilatory support with positive-pressure ventilation has also been examined in small studies showing improved carbon dioxide clearance and clinical scores, but without a clear decrease in the need for intubation.[135,161]

Given that bacterial superinfection is rare in bronchiolitis, antibiotics should only be administered in the setting of proven or highly likely bacterial illness or in suspected sepsis in the unusual toxic child with bronchiolitis. Although pertussis and atypical pneumonias such as Mycoplasma and Chlamydophila may mimic bronchiolitis, significant suspicion for these entities should exist before empiric treatment is considered.

Use of ribavirin should be restricted to immunodeficient children with severe illness, given the lack of evidence in other scenarios.[130,158,159] Surfactant treatment may play a role in young infants requiring ICU care or intubation, although its current role in the ED is not clearly defined.[135]

Given the highly contagious nature of RSV through direct contact and contact with fomites, the importance of hand washing with soap or alcohol-based solutions must be observed by ED personnel and must be stressed to parents. Exposure to second-hand smoke has been found to be a risk factor RSV infection, whereas breastfeeding has been shown to be protective. Palivizumab (Synagis), a monoclonal antibody against RSV given preventatively in 5 monthly doses at the start of the RSV season, may be prescribed for infants at high risk. However, cost effectiveness compared with isolation strategies for those infants at high risk of severe disease has not been well studied, and calls its routine use into question.

Disposition

Admission ideally should be reserved for those at high risk of morbidity and mortality or in whom admission allows for (1) necessary physical observation in the likelihood of serious deterioration requiring immediate medical interventions, and (2) provision of medical interventions and treatment that are not available or practical in the outpatient setting.

Many attempts to define admission criteria are present in the literature. Because bronchiolitis typically worsens and peaks after 3 to 5 days, the natural history of the disease should be taken into account in determining disposition.

Mansbach and colleagues[169] published in 2008 a multicenter cohort study to identify factors associated with safe discharge from the ED in order to create a low-risk model. These factors include:

1. Age ≥ 2 months
2. No history of intubation
3. Eczema
4. Respiratory rate less than normal for age
5. Mild retractions
6. Initial O_2 saturation $\geq 94\%$
7. Few treatments with β-agonists or epinephrine in the first hour
8. Adequate fluid intake.

Infants at high risk of apnea are currently considered a high-risk group and require admission for monitoring. Willwerth and colleagues[170] reviewed admitted bronchiolitis infants over a 5-year period and retrospectively identified a set of risk criteria that predicted the occurrence of apnea in all of the 19 of 691 (2.7%) infants who developed apnea in hospital. These criteria were: (1) born at full term but chronologic age less than 1 month; (2) born preterm at less than 37 weeks but chronologic age less than 48 weeks post conception; or (3) witnessed prior apnea event by parents or a clinician before admission.

In an attempt to identify predictors of bounce-back visits for worsening bronchiolitis within 2 weeks of ED discharge, Norwood and colleagues[171] reviewed 121 of 717 patients with unscheduled return visits, and identified age younger than 2 months, male sex, and history of previous hospitalization as risk factors. Identifying patients at higher risk of return visits or deterioration may be useful to stratify those patients and families in need of the highest level of discharge counseling and instruction, and follow-up with a primary care provider in the following days.

Assessment of physical signs is required to determine need for admission. However, it must be noted that no single physical examination parameter (except perhaps oxygen saturation) has been found to be strongly predictive of severe disease. Studies have instead emphasized constellations of signs and symptoms.

A study in 2011 identified 5 predictors of admission. These factors were then assimilated into a clinical scoring system in which each was equally weighted with 1 point[172]:

1. Duration of symptoms less than 5 days
2. Respiratory rate 50 breaths/min or more
3. Heart rate 155 beats/min or more
4. Oxygen saturation less than 97%
5. Age less than 18 weeks.

The study suggests that patients with scores of 3 or more may require admission or careful monitoring, and scores could be used in conjunction with assessment of other high-risk factors. This study, while providing promising conclusions, has yet to be validated.

PNEUMONIA IN CHILDREN

Pediatric pneumonia is the number one cause of mortality in children worldwide, with an annual incidence of more than 150 million cases per year. More children die of pneumonia than of diarrheal illnesses, malaria, and AIDS,[173] making it a significant global health care concern. In developed countries pneumonia in children, although significantly less likely to cause mortality, remains a common ED presentation.

Assessment

The assessment of a child for pneumonia can be challenging for numerous reasons:

1. Significant overlap in presentation may occur with other common respiratory conditions such as bronchiolitis, asthma, and bronchitis, among others
2. Significant overlap in the presentation between viral, bacterial, and atypical pathogens makes definitive diagnosis challenging given lack of readily available, precise, rapid, noninvasive etiologic testing in the ED setting
3. The extent to which diagnostic testing may truly aid and change the clinical course is often not known
4. An important minority of cases may be caused by atypical pathogens requiring specific testing and treatment beyond standard empiric treatments.

Clinical Presentation

Although the classic presenting symptoms of fever, productive cough, dyspnea and chest pain can assist the ED practitioner in recognizing pneumonia, children may have less typical presentations that require a higher level of suspicion and discernment. Neonates and infants may simply present with lethargy, poor feeding, or irritability. Atypical pneumonias may present with predominantly upper respiratory tract or systemic symptoms such as malaise, headache, vomiting, or rash. Neck pain and, rarely, meningismus may be a manifestation of an upper lobe consolidative process. Abdominal pain is a not uncommon presenting symptom of pneumonia in children, although usually cough, fever, or other symptoms of a URI are present.[174] Fever without a localizable source may be a less common presentation, but is well described.

The World Health Organization guidelines advocate measurement of respiratory rate as an important initial guide to suspecting pneumonia. These guidelines suggest thresholds of RR greater than 60 in infants younger than 2 months, RR greater than 50 in infants 2 to 12 months old, RR greater than 40 in children 1 to 5 years old, and RR greater than 30 in children older than 5 years[175,176] as a simple tool that may help detect as many as 50% to 80% of pneumonias. Respiratory rates should be counted for a full minute when the child is calm. However, studies show the specificity of tachypnea in developed countries is reportedly low in infants under 6 months (39%) compared with older children up to age 5 years (67%).[177] Tachypnea beyond age-specific limits was found in 61% of children under 2 years old and in 26% of those patients older than 2 years in another study of radiographically confirmed pneumonia,[178] underscoring the limits of using tachypnea alone to predict pneumonia.

Other physical findings associated with pneumonia in infants and younger children include nasal flaring, grunting, and retractions, although their specificity for pneumonia is low in infants and younger children, who are more likely to have bronchiolitis. The prevalence of classic pneumonia signs such as crackles (49%), decreased breath sounds (58%), and fever (88%) were documented in a 2008 study of 101 cases of community-acquired pneumonia (CAP).[178] Wheeze may occasionally occur in typical bacterial pneumonia (reported in the literature at 4.9%), but is more likely associated with viral lower respiratory tract infection and *Mycoplasma* (atypical) pneumonia (up to 30%).[179] Absence of all respiratory findings, especially without fever or cough, makes pneumonia highly unlikely, though occult pneumonia (defined as pneumonia in the absence of any noted respiratory and auscultatory findings on examination) has an incidence of 5% to 6%,[176] with absence of auscultatory findings in up to 30%.[180]

For the emergency physician, a careful assessment of presenting signs is crucial to determine the likelihood of diagnosis as well as appropriate treatment and disposition. These signs include hypoxemia, abnormal respiratory rates (respiratory rate >70 or apnea in infants under 2 months, or respiratory rate >50 in children ages 1–4), signs of significantly increased work of breathing, inability to maintain oral hydration, clinical signs of dehydration, signs of sepsis/shock/toxicity, and high fever.[181] Significantly decreased breath sounds or dullness at a lung base may suggest a dense consolidation or effusion/empyema. Features associated with empyema described in a Finnish study included pain on abdominal palpation and tachypnea with greater duration of fever before admission.[182] In contrast to the adult literature, severity scores and indices (eg, CURB-65 score, Pneumonia Severity Index, and so forth) have not to date been validated for use in pediatric pneumonia.

Etiology

Most pediatric pneumonia seen in the ED is caused by respiratory viruses, typical bacterial agents (primarily *Streptococcus pneumoniae*), or atypical bacterial agents (*Mycoplasma* and *Chlamydophila*). Awareness and knowledge of rare but "critically causal" agents is important to properly diagnose and treat these unusual causes, which include tuberculosis, pertussis, *Legionella*, coronavirus/severe acute respiratory syndrome (SARS), H1N1 influenza, hantavirus, varicella, measles, fungi, and potential bioterrorist agents such as anthrax and plague. Workup and treatment beyond the standard empiric approach would be required and is beyond the scope of this review.

The single most important predictor of the causative agent for pneumonia is age. Neonatal pneumonia (<1 month) is unique, as it has a significant incidence of maternally transmitted organisms such as group B *Streptococcus*, gram-negative organisms (*Escherichia coli*, *Haemophilus influenzae*), *Listeria monocytogenes*, anaerobes, and occasionally herpes simplex virus and cytomegalovirus. In the age group between 2 and 12 weeks an organism unique to this age range is *Chlamydophila trachomatis*, which causes an afebrile pneumonitis syndrome characterized by a well-appearing child presenting with cough, tachypnea, and interstitial infiltrates on CXR. The incidence of this disease has declined significantly with prenatal screening for this vertically transmitted organism from mothers. Other bacteria commonly seen in the first 3 to 4 months include *H influenzae* (nontypable or Type B), *Moraxella catarrhalis*, *Streptococcus pyogenes*, *Staphylococcus aureus* and, rarely, *Bordetella pertussis*.

In younger children, especially under the age of 2 years, viral causes predominate. RSV is the most common, followed by parainfluenza, adenovirus, rhinovirus, human metapneumovirus, and influenza viruses. Bacterial causes, mainly *S pneumoniae*, is common, especially in children who require hospitalization. Between the age of 2 and 5 years, the incidence of pneumococcal and atypical organisms rises. In school-aged children, there is a greater increase in the incidence of *Mycoplasma* and *Chlamydophila* pneumonia, while *S pneumoniae* remains the most common bacterial cause. Viral agents remain an important cause in this age group. Tuberculosis accounts for a very small percentage of pediatric CAP.

Classic pneumococcal pneumonia presents with sudden onset of high fever and rigors with a productive cough, focal pleuritic chest pain, mild to moderate systemic toxicity (lethargy, malaise, nausea, vomiting), and focal chest findings on examination. Unfortunately, only a small minority of patients who have a confirmed pneumococcal pneumonia present with these findings. Initial ED presentations may be subtle or atypical. WBC and C-reactive protein (CRP) may be helpful in more severe disease but are nonspecific for milder cases.[144] CXR is significantly limited given that pneumococcus may present as a bronchopneumonia instead of lobar infiltrate.

Features that may be more common in pneumonia caused by Mycoplasma or Chlamydophila include a more insidious onset with constitutional symptoms of malaise, myalgias, pharyngitis, headache, low-grade fever, and a dry cough that progressively worsens. Bullous myringitis and rashes such as erythema nodosum or a generalized maculopapular eruption occasionally occur with Mycoplasma infection.

Viral pneumonias are most common in those younger than 5 years, often presenting in the fall or winter, and usually associated with a viral prodrome such as coryza, pharyngitis, low-grade fever, and dry cough. Viral pneumonias account for the majority of pneumonias in children younger than 2 years in North America. Radiographically, perihilar predominance with peribronchial thickening, hyperinflation, and interstitial involvement is most often seen; however, lobar infiltrates can also be seen.[183] Coinfection with viral and bacterial agents is fairly common, especially in those under the age of 5 years, often ranging from 20% to 35% in many studies.[178,184]

Staphylococcal pneumonia is rare but is associated with more severe illness, especially in the setting of viral coinfection. Reports suggest a rising incidence with the increased prevalence of methicillin-resistant Staphylococcus aureus (MRSA) in the community and in hospital settings.[185] Risk factors for staphylococcal pneumonia include younger age (<1 year old), complicated CXR appearance (effusion/empyema, cavitating or necrotizing infiltrate, lung abscess), toxic appearance, known MRSA contacts or history of community-acquired MRSA, and viral coinfection (notably influenza A).[186,187] Presentation in the ED with hemoptysis, hypotension, and leukopenia should also heighten suspicion for the organism.[186]

Investigations and Workup

Well-appearing children with a clinical diagnosis of pneumonia require no specific workup, as outcome with empiric therapy is very favorable. Circumstances that warrant more rigorous efforts to identify a specific etiologic agent include:

1. The ill child requiring intensive care (ie, those with evidence of hypotension, sepsis, shock, hypoxemia <92%, hypovolemia, respiratory distress, altered mental status) or age <3 months (at higher risk of hypoxemia, apnea, and mortality than older children)[175,188]
2. Significant comorbidities including immunocompromise, underlying cardiopulmonary disease (eg, cystic fibrosis) or neuromuscular/neurologic impairment
3. Evidence of complicated pneumonia on CXR (significant effusion/empyema, pneumatocele, lung abscess)
4. Patients failing treatment, having persistent fever or prolonged clinical courses, or showing clinical deterioration[189]
5. Suspected resistant microbes or rare etiologies (eg, varicella, SARS, fungi, tuberculosis)[189]
6. Unexplained community outbreaks caused by an unclear organism.

Knowledge of local epidemiologic data is important to recognize the possibility of community outbreaks or rising antibiotic resistance patterns. The recent outbreaks of SARS in 2002 to 2003 and of H1N1 in 2008 to 2009 serve as poignant reminders that vigilance is key, and stringent infection control precautions are crucial to minimizing the spread of disease. Appropriate contact, droplet, and airborne precautions must be used. Household contact counseling, testing and treatment may be indicated in outbreaks of serious respiratory infections.

Clinical diagnosis of pneumonia in children is challenging, and physician judgment based on physical findings alone has been shown to have limited predictive power. In a study of 2071 children undergoing CXR in a pediatric ED for suspicion of pneumonia, 7% showed definite pneumonia while 15% showed definite or probable pneumonia.[190] Among the group judged by clinicians to have a high likelihood of pneumonia (>75%), CXR revealed definite consolidation in 30.6% and definite or probable consolidation in 52.8%. In the low-likelihood (<5% clinician suspicion) category, 4.3% showed definite and 10.0% showed definite or probable pneumonia. Another study in 2007 showed a prevalence rate of only 41.2% of positive or equivocal pneumonia in patients with clinical signs of pneumonia.[176] Although not addressing the issue of sensitivity of CXR to the diagnosis, these studies highlight the potential limitations of diagnosis and treatment decisions based on purely clinical grounds.

Many studies use radiographic criteria as the gold standard in the diagnosis of pneumonia, but evidence suggests that CXR lacks sensitivity in making the diagnosis, and lacks specificity in differentiating potential causes.[191] CXR has been shown to have limited specificity in differentiating typical bacterial from atypical bacterial and viral pneumonias. Although lobar consolidation and effusion are more commonly seen with typical bacterial causes, atypical agents such as *Mycoplasma* may present with lobar infiltrates as well as the more classic interstitial pattern and hilar adenopathy.[181] In 2002, Virkki and colleagues[183] evaluated 254 cases of CAP in which etiology was determined in 85%, and compared with CXR findings. Although the classic alveolar/lobar pattern was significantly correlated with a bacterial cause in 78% (P<.001), the interstitial pattern traditionally associated with atypical bacteria and viral infections was less specific, with 50% caused by bacteria (typical and atypical) and 50% caused by viruses. Variability among guidelines regarding the necessity of CXR exists. It has been shown that antimicrobial choice as well as overall outcome is not affected with the use of CXR in children 2 months to 5 years of age with mild disease.[140] As a result, they should not be considered mandatory in these cases.

Although CXR is often ordered in the large number of children with wheezing seen in EDs, the incidence of radiographic pneumonia is very low (3.7%–4.9%) unless fever (>38°C), abdominal pain, or significant hypoxemia (<92%) is present.[179] Moreover, atelectasis may often mimic early consolidation. In those under the age of 2 years with wheezing and crackles, viral bronchiolitis is the most likely diagnosis, with bacterial superinfection being very rare in mild cases.

Ultrasonography has recently emerged as a valuable tool in the diagnosis of pneumonia. Most studies in the adult literature on lung ultrasonography suggest higher sensitivity than CXR, better delineation of complications (such as loculated effusion, empyema, abscess, necrosis, and pneumatocele), and rapid performance times (usually less than 5 minutes).[192,193] Ultrasonography in children has compared very favorably with computed tomography (CT) scanning with respect to diagnosis, complications, and guidance of thoracocentesis, without radiation exposure and risk.[194] Furthermore, ultrasonography is less likely to require patient sedation in comparison with CT scanning. Given these advantages, ED clinicians should be aware of its evolving role.

CBC and differential can sometimes be helpful in suggesting a bacterial cause of pneumonia. A European study reported that *S pneumoniae* pneumonia was more commonly associated with WBC of greater than 15,000 to 20,000/mm^3, and a mean of 25,000/mm^3 if there was also a concomitant bacteremia.[144] However, invasive viral disease such as adenovirus or even influenza may cause similar WBC elevations, so interpretation should be done with caution in consideration of the overall clinical picture. Acute phase reactants such as erythrocyte sedimentation rate and CRP have shown suboptimal utility as sole determinants to distinguish bacterial from viral causes, due to limited specificities.[181,194] Although a procalcitonin level greater than 1.0 ng/mL was helpful in distinguishing bacterial from viral CAP in a recent study,[178] it was unable to distinguish pneumococcal from atypical bacterial pneumonia.

Blood cultures can be highly specific for the etiologic organism and can identify antimicrobial sensitivity patterns important to later care, but play little to no role in initial ED management. Two ED-based studies have shown that bacteremia occurs in only 2% to 3% of patients with radiographic CAP.[195,196] Shah and colleagues[195] reported higher yields of up to 13% in a subset of patients with complicated pneumonia. Due to the overall low yield, the use of blood cultures should be individualized to patients with suspected bacteremia, more ill patients, or patients with complications.

Bacterial serology from serum or urine samples is currently neither widely available nor practical in most EDs. Sensitivity and specificity is low, therefore testing is not recommended by most recent guidelines.[175,181,189,194,197] Cold agglutinin testing, although easy to perform, was shown to have a positive predictive value of only 70%.[181] *Mycoplasma* IgM detection via enzyme-linked immunosorbent assay is sensitive and may be considered in children older than 2 years.[189] Urine for pneumococcal antigen has been shown to lack high specificity in children. *Legionella* antigen testing in the urine may be considered for more severe cases requiring admission to the ICU or when clinical suspicion is high. Nasopharyngeal testing for pertussis and skin testing for tuberculosis should be done when these entities are suspected. Further testing should be based on clinical suspicion.

Rapid viral testing is now available in many settings, and can allow early diagnosis of influenza and RSV. Early identification allows treatment decisions with antivirals (which are rarely indicated), infectious precaution advice, and isolation as inpatients. Disadvantages include cost and low benefit/expense ratio in cases where clinical diagnosis is already clear and the necessity of obtaining specific etiologic diagnosis is low. The overall utility is generally low and should not be routine.[198] Testing may be considered in those with severe illness warranting hospitalization.

Sputum for Gram stain and culture may be feasible for older school-aged children capable of producing more reliable sputum specimens, and may be done for those requiring hospitalization for severe disease.[194,199] Limitations include frequent poor-quality specimens (especially in younger children) and difficulties in culturing organisms such as *Mycoplasma*, *Chlamydophila*, *Legionella*, *Moraxella*, and tuberculosis. Nasopharyngeal and throat cultures have poor reliability in predicting the etiology of pneumonia and are not recommended.

Treatment

Treatment regimens in suspected bacterial CAP take into account the age of the child, treatment setting, severity, special circumstances in each case, and local patterns of organisms and antibiotic susceptibilities.[175,181,189,194,197,199] Consideration for withholding antibiotics should be given for those non-ill children with clinical presentations

Table 2
Empiric antibiotic therapy for suspected bacterial community-acquired pneumonia

Age	Outpatient Treatment	Inpatient Treatment
Neonate	Not recommended > Admit	Ampicillin 50–200 mg/kg/d IV div q 6–12 h plus Cefotaxime 150–200 mg/kg/d IV div q 6 h–q 8 h If ill, add gentamycin 7.5 mg/kg/d IV div q 8 h If HSV likely, add acyclovir 500 mg/m²/dose IV q 8 h

1–4 months	If afebrile pneumonitis
	  Clarithromycin 15 mg/kg/d PO div BIDᵃ or
	  Erythromycin 40 mg/kg/d PO div q 6 h
	
	Amoxicillin 90 mg/kg/d PO div BID–TIDᵇ,ᶜ
	
	If febrile or hypoxic > Admit
		If afebrile pneumonitis
		  Clarithromycin 15 mg/kg/d PO/IV div BIDᵃ or
		  Erythromycin 40 mg/kg/d PO or 20 mg/kg/d IV div q 6 h
		
		If febrile, cefotaxime 150–200 mg/kg/d IV div q 8 h
		  or cefuroxime IV 150 mg/kg/d IV div q 8 h
		
		If ill or MRSA suspected, add vancomycin 40–60 mg/kg/d IV div q 6–8 h or clindamycin 40 mg/kg/d IV div q 6–8 h
		
		If MSSA suspected, cloxacillin 150–200 mg/kg/d IV div q 6 h

4 months to 5 years	Amoxicillin 90 mg/kg/d PO div BID–TIDᵇ,ᶜ
	
	If atypical suspected add Macrolide PO (doses as above)
	
	Second-line alternatives:
	Amoxicillin-clavulanic acid 90 mg/kg/d PO div BID or TIDᵇ,ᶜ
	Cefuroxime axetil 30 mg/kg/d PO div BID
		Ceftriaxone 50–100 mg/kg/d IV div q 12–24 h or
		Cefotaxime 150–200 mg/kg/d IV div q 8 h or
		Cefuroxime 150 mg/kg/d IV div q 8 h
		
		If *Streptococcus pneumoniae* likely,
		  Ampicillin 150–200 mg/kg/d IV div q 8 h–q 6 h
		
		If severely ill,
		  add vancomycin 40–60 mg/kg/d IV div q 6–8 h or cloxacillin 150–200 mg/kg/d IV div q 6 h
		  or if pleural effusion, clindamycin 40 mg/kg/d IV div q 6–8 h
		
		If atypical suspected: Macrolide IV or PO (doses as above)ᵃ

(continued on next page)

Table 2 (continued)		
Age	**Outpatient Treatment**	**Inpatient Treatment**
5–18 years	Azithromycin 10 mg/kg/d, Day 1 + 5 mg/kg/d, Days 2–5 or Clarithromycin 15 mg/kg/d div BID or Erythromycin 40 mg/kg/d div q 6 h	Ceftriaxone 50 mg/kg/d IV div q 12 h or q 24 h (max 2 g/d) or Cefuroxime 150 mg/kg/d IV div q 8 h (max 1.5 g/d) or
	If *S pneumoniae* likely Amoxicillin 90 mg/kg/d PO div BID[b,c]	If *S pneumoniae* likely, Ampicillin 150–200 mg/kg/d IV div q 8 h–q 6 h
	Alternatives: Doxycycline[d] 2–4 mg/kg/d PO div BID Amoxicillin-clavulanic acid 90 mg/kg/d PO div BID or TID[b,c] Cefuroxime axetil 30 mg/kg/d PO div BID Levofloxacin[e] 500 mg PO daily or Moxifloxacin[e] 400 mg PO daily	If atypicals suspected Macrolide IV or PO (doses as above) If severely ill, add vancomycin 40–60 mg/kg/d IV div q 6–8 h or cloxacillin 150–200 mg/kg/d IV div q 6 h, or If pleural effusion, clindamycin 40 mg/kg/d IV div q 6–8 h

Abbreviations: BID, twice daily; div, divided (for dosages based on a daily dose, which needs to be then divided into intervals); HSV, herpes simplex virus; IV, intravenous; MRSA, methicillin-resistant *Staphylococcus aureus*; MSSA, methicillin-sensitive *Staphylococcus aureus*; PO, by mouth; q, every; TID, 3 times daily.

[a] Azithromycin: Safety and effectiveness not fully established in infants under 6 months of age. Not approved by US Food and Drug Administration in this age group.

[b] Higher-dose amoxicillin recommended especially if in day-care attendance, recently on antibiotics, or hospitalized in last 3 months, age under 2 years, or area with *S pneumoniae* penicillin resistance greater than 2.0 μg/mL.

[c] Lower-dose amoxicillin 45 mg/kg/d potentially effective in absence of risk factors for resistant *S pneumoniae*.

[d] Avoid if younger than 8 years, because of effects on dentition.

[e] Use only if growth plates are closed.

Data from Refs.[175,181,189,194,199]

consistent with viral illness, given the association between inappropriate antibiotic use and increase in resistant organisms. Suggested empiric antibiotic treatments for CAP are listed in **Table 2**.

Anaerobic coverage should be considered if aspiration is suspected. Antiviral therapy for influenza-related pneumonia should be initiated in high-risk populations within 48 hours of symptom onset. The anti-RSV treatment ribavirin should be limited to high-risk patients as per American Academy of Pediatrics Guidelines.[130]

A large multicenter trial (the PIVOT trial) in 2007, of 246 cases of pediatric CAP comparing oral amoxicillin to IV penicillin followed by oral amoxicillin demonstrated similar outcomes, suggesting IV treatment may not always be necessary for admitted patients with milder cases, thereby saving hospital costs and avoiding IV cannulation.[200] Examining the duration of antibiotic therapy, a 2008 Cochrane systematic review concluded equal efficacy of 3-day versus 5-day treatment regimens in mild CAP in otherwise healthy children 2 months to 5 years of age.[201]

Adjunctive Treatments

Standard supportive care includes oxygen for hypoxemia less than 92%, suctioning of younger infants, and bronchodilators as necessary. IV fluids should be given when necessary but with caution, given the association of SIADH with more severe pneumonias. IV fluid regimens started in the ED may require adjustment in the presence of hyponatremia. Chest physiotherapy has been found to be of no added value and is not routinely recommended. Steroids have no role currently in the treatment of the pneumonia. Noninvasive ventilator support with continuous positive airway pressure or bilevel positive airway pressure may be necessary for those with respiratory failure. Intubation is rarely indicated.

Complications

Complications of pneumonia may include sepsis, respiratory failure, effusion, empyema, abscess, pneumatocele, and infectious spread such as, meningitis, septic arthritis, or osteomyelitis.[175,181] Small free-flowing parapneumonic effusions suspected to be transudative may be given a trial of antibiotics and reassessed for pleurocentesis as necessary. Moderate and large effusions, especially if in respiratory distress, should be considered for prompt pleurocentesis before starting antibiotics, as this may affect culture results.[175] Proven empyemas should be drained and further treatment decisions should be made in consultation with thoracic surgery. Pulmonary

Table 3
Suggested admission criteria for pediatric community-acquired pneumonia

Definite admission	Age <1 month Oxygen saturation ≤92% Signs of significant respiratory distress (tachypnea/apnea, significant work of breathing) Signs of sepsis or toxic appearance Complicated pneumonia on chest radiograph (effusion/empyema, pneumatocele, necrosis, or lung abscess)
Probable admission	Age 1–3 months Oxygen saturation 93%–94% Significant comorbidity (chronic lung disease, congenital heart disease, cystic fibrosis, etc) Significant burden of disease (multilobar or complete lobar consolidation) Immunocompromise (sickle cell disease, human immunodeficiency virus, post-splenectomy, malignancy/recent chemotherapy) Unresolving or worsening illness Significant dehydration/vomiting Inability of parents/caregivers to ensure adequate observation or follow-up
Consider admission	Age 3–6 months Failure of outpatient treatment, especially if any clinical deterioration Larger infiltrate or significant atelectasis on chest radiograph
Outpatient therapy	Non-ill or minimally ill child Uncomplicated mild pneumonia Adequate oxygenation Tolerating feeds well Reliable parents for observation and follow-up

Data from Refs.[175,181,189,194,199]

and infectious disease specialist involvement may be warranted for cases of unresolving infiltrates, abscesses, pneumatoceles, or effusions.

Admission Criteria/Predictors of Poor Outcome

Worldwide, significantly at-risk groups include neonates, human immunodeficiency virus (HIV)-related pneumonia (3–8 times higher case fatality rates compared with non-HIV infected), and severely malnourished children.[188] Significant hypoxemia is also associated with a 2- to 5-fold increase in risk of death.[202] Predictors of antibiotic treatment failure include young age, immunocompromised state (eg, HIV or malnutrition), presence of empyema, prior antibiotic use, poor adherence to treatment, and antibiotic resistance.[188]

Admission criteria based on published guidelines and literature reviews have been proposed, though they have not been vigorously studied. Such criteria should be used with clinical judgment while taking into account modifying factors. Suggested admission criteria are listed in **Table 3**.

Other options for less ill or complicated patients include admission to a short-stay or observation unit for children in whom rapid clinical response is expected, or once-daily IV or IM antibiotics such as ceftriaxone with daily follow-up by an intensive ambulatory care service, as exists in some major hospitals.

Follow-Up

Forty-eight-hour follow-up is strongly recommended for all children diagnosed with pneumonia,[174] especially if any signs of deterioration occur. The World Health Organization definition of clinical improvement requires "slower breathing, less fever, eating better."[202] In children with clinical improvement, follow-up radiography is suggested in cases of complicated pneumonia, round pneumonia, congenital abnormalities, lobar collapse, complicated courses, or persistent clinical abnormalities.[181,189] A recent radiographic follow-up study demonstrated that residual or new changes on CXR could be seen in 30% of cases after 3 to 7 weeks but did not affect management.[203]

SUMMARY

Common respiratory illnesses including asthma, croup, bronchiolitis, and pneumonia will undoubtedly continue to make up the bulk of pediatric respiratory problems presenting to EDs. Given their potential to cause life-threatening illness, emergency clinicians will need to continue to maintain and update their knowledge on current recommendations for these illnesses. Underuse of some key therapies and overutilization of unproven therapies and low-utility diagnostic tests are several important areas that can be improved through improved education and knowledge of published clinical practice guidelines.

REFERENCES

1. American Lung Association, Epidemiology and Statistics Unit. Trends in asthma morbidity and mortality. Washington, DC. Available at: http://www.lungusa.org/finding-cures/our-research/trend-reports/asthma-trend-report.pdf. Accessed April 13, 2011.
2. Global Initiative for Asthma. Global strategy for asthma management and prevention. Bethesda (MD): Global Initiative for Asthma; 2010.
3. National Heart, Lung, and Blood Institute (US). Expert panel report 3: guidelines for the diagnosis and management of asthma. Bethesda (MD): National Heart,

Lung, and Blood Institute, U.S. Department of Health and Human Services, National Institutes of Health; 2007.

4. Busse WW, Lemanske RF. Asthma. N Engl J Med 2001;344(5):350–62.

5. Stevenson D, Szczeklik A. Clinical and pathologic perspectives on aspirin sensitivity and asthma. J Allergy Clin Immunol 2006;118(4):773–86 [quiz: 787–8].

6. Global Initiative for Asthma. Global strategy for the diagnosis and management of asthma in children 5 years and younger. Bethesda (MD): Global Initiative for Asthma; 2009.

7. Brand PL, Baraldi E, Bisgaard H, et al. Definition, assessment and treatment of wheezing disorders in preschool children: an evidence-based approach. Eur Respir J 2008;32(4):1096–110.

8. Panickar J, Lakhanpaul M, Lambert P, et al. Oral prednisolone for preschool children with acute virus-induced wheezing. N Engl J Med 2009;360(4): 329–38.

9. British Thoracic Society and the Scottish Intercollegiate Guidelines Network. British guideline on the management of asthma. London, England: The British Thoracic Society; 2009.

10. Ducharme F, Chalut D, Plotnick L, et al. The pediatric respiratory assessment measure: a valid clinical score for assessing acute asthma severity from toddlers to teenagers. J Pediatr 2008;152(4):476–80, 480.e471.

11. Chalut DS, Ducharme FM, Davis GM. The Preschool Respiratory Assessment Measure (PRAM): a responsive index of acute asthma severity. J Pediatr 2000;137(6):762–8.

12. Gorelick M, Stevens M, Schultz T, et al. Performance of a novel clinical score, the Pediatric Asthma Severity Score (PASS), in the evaluation of acute asthma. Acad Emerg Med 2004;11(1):10–8.

13. Gouin S, Robidas I, Gravel J, et al. Prospective evaluation of two clinical scores for acute asthma in children 18 months to 7 years of age. Acad Emerg Med 2010;17(6):598–603.

14. Goldberg R, Chan L, Haley P, et al. Critical pathway for the emergency department management of acute asthma: effect on resource utilization. Ann Emerg Med 1998;31(5):562–7.

15. Eid N, Yandell B, Howell L, et al. Can peak expiratory flow predict airflow obstruction in children with asthma? Pediatrics 2000;105(2):354–8.

16. Gorelick M, Stevens M, Schultz T, et al. Difficulty in obtaining peak expiratory flow measurements in children with acute asthma. Pediatr Emerg Care 2004;20(1):22–6.

17. Rodrigo G, Rodriquez Verde M, Peregalli V, et al. Effects of short-term 28% and 100% oxygen on $PaCO_2$ and peak expiratory flow rate in acute asthma: a randomized trial. Chest 2003;124(4):1312–7.

18. Camargo CA, Spooner CH, Rowe BH. Continuous versus intermittent beta-agonists in the treatment of acute asthma. Cochrane Database Syst Rev 2003;4:CD001115.

19. Papo MC, Frank J, Thompson AE. A prospective, randomized study of continuous versus intermittent nebulized albuterol for severe status asthmaticus in children. Crit Care Med 1993;21(10):1479–86.

20. Cates CCJ, Bara A, Crilly JA, et al. Holding chambers versus nebulisers for beta-agonist treatment of acute asthma. Cochrane Database Syst Rev 2003;3: CD000052.

21. Closa RM, Ceballos JM, Gmez-Pap A, et al. Efficacy of bronchodilators administered by nebulizers versus spacer devices in infants with acute wheezing. Pediatr Pulmonol 1998;26(5):344–8.

22. Wildhaber JH, Devadason SG, Hayden MJ, et al. Aerosol delivery to wheezy infants: a comparison between a nebulizer and two small volume spacers. Pediatr Pulmonol 1997;23(3):212–6.

23. Rubilar L, Castro Rodriguez JA, Girardi G. Randomized trial of salbutamol via metered-dose inhaler with spacer versus nebulizer for acute wheezing in children less than 2 years of age. Pediatr Pulmonol 2000;29(4):264–9.

24. Doan Q, Shefrin A, Johnson D. Cost-effectiveness of metered-dose inhalers for asthma exacerbations in the pediatric emergency department. Pediatrics 2011; 127(5):e1105–11 peds.2010-2963.

25. Asmus MJ, Hendeles L. Levalbuterol nebulizer solution: is it worth five times the cost of albuterol? Pharmacotherapy 2000;20(2):123–9.

26. Milgrom H, Skoner DP, Bensch G, et al. Low-dose levalbuterol in children with asthma: safety and efficacy in comparison with placebo and racemic albuterol. J Allergy Clin Immunol 2001;108(6):938–45.

27. Nelson HS, Bensch G, Pleskow WW, et al. Improved bronchodilation with levalbuterol compared with racemic albuterol in patients with asthma. J Allergy Clin Immunol 1998;102(6):943–52.

28. Gawchik SM, Saccar CL, Noonan M, et al. The safety and efficacy of nebulized levalbuterol compared with racemic albuterol and placebo in the treatment of asthma in pediatric patients. J Allergy Clin Immunol 1999;103(4):615–21.

29. Carl J, Myers T, Kirchner HL, et al. Comparison of racemic albuterol and levalbuterol for treatment of acute asthma. J Pediatr 2003;143(6):731–6.

30. Tripp K, McVicar W, Nair P, et al. A cumulative dose study of levalbuterol and racemic albuterol administered by hydrofluoroalkane-134a metered-dose inhaler in asthmatic subjects. J Allergy Clin Immunol 2008;122(3):544–9.

31. Lam S, Chen J. Changes in heart rate associated with nebulized racemic albuterol and levalbuterol in intensive care patients. Am J Health Syst Pharm 2003; 60(19):1971–5.

32. Plotnick LH, Ducharme FM. Combined inhaled anticholinergics and beta2-agonists for initial treatment of acute asthma in children. Cochrane Database Syst Rev 2000;4:CD000060.

33. Rodrigo GJ, Castro Rodriguez JA. Anticholinergics in the treatment of children and adults with acute asthma: a systematic review with meta-analysis. Thorax 2005;60(9):740–6.

34. Rowe BH, Edmonds ML, Spooner CH, et al. Corticosteroid therapy for acute asthma. Respir Med 2004;98(4):275–84.

35. Fiel S, Vincken W. Systemic corticosteroid therapy for acute asthma exacerbations. J Asthma 2006;43(5):321–31.

36. Smith M, Iqbal Shaikh Mohammed SI, Rowe Brian H, et al. Corticosteroids for hospitalised children with acute asthma. Cochrane Database Syst Rev 2003;1. Available at: http://www.mrw.interscience.wiley.com/cochrane/clsysrev/articles/CD002886/frame.html. Accessed May 1, 2011.

37. Becker JM, Arora A, Scarfone RJ, et al. Oral versus intravenous corticosteroids in children hospitalized with asthma. J Allergy Clin Immunol 1999;103(4): 586–90.

38. Barnett PL, Caputo GL, Baskin M, et al. Intravenous versus oral corticosteroids in the management of acute asthma in children. Ann Emerg Med 1997;29(2): 212–7.

39. Kravitz J, Dominici P, Ufberg J, et al. Two days of dexamethasone versus 5 days of prednisone in the treatment of acute asthma: a randomized controlled trial. Ann Emerg Med 2011;58(2):200–4.

40. Greenberg R, Kerby G, Roosevelt G. A comparison of oral dexamethasone with oral prednisone in pediatric asthma exacerbations treated in the emergency department. Clin Pediatr 2008;47(8):817–23.
41. Shefrin R. Use of dexamethasone and prednisone in acute asthma exacerbations in pediatric patients. Can Fam Physician 2009;55(7):704–6.
42. Altamimi M. Single-dose oral dexamethasone in the emergency management of children with exacerbations of mild to moderate asthma. Pediatr Emerg Care 2006;22(12):786–93.
43. Gordon S, Tompkins T, Dayan P. Randomized trial of single-dose intramuscular dexamethasone compared with prednisolone for children with acute asthma. Pediatr Emerg Care 2007;23(8):521–7.
44. Gries DM, Moffitt DR, Pulos E, et al. A single dose of intramuscularly administered dexamethasone acetate is as effective as oral prednisone to treat asthma exacerbations in young children. J Pediatr 2000;136(3):298–303.
45. FitzGerald JM, Becker A, Sears MR, et al. Doubling the dose of budesonide versus maintenance treatment in asthma exacerbations. Thorax 2004;59(7):550–6.
46. Edmonds ML, Camargo CA, Pollack CV, et al. Early use of inhaled corticosteroids in the emergency department treatment of acute asthma. Cochrane Database Syst Rev 2003;3:CD002308.
47. Schuh S, Dick P, Stephens D, et al. High-dose inhaled fluticasone does not replace oral prednisolone in children with mild to moderate acute asthma. Pediatrics 2006;118(2):644–50.
48. Schuh S, Reisman J, Alshehri M, et al. A comparison of inhaled fluticasone and oral prednisone for children with severe acute asthma. N Engl J Med 2000; 343(10):689–94.
49. Upham BD, Mollen CJ, Scarfone RJ, et al. Nebulized budesonide added to standard pediatric emergency department treatment of acute asthma: a randomized, double-blind trial. Acad Emerg Med 2011;18(7):665–73.
50. Spivey WH, Skobeloff EM, Levin RM. Effect of magnesium chloride on rabbit bronchial smooth muscle. Ann Emerg Med 1990;19(10):1107–12.
51. Ciarallo L, Sauer AH, Shannon MW. Intravenous magnesium therapy for moderate to severe pediatric asthma: results of a randomized, placebo-controlled trial. J Pediatr 1996;129(6):809–14.
52. Noppen M, Vanmaele L, Impens N, et al. Bronchodilating effect of intravenous magnesium sulfate in acute severe bronchial asthma. Chest 1990;97(2):373–6.
53. Rowe BH, Bretzlaff JA, Bourdon C, et al. Intravenous magnesium sulfate treatment for acute asthma in the emergency department: a systematic review of the literature. Ann Emerg Med 2000;36(3):181–90.
54. Rowe BH, Bretzlaff JA, Bourdon C, et al. Magnesium sulfate for treating exacerbations of acute asthma in the emergency department. Cochrane Database Syst Rev 2000;2:CD001490.
55. Gallegos-Solorzano MC, Perez-Padilla R, Hernandez-Zenteno RJ. Usefulness of inhaled magnesium sulfate in the coadjuvant management of severe asthma crisis in an emergency department. Pulm Pharmacol Ther 2010;23(5):432–7.
56. Hughes R, Goldkorn A, Masoli M, et al. Use of isotonic nebulised magnesium sulphate as an adjuvant to salbutamol in treatment of severe asthma in adults: randomised placebo-controlled trial. Lancet 2003;361(9375):2114–7.
57. Bessmertny O, DiGregorio RV, Cohen H, et al. A randomized clinical trial of nebulized magnesium sulfate in addition to albuterol in the treatment of acute mild-to-moderate asthma exacerbations in adults. Ann Emerg Med 2002; 39(6):585–91.

58. Blitz M, Blitz S, Beasely R, et al. Inhaled magnesium sulfate in the treatment of acute asthma. Cochrane Database Syst Rev 2005;4. Available at: http://www.mrw.interscience.wiley.com/cochrane/clsysrev/articles/CD003898/frame.html. Accessed May 1, 2011.

59. Harmanci K, Bakirtas A, Turktas I, et al. Oral montelukast treatment of preschool-aged children with acute asthma. Ann Allergy Asthma Immunol 2006;96(5): 731–5.

60. Nelson K, Smith S, Trinkaus K, et al. Pilot study of oral montelukast added to standard therapy for acute asthma exacerbations in children aged 6 to 14 years. Pediatr Emerg Care 2008;24(1):21–7.

61. Dockhorn RJ, Baumgartner RA, Leff JA, et al. Comparison of the effects of intrave-nous and oral montelukast on airway function: a double blind, placebo controlled, three period, crossover study in asthmatic patients. Thorax 2000;55(4):260–5.

62. Camargo C, Smithline H, Malice MP, et al. A randomized controlled trial of intra-venous montelukast in acute asthma. Am J Respir Crit Care Med 2003;167(4): 528–33.

63. Gupta VK, Cheifetz IM. Heliox administration in the pediatric intensive care unit: an evidence-based review. Pediatr Crit Care Med 2005;6(2):204–11.

64. Kim I, Phrampus E, Venkataraman S, et al. Helium/oxygen-driven albuterol nebulization in the treatment of children with moderate to severe asthma exac-erbations: a randomized, controlled trial. Pediatrics 2005;116(5):1127–33.

65. Lee D, Hsu CW, Lee H, et al. Beneficial effects of albuterol therapy driven by he-liox versus by oxygen in severe asthma exacerbation. Acad Emerg Med 2005; 12(9):820–7.

66. Rivera M, Kim T, Stewart G, et al. Albuterol nebulized in heliox in the initial ED treatment of pediatric asthma: a blinded, randomized controlled trial. Am J Emerg Med 2006;24(1):38–42.

67. Travers A, Jones AP, Kelly K, et al. Intravenous beta2-agonists for acute asthma in the emergency department. Cochrane Database Syst Rev 2001;2:CD002988:

68. Mitra A, Bassler D, Goodman K, et al. Intravenous aminophylline for acute severe asthma in children over two years receiving inhaled bronchodilators. Co-chrane Database Syst Rev 2005;2:CD001276.

69. Ream RS, Loftis LL, Albers GM, et al. Efficacy of IV theophylline in children with severe status asthmaticus. Chest 2001;119(5):1480–8.

70. Akingbola O, Simakajornboon N, Hadley E Jr, et al. Noninvasive positive-pressure ventilation in pediatric status asthmaticus. Pediatr Crit Care Med 2002;3(2):181–4.

71. Bernet V, Hug M, Frey B. Predictive factors for the success of noninvasive mask ventilation in infants and children with acute respiratory failure. Pediatr Crit Care Med 2005;6(6):660–4.

72. Carroll C, Schramm C. Noninvasive positive pressure ventilation for the treat-ment of status asthmaticus in children. Ann Allergy Asthma Immunol 2006; 96(3):454–9.

73. Essouri S, Chevret L, Durand P, et al. Noninvasive positive pressure ventilation: five years of experience in a pediatric intensive care unit. Pediatr Crit Care Med 2006;7(4):329–34.

74. Padman R, Lawless ST, Kettrick RG. Noninvasive ventilation via bilevel positive airway pressure support in pediatric practice. Crit Care Med 1998;26(1): 169–73.

75. Thill P, McGuire J, Baden H, et al. Noninvasive positive-pressure ventilation in children with lower airway obstruction. Pediatr Crit Care Med 2004;5(4):337–42.

76. Ram FS, Wellington S, Rowe B, et al. Non-invasive positive pressure ventilation for treatment of respiratory failure due to severe acute exacerbations of asthma. Cochrane Database Syst Rev 2005;3:CD004360.
77. Brown RH, Wagner EM. Mechanisms of bronchoprotection by anesthetic induction agents: propofol versus ketamine. Anesthesiology 1999;90(3):822–8.
78. Allen J, Macias C. The efficacy of ketamine in pediatric emergency department patients who present with acute severe asthma. Ann Emerg Med 2005;46(1): 43–50.
79. Howton JC, Rose J, Duffy S, et al. Randomized, double-blind, placebo-controlled trial of intravenous ketamine in acute asthma. Ann Emerg Med 1996;27(2):170–5.
80. Green S, Roback M, Krauss B. Anticholinergics and ketamine sedation in children: a secondary analysis of atropine versus glycopyrrolate. Acad Emerg Med 2010;17(2):157–62.
81. Green SM, Roback MG, Kennedy RM, et al. Clinical practice guideline for emergency department ketamine dissociative sedation: 2011 update. Ann Emerg Med 2011;57(5):449–61.
82. Bellomo R, McLaughlin P, Tai E, et al. Asthma requiring mechanical ventilation. A low morbidity approach. Chest 1994;105(3):891–6.
83. Cox RG, Barker GA, Bohn DJ. Efficacy, results, and complications of mechanical ventilation in children with status asthmaticus. Pediatr Pulmonol 1991; 11(2):120–6.
84. Darioli R, Perret C. Mechanical controlled hypoventilation in status asthmaticus. Am Rev Respir Dis 1984;129(3):385–7.
85. Dworkin G, Kattan M. Mechanical ventilation for status asthmaticus in children. J Pediatr 1989;114(4):545–9.
86. Hickling KG, Walsh J, Henderson S, et al. Low mortality rate in adult respiratory distress syndrome using low-volume, pressure-limited ventilation with permissive hypercapnia: a prospective study. Crit Care Med 1994;22(10):1568–78.
87. Menitove SM, Goldring RM. Combined ventilator and bicarbonate strategy in the management of status asthmaticus. Am J Med 1983;74(5):898–901.
88. Sin D, Bell N, Svenson L, et al. The impact of follow-up physician visits on emergency readmissions for patients with asthma and chronic obstructive pulmonary disease: a population-based study. Am J Med 2002;112(2):120–5.
89. Zeiger RS, Heller S, Mellon MH, et al. Facilitated referral to asthma specialist reduces relapses in asthma emergency room visits. J Allergy Clin Immunol 1991;87(6):1160–8.
90. Zorc J, Scarfone R, Li Y, et al. Scheduled follow-up after a pediatric emergency department visit for asthma: a randomized trial. Pediatrics 2003;111(3):495–502.
91. Baren J, Boudreaux E, Brenner B, et al. Randomized controlled trial of emergency department interventions to improve primary care follow-up for patients with acute asthma. Chest 2006;129(2):257–65.
92. Sin D, Man SF. Low-dose inhaled corticosteroid therapy and risk of emergency department visits for asthma. Arch Intern Med 2002;162(14):1591–5.
93. Edmonds M, Brenner Barry E, Camargo Carlos A, et al. Inhaled steroids for acute asthma following emergency department discharge. Cochrane Database Syst Rev 2000;3. Available at: http://www.mrw.interscience.wiley.com/cochrane/clsysrev/articles/CD002316/frame.html. Accessed May 1, 2011.
94. Cowie RL, Revitt SG, Underwood MF, et al. The effect of a peak flow-based action plan in the prevention of exacerbations of asthma. Chest 1997;112(6): 1534–8.

95. Cherry J. Clinical practice. Croup. N Engl J Med 2008;358(4):384–91.
96. Segal A, Crighton E, Moineddin R, et al. Croup hospitalizations in Ontario: a 14-year time-series analysis. Pediatrics 2005;116(1):51–5.
97. Peltola V, Heikkinen T, Ruuskanen O. Clinical courses of croup caused by influenza and parainfluenza viruses. Pediatr Infect Dis J 2002;21(1):76–8.
98. Groblewski J, Shah R, Zalzal G. Microdebrider-assisted supraglottoplasty for laryngomalacia. Ann Otol Rhinol Laryngol 2009;118(8):592–7.
99. Antony R, Al Rawas A, Irwin M. Stridor in a newborn. CMAJ 2005;173(6):601–2.
100. Mancuso RF. Stridor in neonates. Pediatr Clin North Am 1996;43(6):1339–56.
101. Koplewitz B, Springer C, Slasky B, et al. CT of hemangiomas of the upper airways in children. AJR Am J Roentgenol 2005;184(2):663–70.
102. Rahbar R, Litrovnik B, Vargas S, et al. The biology and management of laryngeal neurofibroma. Arch Otolaryngol Head Neck Surg 2004;130(12):1400–6.
103. Durden F, Sobol S. Balloon laryngoplasty as a primary treatment for subglottic stenosis. Arch Otolaryngol Head Neck Surg 2007;133(8):772–5.
104. Spanos W, Brookes J, Smith M, et al. Unilateral vocal fold paralysis in premature infants after ligation of patent ductus arteriosus: vascular clip versus suture ligature. Ann Otol Rhinol Laryngol 2009;118(10):750–3.
105. Strife JL. Upper airway and tracheal obstruction in infants and children. Radiol Clin North Am 1988;26(2):309–22.
106. Westley CR, Cotton EK, Brooks JG. Nebulized racemic epinephrine by IPPB for the treatment of croup: a double-blind study. Am J Dis Child 1978;132(5):484–7.
107. Bjornson CL, Johnson DW. Croup—treatment update. Pediatr Emerg Care 2005; 21(12):863–70 [quiz: 871–3].
108. Sparrow A, Geelhoed G. Prednisolone versus dexamethasone in croup: a randomised equivalence trial. Arch Dis Child 2006;91(7):580–3.
109. Russell K, Liang Y, O'Gorman K, et al. Glucocorticoids for croup. Cochrane Database Syst Rev 2011;1:CD001955.
110. Cetinkaya F, Tfeki B, Kutluk G. A comparison of nebulized budesonide, and intramuscular, and oral dexamethasone for treatment of croup. Int J Pediatr Otorhinolaryngol 2004;68(4):453–6.
111. Geelhoed GC, Macdonald WB. Oral dexamethasone in the treatment of croup: 0.15 mg/kg versus 0.3 mg/kg versus 0.6 mg/kg. Pediatr Pulmonol 1995;20(6):362–8.
112. Dobrovoljac M, Geelhoed G. 27 years of croup: an update highlighting the effectiveness of 0.15 mg/kg of dexamethasone. Emerg Med Australas 2009; 21(4):309–14.
113. Chub Uppakarn S, Sangsupawanich P. A randomized comparison of dexamethasone 0.15 mg/kg versus 0.6 mg/kg for the treatment of moderate to severe croup. Int J Pediatr Otorhinolaryngol 2007;71(3):473–7.
114. Duman M, Ozdemir D, Atasever S. Nebulised L-epinephrine and steroid combination in the treatment of moderate to severe croup. Clin Drug Investig 2005; 25(3):183–9.
115. Klassen TP, Craig WR, Moher D, et al. Nebulized budesonide and oral dexamethasone for treatment of croup: a randomized controlled trial. JAMA 1998; 279(20):1629–32.
116. Geelhoed GC. Budesonide offers no advantage when added to oral dexamethasone in the treatment of croup. Pediatr Emerg Care 2005;21(6):359–62.
117. Bjornson C, Russell Kelly F, Vandermeer B, et al. Nebulized epinephrine for croup in children. Cochrane Database Syst Rev 2011;2. Available at: http://www.mrw. interscience.wiley.com/cochrane/clsysrev/articles/CD006619/frame.html. Accessed May 1, 2011.

118. Taussig LM, Castro O, Beaudry PH, et al. Treatment of laryngotracheobronchitis (croup). Use of intermittent positive-pressure breathing and racemic epinephrine. Am J Dis Child 1975;129(7):790–3.
119. Scolnik D, Coates A, Stephens D, et al. Controlled delivery of high vs low humidity vs mist therapy for croup in emergency departments: a randomized controlled trial. JAMA 2006;295(11):1274–80.
120. Neto G, Kentab O, Klassen T, et al. A randomized controlled trial of mist in the acute treatment of moderate croup. Acad Emerg Med 2002;9(9):873–9.
121. Moore M, Little P. Humidified air inhalation for treating croup. Cochrane Database Syst Rev 2006;(3). Available at: http://www.mrw.interscience.wiley.com/cochrane/clsysrev/articles/CD002870/frame.html. Accessed May 1, 2011.
122. Weber JE, Chudnofsky CR, Younger JG, et al. A randomized comparison of helium-oxygen mixture (Heliox) and racemic epinephrine for the treatment of moderate to severe croup. Pediatrics 2001;107(6):E96.
123. Terregino CA, Nairn SJ, Chansky ME, et al. The effect of heliox on croup: a pilot study. Acad Emerg Med 1998;5(11):1130–3.
124. Vorwerk C, Coats T. Heliox for croup in children. Cochrane Database Syst Rev 2010;2:CD006822.
125. Everard M. Acute bronchiolitis and croup. Pediatr Clin North Am 2009;56(1):119–33.
126. Ducharme FM. Management of acute bronchiolitis. BMJ 2011;342:d1658.
127. Mansbach JM, McAdam AJ, Clark S, et al. Prospective multicenter study of the viral etiology of bronchiolitis in the emergency department. Acad Emerg Med 2008;15(2):111–8.
128. Midulla F, Scagnolari C, Bonci E, et al. Respiratory syncytial virus, human bocavirus and rhinovirus bronchiolitis in infants. Arch Dis Child 2010;95(1):35–41.
129. Miron D, Srugo I, Kra-Oz Z, et al. Sole pathogen in acute bronchiolitis—is there a role for other organisms apart from RSV? Pediatr Infect Dis J 2010;2010(29):e7–10.
130. American Academy of Pediatrics Subcommittee on Diagnosis and Management of Bronchiolitis. Diagnosis and management of bronchiolitis. Pediatrics 2006;118(4):1774–93.
131. Shay DK, Holman RC, Newman RD, et al. Bronchiolitis-associated hospitalizations among US children, 1980-1996. JAMA 1999;282(15):1440–6.
132. Shay DK, Holman RC, Roosevelt GE, et al. Bronchiolitis-associated mortality and estimates of respiratory syncytial virus-associated deaths among US children, 1979-1997. J Infect Dis 2001;183(1):16–22.
133. Swingler GH, Hussey GD, Zwarenstein M. Duration of illness in ambulatory children diagnosed with bronchiolitis. Arch Pediatr Adolesc Med 2000;154(10):997–1000.
134. Petruzella FD, Gorelick MH. Duration of illness in infants with bronchiolitis evaluated in the emergency department. Pediatrics 2010;126(2):285–90.
135. Bialy L, Foisy M, Smith M, et al. The Cochrane library and the treatment of bronchiolitis in children: an overview of reviews. Evid Base Child Health 2011;6(1):258–75.
136. Goutzamanis J. Bronchiolitis. In: Frank LR, Jobe KA, editors. Admission & discharge decisions in emergency medicine. Philadelphia: Hanley & Belfus, Inc; 2002. p. 246–50.
137. Everard M. What link between early respiratory viral infections and atopic asthma? Lancet 1999;354(9178):527–8.
138. Gern JE. Viral respiratory infection and the link to asthma. Pediatr Infect Dis J 2008;27(10):S97–103.

139. Stein RT, Sherrill D, Morgan WJ, et al. Respiratory syncytial virus in early life and risk of wheeze and allergy by age 13 years. Lancet 1999;354(9178): 541–5.

140. Swingler GH, Hussey GD, Zwarenstein M. Randomised controlled trial of clinical outcome after chest radiograph in ambulatory acute lower-respiratory infection in children. Lancet 1998;351(9100):404–8.

141. Schuh S, Lalani A, Allen U, et al. Evaluation of the utility of radiography in acute bronchiolitis. J Pediatr 2007;150(4):429–33.

142. Mahabee-Gittens EM, Bachman DT, Shapiro ED, et al. Chest radiographs in the pediatric emergency department for children ≤18 months of age with wheezing. Clin Pediatr 1999;38(7):395–9.

143. Purcell K, Fergie J. Lack of usefulness of an abnormal white blood cell count for predicting a concurrent serious bacterial infection in infants and young children hospitalized with respiratory syncytial virus lower respiratory tract infection. Pediatr Infect Dis J 2007;2007(26):311–5.

144. Peltola V, Mertsola J, Ruuskanen O. Comparison of total white blood cell count and serum C-reactive protein levels in confirmed bacterial and viral infections. J Pediatr 2006;149(5):721–4.

145. Liebelt EL, Qi K, Harvey K. Diagnostic testing for serious bacterial infections in infants aged 90 days or younger with bronchiolitis. Arch Pediatr Adolesc Med 1999;153(5):525–30.

146. Antanow J, Hansen K, McKinstry CA. Sepsis evaluations in hospitalized infants with bronchiolitis. Pediatr Infect Dis J 1998;17(3):231–6.

147. Thorburn K, Harigopal S, Reddy V, et al. High incidence of pulmonary bacterial co-infection in children with severe respiratory syncytial virus (RSV) bronchiolitis. Thorax 2006;61(7):611–5.

148. Bilavsky E, Shouval D, Yarden-Bilavsky H. A prospective study of the risk for serious bacterial infections in hospitalized febrile infants with or without bronchiolitis. Pediatr Infect Dis J 2008;27(3):269–82.

149. Duttweiler L, Nadal D, Frey B. Pulmonary and systemic bacterial co-infections in severe RSV bronchiolitis. Arch Dis Child 2004;89(12):1155–7.

150. Hartling L, Bialy Liza M, Vandermeer B, et al. Epinephrine for bronchiolitis. Cochrane Database Syst Rev 2011;(6). Available at: http://www.mrw.interscience.wiley.com/cochrane/clsysrev/articles/CD003123/frame.html. Accessed April 13, 2011.

151. Hartling L, Fernandes RM, Bialy L, et al. Steroids and bronchodilators for acute bronchiolitis in the first two years of life: systematic review and meta-analysis. BMJ 2011;342:d1714.

152. Chavasse Richard JPG, Seddon P, Bara A, et al. Short acting beta2-agonists for recurrent wheeze in children under two years of age. Cochrane Database Syst Rev 2002;2. Available at: http://www.mrw.interscience.wiley.com/cochrane/clsysrev/articles/CD002873/frame.html. Accessed April 13, 2011.

153. Everard M, Bara A, Kurian M, et al. Anticholinergic drugs for wheeze in children under the age of two years. Cochrane Database Syst Rev 2005;3. Available at: http://www.mrw.interscience.wiley.com/cochrane/clsysrev/articles/CD001279/frame.html. Accessed April 13, 2011.

154. Fernandes Ricardo M, Bialy Liza M, Vandermeer B, et al. Glucocorticoids for acute viral bronchiolitis in infants and young children. Cochrane Database Syst Rev 2010;10. Available at: http://www.mrw.interscience.wiley.com/cochrane/clsysrev/articles/CD004878/frame.html. Accessed April 13, 2011.

155. Zhang L, Mendoza-Sassi Raúl A, Wainwright C, et al. Nebulized hypertonic saline solution for acute bronchiolitis in infants. Cochrane Database Syst Rev

2008;4. Available at: http://www.mrw.interscience.wiley.com/cochrane/clsysrev/articles/CD006458/frame.html. Accessed April 13, 2011.

156. Liet JM, Ducruet T, Gupta V, et al. Heliox inhalation therapy for bronchiolitis in infants. Cochrane Database Syst Rev 2010;4. Available at: http://www.mrw.interscience.wiley.com/cochrane/clsysrev/articles/CD006915/frame.html. Accessed April 13, 2011.

157. Bronchiolitis Guideline Team, Cincinatti Children's Hospital Medical Team. Evidenced-based care guideline for management of bronchiolitis in infants 1 year of age or less with a first time epidose. Cincinnatti (OH): Bronchiolitis Pediatric Evidence-Based Care Guidelines, Cincinnatti Children's Hospital Medical Center. Available at: http://www.cincinnatichildrens.org/service/j/anderseon-center/evidence-based-care/bronchiolitis/. Accessed October 27, 2011.

158. Turner T, Wllkinson F, Harris C. Evidence-based guideline for the management of bronchiolitis. Aust Fam Physician 2008;37(6):6–13.

159. Bronchiolitis in children—a national clinical guideline. Scottish Intercollegiate Guidelines Network; 2006. Available at: http://www.sign.ac.uk/pdf/sign91.pdf. Accessed April 13, 2011.

160. Gadomski Anne M, Brower M. Bronchodilators for bronchiolitis. Cochrane Database Syst Rev 2010;12. Available at: http://www.mrw.interscience.wiley.com/cochrane/clsysrev/articles/CD001266/frame.html. Accessed April 13, 2011.

161. Seiden JA, Scarfone RJ. Bronchiolitis: an evidence-based approach to management. Clin Pediatr Emerg Med 2009;10(2):75–81.

162. Grewal S, Ali S, McConnell DW, et al. A randomized trial of nebulized 3% hypertonic saline with epinephrine in the treatment of acute bronchiolitis in the emergency department. Arch Pediatr Adolesc Med 2009;163(11):1007–12.

163. Corneli HM, Zorc JJ, Mahajan P, et al. A multicenter, randomized, controlled trial of dexamethasone for bronchiolitis. N Engl J Med 2007;357(4):331–9.

164. Plint AC, Johnson DW, Patel H, et al. Epinephrine and dexamethasone in children with bronchiolitis. N Engl J Med 2009;360(20):2079–89.

165. Wark P, McDonald Vanessa M. Nebulised hypertonic saline for cystic fibrosis. Cochrane Database Syst Rev 2009;2. Available at: http://www.mrw.interscience.wiley.com/cochrane/clsysrev/articles/CD001506/frame.html. Accessed April 13, 2011.

166. Chaudhry K, Sinert R. Is nebulized hypertonic saline solution an effective treatment for bronchiolitis in infants? Ann Emerg Med 2010;55(1):120–2.

167. Kuzik BA, Flavin MP, Kent S, et al. Effect of inhaled hypertonic saline on hospital admission rate in children with viral bronchiolitis: a randomized trial. CJEM 2010;12(6):477.

168. Kim IK, Corcoran T. Recent developments in heliox therapy for asthma and bronchiolitis. Clin Pediatr Emerg Med 2009;10(2):68–74.

169. Mansbach JM, Clark S, Christopher NC, et al. Prospective multicenter study of bronchiolitis: predicting safe discharges from the emergency department. Pediatrics 2008;121(4):680–8.

170. Willwerth BM, Harper MB, Greenes DS. Identifying hospitalized infants who have bronchiolitis and are at high risk for apnea. Ann Emerg Med 2006;48(4):441–7.

171. Norwood A, Mansbach JM, Clark S, et al. Prospective multicenter study of bronchiolitis: predictors of an unscheduled visit after discharge from the emergency department. Acad Emerg Med 2010;17(4):376–82.

172. Marlais M, Evans J, Abrahamson E. Clinical predictors of admission in infants with acute bronchiolitis. Arch Dis Child 2011;96(7):648–52.

173. Black RE, Cousens S, Johnson HL, et al. Global, regional, and national causes of child mortality in 2008: a systematic analysis. Lancet 2010;375(9730):1969–87.

174. Homier V, Bellevance C, Xhignesse M. Prevalence of pneumonia in children under 12 years of age who undergo abdominal radiography in the emergency department. CJEM 2007;9(5):347–51.

175. Evidence-Based (EB) Clinical Decision Support Team & Community-Acquired Pneumonia Content Expert Team - Texas Children's Hospital. Community-acquired pneumonia (CAP) clinical guideline. Available at: http://www.bcm.edu/web/pediatrics/documents/rp_archive_21.pdf. Accessed October 27, 2011.

176. Murphy CG, Van De Pol AC, Harper MB, et al. Clinical predictors of occult pneumonia in the febrile child. Acad Emerg Med 2007;14(3):243–9.

177. Shah S, Bachur R, Kim D, et al. Lack of predictive value of tachypnea in the diagnosis of pneumonia in children. Pediatr Infect Dis J 2010;29:406–9.

178. Korppi M, Don M, Valent F, et al. The value of clinical features in differentiating between viral, pneumococcal and atypical bacterial pneumonia in children. Acta Paediatr 2008;97(7):943–7.

179. Mathews B, Shah S, Cleveland RH, et al. Clinical predictors of pneumonia among children with wheezing. Pediatrics 2009;124(1):e29–36.

180. Korppi M. Antibiotic therapy for pneumonia in the pediatric population. Pediatr Health 2007;1(1):77.

181. British Thoracic Society. BTS guidelines for the management of community-acquired pneumonia in childhood. Thorax 2002;57(Suppl 1):i1–24.

182. Lahti E, Peltola V, Virkki R, et al. Development of parapneumonic empyema in children. Acta Paediatr 2007;96(11):1686–92.

183. Virkki R, Juven T, Rikalainen H, et al. Differentiation of bacterial and viral pneumonia in children. Thorax 2002;57(5):438–41.

184. Michelow IC, Olsen K, Lozano J, et al. Epidemiology and clinical characteristics of community-acquired pneumonia in hospitalized children. Pediatrics 2004;113(4):701–7.

185. Carrillo-Marquez M, Hulten K, Hammerman W, et al. *Staphylococcus aureus* pneumonia in children in the era of community-acquired methicillin-resistance at Texas Children's Hospital. Pediatr Infect Dis J 2011;30(7):545–50.

186. Wallin T, Hern H, Frazee B. Community-acquired methicillin-resistant *Staphylococcus aureus*. Emerg Med Clin North Am 2008;26:431–55.

187. Liu C, Bayer A, Cosgrove SE, et al. Clinical practice guidelines by the Infectious Diseases Society of America for the treatment of methicillin-resistant *Staphylococcus aureus* infections in adults and children: executive summary. Clin Infect Dis 2011;52(3):285–92.

188. Graham S, English M, Hazir T, et al. Challenges to improving case management of childhood pneumonia at health facilities in resource-limited settings. Bull World Health Organ 2008;86(5):349–55.

189. Clinical Practice Guidelines Group - Toward Optimized Practice (TOP) Program. Guideline for the diagnosis and management of community acquired pneumonia: pediatric - 2008 Update. Available at: http://www.topalbertadoctors.org/cpgs.php?sid=15&cpg_cats=61. Accessed April 26, 2011.

190. Newman M, Scully K, Kim D. Physician assessment of the likelihood of pneumonia in pediatric emergency department. Pediatr Emerg Care 2010;26(11):817–22.

191. Lynch T, Bialy L, Kellner J. A systematic review on the diagnosis of pediatric bacterial pneumonia: when gold is bronze. PLoS One 2010;5(8):1–7.

192. Cortellaro F, Colombo S, Coen D, et al. Lung ultrasound is an accurate diagnostic tool for the diagnosis of pneumonia in the emergency department. Emerg Med J 2010. [Epub ahead of print].

193. Kurian J, Levin TL, Han BK, et al. Comparison of ultrasound and CT in the evaluation of pneumonia complicated by parapneumonic effusion in children. Am J Roentgenol 2009;193(6):1648–54.
194. Community Acquired Pneumonia Guideline Team, Cincinnati Children's Hospital Medical Center. Evidence-based care guideline for medical management of community acquired pneumonia in children 60 days to 17 years of age. Available at: http://www.cincinnatichildrens.org/service/j/anderson-center/evidence-based-care/community-acquired-pneumonia/. Accessed October 27, 2011.
195. Shah S, Dugan M, Bell L, et al. Blood cultures in the emergency department evaluation of childhood pneumonia. Pediatr Infect Dis J 2011;30:475–9.
196. Hickey RW, Bowman MJ, Smith GA. Utility of blood cultures in pediatric patients found to have pneumonia in the emergency department. Ann Emerg Med 1996; 27(6):721–5.
197. Jadavji T, Law B. A practical guide for the diagnosis and treatment of pediatric pneumonia. CMAJ 1997;156(5):S703.
198. Wilde JA. Rapid diagnostic testing for the identification of respiratory agents in the emergency department. Clin Pediatr Emerg Med 2002;3(3):181–90.
199. Bradley JS, Byington CL, Shah SS, et al. The management of community-acquired pneumonia in infants and children older than 3 months of age: clinical practice guidelines by the Pediatric Infectious Diseases Society and the Infectious Diseases Society of America. Clin Infect Dis 2011;53(7):e25–76.
200. Atkinson M, Lakhanpaul M, Smyth A, et al. Comparison of oral amoxicillin and intravenous benzyl penicillin for community acquired pneumonia in children (PIVOT trial): a multicentre pragmatic randomised controlled equivalence trial. Thorax 2007;62(12):1102–6.
201. Haider Batool A, Lassi Zohra S, Bhutta Zulfiqar A. Short-course versus long-course antibiotic therapy for non-severe community-acquired pneumonia in children aged 2 months to 59 months. Cochrane Database Syst Rev 2008;2. Available at: http://www.mrw.interscience.wiley.com/cochrane/clsysrev/articles/CD005976/frame.html. Accessed June 12, 2011.
202. Ayieko P, English M. Case management of childhood pneumonia in developing countries. Pediatr Infect Dis J 2007;26(5):432–40.
203. Virkki R, Juven T, Mertsola J, et al. Radiographic follow-up of pneumonia in children. Pediatr Pulmonol 2005;40(3):223–7.

Thoracic Emergencies in Immunocompromised Patients

Saleh Fares, MD, MPH, FRCPC[a,b],*, Furqan B. Irfan, MBBS[c]

KEYWORDS

• Emergency • Thoracic • Immunocompromised • Cardiac
• Pulmonary • Esophagus • Great vessels

The immunocompromised patient is at greater risk for frequent as well as serious medical emergencies in comparison with their immunocompetent counterparts. Moreover, diagnosis and assessment of an immunocompromised patient is often difficult, due to vague signs and symptoms.[1] The increased prevalence of immunosuppressed patients over the past few decades can be attributed to human immunodeficiency virus (HIV) disease, transplant medicine, and chemotherapy.[1,2] The prevalence of HIV infection among patients presenting to emergency departments (EDs) in hospitals in the United States is between 2% and 17%.[3,4] By contrast, some emergency medical units in western Kenya and Uganda have a much higher prevalence of HIV infection, ranging between 23% and 50%, respectively.[5,6] With a similar worldwide surge in cancer diagnoses and subsequent increase in chemotherapeutic use,[1] it has become increasingly important for the emergency physician to be aware of the variety of presentations faced by these patients. This article aims to describe a clinical approach to recognizing thoracic emergencies specifically found in immunocompromised patients, in order to enable rapid assessment and appropriate emergency intervention and management.

Due to the very high prevalence of HIV-infected patients as well as patients undergoing cancer therapy, these two sets of disease states are used to illustrate the various emergency illnesses that are likely to present to the ED.[7] Thoracic emergencies in the immunocompromised patient may include cardiovascular events, opportunistic pulmonary and esophageal infections, masses and malignancies, and

The authors have nothing to disclose.
[a] Emergency Medicine, Zayed Military Hospital, PO Box 8313, Abu Dhabi, United Arab Emirates
[b] Harvard-Affiliated Disaster Medicine/EMS Fellowship Program, Department of Emergency Medicine, One Deaconess Road, West Campus Clinical Center, 2nd Floor, Boston, MA 02215, USA
[c] Department of Surgery, Aga Khan University, Stadium Road, PO Box 3500, Karachi 74800, Pakistan
* Corresponding author.
E-mail address: sfares@bidmc.Harvard.edu

Emerg Med Clin N Am 30 (2012) 565–589
doi:10.1016/j.emc.2011.10.007
0733-8627/12/$ – see front matter © 2012 Elsevier Inc. All rights reserved.

emed.theclinics.com

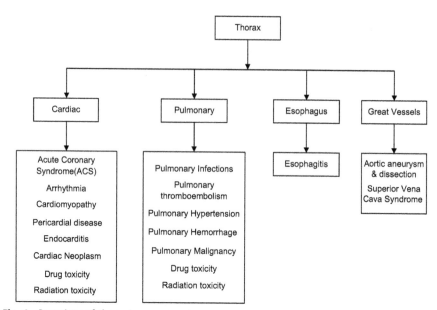

Fig. 1. Overview of thoracic emergencies.

drug-induced and radiation-induced toxicities. An anatomic approach is used to describe thoracic emergencies in this article, with an emphasis on emergencies of particular relevance and frequency in the immunosuppressed state (**Fig. 1**).

IMMUNE SYSTEM

The immune system consists of a network of interdependent cell types, tissues, and organs that collectively form the defense system of the body. It is composed of two major subdivisions: the innate or nonspecific immune system and the acquired or specific immune system.

Innate or nonspecific immunity is the natural immunity with which a person is born, and provides immediate defense against infection. The surface barriers, including the skin and mucous membranes lining the respiratory, digestive, reproductive, and urological tracts, form the first line of defense. Acute inflammation is one of the first responses when surface barriers are breached, and is brought about by humoral and chemical factors (histamine, bradykinin, serotonin, leukotrienes, and prostaglandins) as well as the complement system. Cellular innate response consists of leukocytes (white blood cells) and the phagocytic cells, including neutrophils and macrophages.

Acquired (adaptive) or specific immunity is not present at birth, and develops following exposure to various antigens exhibiting immunologic memory. Lymphocytes originating from stem cells in bone marrow (mainly B cells and T cells) make up the cellular elements of an acquired immune system. Both B and T cells have receptors that are specific for a particular antigen. Killer (cytotoxic) T cells destroy infected cells, cancer cells, and foreign cells. Helper T cells aid other immune cells (B cells, T cells, and macrophages). Suppressor (regulatory) T cells maintain the immune system homeostasis and immunologic tolerance. B cells are involved in the humoral immune response, and on encountering a specific antigen are stimulated to transform into either a plasma cell (which produces antibodies) or memory B cell. Memory B cells are long-lived and on encountering the antigen again, rapidly transform into plasma cells to produce antibodies.[8]

IMMUNODEFICIENCY CONDITIONS AND DISEASES

Patients with immunocompromised or immunodeficient systems are in a state where the immune system fails or is impaired, resulting in an increased risk of infections or opportunistic complications.[2] In the majority of cases immunodeficiency is acquired or secondary, whereas primary immunodeficiency (congenital) disorders are relatively rare.

Acquired immunodeficiency disorders affect patients with a normal immune system, develop later in life, and are the result of external diseases or medications, therapies, and certain physiologic states (**Table 1**). The most common secondary immunodeficiency worldwide is caused by severe malnutrition. A variety of metabolic disorders such as diabetes, alcoholism, and uremia can also cause an acquired immunodeficiency state.[9]

Various classes of drugs can cause secondary immunodeficiency, including anti-inflammatory agents (corticosteroids), immunosuppressant use in transplant medicine (calcineurin inhibitors), and cancer chemotherapy (cytotoxic agents). Autoimmune diseases, neutropenia in cancers (leukemias, lymphomas), and asplenia due to surgery (splenectomy) and hemoglobinopathies are also secondary immunodeficiency conditions, while infectious disease etiology includes HIV infection and AIDS. Pregnancy and extremes of age are physiologic immunodeficiency states. Environmental aspects, such as burn injuries, radiotherapy, and ionizing radiation, can also cause secondary immunodeficiency, all of which may be encountered in the ED.[9]

CARDIAC EMERGENCIES

Cardiac complications and emergencies in HIV/AIDS patients may be a direct consequence of the disease itself as well as its treatment. HIV patients exhibit an increase in coronary artery disease as well as lipid and metabolic derangements, especially those on antiretroviral therapy (ART).[10,11] Protease inhibitors are associated with lipodystrophy, insulin resistance, high levels of low-density lipoprotein, and increased total cholesterol levels.[12,13]

Table 1 Incidence of compromised immune function in groups of emergency department patients	
Condition	Incidence (%)
Old age	10–20
Diabetes	5
Alcoholism	10–20
Drug abuse	5–10
Cancer	5
Transplantation	<1
Malnutrition	2–3
HIV/AIDS	1–10
Immunosuppressive drugs	2–4
Burns	<1
Renal or hepatic failure	2–3
Autoimmune disorders	<1

Abbreviations: AIDS, acquired immunodeficiency syndrome; HIV, human immunodeficiency virus.
Data from Burns MJ, Langdorf MI. The immunocompromised patient. In: Marx JA, editor-in-chief. Rosen's emergency medicine: concepts and clinical practice. 6th edition. Philadelphia: Elsevier, 2011.

Acute Coronary Syndrome

There is some controversy regarding the increased incidence of myocardial infarction (MI) in HIV-infected patients on ART, with some large studies suggesting an association between the incidence of MI and protease inhibitors and nucleoside reverse transcriptase inhibitors (abacavir and didanosine).[11,14–16] Other studies report no association.[10,17,18] Acute coronary syndrome (ACS) in HIV-infected patients commonly presents in relatively young patients in their 40s.[10] A prospective cohort study reported that stress echocardiography may provide prognostic value and risk stratification in HIV-infected patients with coronary artery disease.[19] Treatment is the same standard medical approach as with immunocompetent patients. Unstable angina or non–Q-wave MI should be treated medically in the absence of therapeutic contraindications.[13] Percutaneous coronary intervention is recommended in HIV patients with ACS, but has a higher rate of restenosis. Coronary artery bypass graft surgery is also feasible, especially with multivessel disease.[10]

Arrhythmia

Bradycardias and ventricular arrhythmias have been reported in patients with HIV-associated dilated cardiomyopathy.[13,20] Protease inhibitors and certain drugs used to treat opportunistic infections in HIV-infected patients have been implicated in prolongation of the QT interval resulting in ventricular tachycardia and torsades de pointes.[21] These agents include ganciclovir, amphotericin B, trimethoprim-sulfamethoxazole, and pentamidine.[13,22,23] Management of arrhythmias should follow standard Advanced Cardiac Life Support protocols, along with immediate withdrawal of the inciting drugs and correction of electrolyte imbalances.[13]

Cardiomyopathy

The prevalence of dilated cardiomyopathy among HIV-infected patients has decreased significantly in developed countries since the advent of highly active antiretroviral therapy (HAART).[24,25] However, in developing countries in Africa where HAART is still not widely accessible, cross-sectional studies show a prevalence of HIV-associated cardiomyopathy of 9% to 57%.[26–29] A recent retrospective cohort study suggested that ongoing viral replication in HIV infection is a risk factor for heart failure.[30] Survival rates are much lower for patients with HIV-associated dilated cardiomyopathy than for those with idiopathic dilated cardiomyopathy.[31] The etiology of HIV-associated cardiomyopathy includes autoimmunity (cardiac-specific autoantibodies), nutritional deficiencies, autonomic dysfunction, cardiotoxicity (zidovudine, doxorubicin, foscarnet sodium), and myocarditis.[10,32–35] Left ventricular dysfunction as a result of dilated cardiomyopathy is a late manifestation of HIV-associated heart disease and is associated with low CD4 levels, myocarditis, and an elevation of antiheart antibodies.[36,37] Symptoms include dyspnea, orthopnea, fatigue, lightheadedness, palpitations, and swelling of the lower extremities. Echocardiography for diagnosis should be considered early on in suspected patients. Management of HIV-associated cardiomyopathy and heart failure should follow standard treatment guidelines.[13]

Pericardial Disease

The clinical presentation of acute pericarditis is similar to that of the immunocompetent patient.[37] Purulent pericarditis can occur in immunocompromised patients, including those taking immunosuppressive drugs.[38] Before the advent of HAART, pericardial effusion was one of the most common cardiovascular complications in HIV-infected patients, with an incidence of around 11% per year.[39] However, in developing countries without regular access to HAART, the prevalence of pericardial effusion has in fact increased, mostly attributable to mycobacterial infections.[40] Besides opportunistic infections, pericardial effusion in HIV-infected patients and other immunocompromised conditions can also be due to malignancy (eg, Kaposi sarcoma, non-Hodgkin lymphoma), but most cases are of unknown etiology.[33] Clinical presentation of pericardial effusion can range from asymptomatic pericardial effusion to pericarditis, cardiac tamponade, and constrictive pericarditis.[37] According to prospective echocardiographic studies, the majority of pericardial effusions are small and asymptomatic, with 13% to 42% resolving spontaneously.[39,41] Cardiac tamponade in HIV-infected patients is not common, with an annual incidence of 9% in AIDS patients with pericardial effusion.[39] Pericardiocentesis is recommended only for large and symptomatic effusions, and then only for diagnostic purposes or as therapy for tamponade.[10,13]

Endocarditis

Nonbacterial thrombotic endocarditis (NBTE, also known as marantic endocarditis) occurs in approximately 3% to 5% of AIDS patients (pre-ART era), and is characterized by vegetations on cardiac valves consisting of a fibrinous lattice of platelets and red blood cells, which can lead to embolization.[37] Other immunocompromised conditions also associated with nonbacterial thrombotic endocarditis include neoplastic disease, hypercoagulable diseases, and chronic wasting disease.[42,43] NBTE can lead to systemic embolization of the central nervous system, coronary arteries, spleen, kidney, lungs, and extremities.[37] Diagnosis is by echocardiography and management involves treating the underlying immune condition along with systemic anticoagulation. Unfractionated heparin is recommended in cancer patients with NBTE to prevent recurrent thromboembolism.[44]

Cardiac Neoplasm

Kaposi sarcoma is an AIDS-associated malignancy that is 300 times more common in HIV-infected patients than in patients with other immunocompromised conditions.[45] Before the use of ART, retrospective autopsy studies showed a prevalence of 12% to 28% of disseminated Kaposi sarcoma involving the heart.[46,47] HIV-associated metastatic Kaposi sarcoma lesions are typically small (<1 cm) and involve either the pericardium or subepicardial fat.[33,37] The clinical manifestations are vague and the lesions rarely give rise to complications, with most cases being discovered at autopsy.[33] Rarely, cardiac tamponade and pericardial constriction have been reported.[37,48] However, pericardiocentesis, a high-risk procedure in patients with HIV-associated Kaposi sarcoma, is often not advised. Instead, an early pericardial window is recommended for decompression and diagnosis.[37,48]

Non-Hodgkin lymphoma involving the heart in AIDS patients results mostly from disseminated disease and is intermediate or high grade in most cases.[37] Cardiac lymphoma can lead to various clinical presentations such as congestive heart failure, arrhythmia, and pericardial effusions.[49] Despite chemotherapy, prognosis of cardiac lymphoma is poor.[50] Cardiac surgery has also been reported to be beneficial in obstructive disease.[51] Since the advent of HAART, the incidence of both HIV-associated cardiac Kaposi sarcoma and non-Hodgkin lymphomas has decreased by about 50% in developed countries.[33]

Drug-Induced Cardiac Toxicity

Cardiovascular toxicity associated with chemotherapeutic drugs is well established. The spectrum of drug-related effects ranges from slight changes in blood pressure and electrocardiography (ECG) changes to life-threatening arrhythmias, myocarditis, pericarditis, MI, cardiomyopathy, and congestive heart failure.[52] Risk factors include cumulative drug dosage, the rate and route of administration, the use of concurrent cardiotoxic drugs, previous or coexistent cardiovascular disease, and prior thoracic radiation exposure.[53] Anthracyclines (doxorubicin, daunorubicin, and epirubicin), alkylating agents (cyclophosphamide, busulfan, cisplatin, mitomycin), antimetabolites (5-fluorouracil), antimicrotubule agents (paclitaxel), vinca alkaloids, and monoclonal antibodies (bevacizumab, trastuzumab) all have cardiotoxic potential (**Table 2**).[53–59] Investigations to detect and monitor drug-induced cardiac toxicity include the same measures as for immunocompetent patients.[53,60,61] Endomyocardial biopsy is the most reliable investigation for evaluation of cardiotoxicity,[62] but it is a complex and invasive procedure, limiting its use. The American College of Cardiology and American Heart Association practice guidelines recommend baseline echocardiography and reevaluations of patients receiving cardiotoxic chemotherapy.[63] Prevention and treatment of any presumed drug-induced cardiac toxicity include withdrawal or reduction in dosage of the offending drug, changes in chemotherapy combination regimen, adding cardioprotectants (eg, dexrazoxane), and other standard management protocols for underlying cardiac toxicity (angiotensin-converting enzyme inhibitors and β-blocking agents for chemotherapy-induced heart failure).[53,64]

Radiation Toxicity

Radiation therapy is used to treat many cancers of the thorax, from hematological malignancies to breast, lung, and esophageal cancers. Radiation-induced heart disease is a well-known adverse effect of radiotherapy. The pericardium is most commonly involved. However, all cardiac elements, including the myocardium, cardiac valves, and coronary vessels, are also affected. According to the American Society of Clinical Oncology, patient risk factors for radiation-induced heart disease include previous or concurrent use of chemotherapy (eg, anthracycline), tumor location close to heart border, age less than 18 years, associated cardiac risk factors and disease, and greater than 10 years postradiation therapy.[65] Radiation-based

Table 2
Cardiotoxic drugs in cancer patients

Drugs	Cardiotoxic Effect
Anthracyclines/anthraquinolones Daunorubicin, doxorubicin, epirubicin, idarubicin, mitoxantrone	Left ventricular systolic dysfunction, congestive heart failure
Alkylating agents Cyclophosphamide, ifosfamide, mitomycin, busulfan	Congestive heart failure, myocarditis, pericarditis
Cisplatin	Hypertension, myocardial ischemia, infarction
Antimicrotubules Paclitaxel, vinca alkaloids	Arrhythmias, myocardial ischemia
Antimetabolites Cytarabine, fluorouracil, capecitabine	Myocardial ischemia/infarction, arrhythmias, cardiomyopathy
Monoclonal antibodies Alemtuzumab, cetuximab, trastuzumab, bevacizumab, rituximab	Hypotension, arrhythmias, congestive heart failure
Interleukins and interferons	Hypotension, arrhythmias, cardiomyopathy

risk factors for radiation-induced heart disease include orthovoltage radiation (rarely used since the 1970s), volume of irradiated heart, total dose to the heart of greater than 30 Gy, daily dose fraction of greater than 2 Gy/d, and absence of subcarinal blocking.[65]

Acute pericarditis and pericardial effusion can present anywhere from 2 to 145 months (mean time interval of 58 months) after radiation therapy, and can progress to constrictive pericarditis or cardiac tamponade.[66,67] Cardiac valves as well as coronary arteries and myocardium undergo fibrous thickening because of radiation. This thickening can lead to valvular dysfunction, radiation-induced cardiomyopathy, and radiation-induced coronary artery disease (RICAD), which has a mean interval of development of approximately 82 months after radiotherapy.[53,66,68]

The clinical presentation of patients with RICAD includes angina and MI, dyspnea or heart failure, and sometimes even sudden death.[66] The mechanism for the detection and monitoring of radiation-induced cardiovascular toxicity is similar to modalities described for drug-induced cardiac toxicity, and standard treatment guidelines are followed for radiation-induced cardiac disease as for immunocompetent patients, with consideration given to radiation changes in heart and surrounding organs.[66,69] However, over the past few decades equipment for delivering radiation therapy has improved considerably, resulting in reduced total radiation dosage to surrounding organs and thorax.[61] This reduced dosage should lead to decreased prevalence of all adverse effects from radiotherapy, including cardiotoxicity in patients treated over the past few years.[61]

PULMONARY EMERGENCIES

The incidence of pulmonary emergencies among immunocompromised patients is growing.[70] Although pulmonary infections are the most common presenting complaints, significant noninfectious pulmonary emergencies often coexist, making diagnosis a challenging task for emergency physicians.[70] Acute symptoms suggest bacterial pneumonia, hemorrhage, pulmonary emboli, and pulmonary edema whereas chronic symptoms are suggestive of opportunistic fungal or viral infections, malignancy, or drug toxicity.

Pulmonary Infections

Respiratory infection is the most common pulmonary complication in immunosuppressed patients, accounting for nearly 75% of lung disease.[71] Respiratory infections are associated with about 65% of AIDS-defining illnesses.[72]

Bacterial pneumonia

The incidence of bacterial pneumonia in AIDS patients is 5 times higher than in the general population.[73] Bacterial respiratory infections in immunocompromised patients can be subdivided into community-acquired infection, atypical organisms, mycobacterium, and opportunistic infections (**Box 1**). The most common community-acquired pathogens include *Streptococcus pneumoniae* and *Haemophilus* species, while *Pseudomonas aeruginosa* and *Staphylococcus aureus* also occur with greater frequency and have been reported as community-acquired organisms in HIV-infected patients.[74,75] Gram-negative bacteria are also common in neutropenic and nosocomial infections and include *Klebsiella* species, *Acinetobacter*, *Escherichia coli*, *Enterobacter*, and *Serratia* species.[76] Clinical presentation is usually acute onset of fevers, chills, chest pain, productive cough, and dyspnea.[77] Single or multiple areas of focal consolidation, in segmental or lobar distribution, and parapneumonic effusions are the common chest radiograph findings in HIV-infected patients with pneumonia.[73,78]

Box 1
Bacterial pathogens causing pneumonia in immunocompromised patients

Community acquired

    Streptococcus pneumoniae

    Haemophilus influenzae

    Moraxella catarrhalis

    Staphylococcus aureus

    Pseudomonas aeruginosa

Atypical bacteria

    Legionella species

    Mycoplasma pneumoniae

    Chlamydia species

Mycobacteria

    Mycobacterium tuberculosis

    Mycobacterium avium

    Mycobacterium intracellulare

Opportunistic and nosocomial

    Klebsiella pneumoniae

    Acinetobacter species

    Escherichia coli

    Enterobacter species

    Streptococcus viridians

    Nocardia asteroides

    Rhodococcus equi

    Methicillin-sensitive and methicillin-resistant *Staphylococcus aureus* (MRSA)

Chest radiograph finding of cavitary lesions suggests *P aeruginosa* in HIV-infected patients.[79] After obtaining specimens for Gram stain and cultures, empiric treatment should be started and standard guidelines for pneumonia should be followed, as for immunocompetent patients.[80] The National Institutes of Health (NIH), the Centers for Disease Control and Prevention (CDC), and the HIV Medicine Association (HIVMA) of the Infectious Diseases Society of America recommend that HIV-infected patients with pneumonia should be given a β-lactam (ceftriaxone, cefotaxime, or ampicillin-sulbactam) and a macrolide (azithromycin or clarithromycin). HIV-infected patients with severe pneumonia should receive intravenous β-lactam and either azithromycin or a respiratory fluoroquinolone (moxifloxacin or levofloxacin).[79] HIV-infected patients should not receive macrolide monotherapy because of the risk for drug-resistant *S pneumoniae*.[79]

Pneumocystis pneumonia

Pneumocystis (carinii) jiroveci pneumonia is an opportunistic infection caused by a yeastlike fungus. Previously known as *Pneumocystis carinii* pneumonia (PCP), even though the nomenclature has changed to *jiroveci* the abbreviation PCP is still used for *Pneumocystis* pneumonia. PCP is the most common cause of death in

AIDS patients.[70] In HIV-infected patients, CD4 cell counts of less than 200 cells/μL is the greatest risk factor for developing PCP.[81] The classic presentation in immunocompromised patients is a triad of progressive dyspnea, fever, and cough. Radiographic findings typically demonstrate bilateral interstitial and alveolar infiltrates, mostly over the perihilar region, but may be normal in nearly 30% of cases.[81,82] Computed tomography (CT) findings include perihilar ground-glass opacity and thickening of the interlobular septa.[73]

A firm diagnosis of PCP in the ED is not feasible, but it can be detected in an inpatient setting by the demonstration of trophozoites or cyst forms of *P jiroveci* via microscopy, or by DNA through polymerase chain reaction (PCR) from sputum or bronchoalveolar lavage (BAL).[82] Serum abnormalities that suggest PCP include elevated serum lactate dehydrogenase and hypoxemia.[81,83]

According to the guidelines by the NIH, the CDC, and the HIVMA of the Infectious Diseases Society of America, the drug of choice for PCP is cotrimoxazole (trimethoprim-sulfamethoxazole), given for 21 days.[79] Alternative drugs recommended for the treatment of moderate to severe pneumocystosis (Pao$_2$ <70 mm Hg or arterial-alveolar O$_2$ gradient >35 mm Hg) include clindamycin-primaquine or intravenous pentamidine.[79] The guidelines also recommended that adjunctive therapy with systemic corticosteroids should be initiated early, within 72 hours of starting PCP therapy in HIV patients with moderate to severe disease.[79] In a retrospective study of HIV patients with PCP, hospital survival was approximately 40% in patients requiring intensive care unit admission for hypoxemia and respiratory failure.[84]

Tuberculosis

The rate of pulmonary tuberculosis (TB) has increased significantly since the HIV epidemic in the mid-1980s, and is considered an AIDS-defining disease.[73] In HIV-infected patients, CD4 cell counts between 200 and 400/mm^3 are a strong risk factor for contracting TB.[70] TB is mainly caused by *M tuberculosis* and is transmitted via airborne droplets. After inhalation, the organism either causes primary infection or is walled off by lymphocytes and macrophages in the alveoli, forming granulomas leading to latent TB infection. Latent TB can be reactivated into postprimary TB disease, with immunocompromise being one of the key predisposing factors.[85] Typical symptoms include fatigue, anorexia, weight loss, productive cough, night sweats, and fever, while patients with lower CD4 cell counts may manifest with extrapulmonary symptoms.[70] Disseminated TB is seen not only in AIDS but also in other immunocompromised conditions, including leukemias, as well as in patients taking immune-suppressant medications.[86,87]

Patients suspected of having active TB should be given a mask to wear and placed in isolation once they enter the ED. Health personnel treating the patient should wear protective N95 masks.[88] The findings on chest radiograph vary depending on how advanced the HIV infection is; patients with higher CD4 cell counts (>350 cells/μL) show a typical pattern of upper lobe fibronodular infiltrates with or without cavitation, whereas those with advanced HIV disease demonstrate lower and middle lobe, interstitial and miliary infiltrates, and hilar/mediastinal adenopathy.[89] Cavitations and a miliary (millet seed) pattern are the hallmarks of reactivation TB and miliary/disseminated TB, respectively.[90] Unfortunately, chest radiography is less sensitive in patients with HIV coinfection,[85] and CT will show the characteristic "tree-in-bud" appearance in patients with pulmonary TB.[91]

All patients diagnosed with HIV should be tested for latent TB infection by either interferon-γ release assays or tuberculin skin test.[79] If either test is positive or in patients with symptoms, active TB should be excluded by chest radiography and clinical evaluation. For HIV patients with pulmonary symptoms and an abnormal chest radiograph (or normal chest radiograph and a high clinical suspicion), 3 sputum samples; preferably on consecutive days for TB microscopy and cultures, should be taken.[79,85] In patients with suspected extrapulmonary TB and disseminated disease, needle aspiration or biopsy should be performed. For all TB patients, specimens should be sent for drug-susceptibility testing to commonly used drug regimens (rifampin [RIF], isoniazid [INH], ethambutol [EMB], and pyrazinamide [PZA]).[79] There are no international guidelines recommending the use of serologic diagnostic tests for TB, and after several meta-analyses proving their ineffectiveness, the World Health Organization is due to release a negative policy recommendation on TB serodiagnostics in high-burden countries.[92]

National guidelines recommend that HIV-infected patients should be treated with daily isoniazid for 9 months if (1) they test positive for latent TB infection and have no prior history of treatment, (2) test negative for latent TB infection but are in close contact with pulmonary TB patients, and (3) have a history of untreated/inadequately treated healed TB.[79] HIV-infected patients with suspicion of active TB should be started on an empiric multidrug regimen immediately while awaiting results of investigations.[93] Recommendations for all patients include clinical assessment and baseline investigations to evaluate liver function, renal function, complete blood count, and CD4+ counts.[94] The treatment of TB in patients with HIV coinfection is similar to that for immunocompetent TB patients.[93] The initiation phase is treatment with RIF, INH, PZA, and EMB (RIPE regimen). The initiation phase with RIPE regimen should be administered for 2 months, followed by 4 months of continuous therapy with INH and RIF.[79] All patients treated with INH should receive pyridoxine supplementation, for the prevention of peripheral neuropathy. Recommendations for extrapulmonary TB include a 6- to 9-month regimen: 2 months of RIPE regimen followed by 4 to 7 months of INH and RIF. However, for central nervous system TB disease and bone and joint TB, anti-TB regimen recommendation is for 9 to 12 months.[94] Adjuvant corticosteroid therapy (dexamethasone/prednisone) is also recommended for central nervous system and pericardial TB.[79] Multidrug-resistant TB and extensively drug-resistant TB require longer treatment with second-line drugs.[82]

Fungal pulmonary infections

Fungal pulmonary disease can be caused by endemic or, in the case of immunocompromised patients, by opportunistic fungal pathogens. Endemic fungal pathogens include *Histoplasma capsulatum*, *Coccidioides immitis*, and *Blastomyces dermatitidis*. Although they can occur in immunocompetent patients, they occur with greater frequency and severity in immunocompromised patients. Along with *Pneumocystis* species (discussed earlier), opportunistic pathogens include *Aspergillus* species and *Cryptococcus neoformans*.

Pulmonary histoplasmosis, coccidiomycosis (San Joaquin Valley Fever), and blastomycosis is mostly self-limiting. Symptoms can include dyspnea, cough, fever, headache, malaise, arthralgias, myalgias, abdominal pain, and chills.[70] Chronic pulmonary disease, especially in coccidiomycosis, can cause cavitation, bronchiectasis, and bronchopleural fistulas with pleural empyema.[95]

Immunosuppressed patients are at risk for disseminated disease.[82] Disseminated fungal disease can affect the nervous system as well as cardiovascular, gastrointestinal, dermatologic, and urogenital systems.[70,96,97] Chest radiograph findings may reveal reticulonodular or alveolar infiltrates, hilar lymphadenopathy, cavitations, and pleural effusion.[70] Diagnosis is through cultures, serologic antibodies, antigen detection, and microscopy (for blastomycosis).[98–100] Amphotericin B is the drug of choice, while alternative drugs include triazole antifungals for treatment of histoplasmosis, coc-cidiomycosis, and blastomycosis.[70]

Aspergillosis, caused by the inhalation of *Aspergillus* spores, is an opportunistic infection found in immunosuppressed patients (HIV/AIDS, transplant recipients, diabetics, patients receiving chemotherapy and corticosteroids).[82] Infection can lead to the development of aspergilloma, invasive pulmonary aspergillosis (IPA), chronic necrotizing aspergillosis (CNA), and allergic bronchopulmonary aspergillosis (ABPA). Aspergilloma is a cluster of fungus, known as a fungus ball, which forms inside a preexisting cavity in the lung. ABPA results from a hypersensitivity reaction to the *Aspergillus* species. IPA usually manifests as bronchopneumonia or tracheobronchitis, whereas CNA is a progressive cavitary disease with invasion of lung tissue, presenting with fever, weight loss, malaise, fatigue, and respiratory symptoms lasting weeks or months.[101] Diagnosis is by histopathological examination, microscopy, and cultures.[82] Voriconazole is drug of choice for invasive aspergillosis, while amphotericin B is also effective.[82,102]

Cryptococcosis

Cryptococcosis is an opportunistic infection caused by the yeast *Cryptococcus neoformans*. Disseminated cryptococcosis can present with symptoms of meningitis and meningoencephalitis, and/or pneumonia.[73] Chest radiograph findings can include a nodular or reticulonodular interstitial pattern, hilar lymphadenopathy, masses, and pleural effusions. Diagnosis is made by demonstrating serum cryptococcal antigen in HIV-infected patients.[103] Treatment includes amphotericin B and flucytosine for at least 2 weeks in patients with normal renal function, followed by fluconazole for 8 weeks.[104]

Viral infections

Cytomegalovirus (CMV) disease is a common finding in transplant recipients, AIDS patients, and patients receiving immunosuppressive therapy.[105,106] CMV pneumonia is a life-threatening condition, and results from either reactivation of latent infection or newly acquired infection. The mortality rate of CMV pneumonia is reported as between 31% and 68%, in immunosuppressed (posttransplant) patients with CMV pneumonia.[107,108] CMV pneumonia occurs usually in HIV-infected patients when CD4 count is less than 50 cells/mm^3.[73] Symptoms of CMV pneumonia include fever, anorexia, malaise, myalgias, dyspnea, dry cough, and hypoxemia.[70] Chest radiograph findings may be normal or can reveal a reticulonodular pattern as well as alveolar or interstitial infiltrates.[73]

Demonstration of CMV by histopathology, immunohistochemical analysis, in situ hybridization, cultures, and DNA-PCR tests leads to diagnosis.[70] Newer tests such as CMV pp65 antigen assay and anti-CMV immediate early antigen monoclonal antibody test provide sensitive and quicker results within 6 hours and 3 hours, respectively.[109,110] Intravenous ganciclovir is the drug of choice for the treatment of CMV disease. Patients who have received a bone marrow transplant should receive a combination therapy of CMV immunoglobulins and ganciclovir.[111,112]

Pulmonary Thromboembolism

The incidence of deep vein thrombosis and pulmonary embolism is nearly 10 times greater in HIV/AIDS patients than in the general population.[113] Decreased levels of protein C, protein S, heparin cofactor II, and antithrombin III combined with increased levels of von Willebrand factor, D-dimers, and antiphospholipid antibodies contribute to coagulation abnormalities in HIV infection.[114] Malignancy and immunosuppressive or cytotoxic chemotherapy in cancer patients have been described as risk factors for venous thromboembolism in a population-based case-control study.[115] The clinical presentation is similar to that of immunocompetent patients: pleuritic chest pain, dyspnea, palpitations, and hemoptysis.[116] Diagnosis is made by usual imaging modalities, such as ventilation/perfusion scintigraphy and spiral CT pulmonary angiography. The American Society of Clinical Oncology guidelines recommend short-term and long-term anticoagulation therapy with low molecular weight heparin in cancer patients with venous thromboembolism.[117] An inferior vena cava filter is indicated in cases of recurrent venous thromboembolism despite anticoagulation, or when there exists a contraindication to anticoagulation therapy.[117]

Pulmonary Hypertension

Pulmonary hypertension has an incidence of 1 in 200 in HIV-infected patients, compared with 1 in 200,000 in the general population.[37] Etiology for HIV-associated pulmonary hypertension includes pulmonary infections, thromboembolism, and left ventricular dysfunction.[118] Symptoms include progressive shortness of breath, pedal edema, nonproductive cough, fatigue, syncope, and chest pain.[119] Diagnosis is established by echocardiography and right-sided cardiac catheterization. Management may include the use of pulmonary vasodilators, ART, epoprostenol, calcium-channel blockers, anticoagulation therapy, diuretics, oxygen, and digoxin.[119] HIV-associated pulmonary hypertension is more rapidly progressive than primary pulmonary hypertension, with right-sided heart failure and respiratory failure being the predominant causes of mortality.[120]

Pulmonary Malignancy

Lung cancer accounts for 1.6% to 4.25% of total mortality in HIV-infected patients.[121,122] The AIDS-defining cancers, Kaposi sarcoma and non-Hodgkin lymphoma, are the most common pulmonary malignancies found in the immunocompromised patient.

Kaposi sarcoma is mainly a cutaneous disease, with visceral involvement commonly affecting the lymph nodes as well as gastrointestinal and pulmonary systems.[123] Pulmonary presentation includes dyspnea, nonproductive cough, mild hemoptysis, and stridor.[124] Bronchoalveolar lavage is used to exclude pulmonary infections, and diagnosis is confirmed by direct visualization and biopsy via bronchoscopy, thoracoscopy, mediastinoscopy, or thoracotomy.[125] Chemotherapy regimens form the mainstay of management. In a cohort study, 5-year overall survival in patients with pulmonary Kaposi sarcoma was 49%, compared with 82% in Kaposi sarcoma patients without pulmonary involvement.[126]

In the majority of cases, AIDS-associated non-Hodgkin lymphomas are of B-cell origin, and can be classified according to histologic subtypes: large-cell immunoblastic, small noncleaved cell (Burkitt), and diffuse large cell.[127] Pulmonary involvement in late HIV disease presents fever, night sweats, weight loss, dyspnea, cough, chest pain, and hemoptysis.[128] Diagnosis is made by cytologic examination of pleural fluid in cases of pleural effusions, and by biopsy.[128]

Drug-Induced Pulmonary Toxicity

Chemotherapy and cytotoxic drugs can cause lung toxicity by direct and indirect lung injury.[129] Approximately 10% of patients receiving chemotherapy suffer from an adverse effect on the lungs.[130] Chemotherapeutic pulmonary toxicity is dose dependent, and concurrent administration of radiotherapy or known pulmonary toxic drug, exposure to high concentrations of oxygen, and coexistent lung disease are known risk factors.[129] Common offending agents include busulfan, bleomycin, cyclophosphamide, carmustine, methotrexate, and paclitaxel.[70,129,131] Anti-inflammatory drugs (gold salts, sulfasalazine, and penicillamine) can also cause pulmonary damage.[131]

Drug-induced pulmonary damage has many different histopathologic and clinical manifestations (**Table 3**), with the onset of symptoms varying from minutes and hours to several years after initial drug exposure.[132] Chest radiograph and CT scans, arterial blood gases analysis, and pulmonary function tests are initial investigations for detecting lung toxicity, while the carbon monoxide diffusing capacity test is used for monitoring the disease.[133] Bronchoalveolar lavage, bronchoscopy, and lung biopsy are used for histopathological diagnosis.[132] Discontinuing the offending agent and changing treatment regimen, and treatment of underlying pulmonary disease are the management options.

Radiation Toxicity

Radiation therapy can lead to lung injury.[134] Radiation therapy for the treatment of malignancies of breast, lungs, esophagus, lymphomas, and hematological disorders has been reported to cause pulmonary damage.[135] Risk factors for severity of radiation-induced lung injury include total dosage, dose fractionation schedule, type of radiation, irradiated lung volume, previous radiotherapy courses, previous or concurrent use of chemotherapy, exposure to high concentrations of oxygen, and coexistent lung disease.[134,136]

Radiation-induced lung injury can present in early stages as acute radiation pneumonitis and in the later period as chronic radiation fibrosis.[135] Radiation pneumonitis occurs 4 to 12 weeks after radiation therapy, and symptoms include dyspnea, nonproductive cough, and fever.[135] The condition may resolve over several weeks or may progress and become fulminant, proving fatal. Radiation fibrosis occurs 6 to

Table 3
Pulmonary disease caused by drug toxicity in immunocompromised patients

Pulmonary Disease	Drugs
Hypersensitivity reaction	Methotrexate, procarbazine, azathioprine, 6-mercaptopurine, busulfan
Noncardiogenic pulmonary edema (NCPE)	Cytarabine, gemcitabine, mitomycin-C, sulfasalazine, cyclophosphamide, methotrexate, interleukin-2, vinca alkaloids
Interstitial pneumonitis	Azathioprine, bleomycin, chlorambucil, methotrexate, sulfasalazine, busulfan, cyclophosphamide, melphalan, nitrosoureas, vinca alkaloids
Bronchiolitis obliterans–organizing pneumonia (BOOP)	Bleomycin, cyclophosphamide, methotrexate, mitomycin-C, penicillamine, sulfasalazine
Pleural disease	Methotrexate, procarbazine, carmustine, cyclophosphamide, bleomycin, busulfan, interleukin-2, mitomycin-C, penicillamine, mesalamine, mitomycin
Pulmonary vascular disease	Bleomycin, carmustine, mitomycin-C, cytosine arabinoside, penicillamine, methotrexate, busulfan, nitrosoureas
Simple pulmonary eosinophilia	Bleomycin, etoposide, methotrexate, mitomycin-C, procarbazine, sulfasalazine
Pulmonary edema	Cytosine arabinoside, methotrexate, mitomycin
Pulmonary hemorrhage	Cyclophosphamide, mitomycin, penicillamine

12 months after radiation therapy and presents as progressive dyspnea and persistent dry cough.[137] Radiation-induced lung injury can also occur in a nonirradiated or nonexposed lung, most often following treatment of breast cancer, resulting in bilateral lymphocytic alveolitis or bronchiolitis obliterans–organizing pneumonia (BOOP).[134,136]

Radiation pneumonitis presents radiographically as increased opacities and airspace consolidation within the radiation portal, while findings in radiation fibrosis include volume loss, linear opacities, consolidation, and bronchiectasis with sharp border demarcating the radiation portal.[135,138] Corticosteroids are the mainstay of treatment for radiation pneumonitis and BOOP, while fibrosis is usually irreversible.[134,135]

ESOPHAGEAL EMERGENCIES
Esophagitis

Nearly one-third of HIV-infected patients experiences esophageal disease, with candidiasis being the most common pathogen.[139] Herpes simplex virus and CMV are the major viral pathogens, while less frequent viruses include Epstein-Barr virus, papillomavirus, varicella zoster virus, and HIV virus.[140,141] Radiation therapy with exposure to the esophagus can also cause esophagitis. Doses to the esophagus of greater than 3000 cGy can lead to acute esophagitis within 2 to 4 weeks after exposure, and doses in excess of 5000 cGy can lead to severe esophagitis 4 to 8 months after radiation therapy, resulting in strictures.[142,143]

There are several chemotherapeutic drugs that can cause esophageal damage; the most common include dactinomycin, bleomycin, cytarabine, daunorubicin, 5-flourouracil, methotrexate, and vincristine.[144] Clinical presentation of esophagitis includes odynophagia and dysphagia, as well as the sensation of food passing through or "sticking" retrosternally.[141] Fever, nausea, vomiting, hematemesis, abdominal pain, and oropharyngeal lesions (eg, oral thrush) are associated symptoms.

M tuberculosis can cause erosive esophageal disease, resulting in perforations and fistulas (bronchoesophageal and tracheoesophageal).[141] Barium esophagography (double contrast), esophagoscopy, and endoscopic biopsy, cytology, culture, and immunohistochemical as well as in situ DNA staining are options for diagnosis.[141] Due to the overwhelming majority of esophageal fungal infections caused by Candida, empiric therapy with systemic antifungal medication (oral fluconazole) should be started.[141] Ganciclovir and foscarnet are used for CMV esophagitis and acyclovir for herpes esophagitis.[141] Broad-spectrum antibiotics are required for bacterial esophagitis whereas anti-TB therapy is used for tuberculous esophagitis. Withdrawal or reduction in dose is required in cases of chemotherapy or radiotherapy, whereas perforations, obstructions, strictures, and fistulas require surgical management.

GREAT VESSELS EMERGENCIES
Aortic Aneurysm and Dissection

Aortic aneurysm is dilatation of the aorta (>50% than normal size). Aortic dissection is a tear in the tunica intima leading to longitudinal propagation of blood beneath the tunica intima, tearing the aortic layers apart. Although atherosclerosis and chronic hypertension are the primary causes of aortic aneurysm and dissection,[145] important causes in immunocompromised patients include mycotic aneurysm and autoimmune diseases of the aorta, which weaken the layers of the aortic wall, predisposing the patient to aneurysm formation, rupture, and dissection.

A mycotic aneurysm refers to an infected aneurysm, regardless of etiologic pathogen. These aneurysms occur with increased incidence in immunocompromised conditions such as chronic renal failure and corticosteroid use, as well as in autoimmune diseases causing vasculitis and inflammatory lesions of the aorta (Takayasu arteritis and giant cell arteritis), Behçet disease, Ormond disease, and rheumatoid arthritis.[145,146]

Thoracic aortic aneurysms often present with rupture, as the majority are asymptomatic and are diagnosed late. However, symptoms of heart failure and aortic insufficiency, chest or back pain, and compressive symptoms of hoarseness, dyspnea, wheezing or cough, dysphagia, hemoptysis, or hematemesis can occur depending on the size and location of the aneurysm. A ruptured aortic aneurysm causes severe pain with signs of shock such as hypotension, tachycardia, and loss of consciousness.

Aortic dissection presents as sudden onset of severe, sharp, tearing pain that can be localized to the anterior chest (ascending aortic dissection), back/interscapular region (descending aortic dissection), or radiating to the neck or jaw (aortic arch dissection).[147] Syncope and pulse deficits along with signs and symptoms of cardiac tamponade, cardiac failure, and aortic regurgitation, as well as stroke are among the varying presentations of aortic dissection.[145]

Investigations and treatment of aortic aneurysm and dissection are similar in immunocompromised and immunocompetent patients. Chest radiography can reveal widened mediastinum, pleural effusions, abnormal configuration of aortic contours, and tracheal displacement.[148] Spiral CT, transesophageal echocardiography, magnetic resonance imaging (MRI), angiography, and intravascular ultrasonography are the imaging modalities currently in use for diagnosing aortic aneurysm and dissection.[145] Management of an aortic dissection, especially in the ED, involves hemodynamic stabilization and tight control of blood pressure.[147] Emergency surgical intervention is required for ascending aortic dissections whereas descending aortic dissections can be managed medically, with surgery reserved for recurrent pain and complications.[148]

Superior Vena Cava Syndrome

Compression of the superior vena cava (SVC) can occur by way of extrinsic tumors and masses, infiltration of vessel wall, or intraluminal thrombosis.[149] Lung cancer accounts for 65% to 70% of cases,[150,151] followed by lymphoma, breast cancer, and other thoracic masses.[152] A meta-analysis of cancer incidence in population-based cohort studies on immunocompromised HIV/AIDS patients and transplant recipients reported an increased incidence of cancers (lung cancer, Kaposi sarcoma, and non-Hodgkin lymphoma) as a result of immune deficiency.[153] Compression of SVC has been reported after initiation of pulmonary TB treatment in an HIV-infected patient.[154]

SVC compression leads to progressive or sudden-onset dyspnea, dysphagia, facial, laryngeal, and upper extremity edema, vision, voice, and mental changes, cyanosis, and plethora. Chest radiograph findings include mediastinal widening, pleural effusion, and mediastinal mass.[155] Nuclear scintigraphy, CT angiography, and contrast venography are used for diagnosing SVC obstruction, while sputum cytology, bronchoscopy/mediastinoscopy, and CT-guided biopsy may reveal histologic etiology.[155] Initial management includes head elevation, supplemental oxygen, corticosteroids, and diuretics, while chemotherapy and radiotherapy are employed for the treatment of malignancy.[152] Balloon angioplasty and endoluminal stents are used to relieve compression, and thrombolytic therapy is initiated in cases of thrombosis.[149,155]

CLINICAL APPROACH TO THE IMMUNOCOMPROMISED PATIENT

An immunocompromised patient presenting to the ED with thoracic symptoms can be challenging not only because of the various systems and differential diagnoses to consider but also because of the potential for increased complications and rapid deterioration. Symptoms in immunocompromised patients can often be diminished and atypical, which may result in a false sense of security to the emergency physician.[1] Although in most cases the patient's immunosuppressed state will be obvious, the less recognizable causes of immune dysfunction will become apparent after taking a thorough history. History should include the current symptoms and duration of illness (acute or chronic), a review of the immunocompromised condition and immune status, past infections and medical history, alcohol and medications history (eg, immunosuppressive drugs and chemotherapy), occupational, travel, and social history (eg, risk of HIV infection), family history (eg, primary immunodeficiencies), and a review of systems.

Physical examination should be diligent and complete, as even subtle signs (eg, fever) might reveal clues to significant underlying pathology. Particular attention must be paid to the use of personal protective equipment. General physical examination with close inspection of the patient's nails may reveal signs of cyanotic disease, while palpable lymph nodes could reveal lymphadenopathy. The patient's skin and both ends of the gastrointestinal system, the oral cavity and anorectal region, are particularly important for any visible signs of disseminated disease. Previous or current ports of entry or barrier compromise (indwelling line ventriculoperitoneal shunt, urinary catheter) should be carefully inspected for signs of infection. Cardiopulmonary examination, especially in the context of thoracic emergencies, is obviously important. Vital signs and, especially, tachypnea are important indicators of disease severity in HIV-infected patients presenting with sepsis.[156] Auscultation of chest may indicate pneumonia (crackles), endocarditis and cardiomyopathy (murmurs), and pericarditis (pericardial friction rub). A localized wheeze may suggest a tumor. A gastrointestinal examination could reveal hepatosplenomegaly or masses. A neurologic examination for any deficits and ophthalmologic examination could reveal greater involvement and disseminated disease. Other examinations should be performed and tailored according to the patient's complaints and suggestive findings.

Investigations that should be performed in all immunocompromised patients presenting to the ED include complete blood count, electrolytes, blood urea nitrogen, and creatinine, liver function tests, urinalysis, and blood gas. Samples of sputum, blood, urine, and any indwelling lines should be taken for Gram stain and cultures before the administration of antibiotics.

Other tests depend on patient's symptoms and signs; for example, creatinine kinase and troponins should be ordered if there is chest pain, dyspnea, or any other symptom suggesting cardiopulmonary pathology. An upright and lateral chest radiograph is essential, as up to 17% of immunocompromised patients have been reported to have clinically silent pneumonia.[157] However, because nearly 10% of symptomatic immunocompromised patients may have normal chest radiographs, a chest CT scan should be performed after encountering such patients.[70] Furthermore, CT scans allow classic findings (eg, aspergilloma), in some cases leading to diagnosis, and also reveal the location and extent of disease. Other imaging studies include MRI and angiography. After an initial assessment, other investigations should be ordered as the results of tests come in. Depending on the working and differential diagnosis, arrangements should be made for inpatient admission to a ward or intensive and special care unit.

SUMMARY

Thoracic emergencies in immunocompromised patients encompass diverse conditions involving primarily cardiac, pulmonary, gastrointestinal, and vascular systems.

The increased prevalence can be attributed to either the disease states themselves that cause the immunosuppression (such as HIV/AIDS) or as a direct consequence of therapy to treat a variety of conditions (eg, cancer). Overlapping and subtle signs and symptoms in patients with suppressed immune systems pose a challenge in the ED. Because of the potentially catastrophic consequences of delayed diagnosis and treatment in these patients, the emergency physician must keep a high level of vigilance even with minor symptoms; all systems should be considered in the differential and working diagnosis. While management remains the same in most cases, empiric therapy should be started earlier in the ED, based on clinical assessment.

REFERENCES

1. Mendelson M. Fever in the immunocompromised host. Emerg Med Clin North Am 1998;16(4):761–79, vi.
2. Pizzo PA. Fever in immunocompromised patients. N Engl J Med 1999;341(12): 893–900.
3. Rothman RE. Current Centers for Disease Control and Prevention guidelines for HIV counseling, testing, and referral: critical role of and a call to action for emergency physicians. Ann Emerg Med 2004;44(1):31–42.
4. Rothman RE, Ketlogetswe KS, Dolan T, et al. Preventive care in the emergency department: should emergency departments conduct routine HIV screening? a systematic review. Acad Emerg Med 2003;10(3):278–85.
5. Waxman MJ, Kimaiyo S, Ongaro N, et al. Initial outcomes of an emergency department rapid HIV testing program in western Kenya. AIDS Patient Care STDS 2007;21(12):981–6.
6. Nakanjako D, Kamya M, Daniel K, et al. Acceptance of routine testing for HIV among adult patients at the medical emergency unit at a national referral hospital in Kampala, Uganda. AIDS Behav 2007;11(5):753–8.
7. Marco CA, Rothman RE. HIV infection and complications in emergency medicine. Emerg Med Clin North Am 2008;26(2):367–87, viii–ix.
8. Janeway CA, Travers P, Walport M, et al. Immunobiology. 5th edition. New York and London: Garland Science; 2001.
9. Chinen J, Shearer WT. Secondary immunodeficiencies, including HIV infection. J Allergy Clin Immunol 2010;125(2 Suppl 2):S195–203.
10. Mishra RK. Cardiac emergencies in patients with HIV. Emerg Med Clin North Am 2010;28(2):273–82.
11. Holmberg SD, Moorman AC, Williamson JM, et al. Protease inhibitors and cardiovascular outcomes in patients with HIV-1. Lancet 2002;360(9347):1747–8.
12. Mulligan K, Grunfeld C, Tai VW, et al. Hyperlipidemia and insulin resistance are induced by protease inhibitors independent of changes in body composition in patients with HIV infection. J Acquir Immune Defic Syndr 2000; 23(1):35–43.
13. Barbaro G, Fisher SD, Giancaspro G, et al. HIV-associated cardiovascular complications: a new challenge for emergency physicians. Am J Emerg Med 2001;19(7):566–74.
14. Mary-Krause M, Cotte L, Simon A, et al. Increased risk of myocardial infarction with duration of protease inhibitor therapy in HIV-infected men. AIDS 2003; 17(17):2479–86.
15. Sabin CA, Worm SW, Weber R, et al. Use of nucleoside reverse transcriptase inhibitors and risk of myocardial infarction in HIV-infected patients enrolled in the D:A:D study: a multi-cohort collaboration. Lancet 2008;371(9622):1417–26.

16. Friis-Moller N, Reiss P, Sabin CA, et al. Class of antiretroviral drugs and the risk of myocardial infarction. N Engl J Med 2007;356(17):1723–35.

17. Klein D, Hurley LB, Quesenberry CP Jr, et al. Do protease inhibitors increase the risk for coronary heart disease in patients with HIV-1 infection? J Acquir Immune Defic Syndr 2002;30(5):471–7.

18. Bozzette SA, Ake CF, Tam HK, et al. Cardiovascular and cerebrovascular events in patients treated for human immunodeficiency virus infection. N Engl J Med 2003;348(8):702–10.

19. Wever Pinzon O, Silva Enciso J, Romero J, et al. Risk stratification and prognosis of human immunodeficiency virus-infected patients with known or suspected coronary artery disease referred for stress echocardiography. Circ Cardiovasc Imaging 2011;4(4):363–70.

20. Barbaro G, Di Lorenzo G, Grisorio B, et al. Clinical meaning of ventricular ectopic beats in the diagnosis of HIV-related myocarditis: a retrospective analysis of Holter electrocardiographic recordings, echocardiographic parameters, histopathological and virologic findings. Cardiologia 1996;41(12):1199–207.

21. Anson BD, Weaver JG, Ackerman MJ, et al. Blockade of HERG channels by HIV protease inhibitors. Lancet 2005;365(9460):682–6.

22. Girgis I, Gualberti J, Langan L, et al. A prospective study of the effect of I.V. pentamidine therapy on ventricular arrhythmias and QTc prolongation in HIV-infected patients. Chest 1997;112(3):646–53.

23. Lopez JA, Harold JG, Rosenthal MC, et al. QT prolongation and torsades de pointes after administration of trimethoprim-sulfamethoxazole. Am J Cardiol 1987;59(4):376–7.

24. Bijl M, Dieleman JP, Simoons M, et al. Low prevalence of cardiac abnormalities in an HIV-seropositive population on antiretroviral combination therapy. J Acquir Immune Defic Syndr 2001;27(3):318–20.

25. Torre D, Pugliese A, Orofino G. Effect of highly active antiretroviral therapy on ischemic cardiovascular disease in patients with HIV-1 infection. Clin Infect Dis 2002;35(5):631–2.

26. Niakara A, Drabo YJ, Kambire Y, et al. [Cardiovascular diseases and HIV infection: study of 79 cases at the National Hospital of Ouagadougou (Burkina Faso).] Bull Soc Pathol Exot 2002;95(1):23–6.

27. Hakim JG, Matenga JA, Siziya S. Myocardial dysfunction in human immunodeficiency virus infection: an echocardiographic study of 157 patients in hospital in Zimbabwe. Heart 1996;76(2):161–5.

28. Nzuobontane D, Blackett KN, Kuaban C. Cardiac involvement in HIV infected people in Yaounde, Cameroon. Postgrad Med J 2002;78(925):678–81.

29. Bouramoue C, Ekoba J. The heart and AIDS. Med Trop (Mars) 1996;56(Suppl 3): 33–9 [in French].

30. Butt AA, Chang CC, Kuller L, et al. Risk of heart failure with human immunodeficiency virus in the absence of prior diagnosis of coronary heart disease. Arch Intern Med 2011;171(8):737–43.

31. Felker GM, Thompson RE, Hare JM, et al. Underlying causes and long-term survival in patients with initially unexplained cardiomyopathy. N Engl J Med 2000;342(15):1077–84.

32. Gluck T, Degenhardt E, Scholmerich J, et al. Autonomic neuropathy in patients with HIV: course, impact of disease stage, and medication. Clin Auton Res 2000; 10(1):17–22.

33. Barbaro G, Silva EF. Cardiovascular complications in the acquired immunodeficiency syndrome. Rev Assoc Med Bras 2009;55(5):621–30.

34. Currie PF, Goldman JH, Caforio AL, et al. Cardiac autoimmunity in HIV related heart muscle disease. Heart 1998;79(6):599–604.
35. Miller TL, Orav EJ, Colan SD, et al. Nutritional status and cardiac mass and function in children infected with the human immunodeficiency virus. Am J Clin Nutr 1997;66(3):660–4.
36. Herskowitz A, Willoughby SB, Vlahov D, et al. Dilated heart muscle disease associated with HIV infection. Eur Heart J 1995;16(Suppl O):50–5.
37. Rerkpattanapipat P, Wongpraparut N, Jacobs LE, et al. Cardiac manifestations of acquired immunodeficiency syndrome. Arch Intern Med 2000;160(5):602–8.
38. Sweet DD, Isac G, Morrison B, et al. Purulent pericarditis in a patient with rheumatoid arthritis treated with etanercept and methotrexate. CJEM 2007;9(1): 40–2.
39. Heidenreich PA, Eisenberg MJ, Kee LL, et al. Pericardial effusion in AIDS. Incidence and survival. Circulation 1995;92(11):3229–34.
40. Ntsekhe M, Hakim J. Impact of human immunodeficiency virus infection on cardiovascular disease in Africa. Circulation 2005;112(23):3602–7.
41. Silva-Cardoso J, Moura B, Martins L, et al. Pericardial involvement in human immunodeficiency virus infection. Chest 1999;115(2):418–22.
42. Rosen P, Armstrong D. Nonbacterial thrombotic endocarditis in patients with malignant neoplastic diseases. Am J Med 1973;54(1):23–9.
43. Lopez JA, Ross RS, Fishbein MC, et al. Nonbacterial thrombotic endocarditis: a review. Am Heart J 1987;113(3):773–84.
44. el-Shami K, Griffiths E, Streiff M. Nonbacterial thrombotic endocarditis in cancer patients: pathogenesis, diagnosis, and treatment. Oncologist 2007;12(5): 518–23.
45. Iscovich J, Boffetta P, Franceschi S, et al. Classic Kaposi sarcoma: epidemiology and risk factors. Cancer 2000;88(3):500–17.
46. Silver MA, Macher AM, Reichert CM, et al. Cardiac involvement by Kaposi's sarcoma in acquired immune deficiency syndrome (AIDS). Am J Cardiol 1984;53(7):983–5.
47. Lewis W. AIDS: cardiac findings from 115 autopsies. Prog Cardiovasc Dis 1989; 32(3):207–15.
48. Vijay V, Aloor RK, Yalla SM, et al. Pericardial tamponade from Kaposi's sarcoma: role of early pericardial window. Am Heart J 1996;132(4):897–9.
49. Aboulafia DM, Bush R, Picozzi VJ. Cardiac tamponade due to primary pericardial lymphoma in a patient with AIDS. Chest 1994;106(4):1295–9.
50. Duong M, Dubois C, Buisson M, et al. Non-Hodgkin's lymphoma of the heart in patients infected with human immunodeficiency virus. Clin Cardiol 1997;20(5): 497–502.
51. Horowitz MD, Cox MM, Neibart RM, et al. Resection of right atrial lymphoma in a patient with AIDS. Int J Cardiol 1992;34(2):139–42.
52. Gharib MI, Burnett AK. Chemotherapy-induced cardiotoxicity: current practice and prospects of prophylaxis. Eur J Heart Fail 2002;4(3):235–42.
53. Yeh ET, Tong AT, Lenihan DJ, et al. Cardiovascular complications of cancer therapy: diagnosis, pathogenesis, and management. Circulation 2004; 109(25):3122–31.
54. Braverman AC, Antin JH, Plappert MT, et al. Cyclophosphamide cardiotoxicity in bone marrow transplantation: a prospective evaluation of new dosing regimens. J Clin Oncol 1991;9(7):1215–23.
55. Labianca R, Beretta G, Clerici M, et al. Cardiac toxicity of 5-fluorouracil: a study on 1083 patients. Tumori 1982;68(6):505–10.

56. Yancey RS, Talpaz M. Vindesine-associated angina and ECG changes. Cancer Treat Rep 1982;66(3):587–9.
57. Rowinsky EK, McGuire WP, Guarnieri T, et al. Cardiac disturbances during the administration of taxol. J Clin Oncol 1991;9(9):1704–12.
58. Roca E, Bruera E, Politi PM, et al. Vinca alkaloid-induced cardiovascular autonomic neuropathy. Cancer Treat Rep 1985;69(2):149–51.
59. Lejonc JL, Vernant JP, Macquin J, et al. Myocardial infarction following vinblastine treatment. Lancet 1980;2(8196):692.
60. Cardinale D, Sandri MT, Colombo A, et al. Prognostic value of troponin I in cardiac risk stratification of cancer patients undergoing high-dose chemotherapy. Circulation 2004;109(22):2749–54.
61. Galderisi M, Marra F, Esposito R, et al. Cancer therapy and cardiotoxicity: the need of serial Doppler echocardiography. Cardiovasc Ultrasound 2007;5:4.
62. Mason JW, Bristow MR, Billingham ME, et al. Invasive and noninvasive methods of assessing adriamycin cardiotoxic effects in man: superiority of histopathologic assessment using endomyocardial biopsy. Cancer Treat Rep 1978;62(6):857–64.
63. Cheitlin MD, Armstrong WF, Aurigemma GP, et al. ACC/AHA/ASE 2003 guideline update for the clinical application of echocardiography: summary article: a report of the American College of Cardiology/American Heart Association Task Force on Practice Guidelines (ACC/AHA/ASE Committee to Update the 1997 Guidelines for the Clinical Application of Echocardiography). Circulation 2003;108(9): 1146–62.
64. Cardinale D, Colombo A, Cipolla CM. Prevention and treatment of cardiomyopathy and heart failure in patients receiving cancer chemotherapy. Curr Treat Options Cardiovasc Med 2008;10(6):486–95.
65. Carver JR, Shapiro CL, Ng A, et al. American Society of Clinical Oncology clinical evidence review on the ongoing care of adult cancer survivors: cardiac and pulmonary late effects. J Clin Oncol 2007;25(25):3991–4008.
66. Yusuf SW, Sami S, Daher IN. Radiation-induced heart disease: a clinical update. Cardiol Res Pract 2011;2011:317659.
67. Stewart JR, Fajardo LF, Gillette SM, et al. Radiation injury to the heart. Int J Radiat Oncol Biol Phys 1995;31(5):1205–11.
68. Veinot JP, Edwards WD. Pathology of radiation-induced heart disease: a surgical and autopsy study of 27 cases. Hum Pathol 1996;27(8):766–73.
69. Bovelli D, Plataniotis G, Roila F. Cardiotoxicity of chemotherapeutic agents and radiotherapy-related heart disease: ESMO Clinical Practice Guidelines. Ann Oncol 2010;21(Suppl 5):v277–82.
70. Belleza WG, Browne B. Pulmonary considerations in the immunocompromised patient. Emerg Med Clin North Am 2003;21(2):499–531, x–xi.
71. Rosenow EC 3rd, Wilson WR, Cockerill FR 3rd. Pulmonary disease in the immunocompromised host. 1. Mayo Clin Proc 1985;60(7):473–87.
72. Meduri GU, Stein DS. Pulmonary manifestations of acquired immunodeficiency syndrome. Clin Infect Dis 1992;14(1):98–113.
73. Franquet T. Respiratory infection in the AIDS and immunocompromised patient. Eur Radiol 2004;14(Suppl 3):E21–33.
74. Levine SJ, White DA, Fels AO. The incidence and significance of *Staphylococcus aureus* in respiratory cultures from patients infected with the human immunodeficiency virus. Am Rev Respir Dis 1990;141(1):89–93.
75. Afessa B, Green B. Bacterial pneumonia in hospitalized patients with HIV infection: the Pulmonary Complications, ICU Support, and Prognostic

Factors of Hospitalized Patients with HIV (PIP) Study. Chest 2000;117(4): 1017–22.

76. Oh YW, Effmann EL, Godwin JD. Pulmonary infections in immunocompromised hosts: the importance of correlating the conventional radiologic appearance with the clinical setting. Radiology 2000;217(3):647–56.

77. Selwyn PA, Pumerantz AS, Durante A, et al. Clinical predictors of *Pneumocystis carinii* pneumonia, bacterial pneumonia and tuberculosis in HIV-infected patients. AIDS 1998;12(8):885–93.

78. Gil Suay V, Cordero PJ, Martinez E, et al. Parapneumonic effusions secondary to community-acquired bacterial pneumonia in human immunodeficiency virus-infected patients. Eur Respir J 1995;8(11):1934–9.

79. Kaplan JE, Benson C, Holmes KH, et al. Guidelines for prevention and treatment of opportunistic infections in HIV-infected adults and adolescents: recommendations from CDC, the National Institutes of Health, and the HIV Medicine Association of the Infectious Diseases Society of America. MMWR Recomm Rep 2009;58(RR-4):1–207 [quiz: CE201–4].

80. Mandell LA, Wunderink RG, Anzueto A, et al. Infectious Diseases Society of America/American Thoracic Society consensus guidelines on the management of community-acquired pneumonia in adults. Clin Infect Dis 2007;44(Suppl 2): S27–72.

81. Singhal R, Mirdha BR, Guleria R. Human pneumocystosis. Indian J Chest Dis Allied Sci 2005;47(4):273–83.

82. Corti M, Palmero D, Eiguchi K. Respiratory infections in immunocompromised patients. Curr Opin Pulm Med 2009;15(3):209–17.

83. Quist J, Hill AR. Serum lactate dehydrogenase (LDH) in *Pneumocystis carinii* pneumonia, tuberculosis, and bacterial pneumonia. Chest 1995;108(2):415–8.

84. Curtis JR, Yarnold PR, Schwartz DN, et al. Improvements in outcomes of acute respiratory failure for patients with human immunodeficiency virus-related *Pneumocystis carinii* pneumonia. Am J Respir Crit Care Med 2000;162(2 Pt 1):393–8.

85. Wang E, Sohoni A. Tuberculosis: a primer for the emergency physician. Emerg Med Rep 2007;28(1).

86. Chiu YS, Wang JT, Chang SC, et al. *Mycobacterium tuberculosis* bacteremia in HIV-negative patients. J Formos Med Assoc 2007;106(5):355–64.

87. Shima T, Yoshimoto G, Miyamoto T, et al. Disseminated tuberculosis following second unrelated cord blood transplantation for acute myelogenous leukemia. Transpl Infect Dis 2009;11(1):75–7.

88. Golden MP, Vikram HR. Extrapulmonary tuberculosis: an overview. Am Fam Physician 2005;72(9):1761–8.

89. Perlman DC, el-Sadr WM, Nelson ET, et al. Variation of chest radiographic patterns in pulmonary tuberculosis by degree of human immunodeficiency virus-related immunosuppression. The Terry Beirn Community Programs for Clinical Research on AIDS (CPCRA). The AIDS Clinical Trials Group (ACTG). Clin Infect Dis 1997;25(2):242–6.

90. Jeong YJ, Lee KS. Pulmonary tuberculosis: up-to-date imaging and management. AJR Am J Roentgenol 2008;191(3):834–44.

91. Rossi SE, Franquet T, Volpacchio M, et al. Tree-in-bud pattern at thin-section CT of the lungs: radiologic-pathologic overview. Radiographics 2005;25(3):789–801.

92. Morris K. WHO recommends against inaccurate tuberculosis tests. Lancet 2011;377(9760):113–4.

93. Benson CA, Kaplan JE, Masur H, et al. Treating opportunistic infections among HIV-infected adults and adolescents: recommendations from CDC, the National

Institutes of Health, and the HIV Medicine Association/Infectious Diseases Society of America. MMWR Recomm Rep 2004;53(RR-15):1–112.

94. Treatment of tuberculosis. MMWR Recomm Rep 2003;52(RR-11):1–77.

95. Bayer AS. Fungal pneumonias; pulmonary coccidioidal syndromes (Part I). Primary and progressive primary coccidioidal pneumonias—diagnostic, therapeutic, and prognostic considerations. Chest 1981;79(5):575–83.

96. Chapman SW, Lin AC, Hendricks KA, et al. Endemic blastomycosis in Mississippi: epidemiological and clinical studies. Semin Respir Infect 1997;12(3):219–28.

97. Kauffman CA. Histoplasmosis: a clinical and laboratory update. Clin Microbiol Rev 2007;20(1):115–32.

98. Chapman SW, Dismukes WE, Proia LA, et al. Clinical practice guidelines for the management of blastomycosis: 2008 update by the Infectious Diseases Society of America. Clin Infect Dis 2008;46(12):1801–12.

99. Wheat LJ, Kohler RB, Tewari RP. Diagnosis of disseminated histoplasmosis by detection of Histoplasma capsulatum antigen in serum and urine specimens. N Engl J Med 1986;314(2):83–8.

100. Wheat LJ. Improvements in diagnosis of histoplasmosis. Expert Opin Biol Ther 2006;6(11):1207–21.

101. Zmeili OS, Soubani AO. Pulmonary aspergillosis: a clinical update. QJM 2007; 100(6):317–34.

102. Herbrecht R, Denning DW, Patterson TF, et al. Voriconazole versus amphotericin B for primary therapy of invasive aspergillosis. N Engl J Med 2002;347(6): 408–15.

103. Powderly WG, Cloud GA, Dismukes WE, et al. Measurement of cryptococcal antigen in serum and cerebrospinal fluid: value in the management of AIDS-associated cryptococcal meningitis. Clin Infect Dis 1994;18(5):789–92.

104. Perfect JR, Dismukes WE, Dromer F, et al. Clinical practice guidelines for the management of cryptococcal disease: 2010 update by the infectious diseases society of America. Clin Infect Dis 2010;50(3):291–322.

105. Florescu DF, Kalil AC. Cytomegalovirus infections in non-immunocompromised and immunocompromised patients in the intensive care unit. Infect Disord Drug Targets 2011. [Epub ahead of print].

106. Ljungman P, Griffiths P, Paya C. Definitions of cytomegalovirus infection and disease in transplant recipients. Clin Infect Dis 2002;34(8):1094–7.

107. Gasparetto EL, Ono SE, Escuissato D, et al. Cytomegalovirus pneumonia after bone marrow transplantation: high resolution CT findings. Br J Radiol 2004; 77(921):724–7.

108. Konoplev S, Champlin RE, Giralt S, et al. Cytomegalovirus pneumonia in adult autologous blood and marrow transplant recipients. Bone Marrow Transplant 2001;27(8):877–81.

109. Dodt KK, Jacobsen PH, Hofmann B, et al. Development of cytomegalovirus (CMV) disease may be predicted in HIV-infected patients by CMV polymerase chain reaction and the antigenemia test. AIDS 1997;11(3):F21–8.

110. Anti-cytomegalovirus (CMV) immediate early antigen monoclonal antibody, unconjugated, clone 3G9.2: from CHEMICON.

111. Reed EC, Bowden RA, Dandliker PS, et al. Treatment of cytomegalovirus pneumonia with ganciclovir and intravenous cytomegalovirus immunoglobulin in patients with bone marrow transplants. Ann Intern Med 1988;109(10): 783–8.

112. Emanuel D, Cunningham I, Jules-Elysee K, et al. Cytomegalovirus pneumonia after bone marrow transplantation successfully treated with the combination of

ganciclovir and high-dose intravenous immune globulin. Ann Intern Med 1988; 109(10):777–82.

113. Saber AA, Aboolian A, LaRaja RD, et al. HIV/AIDS and the risk of deep vein thrombosis: a study of 45 patients with lower extremity involvement. Am Surg 2001;67(7):645–7.

114. Klein SK, Slim EJ, de Kruif MD, et al. Is chronic HIV infection associated with venous thrombotic disease? A systematic review. Neth J Med 2005;63(4):129–36.

115. Heit JA, Silverstein MD, Mohr DN, et al. Risk factors for deep vein thrombosis and pulmonary embolism: a population-based case-control study. Arch Intern Med 2000;160(6):809–15.

116. Lee AY, Levine MN. Management of venous thromboembolism in cancer patients. Oncology (Williston Park) 2000;14(3):409–17, 421 [discussion: 422, 425–406].

117. Lyman GH, Khorana AA, Falanga A, et al. American Society of Clinical Oncology guideline: recommendations for venous thromboembolism prophylaxis and treatment in patients with cancer. J Clin Oncol 2007;25(34):5490–505.

118. Barbaro G. Cardiovascular manifestations of HIV infection. J R Soc Med 2001; 94(8):384–90.

119. Mehta NJ, Khan IA, Mehta RN, et al. HIV-Related pulmonary hypertension: analytic review of 131 cases. Chest 2000;118(4):1133–41.

120. Mesa RA, Edell ES, Dunn WF, et al. Human immunodeficiency virus infection and pulmonary hypertension: two new cases and a review of 86 reported cases. Mayo Clin Proc 1998;73(1):37–45.

121. Shiels MS, Cole SR, Kirk GD, et al. A meta-analysis of the incidence of non-AIDS cancers in HIV-infected individuals. J Acquir Immune Defic Syndr 2009;52(5): 611–22.

122. Cadranel J, Garfield D, Lavole A, et al. Lung cancer in HIV infected patients: facts, questions and challenges. Thorax 2006;61(11):1000–8.

123. Cadranel J, Naccache J, Wislez M, et al. Pulmonary malignancies in the immunocompromised patient. Respiration 1999;66(4):289–309.

124. Meduri GU, Stover DE, Lee M, et al. Pulmonary Kaposi's sarcoma in the acquired immune deficiency syndrome. Clinical, radiographic, and pathologic manifestations. Am J Med 1986;81(1):11–8.

125. Cadranel JL, Kammoun S, Chevret S, et al. Results of chemotherapy in 30 AIDS patients with symptomatic pulmonary Kaposi's sarcoma. Thorax 1994;49(10): 958–60.

126. Palmieri C, Dhillon T, Thirlwell C, et al. Pulmonary Kaposi sarcoma in the era of highly active antiretroviral therapy. HIV Med 2006;7(5):291–3.

127. Sandler AS, Kaplan L. AIDS lymphoma. Curr Opin Oncol 1996;8(5):377–85.

128. Eisner MD, Kaplan LD, Herndier B, et al. The pulmonary manifestations of AIDS-related non-Hodgkin's lymphoma. Chest 1996;110(3):729–36.

129. Joos L, Tamm M. Breakdown of pulmonary host defense in the immunocompromised host: cancer chemotherapy. Proc Am Thorac Soc 2005;2(5):445–8.

130. Rosenow EC 3rd, Limper AH. Drug-induced pulmonary disease. Semin Respir Infect 1995;10(2):86–95.

131. Rossi SE, Erasmus JJ, McAdams HP, et al. Pulmonary drug toxicity: radiologic and pathologic manifestations. Radiographics 2000;20(5):1245–59.

132. Flieder DB, Travis WD. Pathologic characteristics of drug-induced lung disease. Clin Chest Med 2004;25(1):37–45.

133. Dimopoulou I, Efstathiou E, Samakovli A, et al. A prospective study on lung toxicity in patients treated with gemcitabine and carboplatin: clinical, radiological and functional assessment. Ann Oncol 2004;15(8):1250–5.

134. Prakash UB. Radiation-induced injury in the "nonirradiated" lung. Eur Respir J 1999;13(4):715–7.
135. Davis SD, Yankelevitz DF, Henschke CI. Radiation effects on the lung: clinical features, pathology, and imaging findings. AJR Am J Roentgenol 1992;159(6): 1157–64.
136. Poletti V, Salvucci M, Zanchini R, et al. The lung as a target organ in patients with hematologic disorders. Haematologica 2000;85(8):855–64.
137. Makimoto T, Tsuchiya S, Hayakawa K, et al. Risk factors for severe radiation pneumonitis in lung cancer. Jpn J Clin Oncol 1999;29(4):192–7.
138. Choi YW, Munden RF, Erasmus JJ, et al. Effects of radiation therapy on the lung: radiologic appearances and differential diagnosis. Radiographics 2004;24(4): 985–97 [discussion: 998].
139. Bonacini M, Young T, Laine L. The causes of esophageal symptoms in human immunodeficiency virus infection. A prospective study of 110 patients. Arch Intern Med 1991;151(8):1567–72.
140. Tilbe KS, Lloyd DA. A case of viral esophagitis. J Clin Gastroenterol 1986;8(4): 494–5.
141. Dieterich DT, Wilcox CM. Diagnosis and trej, atment of esophageal diseases associated with HIV infection. Practice Parameters Committee of the American College of Gastroenterology. Am J Gastroenterol 1996;91(11):2265–9.
142. Lepke RA, Libshitz HI. Radiation-induced injury of the esophagus. Radiology 1983;148(2):375–8.
143. Collazzo LA, Levine MS, Rubesin SE, et al. Acute radiation esophagitis: radiographic findings. AJR Am J Roentgenol 1997;169(4):1067–70.
144. Feldman M, Friedman LS, Sleisenger MH, editors. Sleisenger and Fordtran's gastrointestinal and liver disease. 8th edition. Philadelphia (PA): Saunders Elsevier; 2006.
145. Erbel R, Alfonso F, Boileau C, et al. Diagnosis and management of aortic dissection. Eur Heart J 2001;22(18):1642–81.
146. Chan YC, Morales JP, Taylor PR. The management of mycotic aortic aneurysms: is there a role for endoluminal treatment? Acta Chir Belg 2005;105(6):580–7.
147. Khan IA, Nair CK. Clinical, diagnostic, and management perspectives of aortic dissection. Chest 2002;122(1):311–28.
148. Ramanath VS, Oh JK, Sundt TM 3rd, et al. Acute aortic syndromes and thoracic aortic aneurysm. Mayo Clin Proc 2009;84(5):465–81.
149. Zojer N, Ludwig H. Hematological emergencies. Ann Oncol 2007;18(Suppl 1): i45–8.
150. Flounders JA. Oncology emergency modules: superior vena cava syndrome. Oncol Nurs Forum 2003;30(4):E84–90.
151. Ahmann FR. A reassessment of the clinical implications of the superior vena caval syndrome. J Clin Oncol 1984;2(8):961–9.
152. Krimsky WS, Behrens RJ, Kerkvliet GJ. Oncologic emergencies for the internist. Cleve Clin J Med 2002;69(3):209–10, 213–204, 216–207 passim.
153. Grulich AE, van Leeuwen MT, Falster MO, et al. Incidence of cancers in people with HIV/AIDS compared with immunosuppressed transplant recipients: a meta-analysis. Lancet 2007;370(9581):59–67.
154. Minguez C, Roca B, Gonzalez-Mino C, et al. Superior vena cava syndrome during the treatment of pulmonary tuberculosis in an HIV-1 infected patient. J Infect 2000;40(2):187–9.
155. Thomas CR Jr, Edmondson EA. Common emergencies in cancer medicine: cardiovascular and neurologic syndromes. J Natl Med Assoc 1991;83(11):1001–17.

156. Jacob ST, Moore CC, Banura P, et al. Severe sepsis in two Ugandan hospitals: a prospective observational study of management and outcomes in a predominantly HIV-1 infected population. PLoS One 2009;4(11):e7782.
157. Donowitz GR, Harman C, Pope T, et al. The role of the chest roentgenogram in febrile neutropenic patients. Arch Intern Med 1991;151(4):701–4.

Index

Note: Page numbers of article titles are in **boldface** type.

Emerg Med Clin N Am 30 (2012) 591–599
doi:10.1016/S0733-8627(12)00012-0
0733-8627/12/$ – see front matter © 2012 Elsevier Inc. All rights reserved.

emed.theclinics.com

EmergencyMed **Advance**

All the latest emergency medicine news and research you need, all in one place

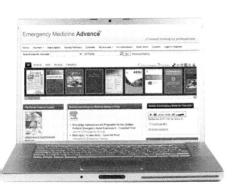

EmergencyMedAdvance.com is a new essential online resource offering valued high-quality content and news for the global community of Emergency Medicine professionals to save time and stay current—from physicians and nurses to EMTs.

Stay current
- Emergency Medicine news
- Upcoming meetings and events

Save time
- Access relevant articles in press from 16 participating journals
- Search across 500+ health sciences journals
- Learn how to submit a manuscript

And more...
- Journals' profiles
- Personalized search results
- Emergency Medicine bookstore
- Sign up for free e-Alerts
- Emergency Medicine jobs

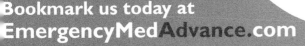

Printed and bound by CPI Group (UK) Ltd, Croydon, CR0 4YY

03/10/2024

01040458-0013